GW00468373

Atlas of Medical Anatomy

JAN LANGMAN, M.D., Ph.D.

Professor and Chairman, Department of Anatomy,
University of Virginia

M. W. WOERDEMAN, M.D., Ph.D., D.Sc.h.c.

Professor of Anatomy and Embryology Emeritus;
Formerly Director of the Department of Anatomy,
The University of Amsterdam

1978
W. B. SAUNDERS COMPANY · Philadelphia · London · Toronto

W. B. Saunders Company: West Washington Square
Philadelphia, PA   19105

1 St. Anne's Road
Eastbourne, East Sussex BN21 3UN, England

1 Goldthorne Avenue
Toronto, Ontario M8Z 5T9, Canada

Atlas of Medical Anatomy   ISBN   0-7216-5626-9

© 1978 by W. B. Saunders Company.   Copyright under the International Copyright
Union.   All rights reserved.   This book is protected by copyright.   No part of it may
be reproduced, stored in a retrieval system, or transmitted in any form or by any means,
electronic, mechanical, photocopying, recording, or otherwise, without written permis-
sion from the publisher.   Made in the United States of America.   Press of W. B.
Saunders Company.   Library of Congress catalog card number 75-22735.

Last digit is the print number: 9   8   7   6   5   4   3   2   1

PREFACE

This anatomical atlas presents approximately one thousand illustrations arranged in regional order to correspond to modern courses in anatomy. Each section of the book is an independent unit, and within each section the illustrations are organized to follow the dissection as closely as possible. The Thorax is the first section presented, but the dissection may start equally well with the Upper Limb or the Head and Neck.

We have selected the title Atlas of Medical Anatomy because the book was written with the training of medical students most in mind. This is reflected in the selection of illustrations; most were prepared from adult specimens, but some are from the newborn. In some regions the anatomical structures in the newborn are different from those in the adult, and it is important to realize that topographical relations change with age.

Certain areas of gross anatomy are difficult for the medical student to understand even when they are represented in three-dimensional illustrations. For this reason we have added schematic drawings that either simplify the anatomical relations or explain them by making use of the simple relations seen in the embryo. The simplicity of the structures found during development frequently helps the student understand the complicated topography in the adult.

In some chapters we have presented photographs of the surface anatomy in an attempt to bridge the gap between the dissected specimen and the patient. Similarly, a number of radiographs have been presented. Both the photographs and the radiographs emphasize that a thorough knowledge of anatomical structures and their interrelationships is an absolute requirement for understanding and interpreting data obtained by clinical examination.

Portrait painters and sculptors study anatomy to create an accurate surface impression of the underlying structures; kinesiologists examine the muscles, bones and joints to analyze and prescribe the most efficient movements. Students of medicine frequently study anatomy with a ferocious appetite for detail—every small blood vessel, every little groove on a bone, each peritoneal ligament and every foramen in the base of the skull is to be learned. How disappointing to discover when entering the clinic and applying this knowledge that the details of many complicated structures are not used at all. For this reason a short text pointing out the clinical importance and interrelations of many structures has been added to the illustrations. Since this atlas does not pretend to be and should not replace a textbook, many descriptive facts found in most textbooks have been deleted. We feel that when the student can see and feel the many anatomical features during the course of dissection, it is most important for him to understand their medical application and clinical importance. We hope that the illustrations in this atlas will help the student to obtain a thorough, three-dimensional knowledge of anatomy and that the text notes will help him with the clinical application of his anatomical knowledge.

MARTIN W. WOERDEMAN, M.D., Ph.D., D.Sc.h.c.
JAN LANGMAN, M.D., Ph.D.

ACKNOWLEDGMENTS

The publication of an anatomical atlas is a monumental task involving the dissection of numerous specimens, the preparation of several thousand illustrations, the logical arrangement of the material and finally, an extraordinary amount of organization for the printing of the illustrations and text. The greatest collaborative effort over a prolonged period of time is required to bring such a large work to its final form. We are therefore deeply indebted to our many co-workers, varying from artists to secretaries and from colleagues in anatomy to a host of medical students. We hope they will forgive us that we cannot express our thanks to all of them personally and that we must restrict ourselves here to the main contributors.

This work could not have been accomplished without the dedication of the late Mrs. H. L. Blumenthal-Rothschild, the main artist, who prepared the majority of the illustrations. She made her artistic and scientific talents available for this work with the greatest enthusiasm and attracted a number of excellent co-workers. These artists, Mesdames L. M. Binger, W. van Slooten and A. van Hamersveld and Messrs J. Tinkelenberg and Chr. van Huizen, each contributed a substantial number of illustrations to this book. To them we offer our most sincere thanks. Some of the drawings that were in the collection of the Anatomy Department of the University of Amsterdam were generously put at our disposal by its present Chairman, Dr. J. van Limborgh.

We are also greatly indebted to Mr. W. Fairweather, who directed the color work on the illustrations for this atlas and prepared several additional drawings. Numerous hours were spent finding the correct color combinations for each structure. For this arduous work our thanks go particularly to Mrs. Judy Fairweather, who prepared the thousands of color overlays with endless patience, great enthusiasm and skill.

We also wish to express our great appreciation to the Saunders Company, who undertook the task of publishing this book. In particular our thanks go to Mr. John Hanley, who stimulated and encouraged us continuously in the preparation of this book. We are also indebted to Miss Ruth Goddard, who edited the text and checked the thousands of labels in the illustrations, to Miss Lorraine Battista, who composed this book page by page, and to Mr. Grant Lashbrook, who checked and frequently improved our artwork.

A number of our colleagues helped us with the laborious task of checking the illustrations and text. We wish to thank them for the many excellent suggestions they made to improve this book.

Finally, we especially wish to thank our companions in life, Mrs. Hanna Woerdeman and Mrs. Ina Langman, for their wonderful encouragement and devotion.

Amsterdam, Holland   MARTIN W. WOERDEMAN

Charlottesville, Virginia   JAN LANGMAN

CONTENTS

CONTENTS

CONTENTS

CONTENTS

BACK

THORAX

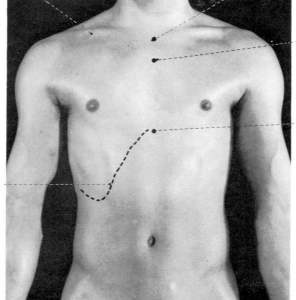

A. Anterior surface of the thorax in a male.

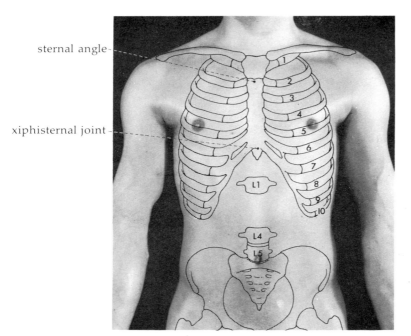

B. Anterior view of the thorax.
The bony skeleton is superimposed.

The following landmarks are important in the physical examination of the thorax. They can all be easily palpated and are helpful as reference points in determining the position of the heart and lungs.

¶ *Suprasternal notch*: the midline depression bordered by the superior margin of the sternum and the medial ends of the clavicles. Deep to the depression the tracheal cartilages can be felt. By moving the finger slightly upwards the cricoid cartilage of the larynx can be palpated.

¶ *Sternal angle*: the angle between the manubrium and the body of the sternum. At this level the second costal cartilage joins the lateral border of the sternum. The sternal angle is an important landmark when counting the ribs and intercostal spaces.

¶ *Xiphisternal joint*: the joint between the body of the sternum and the xiphoid process. The cartilage of the seventh rib attaches to the sternum just above the joint; occasionally it is attached to the xiphoid process. Palpation of the *inferior tip of the xiphoid process* may be painful.

¶ *Costal margin*: the lower boundary of the thorax, formed by the cartilages of the seventh, eighth, ninth and tenth ribs.

¶ *Clavicle*: one of the few bones whose entire length lies immediately under the skin.

¶ *Ribs*: The ribs can best be palpated and counted by first determining the position of the second rib, which is easily identifiable because it attaches to the sternum at the sternal angle. Counting of the ribs is easiest in the midclavicular line. The first rib cannot be felt since it lies deep to the clavicle. Similarly, the eleventh and twelfth ribs are difficult to palpate. The number of each intercostal space corresponds to the number of the rib forming its upper boundary. (For bony components of the thorax see T9 and T10.)

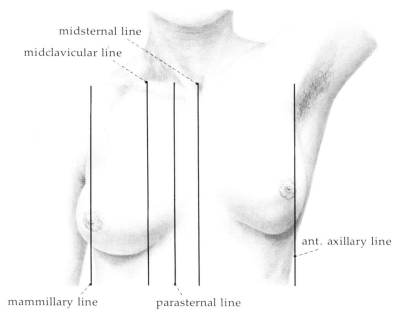

midsternal line

midclavicular line

ant. axillary line

mammillary line   parasternal line

A. Anterior view of the thorax in a female.
Orientation lines are indicated.

Subcutaneous fat tissue and the mammary glands make palpation of the bony landmarks and auscultation and percussion of the heart and lungs more difficult in the female than in the male. The following *orientation lines* may be helpful in physical diagnosis:

1. *Midsternal line*: lies in the median plane of the sternum.

2. *Parasternal line*: is drawn about half an inch from the lateral border of the sternum.

3. *Midclavicular line*: runs vertically down from the midpoint of the clavicle.

4. *Anterior axillary line*: runs vertically down from the anterior axillary fold.

5. *Mammillary or nipple line*: is not of much value considering individual variations and the changes in the position of the nipple that occur with age.

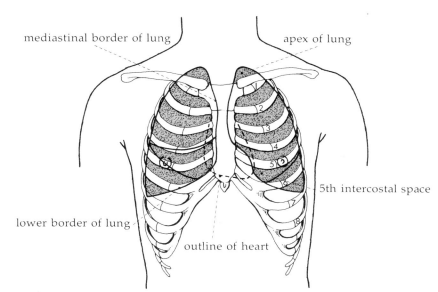

mediastinal border of lung   apex of lung

5th intercostal space

lower border of lung

outline of heart

B. Schematic drawing of the anterior aspect of the thorax.
The outline of the heart and lungs is superimposed.

Note also the following important points:

¶ The top or apex of the lung extends above the first rib and clavicle into the neck, where it forms a dome. Deep wounds above the clavicle may penetrate into the apex of the lung.

¶ On the right side of the sternum the heart is covered anteriorly by the right lung; on the left side, it is covered anteriorly by the lung except in parts of the fourth and fifth intercostal spaces and behind the fourth and fifth ribs (see B).

¶ The apex of the heart, formed by the left ventricle, lies behind the *fifth intercostal space*. The beat of the heart (*apex beat*) can be felt in this space 3½ inches from the midsternal line. When the heart is enlarged, the apex beat may be felt in the midclavicular or even in the anterior axillary line.

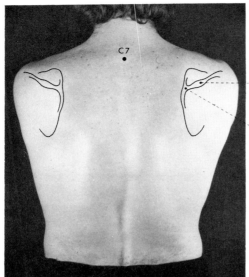

A. Posterior view of the thorax in a male.

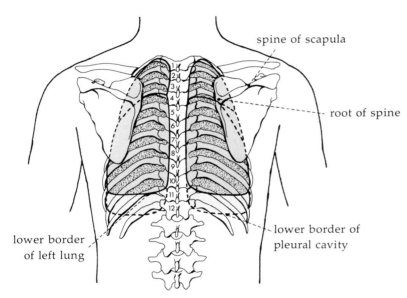

B. Schematic drawing of the posterior aspect of the thorax.
The bony points, lungs and pleura are superimposed.

In examining the posterior aspect of the thorax only a few bony landmarks and orientation lines are used as reference points.

¶ *The vertebra prominens.* This is the seventh cervical vertebra. Its spinous process, contrary to that of the other cervical vertebrae, can be palpated easily by moving the fingers downward along the midline of the posterior aspect of the neck. The first spinous process that is easily distinguishable is that of the seventh cervical vertebra (C7).

¶ *The spinous processes of the thoracic vertebrae.* Once the spinous process of C7 has been determined, it is easy to palpate the spines of the thoracic vertebrae by moving the fingers downward along the vertebral column.

¶ *The spine of the scapula.* This is an easily palpable subcutaneous part of the scapula. The root of the spine lies at the level of the spinous process of the third thoracic vertebra (T3). This landmark is of little value since the scapula can move considerable distances along the posterior body wall. Its relationship to the spine is valid only if the arms are hanging at the sides.

¶ *The scapular line,* which runs vertically downward from the inferior angle of the scapula when the arms are hanging at the sides.

¶ *The posterior axillary line,* which runs vertically downward from the posterior axillary fold (see T12 A).

Note also:

¶ The lower border of the pleural cavity extends at least the width of two fingers below the border of the lungs, a fact of great clinical importance. During respiration the lungs move up and down in the pleural cavity (see T26 and T27).

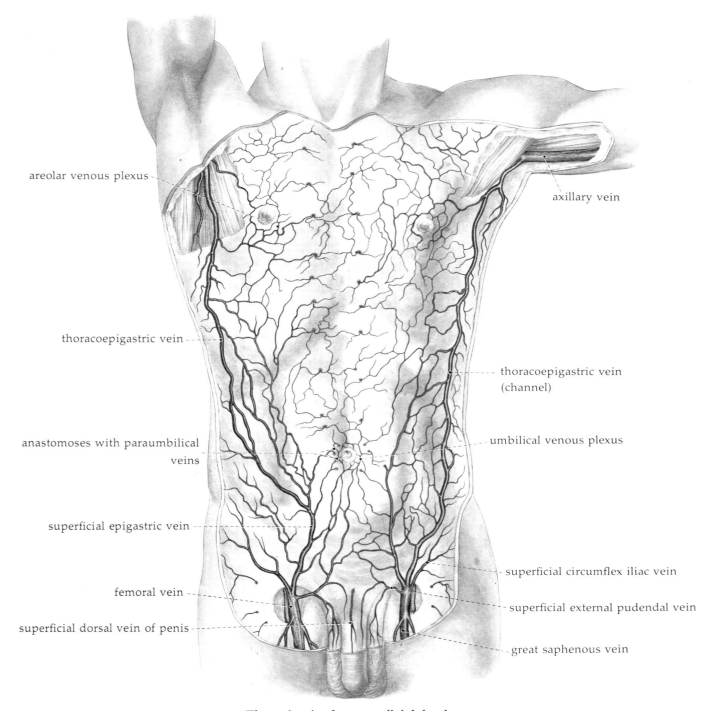

areolar venous plexus

axillary vein

thoracoepigastric vein

thoracoepigastric vein (channel)

anastomoses with paraumbilical veins

umbilical venous plexus

superficial epigastric vein

superficial circumflex iliac vein

femoral vein

superficial external pudendal vein

superficial dorsal vein of penis

great saphenous vein

The veins in the superficial fascia.

¶ The superficial fascia connects the corium of the skin to the underlying deep fascia, which invests the musculature (see T12 *A*). The superficial fascia consists of loose areolar tissue with collagenous and elastic fibers and usually contains considerable fat.

¶ The subcutaneous nerves and the superficial veins are located in the superficial fascia. Under normal conditions few anastomoses exist between the thoracic veins and the epigastric veins of the abdominal wall. Occasionally, however, if the inferior vena cava is obstructed, large anastomoses may develop; the most important channel to bypass the vena cava is the *thoracoepigastric venous channel.*

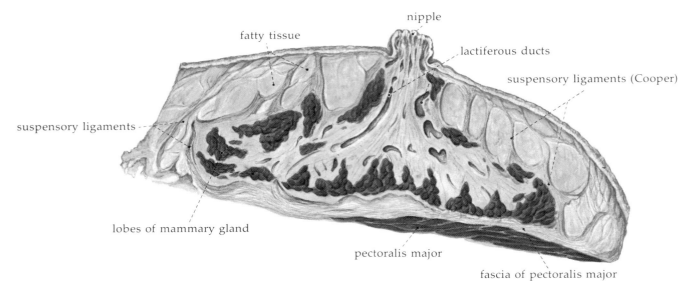

A. Section through the mammary gland.

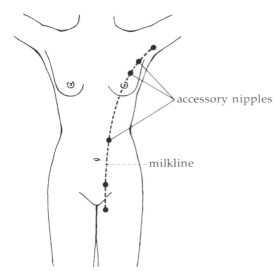

The mammary gland is the most important organ in the superficial fascia of the thorax. Note the following clinically important points:

¶ *Position and attachment.* The breast lies *in* the superficial fascia and rests *on* the deep fascia covering the pectoralis major and serratus anterior muscles. *Fibrous bands*, called *Cooper's suspensory ligaments*, fix the breast to the skin and the underlying fascia. These ligaments are clinically important because the invasion of cancer

B. Schematic drawing of the milkline and accessory nipples. (From Langman, J.: Medical Embryology, 3rd ed. Baltimore, The Williams & Wilkins Co., 1975.)

cells may cause them to retract: on the skin this causes dimpling, and in the nipple area it causes retraction of the nipple. When the tumor invades the fibers inserting into the deep fascia, the breast tissue cannot be moved over the muscles, as in normal women.

¶ *Axillary tail* (Spence). This is a tail-like prolongation of the upper–outer quadrant in an axillary direction. It passes through an opening in the axillary fascia and is thus located deep to the fascia. When the gland is palpated the tail tissue is sometimes confused with enlarged axillary lymph nodes (see T6 *B*).

¶ *Inverted nipple.* Inversion of the nipple is either a congenital condition or the result of the ingrowth of cancer tissue in the suspensory ligaments in the nipple region.

¶ *Ectopic nipple.* Additional nipples (polythelia) may be found anywhere along the length of the so-called milkline, which extends from the axillary region to the inguinal region. Extra nipples are usually not accompanied by breast tissue. Occasionally, however, an extra nipple and functional breast tissue are found in the axillary region (polymastia).

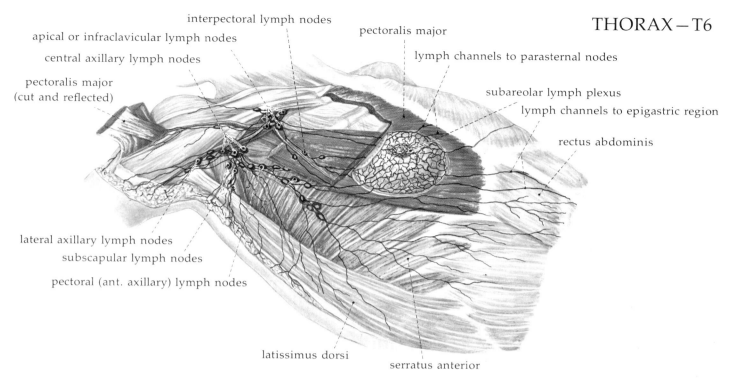

apical or infraclavicular lymph nodes
interpectoral lymph nodes
central axillary lymph nodes
pectoralis major
pectoralis major (cut and reflected)
lymph channels to parasternal nodes
subareolar lymph plexus
lymph channels to epigastric region
rectus abdominis
lateral axillary lymph nodes
subscapular lymph nodes
pectoral (ant. axillary) lymph nodes
latissimus dorsi
serratus anterior

A. Lymph drainage of the female breast.

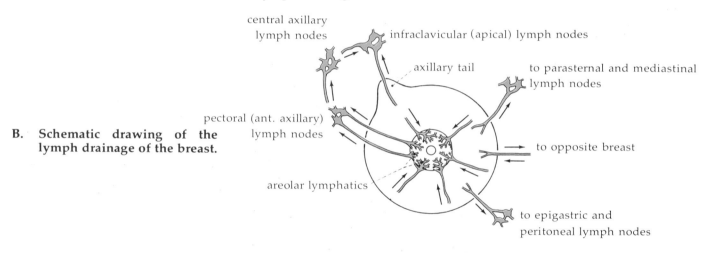

central axillary lymph nodes
infraclavicular (apical) lymph nodes
axillary tail
to parasternal and mediastinal lymph nodes
pectoral (ant. axillary) lymph nodes
to opposite breast
B. Schematic drawing of the lymph drainage of the breast.
areolar lymphatics
to epigastric and peritoneal lymph nodes

The lymph drainage of the breast is extremely important because of the frequent occurrence of cancer in this region and the spread of malignant cells along the lymph vessels.

¶ Most lymphatics of the *glandular* tissue course in a superolateral direction and drain into the pectoral (anterior axillary) nodes. Subsequently they drain into the central axillary nodes located in the fat of the axilla under the axillary tuft of hair and along the inner border of the axillary vein. From here they pass toward the apical or infraclavicular group. Finally, they reach the deep cervical or supraclavicular lymph nodes.

¶ Some lymph vessels, mainly from the medial quadrants of the mammary gland, drain into the parasternal nodes located along the internal thoracic artery. From here, cancer cells may spread to the mediastinal lymph nodes and then to the pleura and lung.

¶ Breast cancer may also spread toward the epigastric region and the peritoneum, thus causing metastases in the liver and the pelvic region.

¶ Occasionally breast cancer spreads across the midline toward the other breast and the lymph nodes in the opposite axilla.

¶ Sometimes cancer cells from the upper and outer quadrants spread directly through the pectoralis muscle to the apical lymph nodes.

¶ The lymphatics which drain the *skin, areola* and *nipple* form rather large channels to the pectoral (anterior axillary) nodes. These are found in the region of the third rib under the anterior axillary fold.

¶ It is important to realize that the axillary lymph nodes also drain the arm. In a radical mastectomy, when many axillary lymph nodes are removed, the lymph drainage of the arm may be severely impeded and severe edema may result.

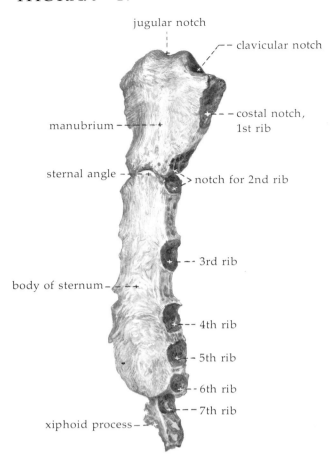

A. Anterolateral view of the sternum.

jugular notch

clavicular notch

manubrium

costal notch, 1st rib

sternal angle

notch for 2nd rib

3rd rib

body of sternum

4th rib

5th rib

6th rib

7th rib

xiphoid process

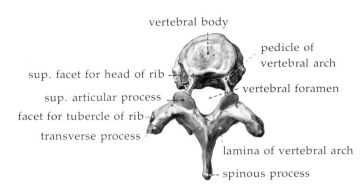

B. Thoracic vertebra seen from above.

vertebral body

pedicle of vertebral arch

sup. facet for head of rib

vertebral foramen

sup. articular process

facet for tubercle of rib

transverse process

lamina of vertebral arch

spinous process

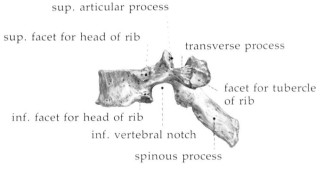

C. Thoracic vertebra seen from the left.

sup. articular process

sup. facet for head of rib

transverse process

facet for tubercle of rib

inf. facet for head of rib

inf. vertebral notch

spinous process

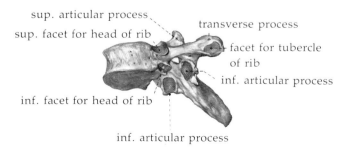

D. Thoracic vertebra seen from the left and below.

sup. articular process

sup. facet for head of rib

transverse process

facet for tubercle of rib

inf. articular process

inf. facet for head of rib

inf. articular process

On the sternum *note:*

¶ The *jugular notch* forming the upper border of the bone. It can easily be palpated.

¶ The joint surfaces for the clavicles and ribs. The first rib lacks a joint surface; its connection with the sternum is a *synchondrosis*. The seventh rib articulates frequently at the xiphisternal junction.

On a *typical* thoracic vertebra *observe:*

¶ The *body*, which has a *weight-bearing* function.

¶ The *arch*, consisting of a *pedicle* and *lamina*. Together the body and the arch surround the vertebral foramen and thus serve as a *protective structure* for the spinal cord.

¶ The three *main vertebral processes* — two transverse processes and one spinous process.

¶ The *articular processes*. Each vertebra has two articular processes that connect it with the vertebra located below and two articular processes that connect it with the vertebra located above.

¶ Each side of the thoracic vertebra has *three articular surfaces for the ribs:* one on its transverse process for the tubercle of the rib, another for the head of the rib (the superior costal facet) and a third one (the inferior costal facet) located at the lower aspect of the body and serving as an articular surface for the head of the next rib. Hence, the head of a rib articulates with two vertebrae, with the exception of the first rib, which does not articulate with C7, and the eleventh and twelfth ribs, which do not articulate with T10 and T11, respectively.

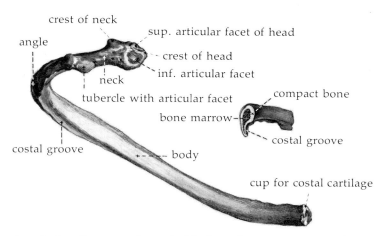

A. Left rib seen from behind and transverse section through a rib.
Note the two articular surfaces of the head: these articulate with two successive vertebrae.

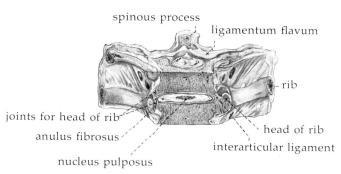

B. Section through the head of a rib and two successive vertebrae.
Note that one rib articulates with two vertebrae.

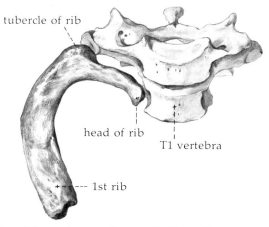

C. Thoracic vertebra with first rib.
The first rib does not articulate with C7.

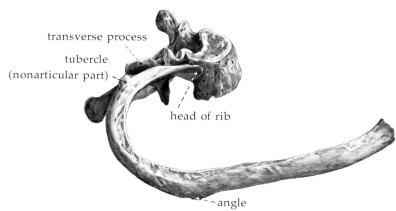

D. Thoracic rib with vertebra.

E. Costovertebral joint.
The rib has a joint with the body as well as with the transverse process of the vertebra.

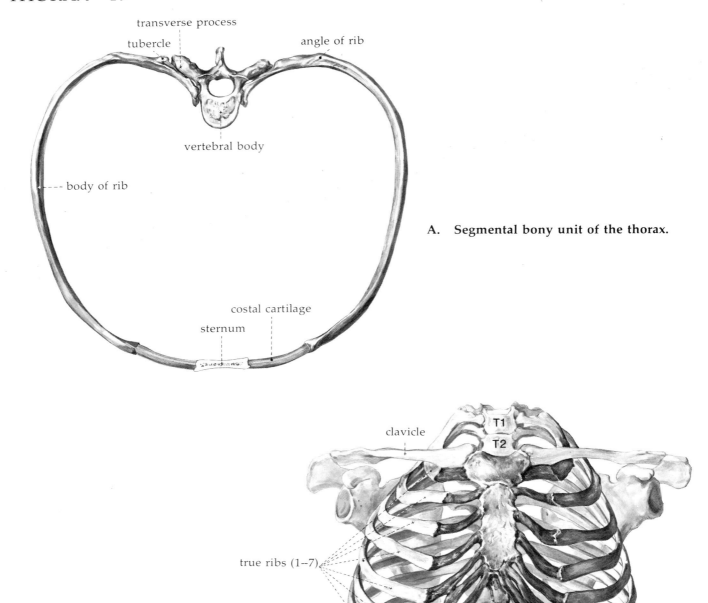

transverse process

tubercle

angle of rib

vertebral body

body of rib

costal cartilage

sternum

A. Segmental bony unit of the thorax.

clavicle

T1

T2

true ribs (1–7)

false ribs (8–10)

T12

L1

L2

floating ribs (11–12)

B. Anterior aspect of the bony thorax.

The following points should be observed:

¶ The upper margin of the manubrium lies opposite the lower border of T2; the sternal angle is located opposite the intervertebral disc between T4 and T5; the xiphisternal joint lies opposite the body of T9.

¶ The bony parts of the ribs have a downward inclination; the cartilaginous parts an upward inclination, with the exception of the first costal cartilage, which has a horizontal position.

¶ Seven pairs of ribs articulate with the sternum; the eighth, ninth and tenth pairs (false ribs) are connected to the cartilaginous components of the higher ribs; the eleventh and twelfth pairs are free or "floating" ribs.

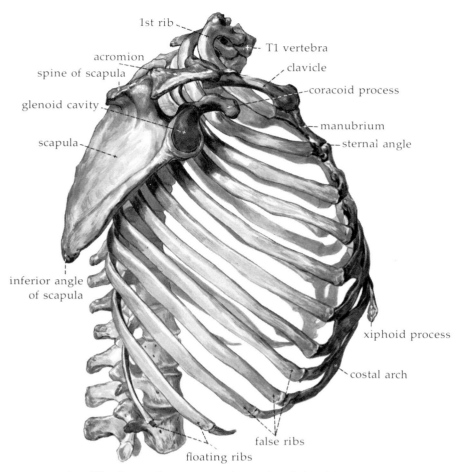

1st rib
T1 vertebra
acromion
clavicle
spine of scapula
coracoid process
glenoid cavity
scapula
manubrium
sternal angle
inferior angle
of scapula
xiphoid process
costal arch
false ribs
floating ribs

A.   The bony thorax seen from the right side.

Note the downward inclination of the bony parts and the upward inclination of the cartilaginous parts of the ribs.

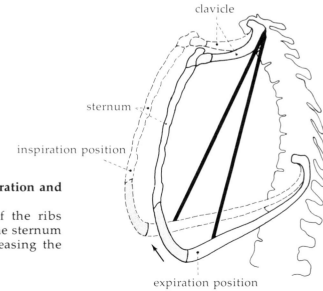

clavicle
sternum
inspiration position
expiration position

B.   Lateral view of the thorax during inspiration and expiration.

During inspiration the sternal ends of the ribs move forward and upward. Similarly, the sternum moves forward and upward, thus increasing the anteroposterior diameter of the chest.

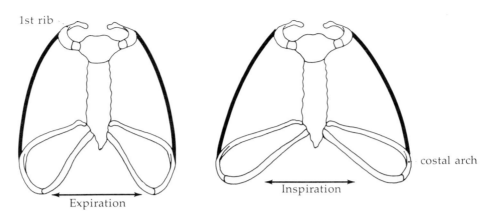

A and B. Position of the bony thorax during expiration and inspiration.
During inspiration the ribs move upward and outward, thereby rotating around the costovertebral axis. In expiration the ribs move downward and inward. Hence, the transverse diameter of the thorax increases during inspiration.

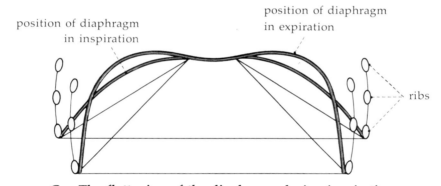

C. The flattening of the diaphragm during inspiration.

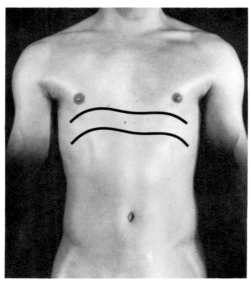

D. Surface view of the thorax with position of the diaphragm superimposed.
The two lines indicate the variability in position of the diaphragm in normal subjects.

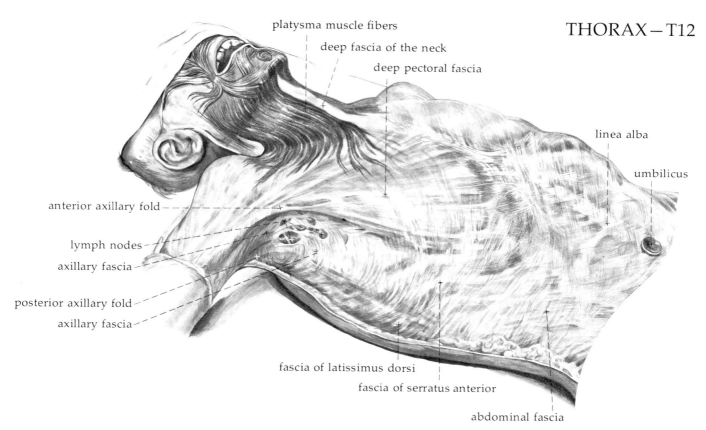

platysma muscle fibers
deep fascia of the neck
deep pectoral fascia
linea alba
umbilicus
anterior axillary fold
lymph nodes
axillary fascia
posterior axillary fold
axillary fascia
fascia of latissimus dorsi
fascia of serratus anterior
abdominal fascia

A. Deep fascia of the thorax.

This fascia forms an investing layer for all the muscles of the thorax; it is shown after removal of the skin and the superficial fascia. Note the opening for the blood vessels and nerves in the fascia of the axillary region. The fascia is not particularly thick— otherwise it might interfere with movement of the muscles.

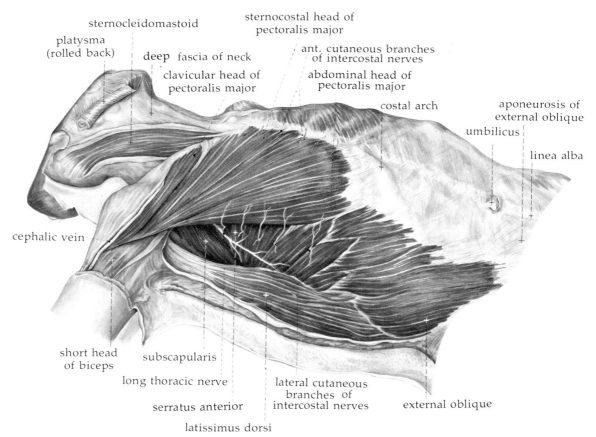

sternocleidomastoid
sternocostal head of pectoralis major
platysma (rolled back)
deep fascia of neck
ant. cutaneous branches of intercostal nerves
clavicular head of pectoralis major
abdominal head of pectoralis major
costal arch
aponeurosis of external oblique
umbilicus
linea alba
cephalic vein
short head of biceps
subscapularis
long thoracic nerve
lateral cutaneous branches of intercostal nerves
external oblique
serratus anterior
latissimus dorsi

B. Position of the superficial thoracic muscles.

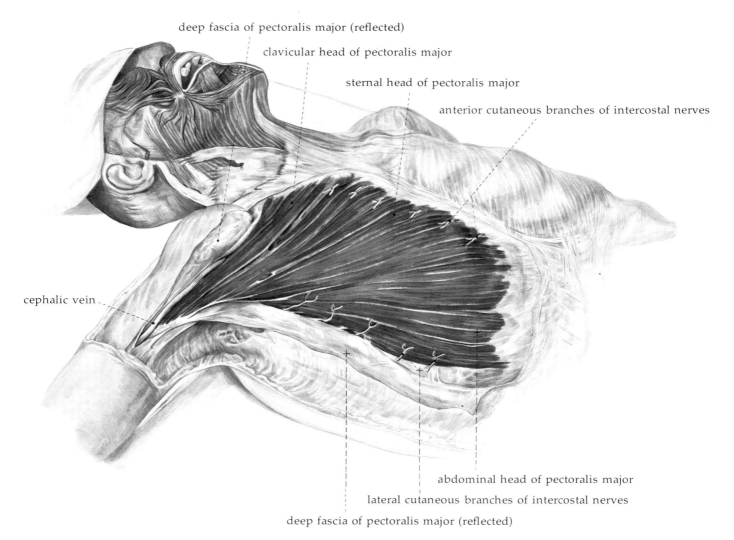

deep fascia of pectoralis major (reflected)

clavicular head of pectoralis major

sternal head of pectoralis major

anterior cutaneous branches of intercostal nerves

cephalic vein

abdominal head of pectoralis major

lateral cutaneous branches of intercostal nerves

deep fascia of pectoralis major (reflected)

Pectoralis major muscle.

Note the cephalic vein and the anterior and lateral cutaneous branches of the intercostal nerves (see T19 *B*). The cephalic vein is frequently used by surgeons as a landmark for the junction between the deltoid and pectoralis major muscles in operations on the shoulder joint.

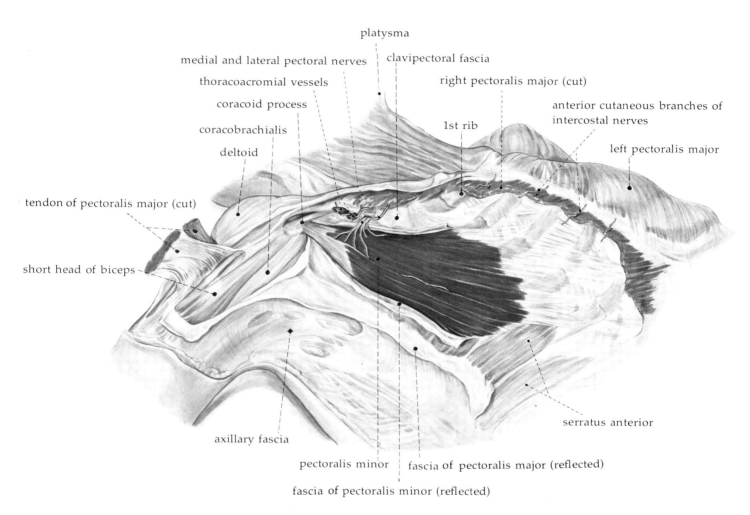

platysma

medial and lateral pectoral nerves

clavipectoral fascia

thoracoacromial vessels

right pectoralis major (cut)

coracoid process

anterior cutaneous branches of intercostal nerves

coracobrachialis

1st rib

deltoid

left pectoralis major

tendon of pectoralis major (cut)

short head of biceps

serratus anterior

axillary fascia

pectoralis minor

fascia of pectoralis major (reflected)

fascia of pectoralis minor (reflected)

Pectoralis minor muscle.

Note:

1.   The lateral pectoral nerve, a branch of the lateral cord of the brachial plexus, supplies the upper half of the pectoralis major muscle. The medial pectoral nerve, a branch of the medial cord of the plexus, pierces the pectoralis major muscle. Despite its medial position, the lateral pectoral nerve is called lateral because it is a branch of the lateral cord (see the brachial plexus of the upper limb, UL3).

2.   The thoracoacromial artery and vein.

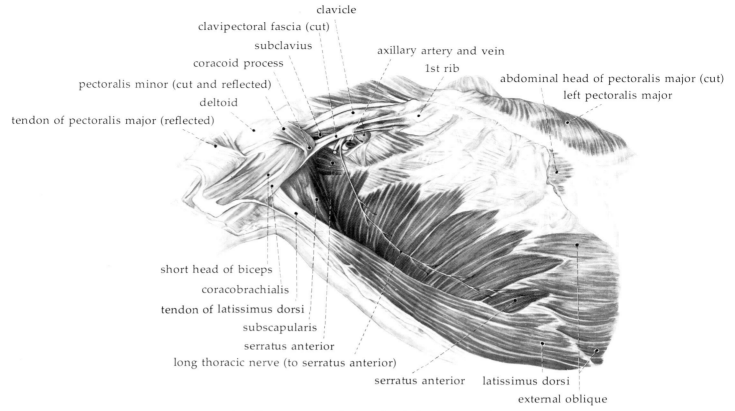

clavicle
clavipectoral fascia (cut)
subclavius
coracoid process
pectoralis minor (cut and reflected)
deltoid
tendon of pectoralis major (reflected)
axillary artery and vein
1st rib
abdominal head of pectoralis major (cut)
left pectoralis major

short head of biceps
coracobrachialis
tendon of latissimus dorsi
subscapularis
serratus anterior
long thoracic nerve (to serratus anterior)
serratus anterior   latissimus dorsi
external oblique

A.   Serratus anterior and subclavius muscles.

Note the nerve to the serratus anterior—the long thoracic nerve—and the axillary artery and vein.

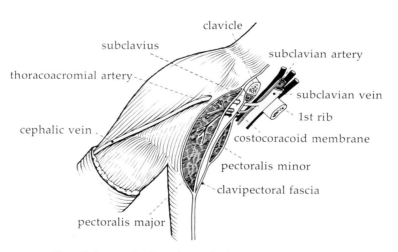

clavicle
subclavius
thoracoacromial artery
subclavian artery
subclavian vein
1st rib
cephalic vein
costocoracoid membrane
pectoralis minor
clavipectoral fascia
pectoralis major

B.   Schematic drawing of clavipectoral fascia.

The clavipectoral fascia is attached to the undersurface of the clavicle. It extends downward and fuses with the deep investing fascia in the axillary region. The subclavius and pectoralis minor muscles are ensheathed by the fascia. The portion between the sheaths of the subclavius and pectoralis muscles is known as the *costocoracoid membrane*. It is penetrated by the cephalic vein, the thoracoacromial artery and the lateral pectoral nerve.

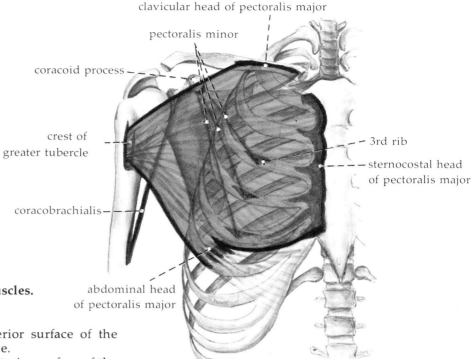

clavicular head of pectoralis major

pectoralis minor

coracoid process

crest of
greater tubercle

3rd rib

sternocostal head
of pectoralis major

coracobrachialis

abdominal head
of pectoralis major

A. Pectoralis major and minor muscles.

Pectoralis major

Origin:

Clavicular portion—anterior surface of the medial half of the clavicle.

Sternocostal portion—anterior surface of the lateral half of the sternum and the adjacent upper six costal cartilages.

Abdominal portion—aponeurosis of the external oblique muscle.

Insertion: Crest of the greater tubercle of the humerus.

Function: Adducts the arm. The clavicular portion also flexes and rotates the arm medially; the sternocostal portion depresses the arm and shoulder. During forced inspiration the muscle elevates the upper ribs.

Pectoralis minor

Origin: Third, fourth and fifth ribs near the costal cartilages.

Insertion: Coracoid process of the scapula.

Function: Depresses the point of the shoulder.

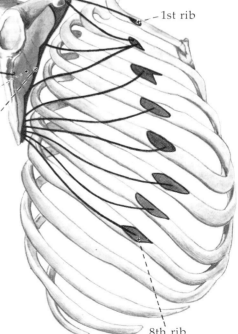

1st rib

costal surface of scapula

medial border of scapula

8th rib

B. Serratus anterior muscle.

Origin: Outer surfaces of the upper eight ribs.

Insertion: Costal aspect of the medial border of the scapula, mainly in the area of the inferior angle.

Function: Rotates the scapula and plays an important role in abduction and elevation of the arm above the horizontal.

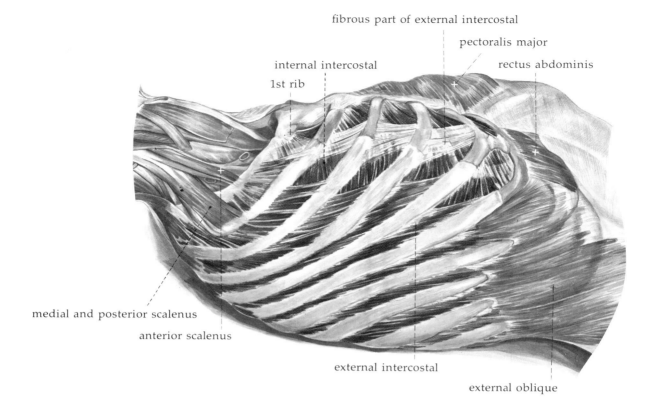

fibrous part of external intercostal

pectoralis major

internal intercostal

rectus abdominis

1st rib

medial and posterior scalenus

anterior scalenus

external intercostal

external oblique

External and internal intercostal muscles.

Intercostal musculature

¶ The *external intercostal muscle fibers* run downward and forward, terminating at the costochondral junction where they become fibrous — the *anterior intercostal membrane*.

¶ The *internal intercostal muscle fibers* run at right angles to the external fibers. They terminate posteriorly at the angle of the ribs, forming the *posterior intercostal membrane*.

¶ The third and innermost layer consists of the *transversus thoracis muscle,* the *subcostal muscle* and usually the *innermost intercostal muscle* (see T20). The latter, if present, may extend from the subcostal muscle to the transversus thoracis muscle.

The role of the musculature in respiration

QUIET INSPIRATION

¶ Because the first rib is attached to the scaleni muscles, the intercostal muscles obtain a fixed base. In quiet respiration the function of the intercostals is minimal and inspiration is mainly the result of contraction of the diaphragm. In deep inspiration the intercostals as well as the subcostal and transversus thoracis muscles become more active.

FORCED INSPIRATION

¶ In forced inspiration the pectoralis major and minor, the serratus anterior and the sternocleidomastoid muscles support the intercostals.

QUIET EXPIRATION

¶ Quiet expiration is brought about by the elastic recoil of the lungs and a relaxation of the intercostal muscles and diaphragm.

FORCED EXPIRATION

¶ The musculature of the abdominal wall contracts, resulting in increased abdominal pressure which pushes the diaphragm upward.

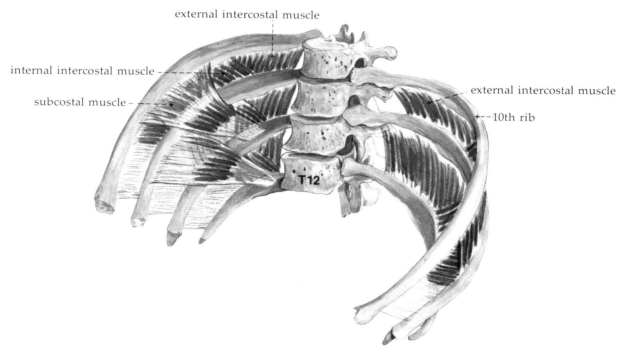

external intercostal muscle

internal intercostal muscle

subcostal muscle

external intercostal muscle

10th rib

T 12

A.   Intercostal and subcostal muscles.

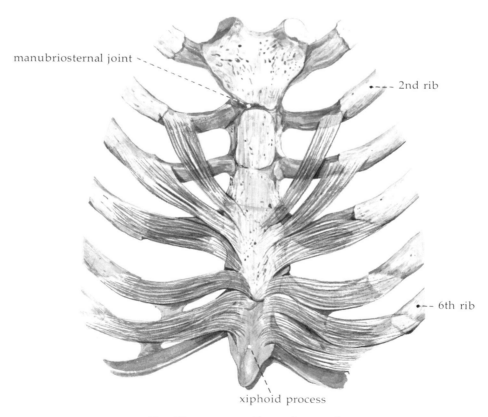

manubriosternal joint

2nd rib

6th rib

xiphoid process

B.   Transversus thoracis muscle.
The sternum is seen from behind.

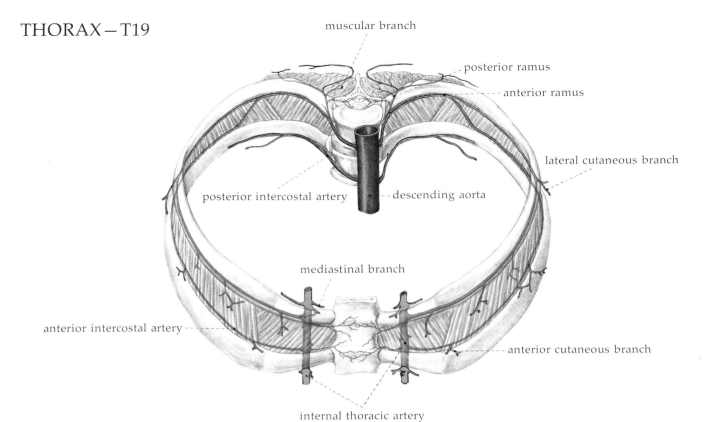

muscular branch

posterior ramus

anterior ramus

lateral cutaneous branch

posterior intercostal artery

descending aorta

mediastinal branch

anterior intercostal artery

anterior cutaneous branch

internal thoracic artery

A.   The intercostal space and its arteries.

Note the connection between the descending aorta and the internal thoracic artery.

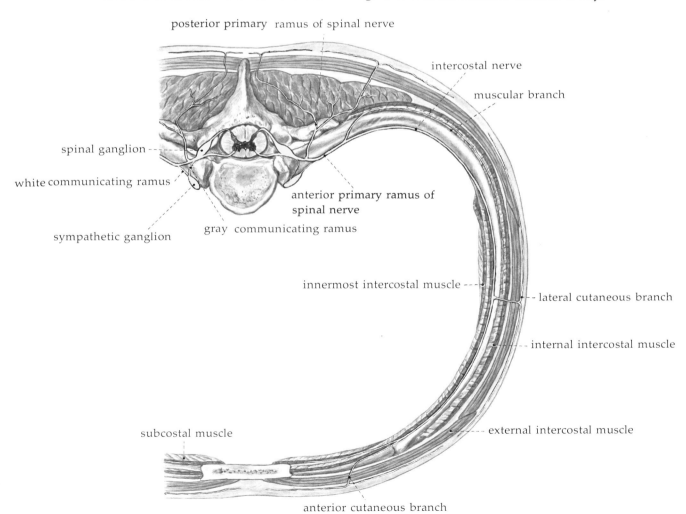

posterior primary ramus of spinal nerve

intercostal nerve

muscular branch

spinal ganglion

white communicating ramus

anterior primary ramus of spinal nerve

sympathetic ganglion

gray communicating ramus

innermost intercostal muscle

lateral cutaneous branch

internal intercostal muscle

external intercostal muscle

subcostal muscle

anterior cutaneous branch

B.   The intercostal nerve and its branches.

In the thoracic region the anterior primary ramus of the spinal nerve is referred to as the intercostal nerve.

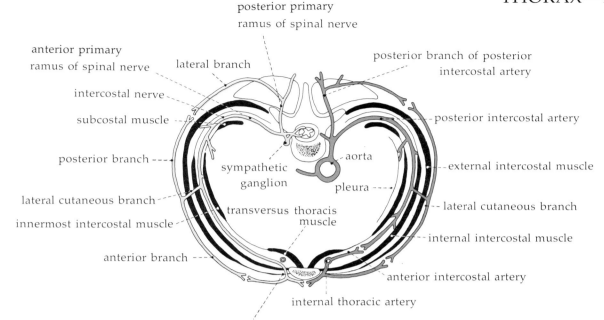

posterior primary
ramus of spinal nerve

anterior primary
ramus of spinal nerve

lateral branch

posterior branch of posterior
intercostal artery

intercostal nerve

subcostal muscle

posterior intercostal artery

posterior branch

aorta

sympathetic
ganglion

external intercostal muscle

pleura

lateral cutaneous branch

lateral cutaneous branch

transversus thoracis
muscle

innermost intercostal muscle

internal intercostal muscle

anterior branch

anterior intercostal artery

internal thoracic artery

anterior cutaneous branch

A.   The intercostal musculature and the position of the artery and nerve.

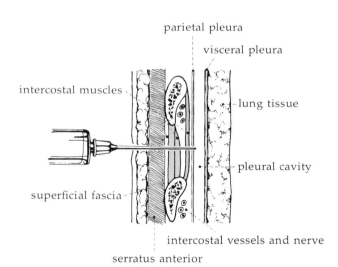

parietal pleura

visceral pleura

intercostal muscles

lung tissue

pleural cavity

superficial fascia

intercostal vessels and nerve

serratus anterior

B.   Puncture of the pleural cavity.

*A number of important clinical
points must be noted:*

¶ The intercostal vein, artery and nerve run in the costal groove or just below the rib. They are located on the inside of the internal intercostal muscle. When a needle is inserted through the intercostal space into the pleural cavity, it should be inserted in the middle of the intercostal space to avoid puncturing the artery or the vein.

¶ The internal thoracic artery runs one finger width laterally from the sternum. It is located between the transversus thoracis muscle and the rib cartilages. A knife pushed into the intercostal space and moved medially toward the sternum will cut the artery and cause severe intrathoracic bleeding.

¶ The *posterior intercostal arteries* originate from the aorta. They communicate with branches of the internal thoracic artery known as the *anterior intercostal arteries.* Hence, blood from the internal thoracic artery can reach the descending aorta by way of the intercostal arteries. This occurs in patients who have a coarctation of the aorta (see T60). Because in such cases little or no blood enters the descending aorta, a collateral circulation between the internal thoracic artery and the descending aorta develops. The intercostal arteries enlarge greatly and can be seen to pulsate. As a result, the lower half of the body receives blood by way of the internal thoracic arteries. On radiographs of the thorax the ribs are seen to be grooved as a result of the pulsations of the intercostal arteries.

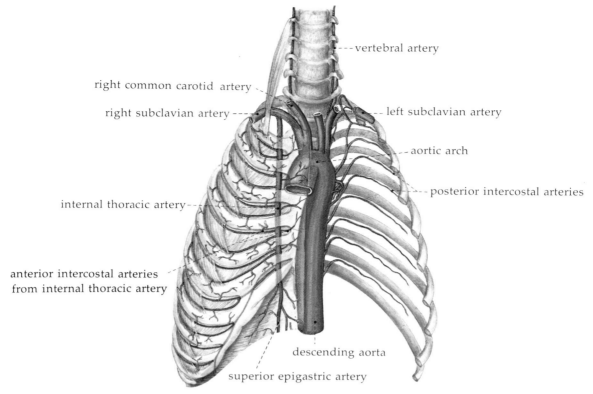

vertebral artery

right common carotid artery

right subclavian artery

left subclavian artery

aortic arch

posterior intercostal arteries

internal thoracic artery

anterior intercostal arteries
from internal thoracic artery

descending aorta

superior epigastric artery

A. Blood supply of the thoracic wall.
Note the origin of the posterior intercostal arteries.

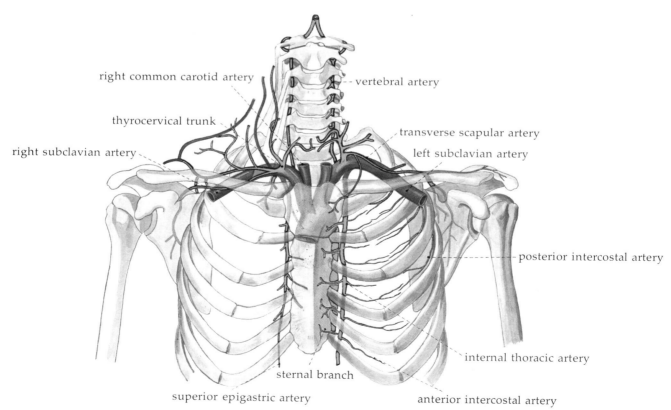

right common carotid artery

vertebral artery

thyrocervical trunk

transverse scapular artery

right subclavian artery

left subclavian artery

posterior intercostal artery

internal thoracic artery

sternal branch

superior epigastric artery

anterior intercostal artery

B. Blood supply of the thoracic wall.
Note the origin and course of the internal thoracic artery and the perforating branches
supplying the mammary gland.

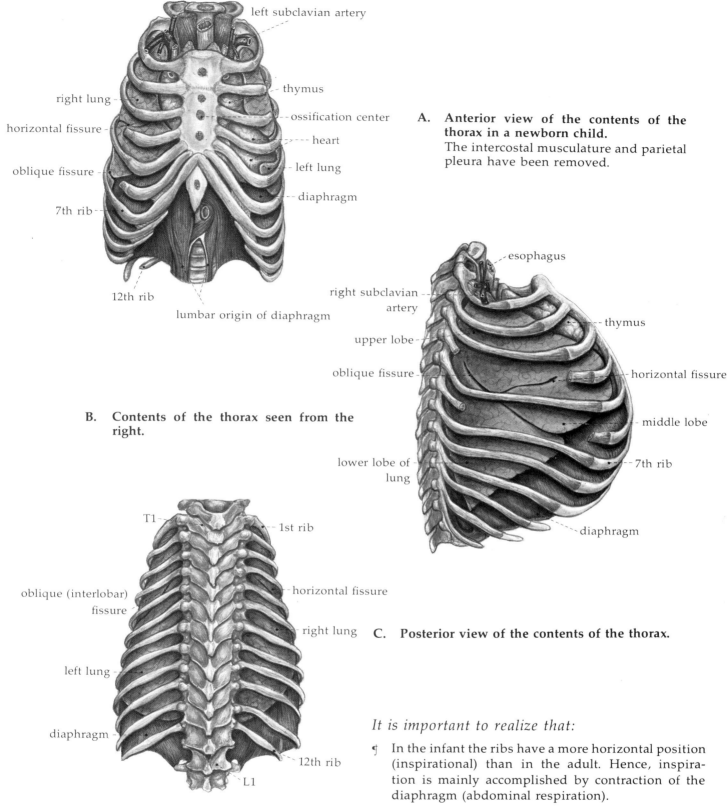

left subclavian artery

right lung

horizontal fissure

oblique fissure

7th rib

12th rib

lumbar origin of diaphragm

thymus

ossification center

heart

left lung

diaphragm

A. Anterior view of the contents of the thorax in a newborn child.
The intercostal musculature and parietal pleura have been removed.

esophagus

right subclavian artery

upper lobe

oblique fissure

lower lobe of lung

thymus

horizontal fissure

middle lobe

7th rib

diaphragm

B. Contents of the thorax seen from the right.

T1

1st rib

oblique (interlobar) fissure

horizontal fissure

right lung

left lung

diaphragm

12th rib

L1

C. Posterior view of the contents of the thorax.

It is important to realize that:

¶ In the infant the ribs have a more horizontal position (inspirational) than in the adult. Hence, inspiration is mainly accomplished by contraction of the diaphragm (abdominal respiration).

¶ The dome of the diaphragm in the infant is higher than it is in the adult. With advancing age the diaphragm becomes flatter.

¶ The thymus in the young infant is large. It is frequently found in front of the pericardial sac and on each side of the body of the sternum.

¶ The pericardium is clearly visible through the third and fourth intercostal spaces. The position of the heart in the infant is higher than that in the adult, owing to the high dome of the diaphragm (see T58).

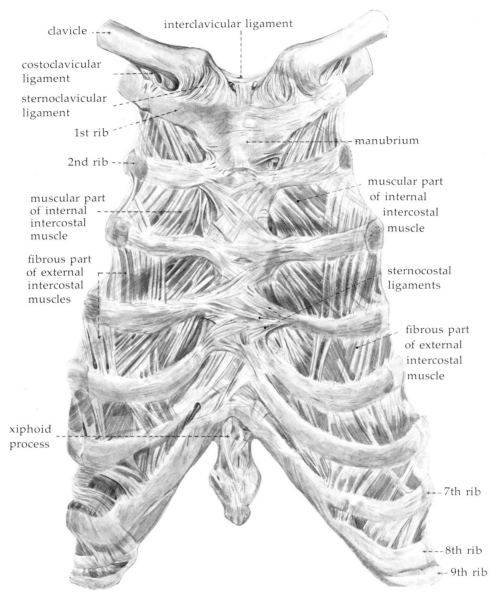

clavicle

interclavicular ligament

costoclavicular ligament

sternoclavicular ligament

1st rib

2nd rib

muscular part of internal intercostal muscle

fibrous part of external intercostal muscles

xiphoid process

manubrium

muscular part of internal intercostal muscle

sternocostal ligaments

fibrous part of external intercostal muscle

7th rib

8th rib

9th rib

A.   Anterior view of the anterior thoracic wall after removal from the body.

Note the fibrous part of the external intercostal muscles and the muscular part of the internal intercostal muscles.

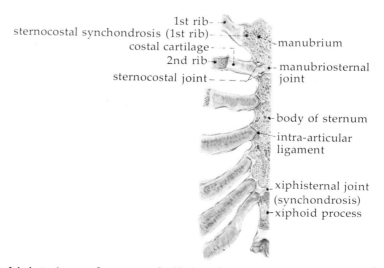

1st rib

sternocostal synchondrosis (1st rib)

costal cartilage

2nd rib

sternocostal joint

manubrium

manubriosternal joint

body of sternum

intra-articular ligament

xiphisternal joint (synchondrosis)

xiphoid process

B.   Sternocostal joints (second to seventh ribs) and synchondrosis of the first rib with the sternum.

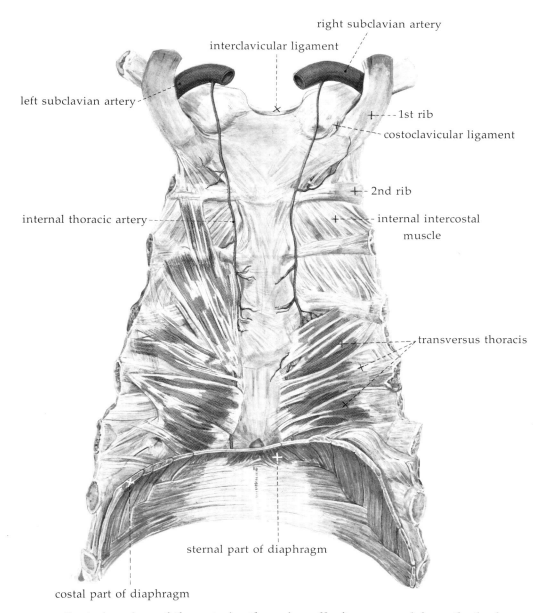

right subclavian artery

interclavicular ligament

left subclavian artery

1st rib

costoclavicular ligament

2nd rib

internal thoracic artery

internal intercostal muscle

transversus thoracis

sternal part of diaphragm

costal part of diaphragm

Posterior view of the anterior thoracic wall after removal from the body.

Note:

¶ The transversus thoracis muscle.

¶ The internal thoracic artery originates from the subclavian artery and subsequently descends between the transversus thoracis and the internal intercostal muscles. Its main branches are: (a) the *pericardiacophrenic artery*, which accompanies the phrenic nerve (see T31); (b) the *musculophrenic artery*, which courses behind the costal attachment of the diaphragm and supplies the lower six intercostal spaces; (c) the *superior epigastric artery* (see A8 *A*), which enters the rectus sheath to anastomose with the inferior epigastric artery; and (d) the *anterior intercostal arteries* (see T20 *A*), with perforating branches to the mammary gland.

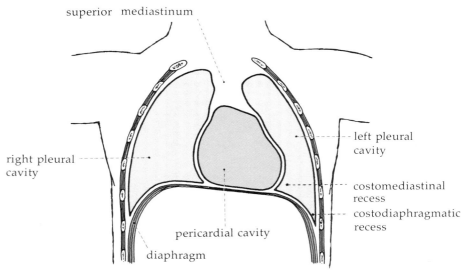

A. Schematic drawing of a frontal section through the thorax.
Note the three serous compartments.

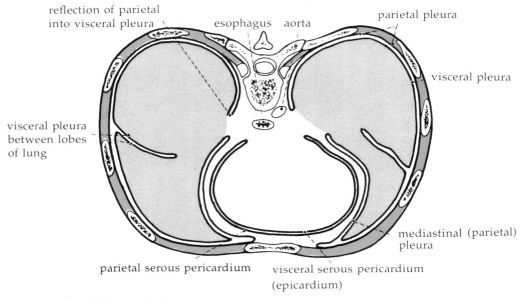

B. Schematic drawing of a transverse section through the thorax.
Note the three serous cavities and the reflection lines of the pleura and pericardium.

It is important to understand the various compartments of the thorax and the relationships of the serous membranes. Keep the following points in mind:

¶ The visceral pleura invests the lung tissue, and the parietal pleura covers the body wall, diaphragm and mediastinum. Between the visceral and parietal pleurae is found the pleural cavity. The reflection line of the parietal pleura into the visceral pleura is located around the hilus of the lung and directly below it as the pulmonary ligament (see T33). Note that the visceral pleura penetrates the fissures between the lobes of the lung.

¶ The visceral layer of the serous membrane of the heart is in intimate contact with the heart muscle and is known as the *epicardium*. The parietal layer forms the inner lining of the *fibrous pericardium*. The space between the parietal layer and the epicardium is the *pericardial cavity*. The parietal layer reflects into the epicardium: (a) around the arterial pole of the heart formed by the aorta and the pulmonary artery; and (b) around the venous pole formed by the superior and inferior venae cavae and the pulmonary veins (see T45 and T57 A).

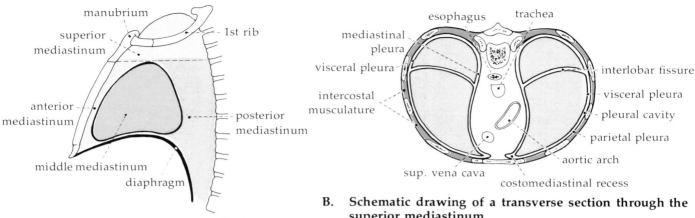

A. Schematic drawing of the mediastinal compartments.

B. Schematic drawing of a transverse section through the superior mediastinum.

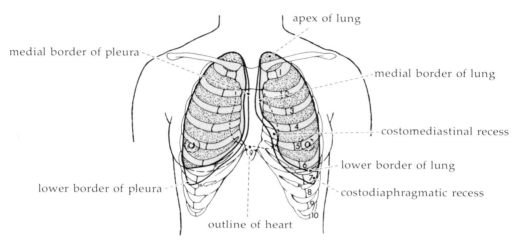

C. Anterior view of the lungs and pleural borders.

The mediastinum is the region between the right and left pleural cavities. It is divided into superior, anterior, middle and posterior sections. The superior mediastinum is the region above the pericardial sac delineated by a plane joining the sternal angle and the intervertebral disc between the fourth and fifth thoracic vertebrae. The anterior mediastinum is the area between the body of the sternum and the pericardial sac; it contains some fat, thymus rests and lymph nodes. The middle mediastinum contains the heart and the root of the great arteries and veins, and the posterior mediastinum lies behind the pericardium, extending downward to the level of the twelfth thoracic vertebra.

In studying the lung and pleural cavity, keep the following points in mind:

¶ The visceral pleura invests the lung and cannot be stripped from the lung tissue.

¶ The parietal pleura is subdivided into four parts: costal, diaphragmatic, mediastinal and cervical. It descends below the lower border of the lungs.

¶ In ordinary breathing the lungs are not completely expanded and hence do not completely fill the pleural cavity. In those areas the parietal and visceral pleura are apposed to each other, preventing the formation of a real cavity. This contact of the pleural layers occurs mainly along the anterior and lower borders. During quiet respiration these potential spaces (recesses) are not used and the two layers remain in apposition. The recesses are known as the right and left *costodiaphragmatic recesses* and the left *costomediastinal recess.* The latter is located at the anterior ends of the fourth and fifth left intercostal spaces. During deep inspiration, the lungs enter the pleural recesses.

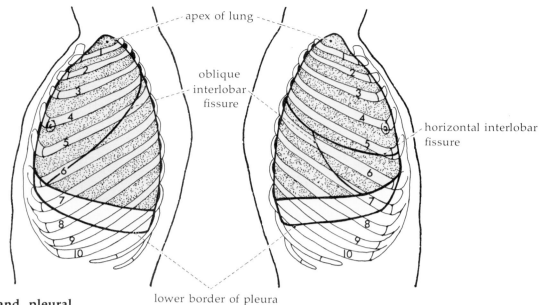

apex of lung

oblique interlobar fissure

horizontal interlobar fissure

lower border of pleura

A. Lung and pleural borders seen from the left.

B. Lung and pleural borders seen from the right.

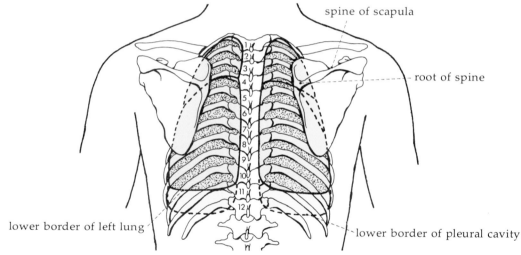

spine of scapula

root of spine

lower border of left lung

lower border of pleural cavity

C. Posterior view of lung and pleural borders.

Under normal conditions the lungs expand freely into the pleural cavities during inspiration. The degree of expansion can be easily determined by percussion and auscultation. The following points are clinically important:

¶ When inflammation of the pleura (pleurisy) occurs, considerable fluid may collect in the pleural cavity. The fluid collects first in the lowest part of the cavity and may be noticed in the posterior costodiaphragmatic recess by percussion and auscultation.

¶ The pleural cavity is sometimes aspirated in a diagnostic or therapeutic procedure. The site is usually slightly *behind the posterior axillary line* in the sixth to eighth intercostal space, depending on the height of the fluid in the pleural cavity. The needle is inserted into the intercostal space a little toward the superior surface of the lower rib to avoid the intercostal artery, vein and nerve (see T20 B).

¶ Below the lower border of the pleural cavity, the diaphragm is in direct contact with the ribs and intercostal musculature. If a needle is passed through the anterior parts of the seventh, eighth, ninth, tenth and eleventh intercostal spaces, it will miss the pleural cavity. After passing through the intercostal musculature, the needle will penetrate the diaphragm and then enter the peritoneal cavity (see A and B and T29).

¶ When the ribs (usually the third to the eighth) are fractured, the fracture itself is of no great importance. Frequently, however, one of the fragments punctures the pleura or the lung. If air enters the pleural cavity, the lung will collapse (pneumothorax).

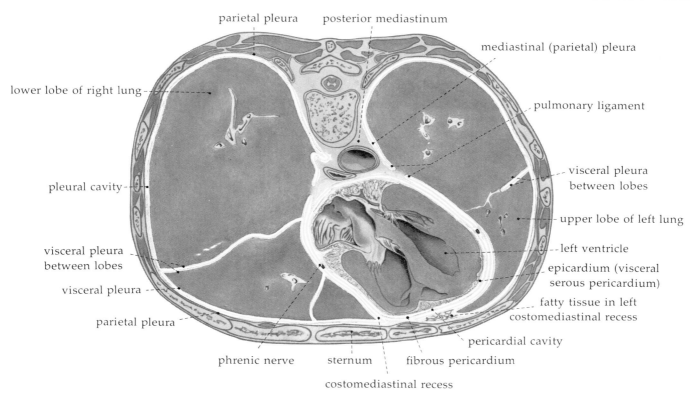

parietal pleura   posterior mediastinum

mediastinal (parietal) pleura

lower lobe of right lung

pulmonary ligament

pleural cavity

visceral pleura
between lobes

upper lobe of left lung

visceral pleura
between lobes

left ventricle

visceral pleura

epicardium (visceral
serous pericardium)

parietal pleura

fatty tissue in left
costomediastinal recess

pericardial cavity

phrenic nerve   sternum   fibrous pericardium

costomediastinal recess

A. Transverse section through the thorax.

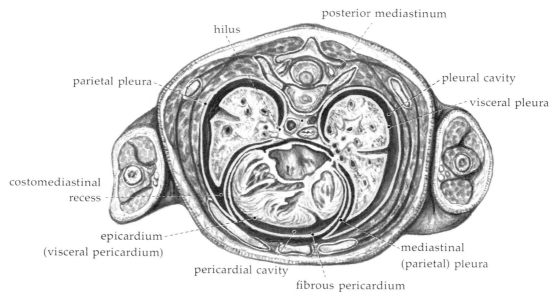

hilus   posterior mediastinum

parietal pleura

pleural cavity

visceral pleura

costomediastinal
recess

epicardium
(visceral pericardium)

mediastinal
(parietal) pleura

pericardial cavity

fibrous pericardium

B. Transverse section through the thorax of a 7-month fetus.

Observe the parietal and visceral pleural lines; note that (a) the visceral pleura is found between the lobes of the lungs; (b) the reflection of the parietal into the visceral pleura is found in the area of the hilus of the lung; (c) the costomediastinal recess is part of the pleural cavity; (d) the epicardium or visceral serous pericardium is directly applied to the muscle of the heart; (e) the phrenic nerves are located between the fibrous pericardium and the mediastinal (parietal) pleura; (f) in a fetus the pleural cavities can be more clearly distinguished than in the adult because the lungs are in a collapsed state.

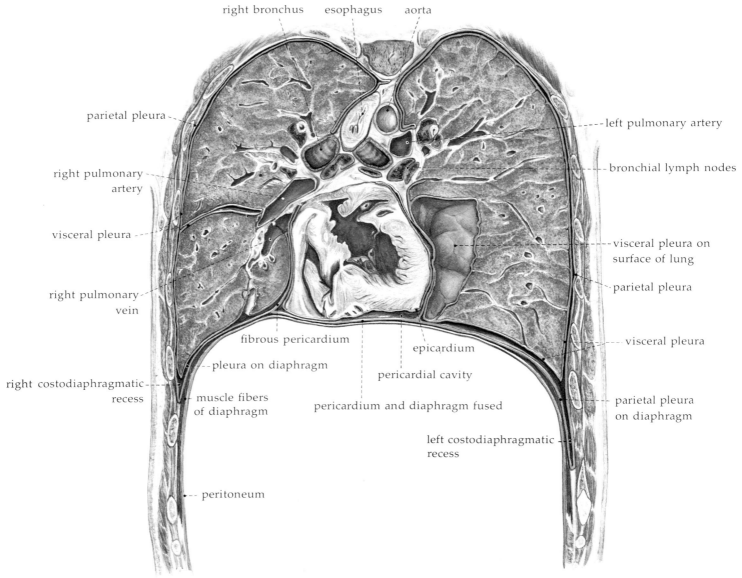

right bronchus   esophagus   aorta

parietal pleura

right pulmonary artery

visceral pleura

right pulmonary vein

right costodiaphragmatic recess

fibrous pericardium

pleura on diaphragm

muscle fibers of diaphragm

peritoneum

left pulmonary artery

bronchial lymph nodes

visceral pleura on surface of lung

parietal pleura

visceral pleura

epicardium

pericardial cavity

pericardium and diaphragm fused

parietal pleura on diaphragm

left costodiaphragmatic recess

Frontal section through the thorax of an adult.
Note the right and left costodiaphragmatic recesses.

¶ The costodiaphragmatic recess is the potential space of the pleural cavity, which becomes larger and smaller during expiration and inspiration, respectively, as the lung moves out and in.

¶ The costomediastinal recess lies at the anterior ends of the fourth and fifth left intercostal spaces. Here the costal and mediastinal layers of the left pleura are in direct contact with each other. During inspiration the left lung expands into the recess in a sternal direction over the heart (see T28 A).

¶ Below the lower border of the pleural cavity, the diaphragm is in direct contact with the ribs and the intercostal musculature.

¶ In the region of the tendinous portion of the diaphragm the fibrous pericardium is fused with the diaphragm.

¶ It is sometimes difficult to separate the fibrous pericardium from the parietal (mediastinal) pleura because the two may be fused together.

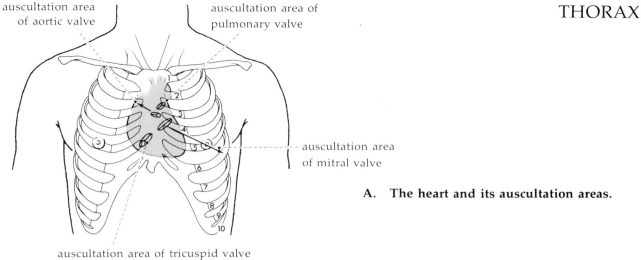

auscultation area of aortic valve

auscultation area of pulmonary valve

auscultation area of mitral valve

auscultation area of tricuspid valve

A. The heart and its auscultation areas.

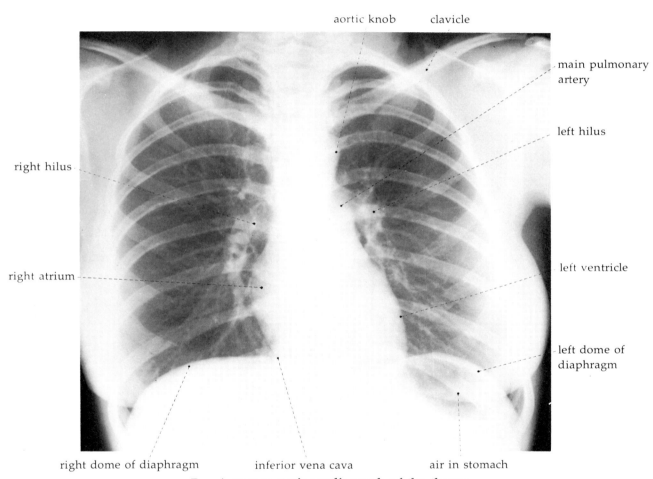

aortic knob   clavicle

main pulmonary artery

left hilus

right hilus

left ventricle

right atrium

left dome of diaphragm

right dome of diaphragm   inferior vena cava   air in stomach

B. Anteroposterior radiograph of the thorax.

¶ The surface markings of the heart valves all lie behind the sternum and are of little practical value. The sounds of the heart valves, however, can be heard with the stethoscope in the following areas:

1. The bicuspid or mitral valve is heard best in the left fifth intercostal space over the area of the apex beat.

2. The tricuspid valve is heard best over the lower right end of the sternum close to the attachment of the fifth rib.

3. The pulmonary valve can be heard over the medial end of the second left intercostal space.

4. The aortic valve can be listened to over the medial end of the second right intercostal space.

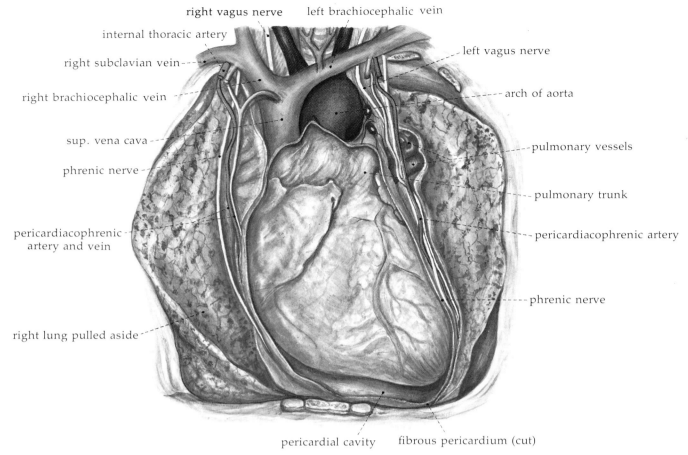

right vagus nerve left brachiocephalic vein

internal thoracic artery

right subclavian vein

left vagus nerve

right brachiocephalic vein

arch of aorta

sup. vena cava

pulmonary vessels

phrenic nerve

pulmonary trunk

pericardiacophrenic artery and vein

pericardiacophrenic artery

phrenic nerve

right lung pulled aside

pericardial cavity   fibrous pericardium (cut)

Anterior view of the thoracic organs.

The fibrous pericardium and parietal pleura have been removed and the lungs have been pulled laterally.

Note:

¶ An important clinical correlation is the location of the reflection line of the fibrous pericardium onto the aorta, pulmonary artery and superior vena cava. If fluid collects in the pericardial cavity when the patient is in a supine position it will be noticed first around the arterial stems (see T58).

¶ The phrenic nerves originate from the anterior primary rami of C4, with occasional contributions from C3 and C5. They provide motor innervation to the diaphragm. Pressure from malignant tumors in the mediastinum or surgical sectioning of the nerve will cause unilateral paralysis of the diaphragm. The dome of the diaphragm will obtain an extreme expiration position and the lower lobe of the lung will become practically immobile.

¶ Keep in mind that the phrenic nerves carry sensory impulses from the central part of the lower aspect of the diaphragm to the central nervous system. Hence, pain impulses are carried by the phrenic nerves from the peritoneum covering the undersurface of the diaphragm and from the pleura covering the central region of the upper surface of the diaphragm, as well as from the pericardium and the mediastinal parietal pleura. Since nerves of the fourth cervical segment also supply the skin of the shoulder, pain may be felt over the shoulder when inflammatory conditions such as pleurisy, liver abscess, cholecystitis and gastric ulcer develop in close contact with the central portion of the diaphragm. Pain referred from the thoracic and abdominal viscera to parts of the body wall is called *referred pain.* A ruptured spleen and gastric air bubbles also may cause pain over the shoulder.

¶ The *pericardiacophrenic arteries* are branches of the internal thoracic arteries. They supply the pericardium and part of the diaphragm.

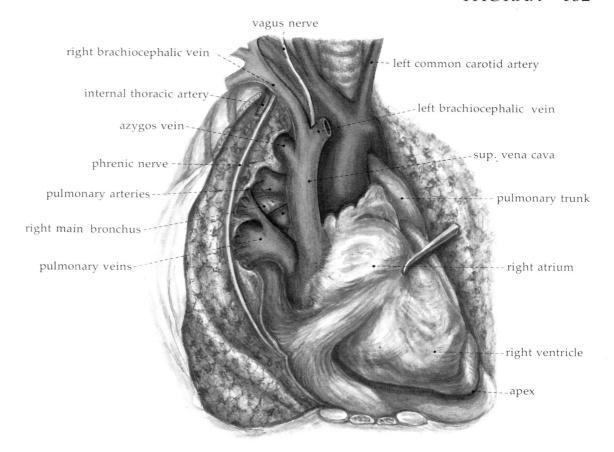

vagus nerve

right brachiocephalic vein

internal thoracic artery

azygos vein

phrenic nerve

pulmonary arteries

right main bronchus

pulmonary veins

left common carotid artery

left brachiocephalic vein

sup. vena cava

pulmonary trunk

right atrium

right ventricle

apex

Retrocardiac view exposing the root of the right lung.

¶ At the root of the lung note: (a) the pulmonary veins, (b) the pulmonary artery, (c) the right bronchus, and (d) the phrenic nerve.

¶ The azygos vein enters the superior vena cava. This vein creates a slight groove on the surface of the lung. Sometimes the vein is deeply embedded in the lung and located between two lobes. On an anteroposterior radiograph, the lumen of the azygos vein may then show as a round hole, which is sometimes confused with a cyst or an abscess.

¶ The intrathoracic course of the inferior vena cava is very short. When the heart is pulled to the left, the diaphragm surrounding the inferior vena cava is pulled with it.

¶ The phrenic nerve, normally embedded between the fibrous pericardium and the parietal pleura, is seen in its position in front of the pulmonary vessels and the bronchus.

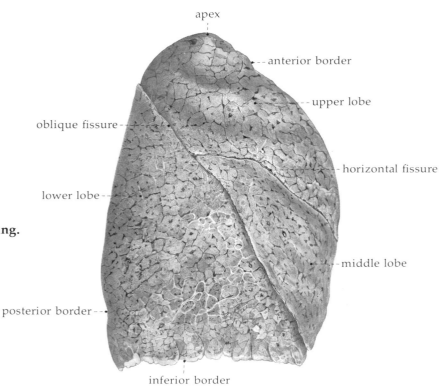

apex

anterior border

upper lobe

oblique fissure

horizontal fissure

lower lobe

middle lobe

posterior border

inferior border

A. Lateral or costal view of the right lung.

upper lobe

groove for azygos vein

groove for superior vena cava

pulmonary artery

bronchial artery

right main bronchus

lymph node

B. Medial surface of the right lung.

pulmonary vein

pulmonary vein

horizontal fissure

cardiac impression

groove for inferior vena cava

pulmonary ligament

middle lobe

lower lobe

oblique fissure

diaphragmatic surface

Observe:

   ¶   The reflection line of the visceral pleura into the parietal pleura. The pulmonary ligament is not a real ligament but merely the reflection line of the parietal pleura into the visceral pleura.

   ¶   Organs adjacent to the lung frequently cause impressions in the spongy lung tissue. On the costal surface note the rib impressions; on the mediastinal surface the impressions of the azygos vein, the heart and the caval veins can be seen.

   ¶   The mottled grayish appearance of the lungs is caused mainly by carbon deposits in the small superficial lymph vessels and alveolar walls.

   ¶   Note the bronchial artery, a direct branch of the descending aorta or of one of the upper intercostal arteries. It supplies the bronchial tree with oxygenated blood.

   ¶   The right lung has three lobes.

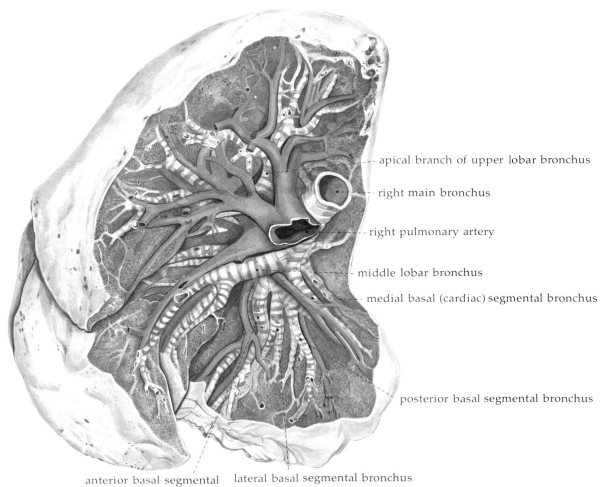

apical branch of upper lobar bronchus

right main bronchus

right pulmonary artery

middle lobar bronchus

medial basal (cardiac) segmental bronchus

posterior basal segmental bronchus

anterior basal segmental bronchus

lateral basal segmental bronchus

Bronchial tree and pulmonary arteries of the right lung.
The pulmonary vein and its branches have been removed.

Note:

¶ Branches of the pulmonary artery accompany the bronchi. Sometimes more than one
artery accompanies a segmental bronchus.

¶ Branches of the pulmonary vein do not accompany the bronchi. They course in the
connective tissue of the intersegmental planes.

¶ A bronchopulmonary segment is the largest subdivision within a lobe. Segments are
separated from each other by connective tissue septa. Surgical removal of a segment in
patients with a cancer or an abscess is possible.

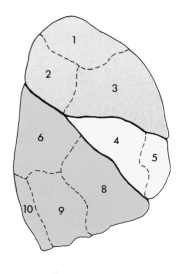
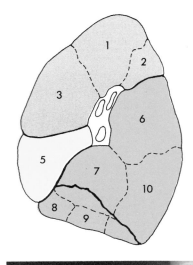

A. Bronchopulmonary segments of the right lung.
Lateral view and medial view.

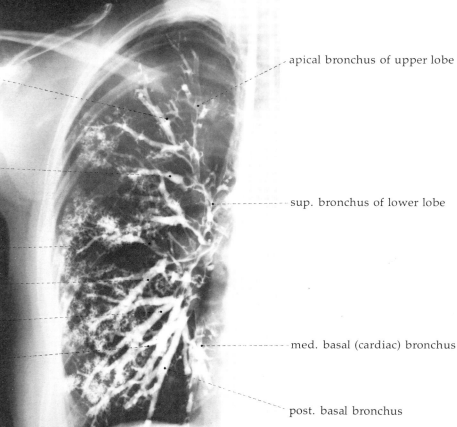

post. bronchus of upper lobe

apical bronchus of upper lobe

ant. bronchus of upper lobe

sup. bronchus of lower lobe

lat. bronchus of middle lobe

med. bronchus of middle lobe

ant. basal bronchus

med. basal (cardiac) bronchus

lat. basal bronchus

post. basal bronchus

B. Bronchogram of the right lung.

¶ The lobes of the lung are subdivided into bronchopulmonary segments, each of them pyramidal in shape with its apex toward the root of the lung and its base toward the surface.

The following segments are recognized in the right lung:

Upper lobe: 1, apical; 2, posterior; 3, anterior
Middle lobe: 4, lateral; 5, medial
Lower lobe: 6, superior; 7, medial basal (cardiac); 8, anterior basal; 9, lateral basal; 10, posterior basal.

¶ In bronchography the tracheobronchial tree is anesthetized, after which a radiopaque contrast medium is introduced through a catheter. Bronchography can provide much useful information, particularly in cases of cancer of the bronchial tree.

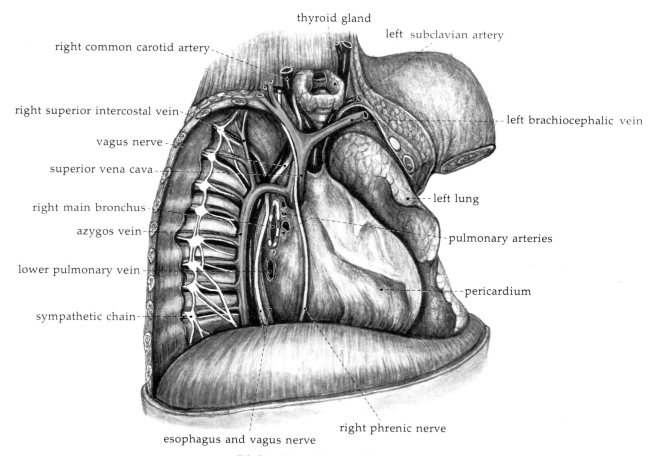

thyroid gland

left subclavian artery

right common carotid artery

right superior intercostal vein

vagus nerve

superior vena cava

right main bronchus

azygos vein

lower pulmonary vein

sympathetic chain

left brachiocephalic vein

left lung

pulmonary arteries

pericardium

right phrenic nerve

esophagus and vagus nerve

Right side of the mediastinum.
The right lung and the mediastinal and costal pleura have been removed.

A number of important observations may be made:

¶ The azygos vein, draining the posterior body wall and the right lung, enters the superi-
or vena cava. It causes a groove on the mediastinal surface of the right lung. The vein is
sometimes embedded in the lung, causing the formation of a separate lobe, which is
referred to as the *azygos lobe*.

¶ The esophagus, accompanied by the vagus nerves, is separated from the posterior
wall of the left atrium only by the fibrous pericardium. If the left atrium is enlarged, it
will produce an indentation of the esophagus. A radiograph of the esophagus may
therefore show whether the left atrium is abnormally large.

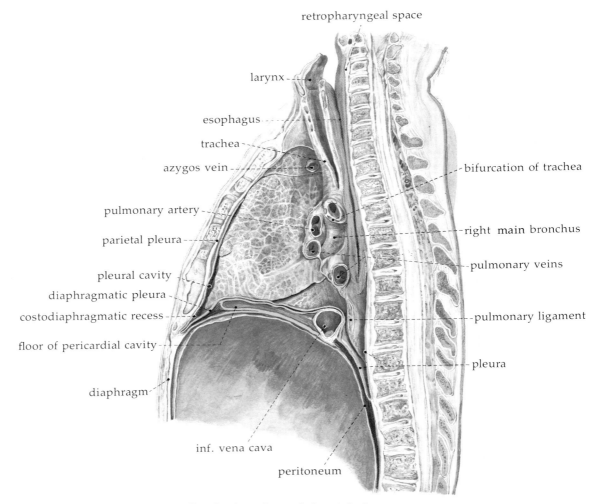

retropharyngeal space

larynx

esophagus

trachea

azygos vein

pulmonary artery

parietal pleura

pleural cavity

diaphragmatic pleura

costodiaphragmatic recess

floor of pericardial cavity

diaphragm

inf. vena cava

peritoneum

bifurcation of trachea

right main bronchus

pulmonary veins

pulmonary ligament

pleura

View of the mediastinal surface of the right lung.
The left lung, heart and great vessels have been removed.

Note:

¶ The parietal pleura covers the anterior, lateral and posterior sections of the thoracic wall and the upper aspect of the diaphragm. The pleural cavity lies between the parietal pleura and the visceral pleura investing the lung tissue. The costodiaphragmatic recess is the space of the pleural cavity into which the lung expands during deep inspiration. The lung also expands into the posterior part of the recess.

¶ When fluid collects in the pleural cavity it is usually first noted in the most posterior (and lowest) part of the costodiaphragmatic recess. An impression of the presence and amount of fluid can be obtained by percussion of the back.

¶ Anteriorly the esophagus is attached to the posterior membranous wall of the trachea by loose connective tissue. Since the trachea and lungbuds develop from the foregut, it is not uncommon to find an open connection between the trachea, mainly in the area of the bifurcation, and the esophagus. This congenital malformation is known as an esophagotracheal fistula. It is usually accompanied by an atresia of the proximal part of the esophagus.

¶ Posteriorly the esophagus adjoins the vertebral column, the prevertebral layer of the deep cervical fascia and the longus colli muscle. Retropharyngeal abscesses may descend into the thorax behind the esophagus (see HN107).

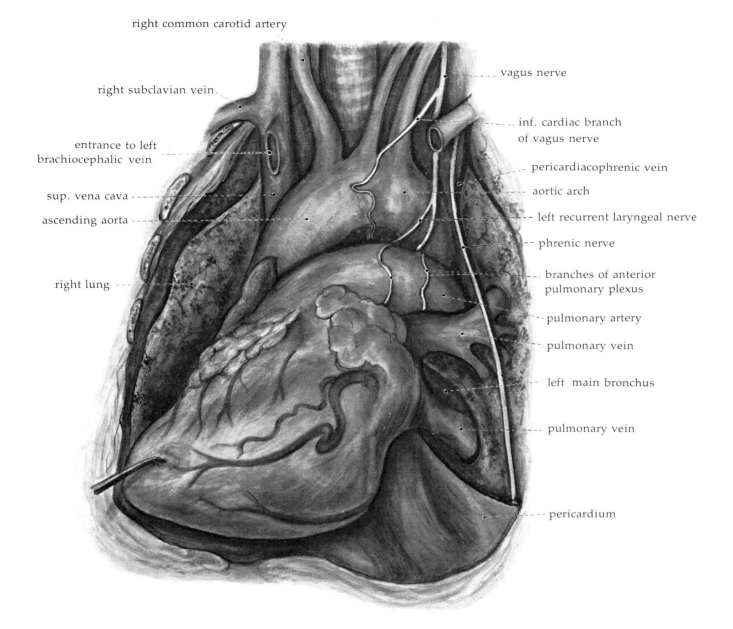

right common carotid artery

right subclavian vein

entrance to left
brachiocephalic vein

sup. vena cava

ascending aorta

right lung

vagus nerve

inf. cardiac branch
of vagus nerve

pericardiacophrenic vein

aortic arch

left recurrent laryngeal nerve

phrenic nerve

branches of anterior
pulmonary plexus

pulmonary artery

pulmonary vein

left main bronchus

pulmonary vein

pericardium

Retrocardiac view exposing the root of the left lung.
Note the vagus nerve with its inferior cardiac and pulmonary branches.

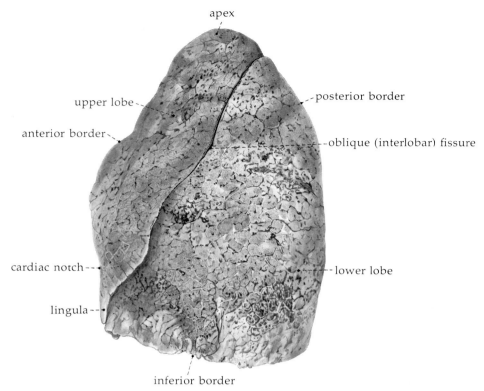

apex

upper lobe

posterior border

anterior border

oblique (interlobar) fissure

cardiac notch

lower lobe

lingula

inferior border

A.   Lateral or costal surface of the left lung.
Note that the left lung has two lobes.

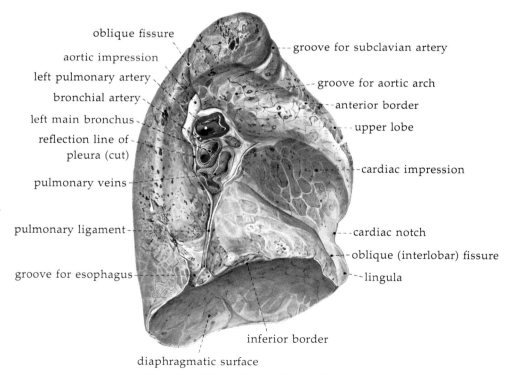

oblique fissure

groove for subclavian artery

aortic impression

left pulmonary artery

groove for aortic arch

bronchial artery

anterior border

left main bronchus

upper lobe

reflection line of
pleura (cut)

pulmonary veins

cardiac impression

pulmonary ligament

cardiac notch

oblique (interlobar) fissure

groove for esophagus

lingula

inferior border

diaphragmatic surface

B.   Medial surface of the left lung.
Note the impressions caused by the esophagus, the descending aorta, the arch of the
aorta, the subclavian artery and the heart.

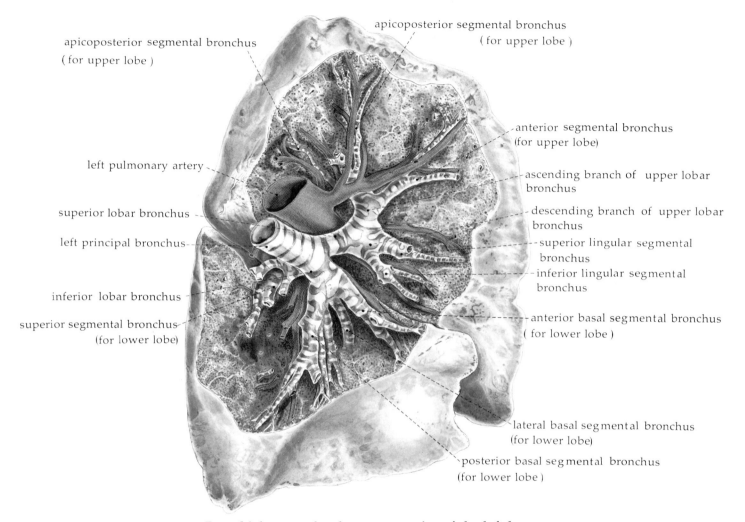

apicoposterior segmental bronchus
(for upper lobe)

apicoposterior segmental bronchus
(for upper lobe)

anterior segmental bronchus
(for upper lobe)

left pulmonary artery

ascending branch of upper lobar
bronchus

descending branch of upper lobar
bronchus

superior lobar bronchus

superior lingular segmental
bronchus

left principal bronchus

inferior lingular segmental
bronchus

inferior lobar bronchus

anterior basal segmental bronchus
(for lower lobe)

superior segmental bronchus
(for lower lobe)

lateral basal segmental bronchus
(for lower lobe)

posterior basal segmental bronchus
(for lower lobe)

Bronchial tree and pulmonary arteries of the left lung.
The pulmonary vein and its branches have been removed.

Note:

The lingula is a small portion of the upper lobe of the left lung located between the cardiac
impression and the oblique fissure. It corresponds to the middle lobe of the right lung.

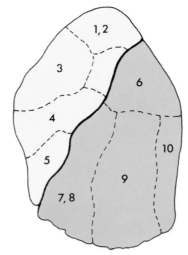
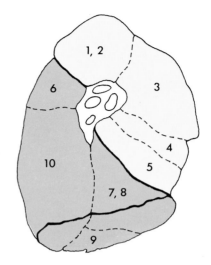

A. Bronchopulmonary segments of the left lung.
Lateral-costal and mediastinal-diaphragmatic views.

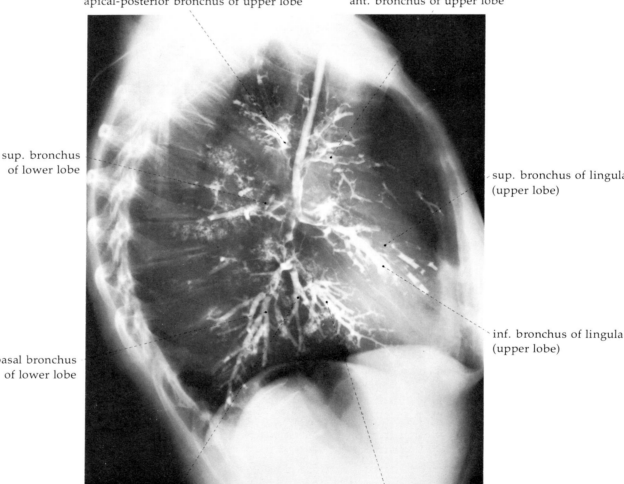

B. Bronchogram of the left lung.

¶ The following segments are recognized in the left lung:

Upper lobe
upper division: 1 and 2, apical-posterior; 3, anterior lower division: 4, superior
lingular; 5, inferior lingular
Lower lobe
6, superior; 7 and 8, anterior-medial basal; 9, lateral basal; 10, posterior basal

¶ Unlike the right lung, which has ten segmental bronchi, the left lung has only eight.
Sometimes it is stated that both lungs have ten segments each. The apical and posterior
bronchi of the left upper lobe usually have a common stem and the two segments are
inseparable. The same is true of the anterior-medial basal segment of the left lower
lobe.

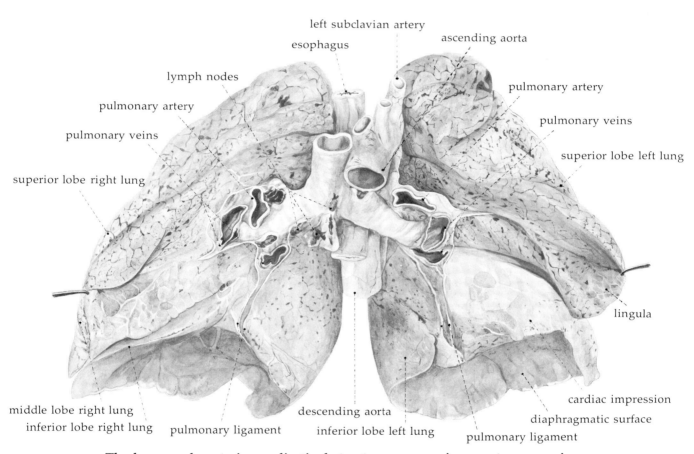

left subclavian artery

esophagus

lymph nodes

pulmonary artery

pulmonary veins

superior lobe right lung

ascending aorta

pulmonary artery

pulmonary veins

superior lobe left lung

lingula

middle lobe right lung

inferior lobe right lung

pulmonary ligament

descending aorta

inferior lobe left lung

cardiac impression

diaphragmatic surface

pulmonary ligament

The lungs and posterior mediastinal structures as seen in an autopsy specimen.

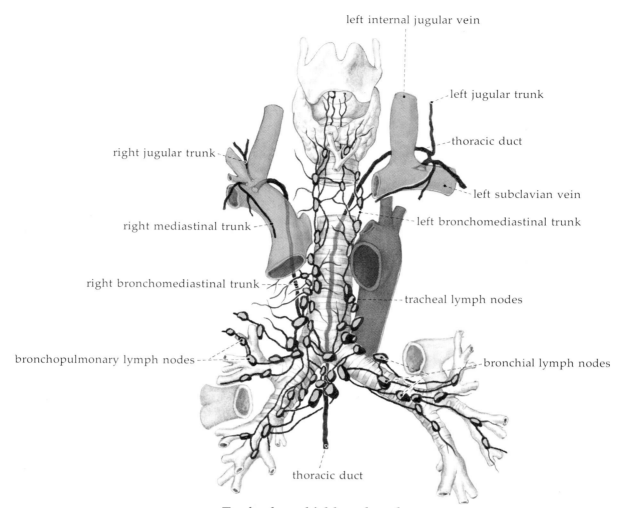

left internal jugular vein

left jugular trunk

thoracic duct

right jugular trunk

left subclavian vein

right mediastinal trunk

left bronchomediastinal trunk

right bronchomediastinal trunk

tracheal lymph nodes

bronchopulmonary lymph nodes

bronchial lymph nodes

thoracic duct

Tracheobronchial lymph nodes.

¶ The lymph vessels of the lung course from the periphery toward the hilus along the bronchi and the arteries. Many lymph nodes are found in the areas of bronchial branching and at the bifurcation of the trachea and roots of the lung (tracheobronchial nodes). On the right side these nodes drain into the bronchomediastinal trunk and on the left side into the thoracic duct.

¶ The lymph nodes are of great clinical importance in patients with bronchial cancers. The cancer cells usually spread rapidly to the tracheobronchial nodes, which frequently fuse together into large masses. In the mediastinum these enlarged and fused lymph nodes may compress the surrounding structures such as the left recurrent laryngeal nerve, which in turn results in paralysis of the left vocal cord. Similarly, the enlarged lymph nodes may compress the superior vena cava, the trachea or the esophagus, thus causing problems in the blood circulation or difficulty with breathing or swallowing.

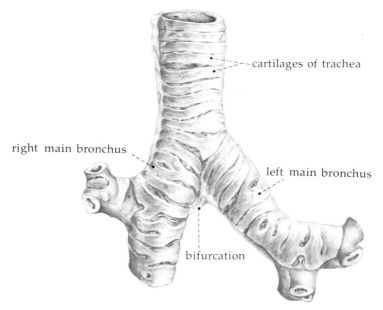

A. Anterior view of bifurcation of the trachea.

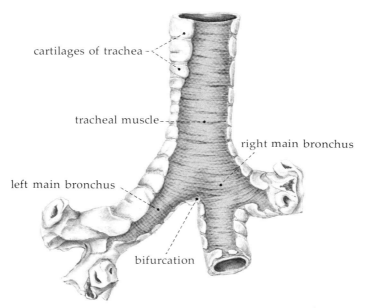

B. Posterior view of bifurcation of the trachea.

Make the following observations:

¶ Because the tracheal and bronchial cartilages are horseshoe-shaped, they provide the support and flexibility of the trachea and main bronchi. Only in the smaller bronchi do they have a ring shape.

¶ The bifurcation of the trachea is located at the level of the fifth thoracic vertebra. The direction of the right main bronchus is more in line with that of the trachea than it is on the left. When foreign bodies such as peanuts, bolts, screws and toys are inhaled, they usually enter the right main bronchus. From there they enter the bronchus of the middle or lower lobe, where they may cause a localized bronchopneumonia and, as a long-term effect, bronchiectasis.

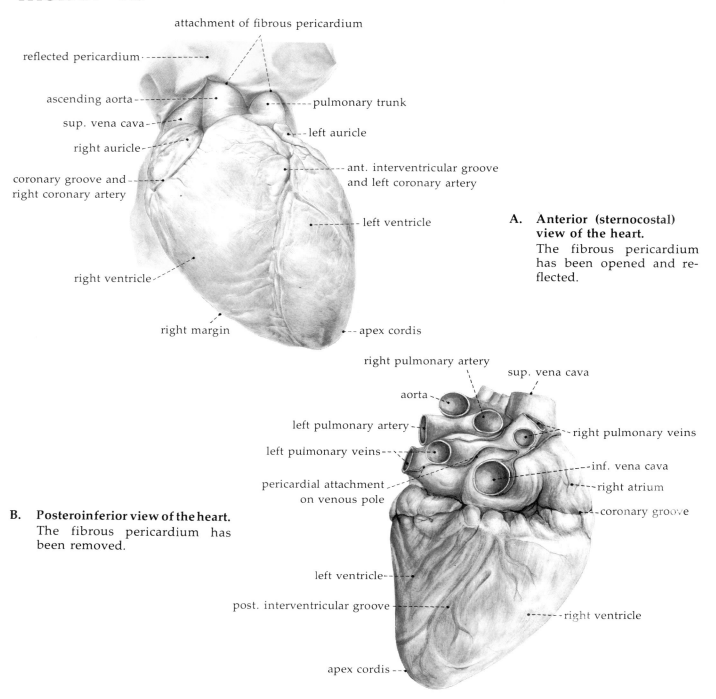

attachment of fibrous pericardium

reflected pericardium

ascending aorta

sup. vena cava

right auricle

coronary groove and
right coronary artery

pulmonary trunk

left auricle

ant. interventricular groove
and left coronary artery

left ventricle

right ventricle

right margin

apex cordis

A. Anterior (sternocostal) view of the heart.
The fibrous pericardium has been opened and reflected.

right pulmonary artery

sup. vena cava

aorta

left pulmonary artery

left pulmonary veins

pericardial attachment
on venous pole

right pulmonary veins

inf. vena cava

right atrium

coronary groove

B. Posteroinferior view of the heart.
The fibrous pericardium has been removed.

left ventricle

post. interventricular groove

right ventricle

apex cordis

The following observations should be made:

¶ The line of attachment of the fibrous pericardium to the vessels at the arterial pole (aorta and pulmonary trunk) as well as at the venous pole (pulmonary veins and caval veins) is clearly visible. At the venous pole the attachment line forms a horizontal T-shaped structure (⊣) with the caval veins at the ends of the crossbar.

¶ A large part of the right ventricle, a small part of the left ventricle and the auricle of the right atrium are clearly visible in the anterior view.

¶ The heart musculature is covered by a shiny layer, the visceral layer of the pericardium or the epicardium. The major arteries are embedded in the epicardium and cannot be distinguished easily. From the epicardium they penetrate with numerous branches into the underlying myocardium.

¶ The apex cordis, formed by the tip of the left ventricle, beats against the wall of the thorax in the fifth intercostal space. Here it can be felt as the apex beat. During contraction the heart rotates around a longitudinal axis that passes through the superior and inferior venae cavae.

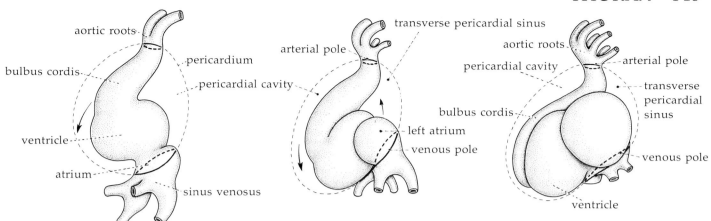

A, B and C. **Schematic drawings showing the formation of the pericardial sac and the transverse sinus.**

The transverse sinus of the pericardial sac is located between the arterial and venous poles. If a finger is placed between the superior vena cava and the ascending aorta and then is inserted behind the aorta and the pulmonary trunk, it will lie in the tunnel-shaped transverse pericardial sinus (see T45 *A* and T57 *A*). (From Langman, J.: Medical Embryology. 3rd ed. Baltimore, The Williams & Wilkins Co., 1975.)

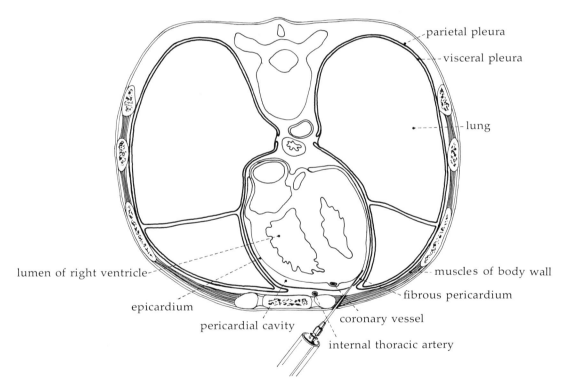

D. **Location of aspiration needle in the pericardial cavity.**

When fluid is present in the pericardial sac, a diagnostic puncture may be performed. The needle is placed half an inch to the left of the xiphoid process and brought into the pericardial cavity in an oblique upward direction. Great care must be taken not to puncture the internal thoracic artery and the anterior interventricular branch of the left coronary artery.

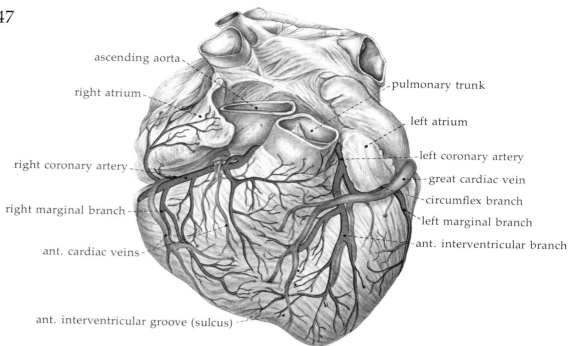

ascending aorta

right atrium

right coronary artery

right marginal branch

ant. cardiac veins

ant. interventricular groove (sulcus)

pulmonary trunk

left atrium

left coronary artery

great cardiac vein

circumflex branch

left marginal branch

ant. interventricular branch

A. Sternocostal (anterior) view of the heart.
The coronary arteries and veins have been dissected.

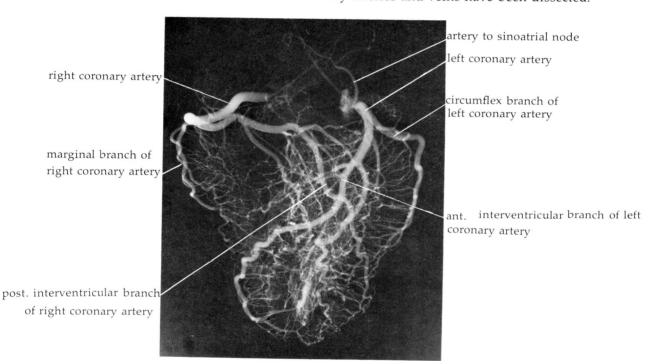

right coronary artery

marginal branch of
right coronary artery

post. interventricular branch
of right coronary artery

artery to sinoatrial node

left coronary artery

circumflex branch of
left coronary artery

ant.   interventricular branch of left
coronary artery

B. Anterior view of the coronary arterial circula-
tion after injection with micropaque. (From
Becker, R. F. et al.: The Anatomical Basis of
Medical Practice. Baltimore, The Williams &
Wilkins Company, 1971.)

A detailed knowledge of the coronary arteries is necessary for an understanding of the results of an obstruction in one of their branches.

The following points are clinically important:

¶ The anterior interventricular branch of the *left* coronary artery supplies most of the wall of the *left* ventricle, but also part of the anterior wall of the *right* ventricle.

¶ Branches of the posterior interventricular branch of the *right* coronary artery supply most of the right ventricle, but also part of the *left* ventricle (see T48).

¶ The left coronary artery supplies the major portion of the interventricular septum from the front; the right coronary artery supplies the remaining part of the interventricular septum from the rear (see T48 *B*).

¶ Of particular clinical importance is a twig from the right coronary artery, which supplies the atrioventricular node and the main bundle of the conducting system in 90 per cent of cases (see T56)

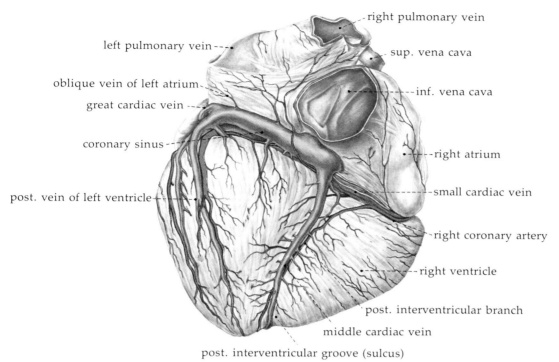

right pulmonary vein

left pulmonary vein

sup. vena cava

oblique vein of left atrium

inf. vena cava

great cardiac vein

coronary sinus

right atrium

post. vein of left ventricle

small cardiac vein

right coronary artery

right ventricle

post. interventricular branch

middle cardiac vein

post. interventricular groove (sulcus)

A. Posterior view of the heart.
The arteries and veins have been dissected.

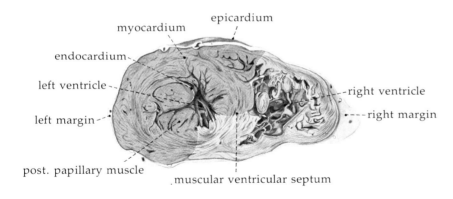

epicardium

myocardium

endocardium

left ventricle

right ventricle

left margin

right margin

post. papillary muscle

muscular ventricular septum

B. Section through the ventricles and the interventricular septum.
The supply areas of the right and left coronary arteries are indicated.

¶ The superficial veins drain by way of the coronary sinus. Much blood, however, returns to the heart by way of the venae cordis minimae, small veins which open directly
into the chambers of the heart. Note also the oblique vein of the left atrium — this is the
remnant of the original left common cardinal vein. Occasionally the oblique vein is
very large, in which case it is part of a persistent left superior vena cava, a relatively
rare abnormality.

¶ The anterior and usually the largest part of the interventricular septum is supplied by
the left coronary artery; the posterior part of the septum is supplied by the right coronary artery. Since the common atrioventricular bundle is located on the right side and in
the posterior part of the membranous interventricular septum, it is supplied by the
right coronary artery. Infarcts caused by obstruction of the right coronary artery are
dangerous, as the conducting system may be affected, and heart block may result.

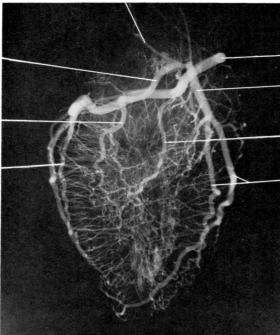

sinoatrial node artery

circumflex branch of
left coronary artery

right coronary artery

ant. interventricular branch of
left coronary artery

marginal branch of
left coronary artery

marginal branch of
right coronary artery

post. interventricular branches
of right coronary artery

branches of ant.
interventricular artery

A. Lateral view of the coronary arterial system after injection with micropaque.
Note the supply of the anterior and posterior myocardial walls. (From Becker, R. F.
et al.: The Anatomical Basis of Medical Practice. Baltimore, The Williams & Wilkins
Company, 1971.)

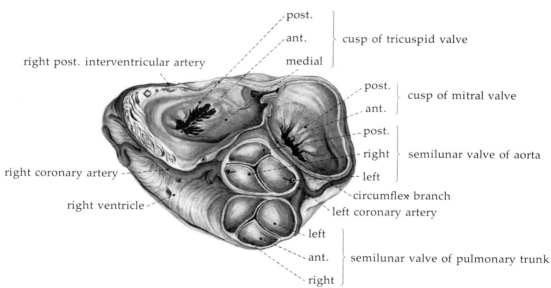

post.

ant. } cusp of tricuspid valve

medial

right post. interventricular artery

post. } cusp of mitral valve

ant.

post.

right } semilunar valve of aorta

left

right coronary artery

circumflex branch
left coronary artery

right ventricle

left

ant. } semilunar valve of pulmonary trunk

right

B. Coronary arteries and their origin from the aorta.
The atria and great vessels have been removed.

¶ Anastomoses between the coronary arteries are important in patients with arteriosclerosis and sudden blockage. Under normal conditions there are always some anastomoses in the myocardium. The participating vessels, however, are small. In a slowly
developing obstruction of a coronary branch, anastomoses may develop to compensate
for the loss of blood resulting from the blockage. A sudden blockage, such as that occurring after an embolus in a coronary artery, is often fatal because anastomoses have
no time to develop.

¶ In patients with severe arteriosclerosis of the coronary arteries a branch from the internal thoracic artery (the pericardiacophrenic artery) or from the omentum is grafted
onto the surface of the heart.

¶ Occasionally an embolus in a very small coronary branch may lead to a fatal outcome.
This usually happens when that branch supplies an essential component of the conducting system.

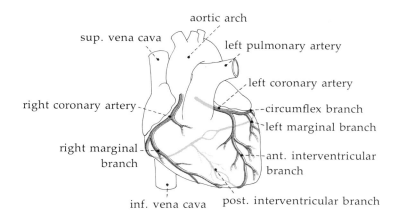

aortic arch
sup. vena cava
left pulmonary artery
left coronary artery
right coronary artery
circumflex branch
left marginal branch
right marginal branch
ant. interventricular branch
inf. vena cava
post. interventricular branch

A.   The course of the coronary arteries.

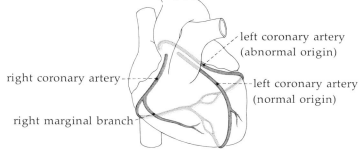

left coronary artery (abnormal origin)
right coronary artery
left coronary artery (normal origin)
right marginal branch

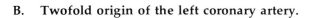

B.   Twofold origin of the left coronary artery.

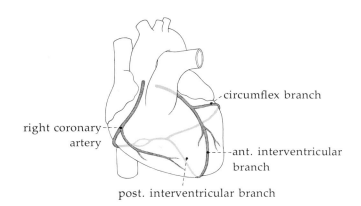

circumflex branch
right coronary artery
ant. interventricular branch
post. interventricular branch

C.   Left coronary artery supplying part of the right territory.

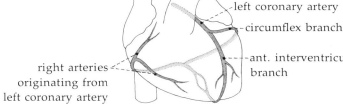

left coronary artery
circumflex branch
ant. interventricular branch
right arteries originating from left coronary artery

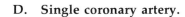

D.   Single coronary artery.

¶ Considerable variation exists in the course and supply area of the coronary arteries: (1) the left circumflex artery sometimes originates directly from the aorta in the right aortic sinus (*B*); (2) the posterior interventricular artery sometimes originates from the left coronary via its circumflex branch (*C*); (3) occasionally a single coronary artery supplies the entire heart (*D*).

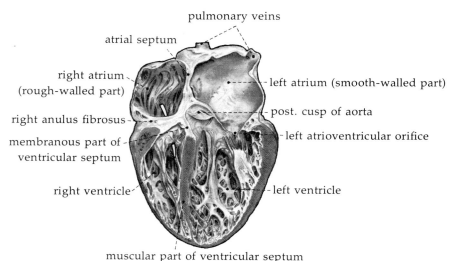

A. Section through the heart of an infant.
Anterior view of the posterior part.

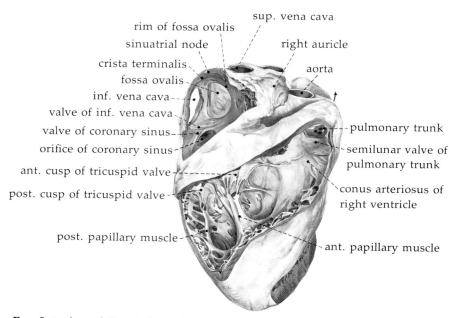

B. Interior of the right atrium and the right ventricle.
The pectinate part of the right atrial wall and a portion of the right
ventricular wall have been removed.

Note the following features:

IN THE RIGHT ATRIUM:

¶   The pectinate or rough-walled part of the atrium (T51 *A*). This portion is derived from
the original primitive heart tube. The smooth-walled part of the atrium is derived from
the sinus venosus.

¶   The fossa ovalis, the thin-walled part of the atrial septum. In patients with an atrial
septal defect, this portion of the wall may be absent, thus permitting blood to flow between the right and left atria (T51 *B*).

¶   The valves of the inferior vena cava and the coronary sinus. In the embryo these valves
guide the blood toward the foramen ovale and into the left atrium.

¶   The crista terminalis and above it the *sinuatrial node* of the conducting system.

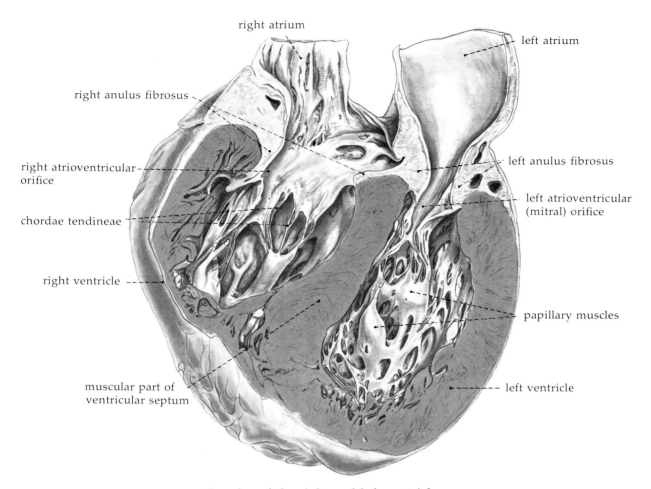

right atrium

left atrium

right anulus fibrosus

right atrioventricular orifice

left anulus fibrosus

left atrioventricular (mitral) orifice

chordae tendineae

right ventricle

papillary muscles

muscular part of ventricular septum

left ventricle

Interior of the right and left ventricles.

IN THE LEFT ATRIUM:

ϟ The smooth-walled part, derived from the pulmonary veins (T51 *A*).

IN THE RIGHT VENTRICLE:

ϟ The thickness of the muscular wall in comparison with that of the left ventricle.

ϟ The anterior cusp with its chordae tendineae and papillary muscle.

ϟ The probe in the right atrioventricular canal (T51 *A*).

ϟ The conus arteriosus of the right ventricle leading into the pulmonary trunk. In some congenital abnormalities the conus may be narrow.

IN THE LEFT VENTRICLE:

ϟ The outflow tract of the aorta and the posterior semilunar valve.

ϟ The atrioventricular canal with the posterior cusp and the posterior papillary muscle (T51 *A*).

ϟ The muscular wall of the left ventricle is twice as thick as that of the right ventricle.

ϟ The fibrous skeleton between the atria and ventricles serves as a base of attachment for the tricuspid and bicuspid (mitral) valves.

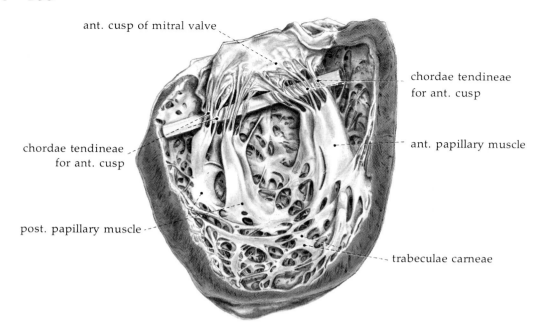

ant. cusp of mitral valve

chordae tendineae
for ant. cusp

chordae tendineae
for ant. cusp

ant. papillary muscle

post. papillary muscle

trabeculae carneae

A. Anterior cusp of the mitral valve with its chordae tendineae and papillary muscles.

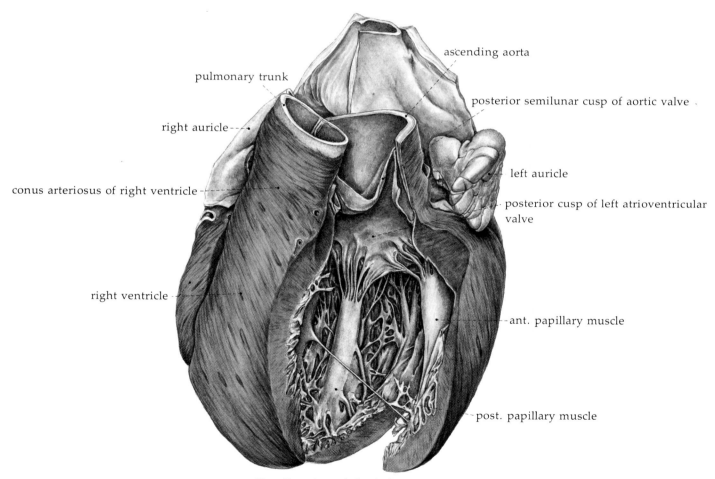

pulmonary trunk

ascending aorta

right auricle

posterior semilunar cusp of aortic valve

conus arteriosus of right ventricle

left auricle

posterior cusp of left atrioventricular
valve

right ventricle

ant. papillary muscle

post. papillary muscle

B. Interior of the left ventricle.

Note:

¶ The outflow tract of the aorta (cut open).

¶ The conus arteriosus of the right ventricle.

¶ Every single cusp of the tricuspid valve and the mitral valve has a double anchor. It has
chordae tendineae to two papillary muscles.

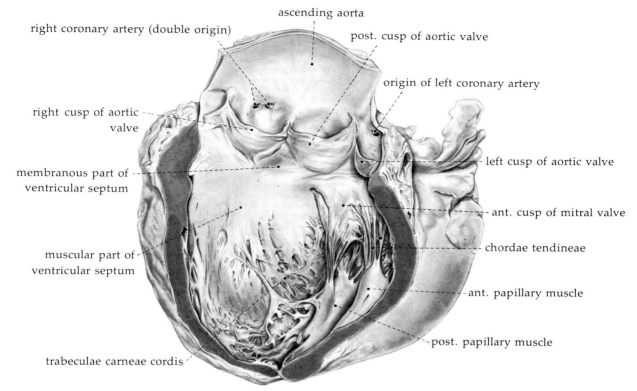

right coronary artery (double origin)

ascending aorta

post. cusp of aortic valve

origin of left coronary artery

right cusp of aortic valve

left cusp of aortic valve

membranous part of ventricular septum

ant. cusp of mitral valve

chordae tendineae

muscular part of ventricular septum

ant. papillary muscle

post. papillary muscle

trabeculae carneae cordis

A. Interior view of the left ventricle and the aorta.

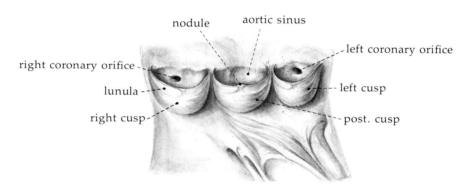

nodule

aortic sinus

right coronary orifice

left coronary orifice

lunula

left cusp

right cusp

post. cusp

B. Cusps (semilunar valves) of the aorta (cut and spread out).

Note:

₵ The origin of the coronary arteries in the aortic sinuses.

₵ The nodules and lunulae in the rim of the aortic cusps.

The semilunar valves of the aorta as well as the cusps of the bicuspid and mitral valves in the left and right atrioventricular canals are frequently affected by rheumatic and infectious diseases. The free edges of the semilunar valves are particularly involved: the rims may become hardened (fibrotic or sclerotic), lose their elasticity and sometimes fuse with each other. Insufficiency and stenosis of the valves result. The bicuspid and tricuspid valves may show similar abnormalities. They may become hardened and sometimes calcified. In addition, the chordae tendineae are also frequently affected: they may become shortened and sometimes fuse together, and they may even rupture. As a result, the valve becomes inoperative and insufficiency follows.

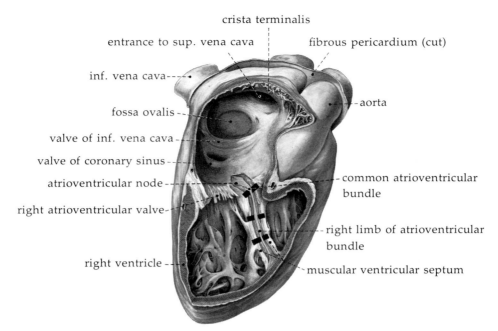

crista terminalis
entrance to sup. vena cava
fibrous pericardium (cut)
inf. vena cava
fossa ovalis
aorta
valve of inf. vena cava
valve of coronary sinus
atrioventricular node
common atrioventricular bundle
right atrioventricular valve
right limb of atrioventricular bundle
right ventricle
muscular ventricular septum

A. Interior view of the right atrium and ventricle in an infant.
Endocardium of ventricular septum is removed.

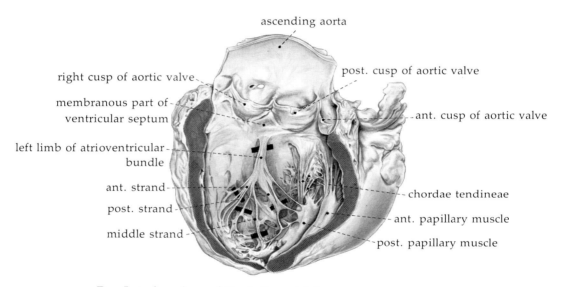

ascending aorta
right cusp of aortic valve
post. cusp of aortic valve
membranous part of ventricular septum
ant. cusp of aortic valve
left limb of atrioventricular bundle
ant. strand
chordae tendineae
post. strand
ant. papillary muscle
middle strand
post. papillary muscle

B. Interior view of the left ventricle.
The left portion of the atrioventricular bundle is shown.

The following important observations should be made:

¶ The pectinate portion of the right atrium, including part of the auricle, has been re-moved to show the atrial septum. In the embryo and fetus the open fossa ovalis permits the blood to flow directly from the right atrium to the left atrium. At the entrance of the inferior vena cava there is a valve, which guides the blood returning from the placenta toward the fossa ovalis.

¶ The crista terminalis forms the borderline between the smooth-walled and the rough-walled portions of the right atrium.

¶ In the tissue of the right atrioventricular ring (right anulus fibrosus) is found the atrio-ventricular node (AV node).

¶ After the atrioventricular bundle passes through the right anulus fibrosus (fibrous ring) it is located on the right side of the membranous portion of the ventricular septum. After dividing, the right bundle descends on the right side of the muscular portion of the ventricular septum and the left bundle descends on the left side.

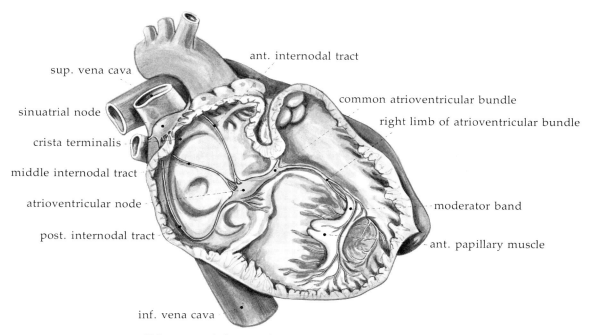

sup. vena cava

ant. internodal tract

sinuatrial node

common atrioventricular bundle

right limb of atrioventricular bundle

crista terminalis

middle internodal tract

atrioventricular node

moderator band

post. internodal tract

ant. papillary muscle

inf. vena cava

Diagram of the conducting system of the heart.

The conducting system and its arterial supply are important for an understanding of abnormalities of the heart rate resulting from a blockage of the coronary arteries. Note:

¶ The *sinuatrial node* (SA node) or *pacemaker* of the heart is located at the upper end of the crista terminalis near the entrance of the superior vena cava. In 55 per cent of hearts it is supplied by a branch of the right coronary artery, and (surprisingly) in the remainder of hearts by the left coronary artery.

¶ The *internodal tracts* are physiologically specialized fibers along which the impulse from the sinuatrial node spreads to the atrioventricular node. Although in histological studies the tracts can be recognized, they cannot be dissected.

¶ The *atrioventricular node* is located in the atrial septum beside the entrance to the coronary sinus. In 90 per cent of cases it is supplied by the right coronary artery.

¶ The atrioventricular bundle is found on the right side of the membranous part of the ventricular septum (posteriorly). It is supplied by the right coronary artery.

¶ The right and left limbs descend subendocardially on the right and left sides of the muscular portion of the ventricular septum and course toward the papillary muscles. In the posterior portion of the septum they are supplied by the right coronary artery, and in the anterior portion by the left coronary artery.

A rather precise diagnosis of the location of an acute coronary blockage can be made by determining which parts of the conducting system are affected.

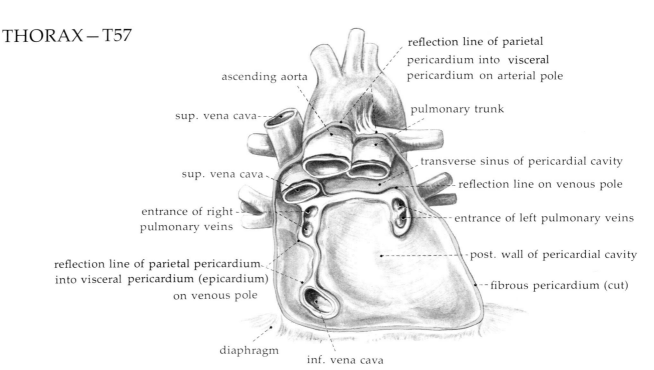

ascending aorta

reflection line of parietal pericardium into visceral pericardium on arterial pole

sup. vena cava

pulmonary trunk

sup. vena cava

transverse sinus of pericardial cavity

reflection line on venous pole

entrance of right pulmonary veins

entrance of left pulmonary veins

reflection line of parietal pericardium into visceral pericardium (epicardium) on venous pole

post. wall of pericardial cavity

fibrous pericardium (cut)

diaphragm

inf. vena cava

A. View at the posterior wall of the pericardial cavity.
The transverse pericardial sinus is shown.

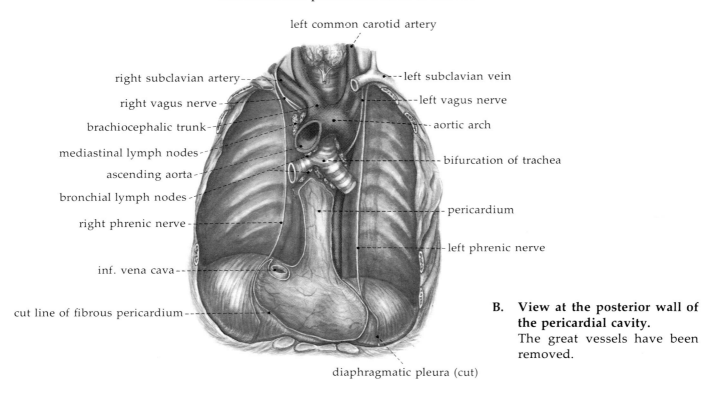

left common carotid artery

right subclavian artery

left subclavian vein

right vagus nerve

left vagus nerve

brachiocephalic trunk

aortic arch

mediastinal lymph nodes

bifurcation of trachea

ascending aorta

bronchial lymph nodes

right phrenic nerve

pericardium

left phrenic nerve

inf. vena cava

cut line of fibrous pericardium

B. View at the posterior wall of the pericardial cavity.
The great vessels have been removed.

diaphragmatic pleura (cut)

Four important structures should be observed:

1. The reflection line of the parietal pericardium into the visceral serous pericardium on the venous pole. This pole is formed by the inferior and superior venae cavae and the right and left pulmonary veins.

2. The reflection line of the parietal pericardium into the visceral pericardium on the arterial pole. This pole is formed by the aorta and the pulmonary trunk.

3. The transverse sinus of the pericardial cavity is located between the arterial and venous poles. Once the fibrous pericardium is opened from the anterior side, a finger can be placed in the transverse sinus behind the aorta and the pulmonary trunk.

4. The posterior midline wall of the pericardial cavity between the pulmonary veins. Behind this portion lie the esophagus and the vagus nerves.

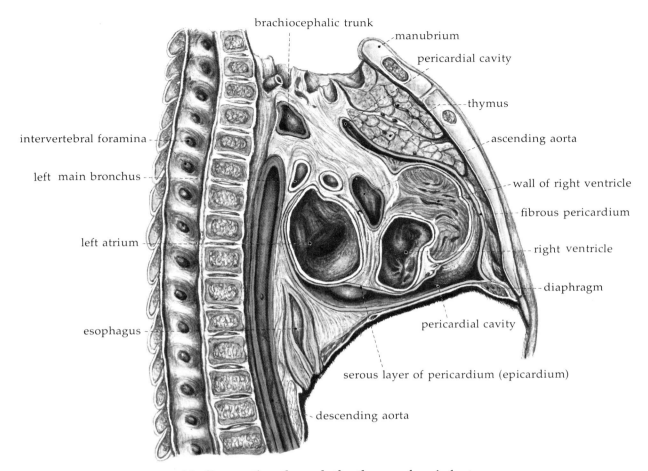

brachiocephalic trunk

manubrium

pericardial cavity

thymus

intervertebral foramina

ascending aorta

left main bronchus

wall of right ventricle

fibrous pericardium

left atrium

right ventricle

diaphragm

esophagus

pericardial cavity

serous layer of pericardium (epicardium)

descending aorta

Median section through the thorax of an infant.
The structures in the anterior, middle and posterior mediastinum are shown.

¶ The thymus is very large in an infant. It is located on the fibrous pericardium behind the body of the sternum.

¶ Note the pericardial cavity behind the thymus. This is part of the sleeve which surrounds the ascending aorta. When fluid collects in the pericardial cavity it is often first detected by physical examination around the arterial pole when the patient is in a supine position.

¶ Note the position of the heart on the diaphragm.

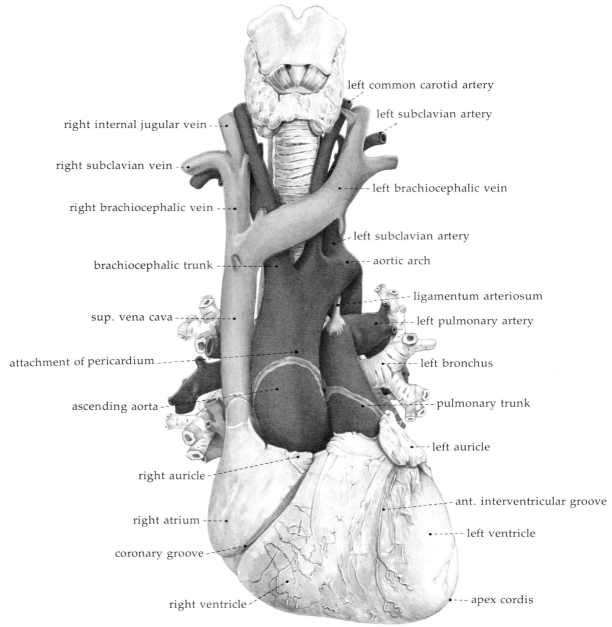

left common carotid artery

left subclavian artery

right internal jugular vein

right subclavian vein

left brachiocephalic vein

right brachiocephalic vein

left subclavian artery

brachiocephalic trunk

aortic arch

ligamentum arteriosum

sup. vena cava

left pulmonary artery

attachment of pericardium

left bronchus

ascending aorta

pulmonary trunk

left auricle

right auricle

ant. interventricular groove

right atrium

left ventricle

coronary groove

right ventricle

apex cordis

Anterior view of the great vessels and trachea.
The esophagus is not visible in this drawing.

It is important to note:

¶ The reflection line of the fibrous pericardium on the aorta, pulmonary artery and superior vena cava.

¶ The ligamentum arteriosum, a remnant of the distal part of the left sixth aortic arch. During fetal life the distal part of this arch forms the ductus arteriosus, an open communication between the pulmonary artery and the aorta. In some cases the ductus remains patent after birth, thus allowing a shunt to form between the aorta and the pulmonary system.

¶ The left brachiocephalic vein, which crosses in front of the arteries originating from the aortic arch.

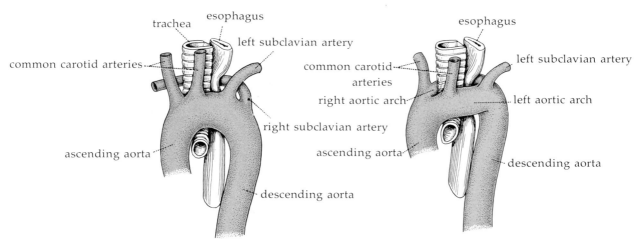

esophagus
trachea
left subclavian artery
common carotid arteries
right aortic arch
right subclavian artery
ascending aorta
descending aorta

A. Abnormal origin of the right subclavian artery.

esophagus
common carotid arteries
left subclavian artery
right aortic arch
left aortic arch
ascending aorta
descending aorta

B. Double aortic arch.

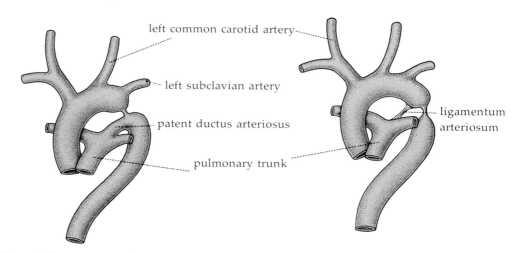

left common carotid artery
left subclavian artery
patent ductus arteriosus
pulmonary trunk
ligamentum arteriosum

C. Coarctation of the aorta (preductal type).   D. Coarctation of the aorta (postductal type).

(From Langman, J.: Medical Embryology, 3rd ed. Baltimore, The Williams and Wilkins Company, 1975.)

¶ Abnormalities of the great arteries are frequently seen. Some of them, such as an abnormal origin of the common carotid arteries or a right aortic arch, usually cause no complaints. Others, however, such as a double aortic arch and an abnormal origin of the right subclavian artery, may cause difficulty in swallowing and breathing. In these cases the esophagus and the trachea may be compressed to a considerable degree.

¶ In patients with a coarctation of the aorta the internal thoracic artery is the main artery carrying blood to the descending aorta. The anterior intercostal branches of the internal thoracic arteries then carry blood to the posterior intercostal arteries of the descending aorta and thus to the lower part of the body (see T20 A). The arteries are large and pulsatile and cause the formation of rather deep grooves in the ribs. These grooves are easily seen on radiographs of the thorax.

THORAX — T61

thyroid gland

left common carotid artery — / — right common carotid artery
left internal jugular vein — / — right internal jugular vein
— right vagus nerve
left subclavian vein — — right subclavian artery
left vagus nerve — — right recurrent laryngeal nerve
left recurrent laryngeal nerve —
left subclavian artery — — sup. vena cava
aortic arch —
descending aorta — — entrance of azygos vein (cut)
intercostal arteries (cut) —
left pulmonary artery — — right main bronchus
— right pulmonary artery
left main bronchus —
— esophagus
coronary sinus — — right atrium
— vagus branches to esophagus
— inf. vena cava
left ventricle — — right ventricle

post. interventricular groove

A. The esophagus in relation to the great vessels, trachea and heart.

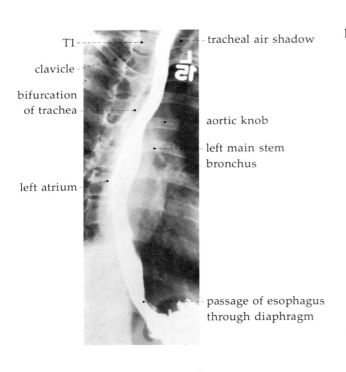

T1 — — tracheal air shadow
clavicle —
bifurcation of trachea —
— aortic knob
— left main stem bronchus
left atrium —
— passage of esophagus through diaphragm

B. Radiography of the esophagus.
Lateral view.

Note the following important points:

¶ There are narrow areas in the esophagus: (a) at its origin immediately below the pharynx; (b) at the aortic arch; (c) at the bifurcation of the trachea; and (d) at its passage through the diaphragm. These areas are clinically important because the mucosa of the narrow parts will be seriously injured if acids or other caustic materials are swallowed.

¶ The esophagus is in contact with the fibrous pericardium in the region of the left atrium. Sharp objects swallowed by accident may pierce the esophagus and enter the left atrium via the pericardium. On the other hand, if the left atrium is enlarged, the esophagus may be pushed to the right (see T58).

¶ The vagus nerves supply the esophagus with its parasympathetic innervation. Because of the rotation of the stomach the right vagus nerve begins to occupy a more posterior position distally and the left vagus nerve a more anterior position.

62

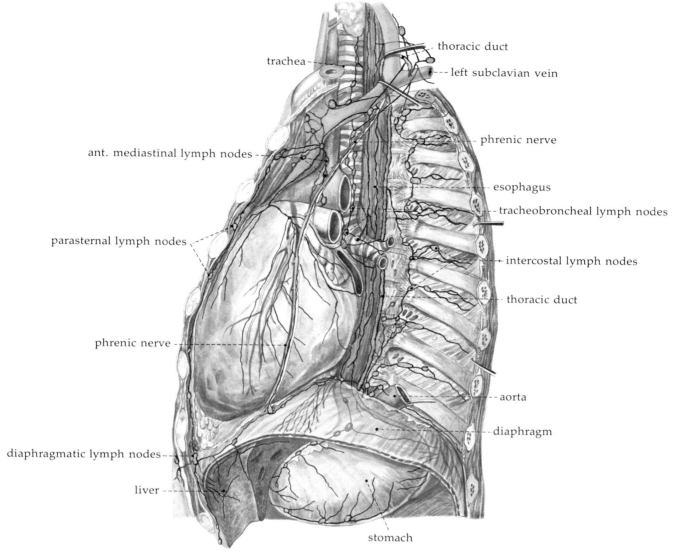

Middle and posterior mediastinum seen from the left.
The descending aorta has been removed.

Note:

¶ The thoracic duct usually enters the thorax through the aortic hiatus in the diaphragm and terminates in the left subclavian vein where the latter joins the jugular vein.

¶ The intercostal nodes drain into the thoracic duct.

¶ The arterial supply of the thoracic part of the esophagus is formed by (a) a branch of the inferior thyroid artery; (b) branches of the descending aorta; and (c) intercostal branches. Close to the diaphragm it is supplied by branches of the left gastric and left inferior phrenic arteries.

The veins of the thoracic part of the esophagus drain into the azygos and hemiazygos veins, and thus into the caval system. Those of the lower part of the esophagus, however, drain into the gastric veins and from there into the portal system. When an obstruction occurs in the venous flow of the portal system, as in cirrhosis of the liver, the venous blood of the lower part of the esophagus is shunted to the azygos vein and to the caval system. As a result many anastomoses develop between the two venous systems in the submucosa of the lower part of the esophagus. These anastomoses may become very large (varicose) and severe bleeding in the esophagus may follow.

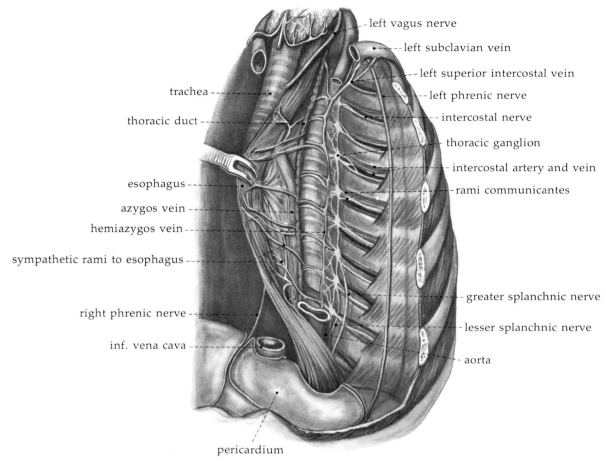

trachea

thoracic duct

esophagus

azygos vein

hemiazygos vein

sympathetic rami to esophagus

right phrenic nerve

inf. vena cava

left vagus nerve

left subclavian vein

left superior intercostal vein

left phrenic nerve

intercostal nerve

thoracic ganglion

intercostal artery and vein

rami communicantes

greater splanchnic nerve

lesser splanchnic nerve

aorta

pericardium

Structures in the posterior mediastinum.
The esophagus is pulled to the right.

Note:

1. The sympathetic chain and its branches innervate the upper two-thirds of the esophagus. The lower part of the esophagus is usually supplied by branches of the greater splanchnic nerve, which originates from the eighth, ninth and tenth sympathetic ganglia. Hence, the esophagus receives parasympathetic branches from the vagus nerve and sympathetic branches from the sympathetic chain.

2. The greater and lesser splanchnic nerves contain preganglionic fibers from white rami communicantes. They end in the celiac and renal ganglia after passing through the diaphragm.

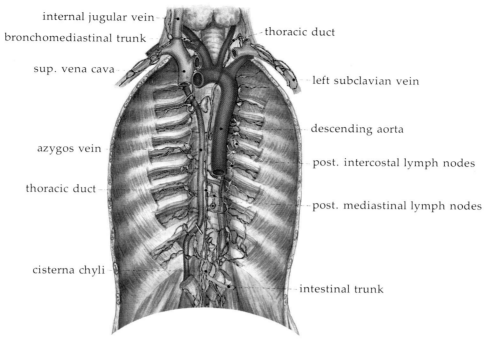

internal jugular vein
bronchomediastinal trunk
sup. vena cava
thoracic duct
left subclavian vein
descending aorta
post. intercostal lymph nodes
azygos vein
thoracic duct
post. mediastinal lymph nodes
cisterna chyli
intestinal trunk

A. Anterior view of the posterior thoracic wall.
Note the relation between the azygos veins, the aorta and the thoracic duct.

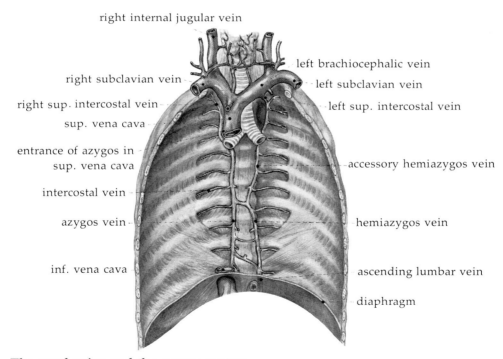

right internal jugular vein
left brachiocephalic vein
right subclavian vein
left subclavian vein
right sup. intercostal vein
left sup. intercostal vein
sup. vena cava
entrance of azygos in
sup. vena cava
accessory hemiazygos vein
intercostal vein
azygos vein
hemiazygos vein
inf. vena cava
ascending lumbar vein
diaphragm

B. The caval veins and the azygos system.
The azygos vein enters the superior vena cava; the hemiazygos vein has several branches that communicate with the azygos vein, but sometimes it continues by way of the accessory hemiazygos and left superior intercostal vein into the left brachiocephalic vein. Originally, the azygos system drained the mesonephros system, but in the adult it drains the posterior body wall (intercostal veins).

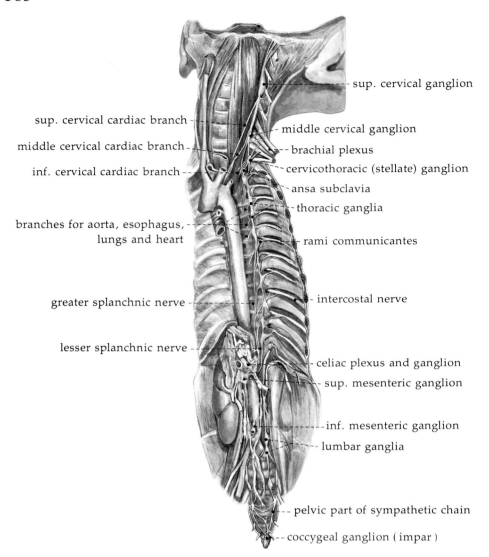

sup. cervical ganglion

sup. cervical cardiac branch

middle cervical cardiac branch

inf. cervical cardiac branch

middle cervical ganglion

brachial plexus

cervicothoracic (stellate) ganglion

ansa subclavia

thoracic ganglia

branches for aorta, esophagus, lungs and heart

rami communicantes

greater splanchnic nerve

intercostal nerve

lesser splanchnic nerve

celiac plexus and ganglion

sup. mesenteric ganglion

inf. mesenteric ganglion

lumbar ganglia

pelvic part of sympathetic chain

coccygeal ganglion (impar)

The left sympathetic chain in a newborn child.

¶ The thoracic portion of the sympathetic trunk is segmentally arranged with the exception of the first thoracic ganglion. This ganglion frequently is fused with the lower cervical ganglion to form the stellate ganglion. Most of the ganglia lie on the heads of the ribs. Inferiorly, however, they lie in front of the eleventh and twelfth thoracic vertebral bodies.

¶ Note the greater and lesser splanchnic nerves.

¶ The cardiac nerves provide the sympathetic innervation to the heart. They have an accelerating, vasodilating and sensory function. Note the superior and middle cardiac nerves originating from the cervical region and the inferior cardiac nerve originating from the upper thoracic region. They reach the atria in the form of a plexus where the sinuatrial node is supplied by the right nerves and the atrioventricular node by the left nerves. Other fibers are distributed to the coronary arteries.

¶ An inadequate blood supply to the myocardium such as that occurring during arteriosclerosis or after the formation of a thrombus may lead to severe pain in the left arm or sometimes in both arms. Pain may also be felt in the neck or the jaw or over the sternum, but it is not felt in the heart. It is thought that the afferent nerve fibers ascend through afferent cardiac branches of the sympathetic nerves to the spinal cord. From there the pain spreads through the cervical branches to the arm and neck and through the thoracic intercostal nerves to skin areas of the thorax.

esophagus and vagus nerves

inf. vena cava and right phrenic nerve   lumbar origin of diaphragm

central tendon   aorta   central tendon

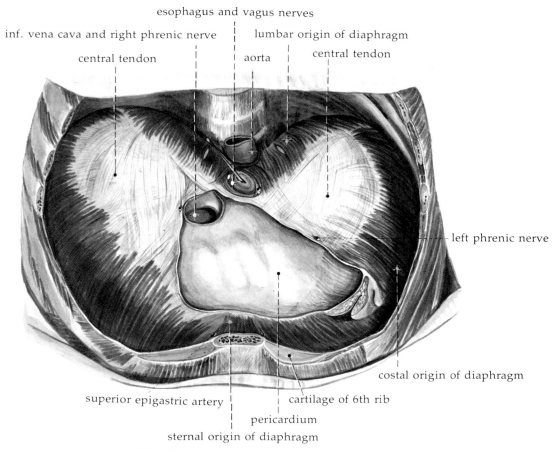

left phrenic nerve

costal origin of diaphragm

superior epigastric artery   cartilage of 6th rib

pericardium

sternal origin of diaphragm

The diaphragm viewed from above.
The diaphragmatic pleura has been removed.

Diaphragmatic openings (apertures):

1. *Aortic opening.* This opening at the lower border of T12 provides passage for the aorta, thoracic duct and azygos vein. It is bounded by fibrous components, and contraction of the diaphragm does not affect the width of the hiatus.

2. *Inferior vena caval opening.* This is located in the tendinous part of the diaphragm. When the diaphragm contracts the tendon is stretched and the flow of venous blood into the thorax is facilitated. The right phrenic nerve accompanies the inferior vena cava to innervate the inferior side of the diaphragm.

3. *Esophageal opening.* This aperture lies in the muscular part of the diaphragm. The decussating fibers probably act as a sphincter for the cardiac end of the stomach and prevent its contents from returning to the esophagus. The vagal nerves as well as branches of the left gastric artery and vein accompany the esophagus.

4. *Other openings.* The superior epigastric vessels and some lymph vessels from the abdominal wall and upper surface of the liver pierce the diaphragm between the sternal and costal origins; the sympathetic trunk passes behind the medial arcuate ligament; the hemiazygos vein pierces the right crus; the splanchnic nerves similarly pierce the crura.

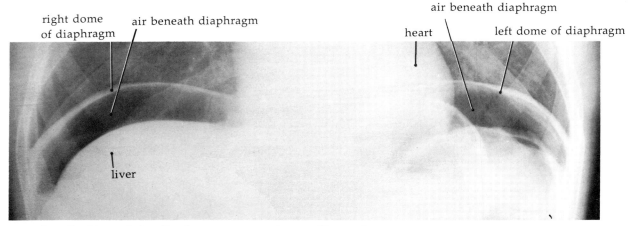

right dome of diaphragm
air beneath diaphragm
air beneath diaphragm
heart
left dome of diaphragm
liver

A. Outline of the diaphragm as seen in a radiograph.
Air has been introduced into the peritoneal cavity. (From Becker, R. F. et al.: The Anatomical Basis of Medical Practice. Baltimore, The Williams & Wilkins Company, 1971.)

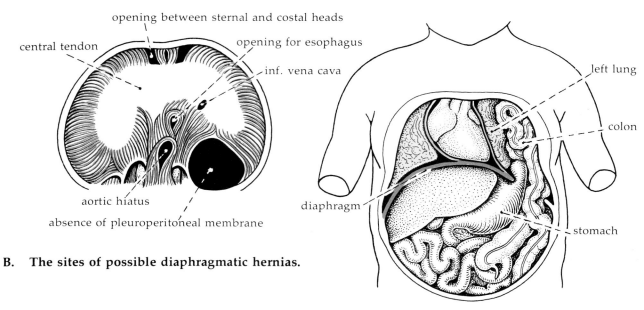

opening between sternal and costal heads
central tendon
opening for esophagus
inf. vena cava
aortic hiatus
absence of pleuroperitoneal membrane

left lung
colon
diaphragm
stomach

B. The sites of possible diaphragmatic hernias.

C. Large congenital diaphragmatic hernia.
This hernia is the result of a defect in the formation of the pleuroperitoneal membrane. (*B* and *C* from Langman, J.: Medical Embryology, 3rd ed. Baltimore, The Williams & Wilkins Company, 1975.)

Diaphragmatic hernias, that is, the herniation of abdominal viscera into the thoracic cavity, are clinically important.

¶   Most congenital hernias are caused by the persistence of the left pleuroperitoneal canal (review the development of the diaphragm in the fetus).

¶   The most frequently acquired hernia is the esophageal hernia. In such cases part of the cardia of the stomach may be found in the thoracic cavity. Usually the hernia is on the left side, since the right side is blocked by the underlying liver.

¶   Occasionally a small hernia occurs between the sternal and costal origins of the diaphragm (foramen of Morgagni).

ABDOMEN

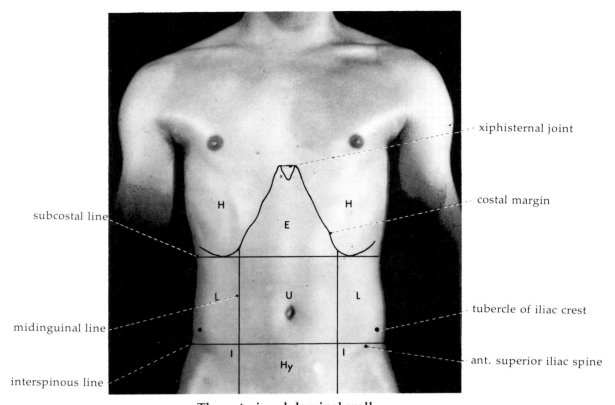

xiphisternal joint

costal margin

subcostal line

midinguinal line

interspinous line

tubercle of iliac crest

ant. superior iliac spine

The anterior abdominal wall.
Important bony points and orientation lines are superimposed.

Only a few bony points are used for orientation in the physical examination of the abdomen:

1. *The xiphisternal joint*, found between the body of the sternum and the xiphoid process.

2. *The costal margin*, formed by the cartilages of the seventh, eighth, ninth and tenth ribs. The level of the lowest part of the costal margin differs considerably between individuals who are short and fat (pyknic), and those who are tall and slender (leptosomatic).

3. *The anterior superior iliac spine* forms a prominence in most patients. When there is much fat, it lies in a depression.

4. *The tubercle of the iliac crest* lies about 2 inches behind the anterior superior iliac spine. By placing the fingers on the spine and moving them along the crest upward and backward, the tubercle can easily be determined.

5. *The pubic symphysis* is the area where the two pubic bones meet in the midline.

To locate the abdominal organs more accurately, a number of orientation lines are used. Several of these are not convenient for clinical purposes, and only the most commonly used are listed here.

1. The *subcostal* line, passing through the lower margin of the costal arch. Its level varies somewhat with body type, posture, respiration and age.

2. The *interspinous* line, passing through the anterior superior iliac spines.

3. *Two vertical lines*, each of which passes through the midpoint of the inguinal ligament, which extends from the anterior superior iliac spine to the pubic symphysis.

With the help of these lines, the abdominal wall is compartmentalized into nine regions. Above the upper horizontal line are the right and left hypochondriac and the central epigastric regions. Between the two horizontal lines are the right and left lumbar (also called lateral abdominal) and umbilical regions. The areas below the lower horizontal line are referred to as the right and left inguinal (or iliac) and the hypogastric regions.

In many hospitals these lines and regions are discarded. Instead, a horizontal and a vertical line is drawn through the umbilicus, and the abdomen is divided into four quadrants.

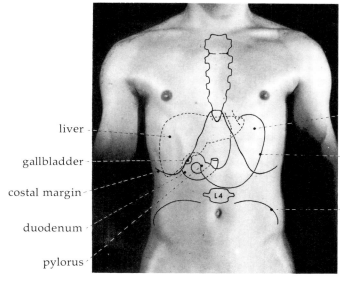

liver

gallbladder

costal margin

duodenum

pylorus

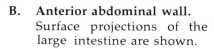

fundus of stomach

greater curvature

iliac crest

A.   Anterior abdominal wall.
The viscera in the upper part of the abdomen are outlined schematically.

B.   Anterior abdominal wall.
Surface projections of the large intestine are shown.

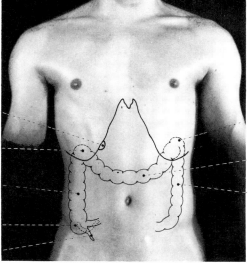

gallbladder

right colic flexure

ascending colon

cecum

vermiform appendix

left colic flexure

transverse colon

descending colon

Palpation of the abdominal wall is an important method of obtaining information about the position and size of the abdominal organs. It is particularly important in patients with enlarged organs or tumors. In a normal person few if any of the abdominal organs can be palpated.

The position of the viscera in the cadaver is about the same as that in the living person during quiet inspiration and in the supine position. The liver, stomach and spleen, however, are somewhat higher owing to the high position of the diaphragm.

¶   The *liver* lies deep in the right hypochondriac region. Its lower border corresponds to that of the right costal margin laterally, and it crosses the epigastric region from the ninth right to the eighth left costal cartilage. The liver is overlapped by the lower borders of both lungs. Under normal conditions the lower border of the liver may be just palpable under the right costal arch during deep inspiration. When enlarged it may protrude the width of one finger to one hand under the arch.

¶   The *stomach* lies mainly to the left of the midline above the umbilicus. Its lower part lies directly under the anterior abdominal wall, and the upper part lies in the hypochondriac area under the left dome of the diaphragm. Normally the stomach cannot be palpated.

¶   The *gallbladder* is attached to the lower surface of the liver and moves with it during respiration. It projects slightly beyond the margin of the liver and lies where the lateral border of the right rectus abdominis muscle crosses the costal arch. Under normal conditions it cannot be felt.

¶   The *cecum, vermiform appendix* and *colon* show great individual variation in position. The right flexure of the colon is sometimes situated below the umbilicus. The left colic flexure is located deep in the left hypochondrium 4 inches from the midline at the level of the eighth costal cartilage. The upper part of the descending colon is separated from the anterior abdominal wall by the jejunum; the lower part lies directly behind the anterior abdominal wall and, when filled, can sometimes be palpated.

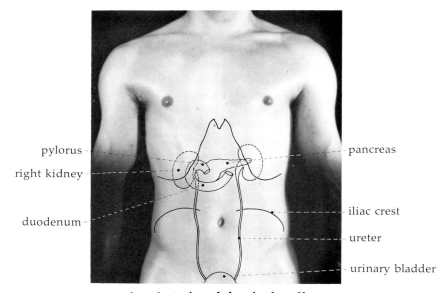

pylorus

right kidney

duodenum

pancreas

iliac crest

ureter

urinary bladder

A.   Anterior abdominal wall.
The position of the duodenum, pancreas, kidneys and ureters are outlined.

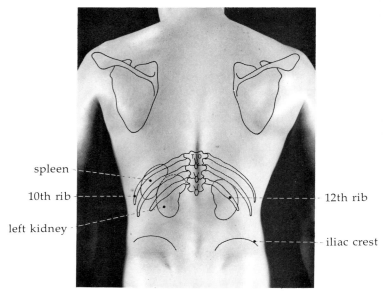

spleen

10th rib

left kidney

12th rib

iliac crest

B.   View of the posterior body wall.
Surface projections of the kidneys and spleen are indicated.

¶   The *pancreas, duodenum* and *ureters* cannot be felt during palpation of the abdomen.

¶   The *bladder* similarly cannot be felt in normal persons. When the bladder is enlarged, for example after hypertrophy of the prostate, it may be felt above the symphysis.

¶   The *spleen* is situated under the left dome of the diaphragm beneath the posterior borders of the ninth, tenth and eleventh ribs. During deep inspiration the spleen descends but usually is not palpable.

¶   The *kidneys* are deeply placed against the posterior abdominal wall. The right kidney, situated somewhat lower than the left, can sometimes be palpated between two hands during deep inspiration. One hand pushes the quadratus lumborum muscle forward while the other is placed on the anterior abdominal wall below the tenth costal cartilage.

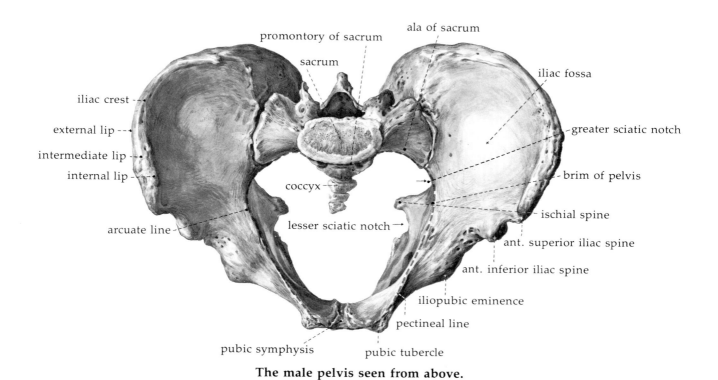

promontory of sacrum
ala of sacrum
sacrum
iliac fossa
iliac crest
external lip
greater sciatic notch
intermediate lip
internal lip
brim of pelvis
coccyx
arcuate line
ischial spine
lesser sciatic notch
ant. superior iliac spine
ant. inferior iliac spine
iliopubic eminence
pectineal line
pubic symphysis
pubic tubercle

The male pelvis seen from above.

Although the main functions of the pelvis are (a) to transmit the weight of the torso to the legs and (b) to serve as a birth canal, it is important to remember that the pelvis also serves as attachment for all the muscles of the abdominal wall.

Particularly important in the study of the abdomen are:

¶ The *iliac crest* with its external, middle and internal lips as attachment areas for several muscles of the abdominal wall.

¶ The *pubic tubercle* and *symphysis* as attachment for the rectus abdominis muscles.

¶ The *pelvic brim*, which forms the dividing line between the *greater* or *false pelvis* and the *lesser* or *true pelvis*. At the same time, it also forms the dividing line between the abdominal and the pelvic cavities. The boundary line of the pelvic brim is formed by: (a) the promontory of the sacrum, (b) the anterior border of the ala of the sacrum, (c) the arcuate line of the ilium, (d) the pectineal line of the pubic bone and the pubic crest (together called the iliopectineal line), and (e) the superior rim of the pubic symphysis. Above the brim is the greater pelvis. Its sides are formed by the iliac fossae, the front by the muscles of the anterior abdominal wall and the back by the lumbar vertebrae.

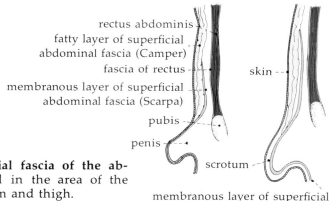

rectus abdominis
fatty layer of superficial
abdominal fascia (Camper)
fascia of rectus
skin
membranous layer of superficial
abdominal fascia (Scarpa)
pubis
penis
scrotum
aponeurosis of external
oblique
membranous layer of superficial
abdominal fascia
inguinal ligament
fascia lata

A. The superficial fascia of the abdominal wall in the area of the penis, scrotum and thigh.

membranous layer of superficial
fascia (Colles)

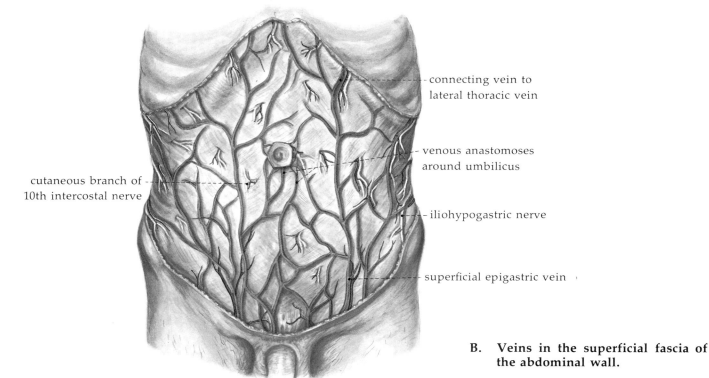

connecting vein to
lateral thoracic vein

venous anastomoses
around umbilicus

cutaneous branch of
10th intercostal nerve

iliohypogastric nerve

superficial epigastric vein

B. Veins in the superficial fascia of the abdominal wall.

The superficial fascia of the abdominal wall contains fat, superficial veins and arteries, and cutaneous nerves. In the upper part of the abdominal wall the superficial fascia consists of one layer, but in the lower part (between the umbilicus and the symphysis) it is divided into two layers: (a) the superficial (fat) layer (formerly known as *Camper's fascia*) and (b) a deeper membranous layer (formerly called *Scarpa's fascia*), which contains no fat. The deep fascia is not to be mistaken for the fascia that invests the underlying muscles, although it is sometimes difficult to separate the two. The deep fascia extends over the spermatic cords, the penis and the scrotum into the perineum. In front of the inguinal ligament, it blends with the fascia lata of the thigh. The fascial arrangement is clinically important (see P20 *B*).

In the superficial fascia there are many veins. Above the umbilicus the flow is directed superiorly, below it inferiorly. Keep the following in mind:

⁋   Under normal conditions small anastomoses exist between the superficial epigastric vein, which drains into the femoral vein, and the lateral thoracic vein, which enters the axillary vein. A few anastomoses also exist around the umbilicus with the paraumbilical veins. These veins run along the ligamentum teres toward the liver to enter the left gastric vein (see A29).

⁋   Anastomoses between the portal and caval systems are of great clinical importance. When the portal vein is obstructed, as for example in cirrhosis of the liver or cardiac failure, the blood of the portal system returns to the heart through the caval system. The sites of anastomoses between the two systems are at the lower end of the esophagus and in the rectum. A third site of development of anastomoses is around the umbilicus through the paraumbilical veins. The superficial veins around the umbilicus then become dilated and radiate from the umbilicus. They resemble writhing snakes, and the symptom is called *caput Medusae*.

74

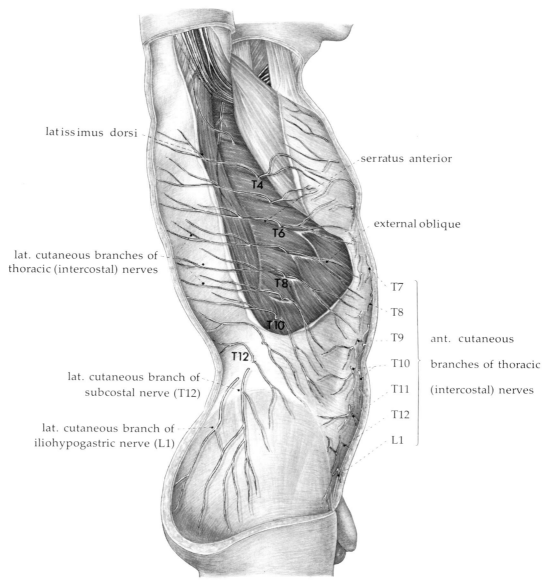

latissimus dorsi

serratus anterior

external oblique

lat. cutaneous branches of
thoracic (intercostal) nerves

T4

T6

T8

T10

T12

T7

T8

T9

T10

T11

T12

L1

ant. cutaneous

branches of thoracic

(intercostal) nerves

lat. cutaneous branch of
subcostal nerve (T12)

lat. cutaneous branch of
iliohypogastric nerve (L1)

Cutaneous innervation of the abdominal wall.

Make the following observations:

¶   The skin of the abdominal wall is almost entirely supplied by cutaneous branches of the thoracic (intercostal) nerves. The region of the umbilicus is innervated by the tenth thoracic nerve. Above the navel the sensory innervation is supplied by T9, T8 and T7; the region below the navel is innervated by T11, T12 and L1 (see also A12 *A*).

¶   The ventral ramus of L1 is distributed through the iliohypogastric and ilioinguinal nerves. Note that the anterior cutaneous branch of the iliohypogastric nerve supplies the skin above the pubis (see A9).

¶   It is important to remember that the cutaneous branches of an intercostal nerve innervate a belt of skin around the body (see T19). The disease herpes zoster, in which a rash appears only in the belt of skin supplied by one or two nerves, demonstrates the girdlelike distribution. The English name for the disease is shingles (from Latin *cingulum*, literally girdle).

¶   Keep in mind that the terminal twigs of the intercostal nerves overlap each other to such an extent that an injury to one nerve does not produce total loss of sensation in the skin area supplied by that particular nerve.

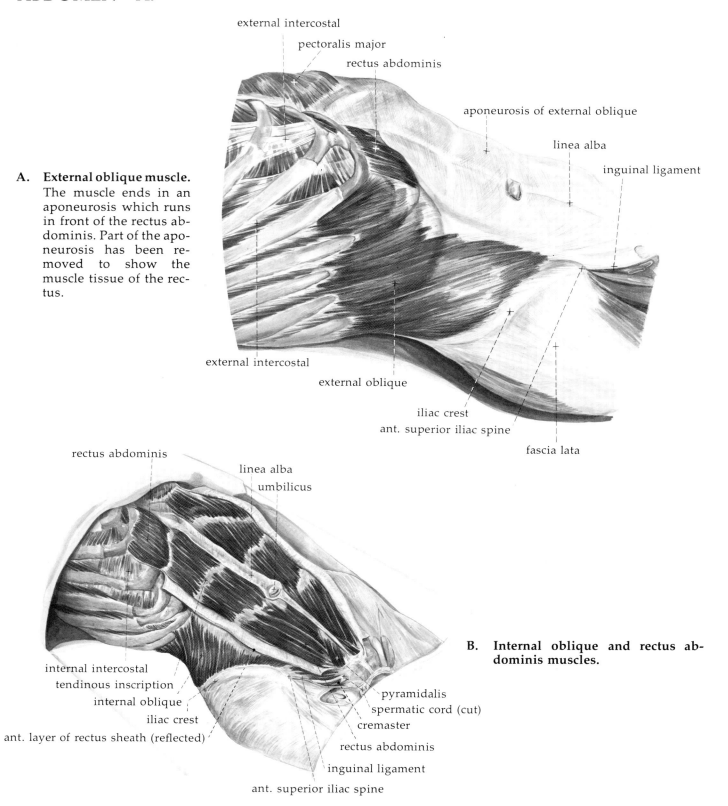

external intercostal

pectoralis major

rectus abdominis

aponeurosis of external oblique

linea alba

inguinal ligament

A. External oblique muscle. The muscle ends in an aponeurosis which runs in front of the rectus abdominis. Part of the aponeurosis has been removed to show the muscle tissue of the rectus.

external intercostal

external oblique

iliac crest

ant. superior iliac spine

fascia lata

rectus abdominis

linea alba

umbilicus

B. Internal oblique and rectus abdominis muscles.

internal intercostal

tendinous inscription

internal oblique

iliac crest

ant. layer of rectus sheath (reflected)

pyramidalis

spermatic cord (cut)

cremaster

rectus abdominis

inguinal ligament

ant. superior iliac spine

¶ The internal oblique ends in an aponeurosis which splits into two layers: (a) an anterior layer which passes in front of the rectus abdominis and is fused with the aponeurosis of the external oblique and (b) a posterior layer which passes behind the rectus abdominis from the costal margin to a point midway between the umbilicus and the symphysis. Below this point, known as the arcuate line, this layer also passes in front of the rectus (see A10 B and C).

¶ Some fibers of the internal oblique continue in the spermatic cord as the cremaster muscle (see A14 B).

¶ The linea alba is wide above the umbilicus but narrow below it. Above the umbilicus it is frequently used in surgery to make vertical incisions to approach the stomach.

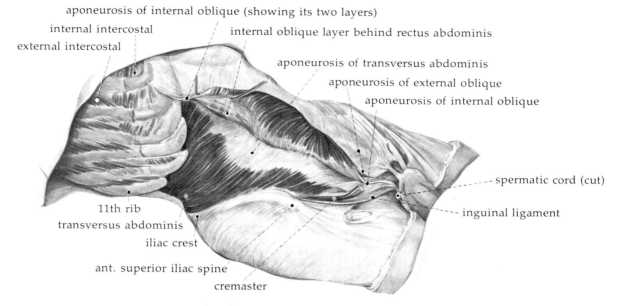

aponeurosis of internal oblique (showing its two layers)
internal intercostal
external intercostal
internal oblique layer behind rectus abdominis
aponeurosis of transversus abdominis
aponeurosis of external oblique
aponeurosis of internal oblique
spermatic cord (cut)
inguinal ligament
11th rib
transversus abdominis
iliac crest
ant. superior iliac spine
cremaster

A. Transversus abdominis muscle.

The external and internal oblique muscles are reflected. The transversus abdominis ends in an aponeurosis which runs behind the rectus abdominis muscle to a point halfway between the umbilicus and the symphysis. Below this point, the arcuate line, it passes in front of the rectus abdominis.

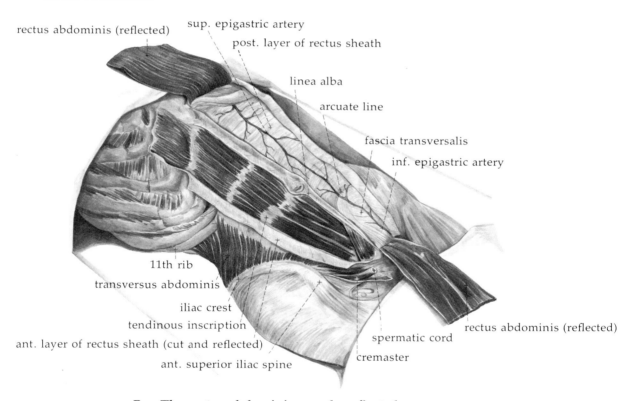

rectus abdominis (reflected)
sup. epigastric artery
post. layer of rectus sheath
linea alba
arcuate line
fascia transversalis
inf. epigastric artery
11th rib
transversus abdominis
iliac crest
tendinous inscription
spermatic cord
rectus abdominis (reflected)
ant. layer of rectus sheath (cut and reflected)
ant. superior iliac spine
cremaster

B. The rectus abdominis muscle reflected.

The posterior wall of the rectus sheath is shown.

Note:

¶ Above the arcuate line the posterior layer of the rectus sheath is formed by the aponeurosis of the transversus abdominis and the posterior layer of the internal oblique aponeurosis. Below the arcuate line the posterior layer of the rectus sheath is formed by the fascia transversalis.

¶ Inside the rectus sheath the superior epigastric artery (the terminal branch of the internal thoracic) and the inferior epigastric artery (a branch of the external iliac) form an anastomosis. Note that the inferior epigastric artery enters the rectus sheath at the arcuate line.

77

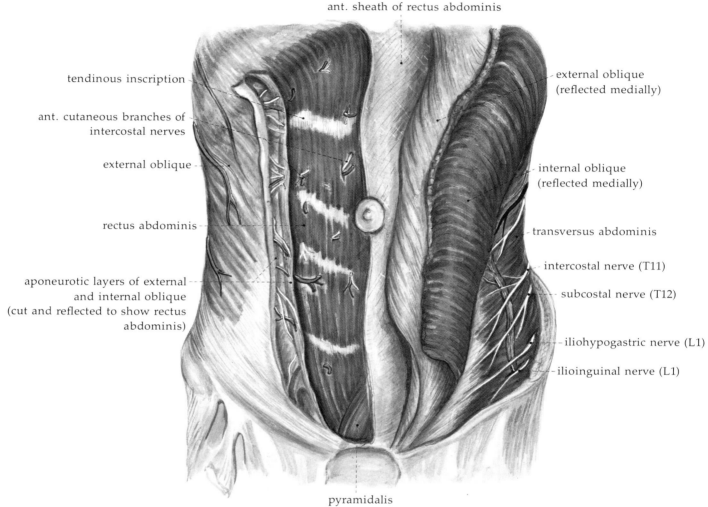

ant. sheath of rectus abdominis

tendinous inscription

ant. cutaneous branches of
intercostal nerves

external oblique

rectus abdominis

aponeurotic layers of external
and internal oblique
(cut and reflected to show rectus
abdominis)

external oblique
(reflected medially)

internal oblique
(reflected medially)

transversus abdominis

intercostal nerve (T11)

subcostal nerve (T12)

iliohypogastric nerve (L1)

ilioinguinal nerve (L1)

pyramidalis

Muscles, nerves and arteries of the anterolateral abdominal wall.

¶ The intercostal, subcostal (T12), iliohypogastric (L1) and ilioinguinal (L1) nerves course between the internal oblique and transversus abdominis muscles. Compare their positions with those of the thoracic intercostal nerves, which course between the internal intercostal and innermost intercostal muscles (see T19).

¶ In making an incision through the musculature of the lateral abdominal wall, it is important to keep in mind: (a) the course and direction of the intercostal nerves (medial and somewhat downward) and (b) the direction of the fibers of the various muscles.

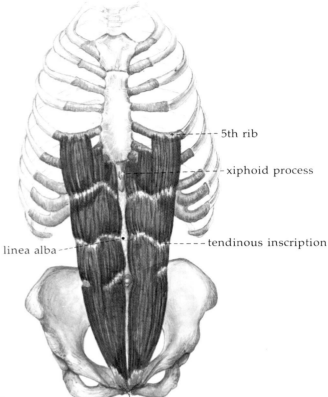

5th rib

xiphoid process

linea alba

tendinous inscription

pubic symphysis

A. The rectus abdominis muscle.
Origin: (1) Cartilage of fifth, sixth and seventh ribs.
(2) Xiphoid process.
Insertion: Front of symphysis and body of pubic bone.

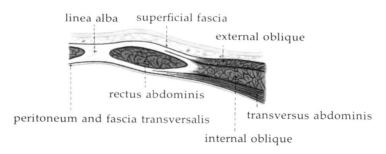

linea alba   superficial fascia

external oblique

rectus abdominis

peritoneum and fascia transversalis

transversus abdominis

internal oblique

B. Transverse section through the rectus abdominis above the arcuate line.
The anterior rectus sheath is formed by the aponeurosis of the external oblique muscle and the anterior layer of the aponeurosis of the internal oblique muscle. The posterior rectus sheath is formed by the posterior layer of the aponeurosis of the internal oblique and the aponeurosis of the transversus abdominis.

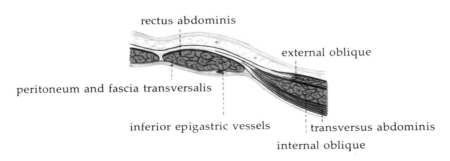

rectus abdominis

external oblique

peritoneum and fascia transversalis

inferior epigastric vessels

transversus abdominis

internal oblique

C. Transverse section through the rectus abdominis below the arcuate line.
The anterior rectus sheath is formed by the aponeuroses of the external oblique, internal oblique and transversus abdominis muscles. The posterior sheath consists of the fascia transversalis. Behind this fascia is the peritoneum.

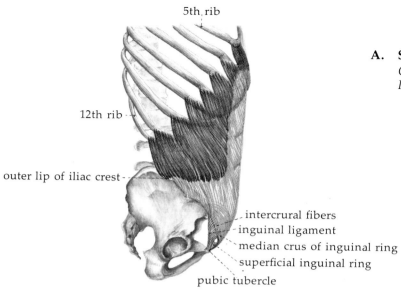

5th rib

12th rib

outer lip of iliac crest

intercrural fibers

inguinal ligament

median crus of inguinal ring

superficial inguinal ring

pubic tubercle

A. Schematic drawing of external oblique muscle.

Origin: Lower eight ribs.

Insertion: (1) Outer lip of the iliac crest. (2) From the anterior superior spine to the pubic tubercle, the aponeurosis forms a free thickened border — the inguinal ligament. (3) The upper fibers pass in front of the rectus abdominis, decussate in the linea alba and cross the median plane; some fibers insert at the body of the pubic bone on the opposite side. The muscle has no attachment to the thoracolumbar fascia and hence has a free edge posteriorly (see A73 *B*).

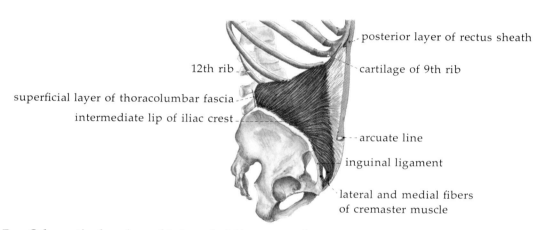

posterior layer of rectus sheath

12th rib

cartilage of 9th rib

superficial layer of thoracolumbar fascia

intermediate lip of iliac crest

arcuate line

inguinal ligament

lateral and medial fibers of cremaster muscle

B.   Schematic drawing of internal oblique muscle.

Origin: (1) Lateral two-thirds of the inguinal ligament; (2) intermediate lip of the iliac crest; (3) superficial layer of the thoracolumbar fascia.

Insertion: (1) Cartilages of the lower four ribs; (2) via the anterior and posterior walls of the rectus sheath into the linea alba; (3) below the arcuate line the fibers pass in front of the rectus abdominis. The lowermost fibers continue to cover the spermatic cord as the cremaster muscle. Fibers passing immediately above the cord contribute to the formation of the conjoined tendon and insert into the pubis (see A15 *A*).

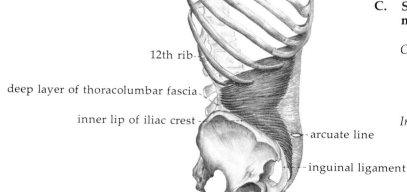

12th rib

deep layer of thoracolumbar fascia

inner lip of iliac crest

arcuate line

inguinal ligament

C.   Schematic drawing of transversus abdominis muscle.

Origin: (1) Inner lip of iliac crest; (2) lateral one-third of the inguinal ligament; (3) lower six costal cartilages; (4) transverse processes of lumbar vertebrae by way of the deep layer of the thoracolumbar fascia (A73 *B*).

Insertion: (1) Linea alba; (2) through the conjoined tendon into the pubic crest and medial part of the pectineal line (see A15 *A*).

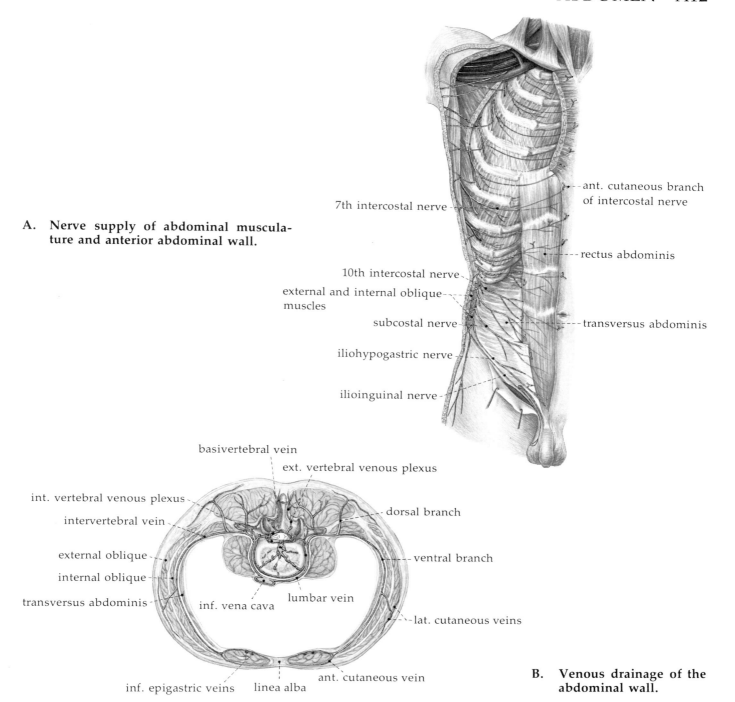

A. Nerve supply of abdominal musculature and anterior abdominal wall.

7th intercostal nerve

ant. cutaneous branch of intercostal nerve

rectus abdominis

10th intercostal nerve

external and internal oblique muscles

subcostal nerve

transversus abdominis

iliohypogastric nerve

ilioinguinal nerve

basivertebral vein

ext. vertebral venous plexus

int. vertebral venous plexus

intervertebral vein

dorsal branch

external oblique

internal oblique

ventral branch

transversus abdominis

inf. vena cava

lumbar vein

lat. cutaneous veins

inf. epigastric veins

linea alba

ant. cutaneous vein

B. Venous drainage of the abdominal wall.

¶ The motor innervation of the ventral abdominal musculature is derived from the intercostal nerves. The nerves are located between the internal oblique and transversus abdominis muscles and course medially and downward. Frequently the nerves connect with each other, thus forming a plexus. The motor function of the iliohypogastric and ilioinguinal nerves with regard to the abdominal muscles is controversial. The cremaster muscle is innervated by the genitofemoral nerve (see P10), which frequently receives a branch from the iliohypogastric nerve.

¶ Blood from the abdominal wall below the umbilicus drains mainly toward the inferior vena cava. Some of it, however, drains by way of the epigastric veins. Note the position of the veins between the muscle layers. Above the umbilicus most of the blood drains toward the superior vena cava through the thoracoepigastric veins (see T4).

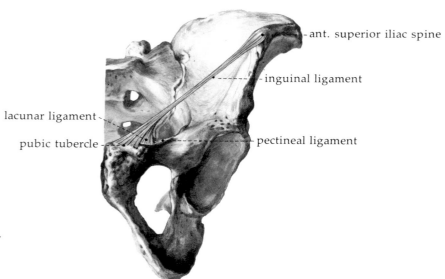

ant. superior iliac spine

inguinal ligament

lacunar ligament

pectineal ligament

pubic tubercle

A. Inguinal ligament and its components.

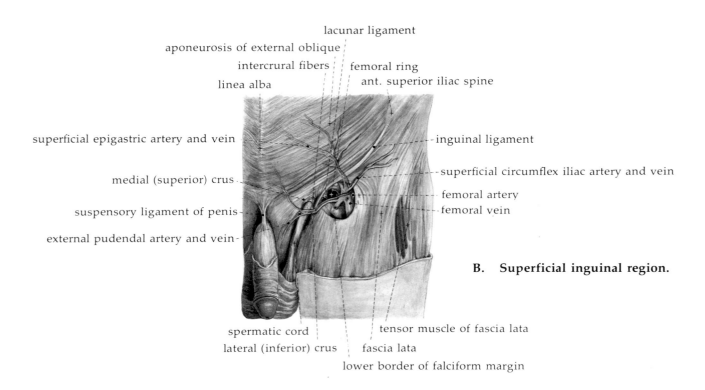

lacunar ligament

aponeurosis of external oblique

intercrural fibers

femoral ring

linea alba

ant. superior iliac spine

superficial epigastric artery and vein

inguinal ligament

superficial circumflex iliac artery and vein

medial (superior) crus

femoral artery

suspensory ligament of penis

femoral vein

external pudendal artery and vein

B. Superficial inguinal region.

spermatic cord

tensor muscle of fascia lata

lateral (inferior) crus

fascia lata

lower border of falciform margin

The inguinal region is clinically important because many hernias occur there. A number of important structures need to be examined carefully:

¶ The *inguinal ligament,* formed by the lower thickened border of the external oblique aponeurosis, extends from the anterior superior iliac spine to the pubic tubercle. Some fibers bend laterally backward — the *lacunar ligament* — and some extend even along the pectineal line — the *pectineal ligament.*

¶ The superficial inguinal ring is the subcutaneous opening of the inguinal canal, that is, the canal through which the spermatic cord passes on its way to the scrotum. The borders of the superficial opening are formed by the *lateral (inferior) crus* and the *medial (superior) crus.* The medial crus is the part of the external oblique aponeurosis that attaches to the pubic crest and symphysis. The two crura are connected by the *intercrural fibers* (see A14 *A*).

¶ From the edges of the superficial inguinal ring arises the *external spermatic fascia* (see A15 *B*), which covers the spermatic cord and the testis. It is much thinner than the external oblique aponeurosis.

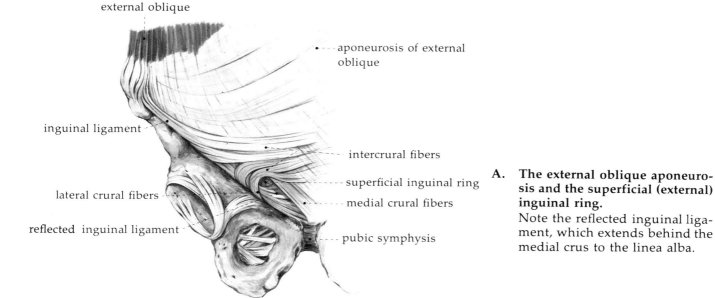

external oblique

aponeurosis of external oblique

inguinal ligament

intercrural fibers

superficial inguinal ring

lateral crural fibers

medial crural fibers

reflected inguinal ligament

pubic symphysis

A. The external oblique aponeurosis and the superficial (external) inguinal ring.
Note the reflected inguinal ligament, which extends behind the medial crus to the linea alba.

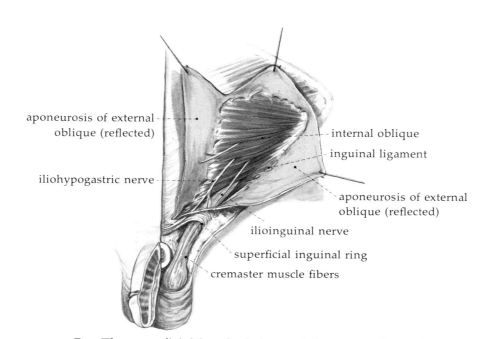

aponeurosis of external oblique (reflected)

internal oblique

inguinal ligament

iliohypogastric nerve

aponeurosis of external oblique (reflected)

ilioinguinal nerve

superficial inguinal ring

cremaster muscle fibers

B. The superficial inguinal ring and the spermatic cord.
Removal of the external oblique aponeurosis opens the anterior wall of the inguinal canal.

¶ The ilioinguinal nerve (L1) passes into the inguinal canal and emerges through the superficial ring to supply the skin of the scrotum. The genital branch of the genitofemoral nerve (L1) follows the same route and innervates the cremaster muscle (see A73 and P10).

¶ When the testis passes through the internal oblique muscle, the latter is prolonged as a saclike covering: the *cremasteric fascia* which contains muscle fibers, the *cremaster muscle*.

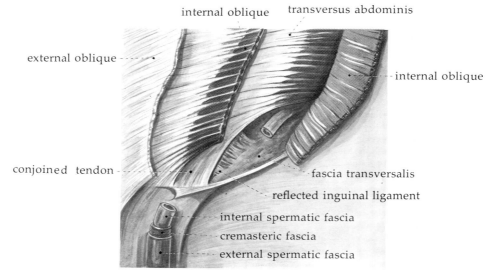

internal oblique   transversus abdominis

external oblique

internal oblique

conjoined tendon

fascia transversalis

reflected inguinal ligament

internal spermatic fascia

cremasteric fascia

external spermatic fascia

A.   Inguinal region after removal of the internal oblique.

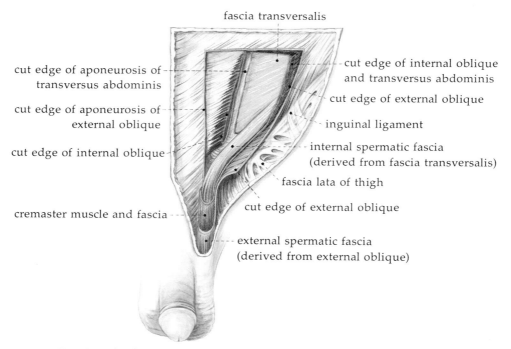

fascia transversalis

cut edge of aponeurosis of transversus abdominis

cut edge of internal oblique and transversus abdominis

cut edge of external oblique

cut edge of aponeurosis of external oblique

inguinal ligament

internal spermatic fascia (derived from fascia transversalis)

cut edge of internal oblique

fascia lata of thigh

cremaster muscle and fascia

cut edge of external oblique

external spermatic fascia (derived from external oblique)

B.   Inguinal region after removal of the transversus abdominis.

¶ The lowest fibers of the internal oblique originate from the lateral half of the inguinal ligament. These fibers arch back over the spermatic cord and form a flattened tendon behind the cord. This tendon forms part of the posterior wall of the inguinal canal and is attached to the pubic crest and pectineal line. Since the tendon is enforced by fibers of the transversus abdominis muscle, it is called the *conjoined tendon* or *falx inguinalis.*

¶ The fibers of the transversus abdominis muscle originate from the most lateral part of the inguinal ligament, that is, above the area of the inguinal canal. Hence, the muscle does not provide a covering for the spermatic cord.

¶ The fascia transversalis is the innermost layer of the abdominal wall with the exception of the parietal peritoneum, which is separated from it by a layer of fat. The fascia is found mainly in the lower part of the abdominal wall where it forms (a) the posterior wall of the rectus sheath below the arcuate line and (b) the posterior wall of the inguinal canal. The fascia also provides a cover for the spermatic cord, the *internal spermatic fascia.* The place where the testis penetrates through the fascia is known as the deep inguinal ring (see A17).

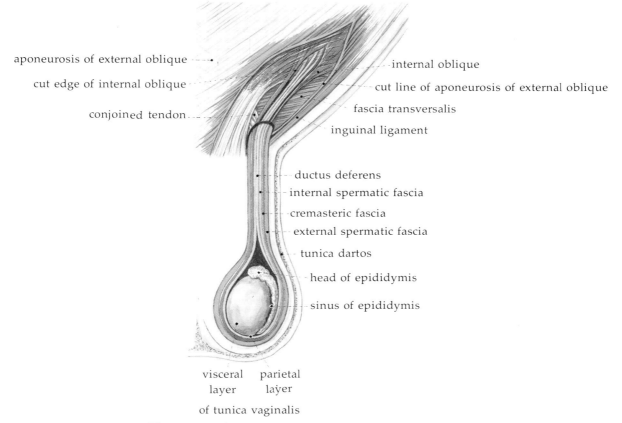

aponeurosis of external oblique

cut edge of internal oblique

conjoined tendon

internal oblique

cut line of aponeurosis of external oblique

fascia transversalis

inguinal ligament

ductus deferens

internal spermatic fascia

cremasteric fascia

external spermatic fascia

tunica dartos

head of epididymis

sinus of epididymis

visceral   parietal
layer   layer
of tunica vaginalis

The spermatic cord and its coverings.

¶ The spermatic cord contains (a) the ductus deferens with its artery, vein and nerve plexus, (b) the testicular artery, (c) the pampiniform plexus of veins, (d) the genital branch of the genitofemoral nerve, and (e) remnants of the processus vaginalis (see P12). On physical examination the cord can easily be felt when it passes over the pubic bone on its way to the scrotum.

¶ The following layers should be recognized as coverings of the spermatic cord and testis.

1. Skin.

2. Tunica dartos—a continuation of the fatty layer of the superficial abdominal fascia.

3. A continuation of the membranous layer of the superficial abdominal fascia.

4. External spermatic fascia—derived from the aponeurosis of the external oblique muscle.

5. Cremasteric fascia and muscle—derived from the internal oblique aponeurosis and muscle.

6. Internal spermatic fascia—derived from the fascia transversalis.

7. A fatty layer—derived from fat between the peritoneum and the fascia transversalis.

8. The parietal and visceral layers of the tunica vaginalis (see P11).

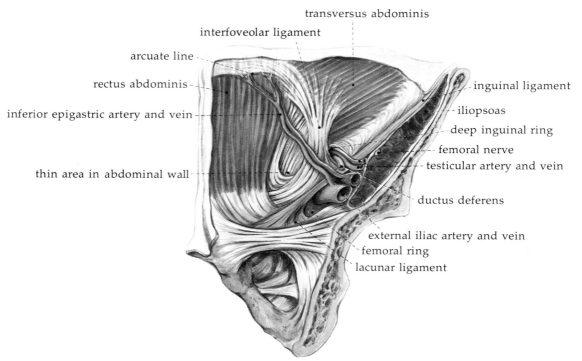

transversus abdominis

interfoveolar ligament

arcuate line

rectus abdominis

inferior epigastric artery and vein

thin area in abdominal wall

inguinal ligament

iliopsoas

deep inguinal ring

femoral nerve

testicular artery and vein

ductus deferens

external iliac artery and vein

femoral ring

lacunar ligament

Posterior view of the inguinal–abdominal and inguinal–femoral regions.
The peritoneum and fascia transversalis have been removed.

Note the following important structures:

⁊   The deep inguinal ring with the ductus deferens, and the testicular artery and vein.

⁊   The inferior epigastric vessels passing medially to the deep inguinal ring toward the rectus abdominis sheath.

⁊   The conjoined tendon is enforced by the *interfoveolar ligament*, a band which is inconstant and connects the lower margin of the transversus abdominis muscle to the superior ramus of the pubis.

Since the conjoined tendon, according to recent information, is clearly distinguishable in only approximately 10 per cent of cases, and the interfoveolar ligament similarly is highly inconstant, the posterior wall of the inguinal canal is frequently formed by the fascia transversalis and fibers of the transversus abdominis only. The region bordered by the lateral margin of the rectus abdominis, the medial part of the inguinal ligament and the epigastric vessels may be very thin. Since the subcutaneous inguinal ring lies in front of this thin spot, a real weak spot exists in the abdominal wall. As a result, this area is subject to herniation. These hernias, which do not pass through the inguinal canal, are known as *direct inguinal hernias.*

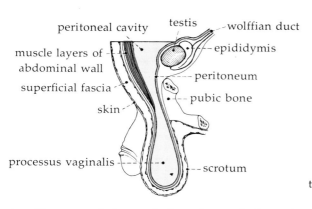

A. Descent of the testis in a fetus of about 7 months.

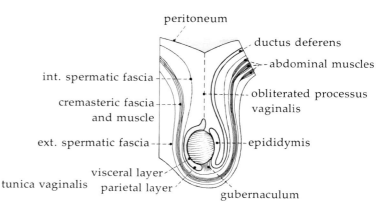

B. Testis has descended and processus vaginalis is closed.

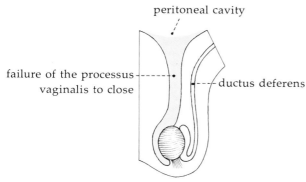

C. Open processus vaginalis.

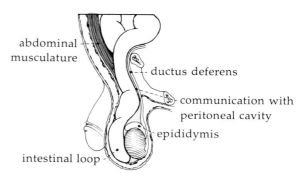

D. Indirect inguinal hernia.

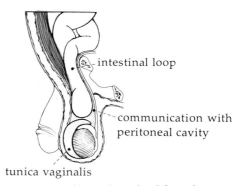

E. Indirect inguinal hernia.

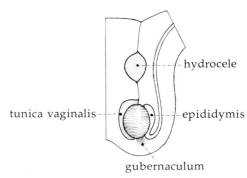

F. Processus vaginalis is partially persistent and has formed a hydrocele.

¶ The testis develops in the lumbar region between the fascia transversalis and the peritoneum. It begins its descent in the third month and during the seventh month it passes through the inguinal canal (A). It is preceded by a peritoneal diverticulum, the *processus vaginalis*. This process of the peritoneum applies itself to the cord and testis. At no time does the processus vaginalis surround them completely. As the testis descends it contacts the fascia transversalis, and the internal and external oblique muscles. It does not force a hole through these layers, but pushes or evaginates them into three coverings. During the eighth month the testis reaches the external inguinal ring, and at the time of birth it is usually in the scrotum (B).

¶ When the processus vaginalis fails to obliterate after birth (C), loops of the intestinal tract or the omentum may enter the process and pass into the scrotum. This condition is known as an *indirect inguinal hernia*. The loops enter the inguinal canal at the deep inguinal ring, pass through the canal and may descend toward the testis (D and E).

¶ Not infrequently, the connection between the peritoneal cavity and the tunica vaginalis obliterates only partially. In such cases a peritoneal cyst remains. At a later age fluid may accumulate in the cavity and the cyst is then known as a hydrocele (F).

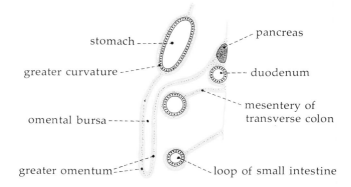

A

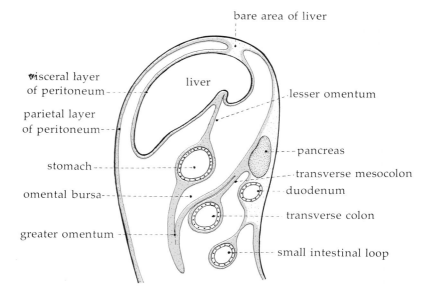

B

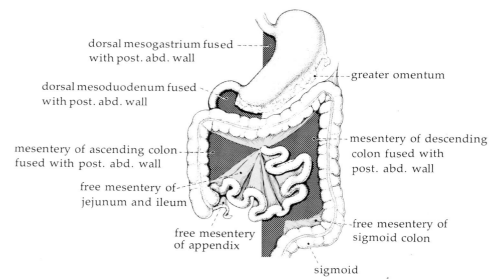

C

A, B and C. Development and position of the greater omentum.

Schematic sagittal section showing the relationship of the greater omentum to the stomach, transverse colon and small intestinal loops in a fetus of 4 months (*A*) and in an adult (*B*). When the greater omentum is removed, those areas of the dorsal mesentery which have fused with the posterior abdominal wall are visible (*C*). (From Langman, J.: Medical Embryology, 3rd ed. Baltimore, The Williams & Wilkins Co., 1975.)

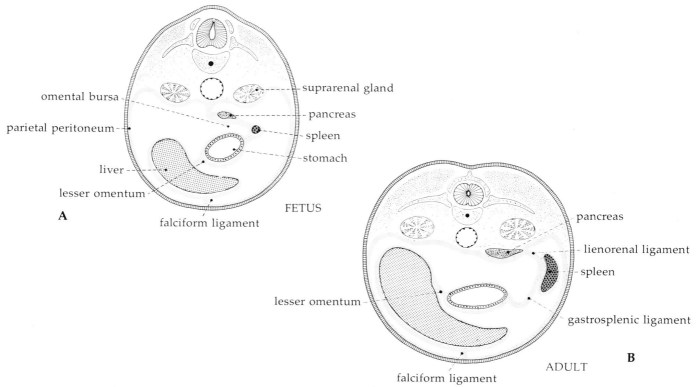

A and B. Transverse sections through the stomach, liver and spleen in a fetus (*A*) and adult (*B*).

Note the formation of the omental bursa, the retroperitoneal position of the pancreas and the position of the spleen. (From Langman, J.: Medical Embryology, 3rd ed. Baltimore. The Williams & Wilkins Co., 1975.)

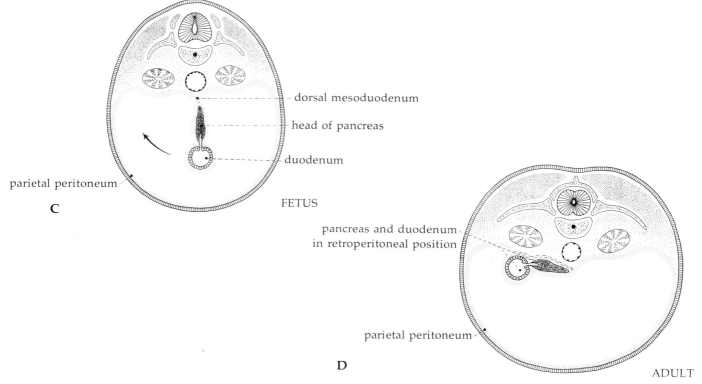

C and D. Transverse sections through the region of the duodenum and pancreas in a fetus (*C*) and adult (*D*).

When the duodenum moves to the right, its dorsal mesentery and the pancreas fuse with the posterior abdominal wall, and the pancreas acquires a retroperitoneal position. (From Langman, J.: Medical Embryology, 3rd ed. Baltimore, The Williams & Wilkins Co., 1975.)

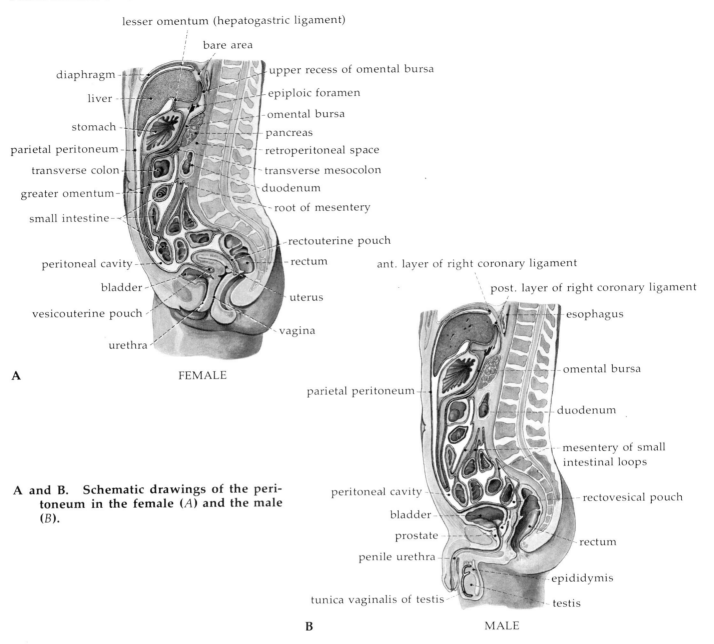

lesser omentum (hepatogastric ligament)

bare area

diaphragm

liver

stomach

parietal peritoneum

transverse colon

greater omentum

small intestine

peritoneal cavity

bladder

vesicouterine pouch

urethra

upper recess of omental bursa

epiploic foramen

omental bursa

pancreas

retroperitoneal space

transverse mesocolon

duodenum

root of mesentery

rectouterine pouch

rectum

uterus

vagina

A   FEMALE

ant. layer of right coronary ligament

post. layer of right coronary ligament

esophagus

omental bursa

parietal peritoneum

duodenum

mesentery of small intestinal loops

peritoneal cavity

rectovesical pouch

bladder

prostate

penile urethra

tunica vaginalis of testis

rectum

epididymis

testis

B   MALE

A and B.   Schematic drawings of the peritoneum in the female (A) and the male (B).

Note:

¶ The inferior side of the diaphragm as well as the anterior abdominal wall is covered by the parietal peritoneum, except in a small area where the diaphragm is in direct contact with the liver.

¶ The liver is covered by peritoneum except at the "bare" area.

¶ The pancreas, most of the duodenum and part of the rectum are located behind the peritoneum.

¶ The four leaves of the greater omentum are separately indicated. Normally they are all fused together. Note the arrow in the omental bursa.

¶ The greater omentum is fused with the wall and the mesentery of the transverse colon.

¶ The relation of the peritoneum on the bladder, uterus and rectum.

¶ In the male the peritoneum extends into the scrotum, covering part of the testis and the epididymis (tunica vaginalis).

¶ In the female, the posterior fornix of the vagina is in contact with the peritoneum.

¶ The peritoneum in the female covers the anterior wall of the body of the uterus but not that of the cervix.

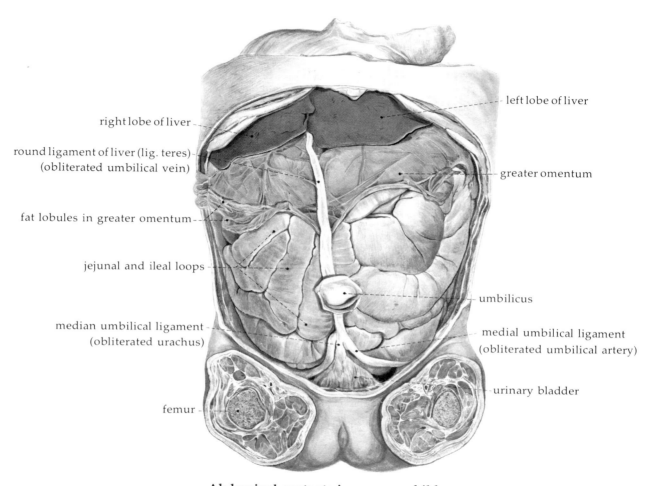

left lobe of liver

right lobe of liver

round ligament of liver (lig. teres)
(obliterated umbilical vein)

greater omentum

fat lobules in greater omentum

jejunal and ileal loops

umbilicus

median umbilical ligament
(obliterated urachus)

medial umbilical ligament
(obliterated umbilical artery)

urinary bladder

femur

Abdominal contents in a young child.
The anterior abdominal wall has been removed.

In a newborn child a number of structures that are not always apparent in an adult are
visible.

- ¶ The remnants of both the umbilical arteries and the umbilical vein are visible. The
  obliterated umbilical vein forms the round ligament of the liver, and the obliterated arteries form the medial umbilical ligaments. These ligaments pass on the lateral side of
  the urinary bladder toward the umbilicus (see also P42).

- ¶ The obliterated urachus forms the median umbilical ligament.

- ¶ The size of the liver is large in comparison with that in the adult. During fetal life
  the liver is one of the most important hematopoietic organs. After birth it loses this
  function.

- ¶ The greater omentum, which in schematic drawings is often represented as a little
  skirt hanging in front of the abdominal contents, in reality usually covers only part of
  the abdominal contents. In the adult it is often fused with the loops of the gut as a result
  of past infections.

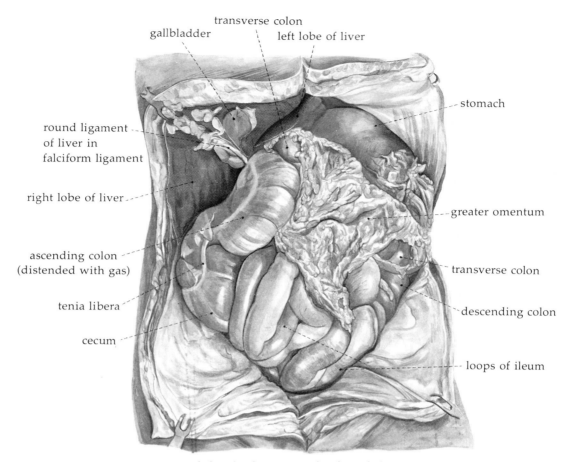

gallbladder

transverse colon

left lobe of liver

stomach

round ligament
of liver in
falciform ligament

right lobe of liver

greater omentum

ascending colon
(distended with gas)

transverse colon

tenia libera

descending colon

cecum

loops of ileum

Abdominal contents in the adult.
The liver has been pulled upward and to the right to show the gallbladder, the round ligament and the ascending colon.

¶ The greater omentum contains many lymph nodes, lymphatic channels and fatty tissue.
It is frequently firmly attached to the stomach, the region of the appendix or the gallbladder by fibrous adhesions. When these organs are inflamed, the greater omentum
is attracted to the site of the infection; its probable function is to prevent the infection
from spreading to the remaining parts of the peritoneal cavity.

¶ In indirect inguinal hernias the greater omentum is frequently the only tissue protruding into the inguinal canal and scrotum.

¶ The right (hepatic) flexure of the ascending colon usually lies under the liver, and the
gallbladder is frequently in direct contact with the ascending colon. This is clinically
important, since in chronic inflammations of the gallbladder it may become fixed to the
wall of the colon. In rare cases a communication may develop between the gallbladder
and the colon, and gallstones may be released into the colon (see A58).

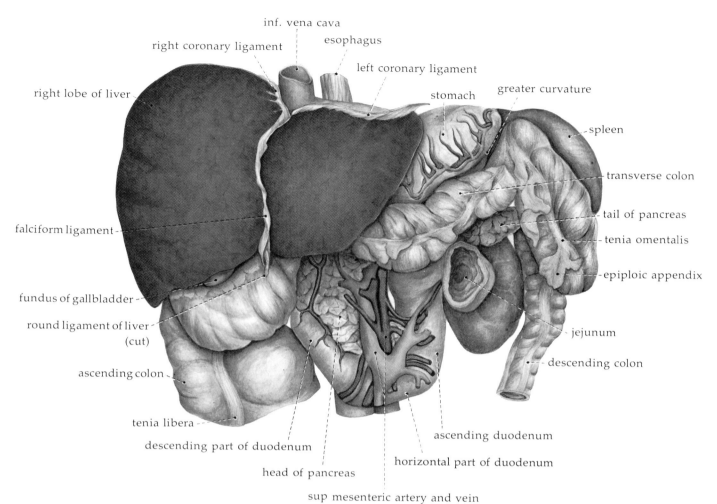

The abdominal organs of the hypochondriac and epigastric regions.
The greater omentum and the small intestinal loops have been removed.

Observe:

§ The falciform ligament on the diaphragmatic surface of the liver forms the dividing line between the right and left lobes. On the visceral surface the fissure for the ligamentum venosum forms the demarcation line between the two lobes. Keep in mind that the anatomic division does not correspond to the functional division between the lobes. The latter division extends forward from the gallbladder and inferior vena cava somewhat to the right of the falciform ligament. Each half has its own arteries, veins and ducts, and the two halves are about equal in weight (see also A51 and A54).

§ The gallbladder protrudes slightly below the anterior border of the right lobe of the liver. The right (hepatic) flexure or the transverse colon is usually in contact with the gallbladder (see also A58).

§ Most of the stomach is hidden behind the liver.

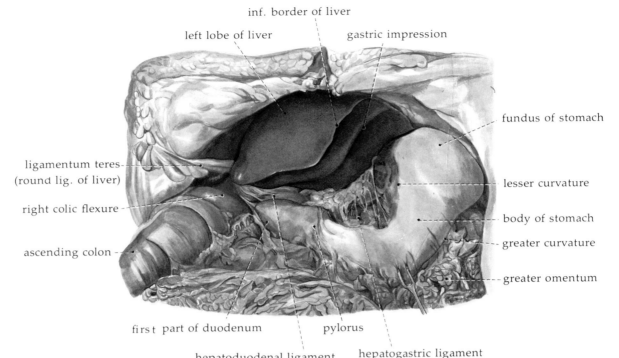

inf. border of liver

left lobe of liver   gastric impression

ligamentum teres
(round lig. of liver)

fundus of stomach

right colic flexure

lesser curvature

ascending colon

body of stomach

greater curvature

greater omentum

first part of duodenum   pylorus

hepatoduodenal ligament   hepatogastric ligament

A. The lesser omentum.
The stomach has been pulled downward and to the left.

gastric impression

lesser omentum

left lobe of liver   lesser curvature

falciform ligament

round ligament of liver   body of stomach

right lobe of liver
(quadrate lobe)

gallbladder (reflected)   greater curvature

epiploic foramen

colic impression on
inf. surface of liver

greater omentum

pylorus

ascending colon   transverse colon   gastrocolic ligament

hepatoduodenal ligament

B. The lesser omentum.
Note the hepatoduodenal ligament and the epiploic foramen.

¶ The lesser omentum is the peritoneal connection between the liver on one side and the stomach and first 3 centimeters of the duodenum on the other side (A20). From the lesser curvature of the stomach and the upper part of the duodenum it runs across to the liver and attaches between the right and left lobes at the porta hepatis and the fissure for the ligamentum venosum (A53 and A54).

¶ The lesser omentum is divided into a thin hepatogastric ligament and a much thicker hepatoduodenal ligament. In the lower rim of the hepatoduodenal ligament are found (a) the bile duct, (b) the portal vein, (c) the hepatic artery, and (d) the lymphatics and autonomic nerves (see A27 and A59 A). By placing the index finger in the epiploic foramen and the thumb on the hepatoduodenal ligament, the bile duct can be palpated between the two fingers.

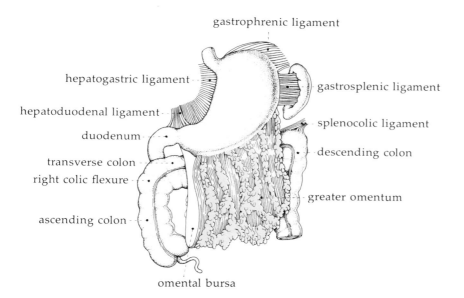

gastrophrenic ligament

hepatogastric ligament

gastrosplenic ligament

hepatoduodenal ligament

splenocolic ligament

duodenum

descending colon

transverse colon

right colic flexure

greater omentum

ascending colon

omental bursa

A. Schematic drawing showing the stomach and its ligaments.

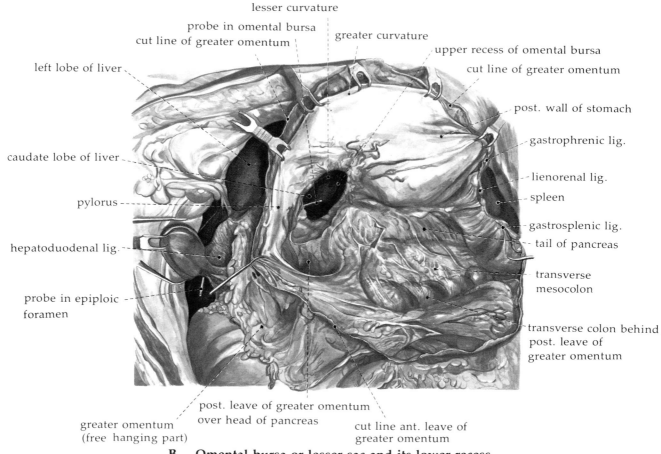

lesser curvature

probe in omental bursa

greater curvature

cut line of greater omentum

upper recess of omental bursa

left lobe of liver

cut line of greater omentum

post. wall of stomach

gastrophrenic lig.

caudate lobe of liver

lienorenal lig.

spleen

pylorus

gastrosplenic lig.

tail of pancreas

hepatoduodenal lig.

transverse mesocolon

probe in epiploic foramen

transverse colon behind post. leave of greater omentum

greater omentum (free hanging part)

post. leave of greater omentum over head of pancreas

cut line ant. leave of greater omentum

B. Omental bursa or lesser sac and its lower recess.
The greater omentum has been cut and the stomach lifted upward.

¶ When the greater omentum is cut close to the major curvature and the stomach lifted upward (as in B), a view is obtained of the posterior wall of the omental bursa (see A19 B). In this region can be seen the pancreas, the transverse mesocolon and the transverse colon. The gastrosplenic ligament (cut) forms the left boundary of the lesser sac (see A and A20 B).

¶ The surgeon gains entrance to the bursa through the epiploic foramen (note the probe) and in this manner can palpate the hepatoduodenal ligament and part of the bursa.

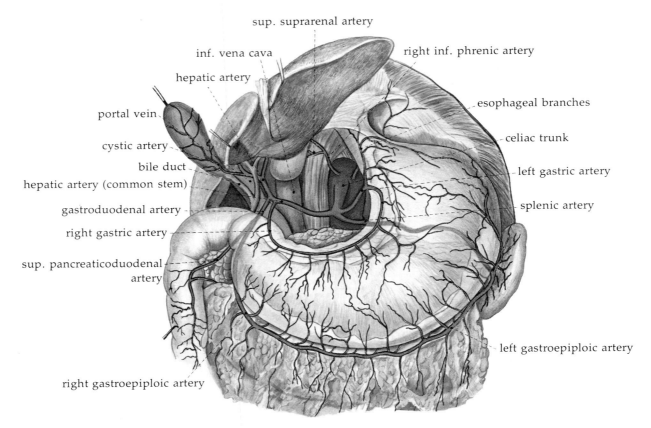

sup. suprarenal artery

inf. vena cava

right inf. phrenic artery

hepatic artery

esophageal branches

portal vein

celiac trunk

cystic artery

bile duct

left gastric artery

hepatic artery (common stem)

splenic artery

gastroduodenal artery

right gastric artery

sup. pancreaticoduodenal artery

left gastroepiploic artery

right gastroepiploic artery

The main branches of the celiac trunk.

The lesser omentum, consisting of the hepatoduodenal and hepatogastric ligaments, has been removed to show the hepatic artery and its relation to the bile duct and portal vein. The liver has been pulled upward and to the right.

Give attention to the following:

¶ The common bile duct, portal vein and hepatic artery course through the hepatoduodenal ligament toward the liver. Although the ligament has been removed, the relationship of the three important structures can be studied:

1. The bile duct – anterior and to the right.
2. The hepatic artery – to the left of the bile duct.
3. The portal vein – posterior to the bile duct and the artery.

¶ After removal of the lesser omentum the celiac trunk can be seen. This large artery arises from the abdominal aorta at the upper border of the pancreas. The main branches are: (a) the splenic artery, (b) the left gastric artery, and (c) the common hepatic artery. Observe also the right inferior phrenic artery and its branch to the right suprarenal gland.

¶ Clinically important branches of the left gastric artery pass upward to the lower part of the esophagus and pierce the diaphragm to enter the thorax. The accompanying veins leave the thorax and, by way of the left gastric vein, become tributaries of the portal vein. Since the remaining part of the esophagus drains by way of the azygos vein, the esophagus is one of the anastomotic areas between the portal and caval venous systems (see A29).

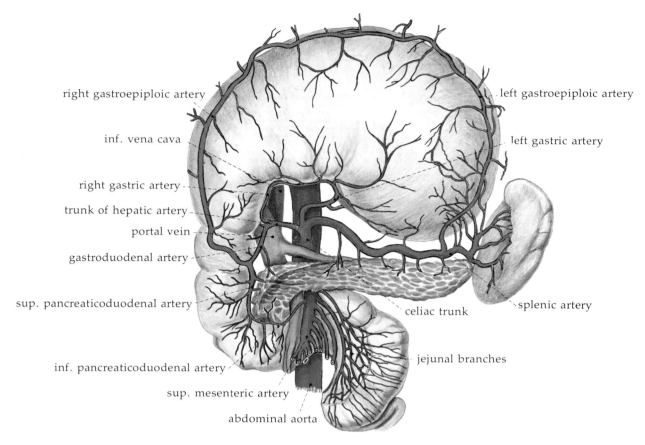

right gastroepiploic artery

inf. vena cava

right gastric artery

trunk of hepatic artery

portal vein

gastroduodenal artery

sup. pancreaticoduodenal artery

inf. pancreaticoduodenal artery

sup. mesenteric artery

abdominal aorta

left gastroepiploic artery

left gastric artery

splenic artery

celiac trunk

jejunal branches

Branches of the celiac trunk and superior mesenteric artery.
The stomach is reflected upward to show the splenic artery.

In this important illustration observe:

¶ The four main arteries supplying the stomach: (a) the left gastric, (b) the right gastric,
(c) the left gastroepiploic, and (d) the right gastroepiploic.

¶ The splenic artery with its branches to the pancreas.

¶ The superior mesenteric artery, which appears at the lower border of the pancreas and
passes in front of the duodenum.

¶ The superior pancreaticoduodenal artery originating from the gastroduodenal artery
and the inferior pancreaticoduodenal artery, a direct branch of the superior mesenteric
artery.

¶ The confluence of the splenic and superior mesenteric veins to form the portal vein.

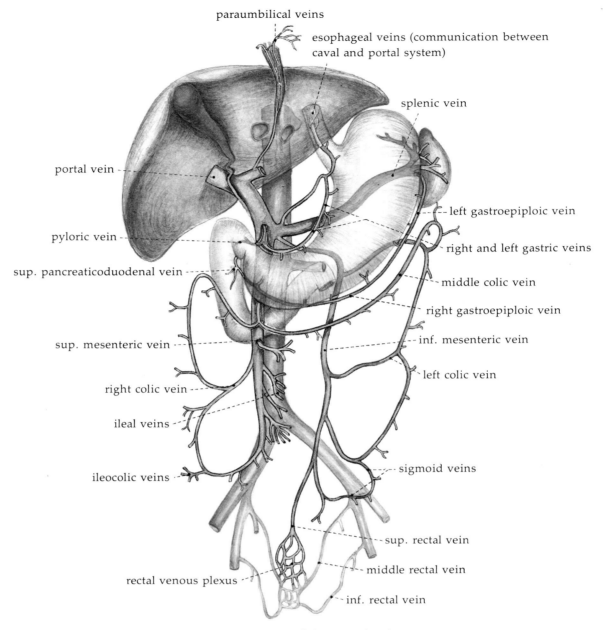

paraumbilical veins

esophageal veins (communication between caval and portal system)

splenic vein

portal vein

left gastroepiploic vein

pyloric vein

right and left gastric veins

sup. pancreaticoduodenal vein

middle colic vein

right gastroepiploic vein

inf. mesenteric vein

sup. mesenteric vein

left colic vein

right colic vein

ileal veins

ileocolic veins

sigmoid veins

sup. rectal vein

middle rectal vein

rectal venous plexus

inf. rectal vein

Drainage area of the portal vein.

¶ The anastomoses between the portal vein and the caval system are important. Under normal circumstances the entire abdominal gastrointestinal tract drains toward the liver by means of the portal system. This includes a small thoracic portion of the esophagus, the upper half of the rectum and sometimes the region of the navel.

¶ When the blood flow in the liver is impeded either by liver disease such as cirrhosis or by cardiac failure, the portal blood seeks other ways to return to the heart. The most important areas of anastomosis between the portal and caval systems are: (a) the lower end of the esophagus, (b) the lower part of the rectum, and (c) by way of the paraumbilical veins and the epigastric veins of the abdominal wall.

¶ The superior mesenteric vein is the largest contributor to the portal vein; the inferior mesenteric vein empties into either the superior mesenteric or the splenic, or directly into the portal vein.

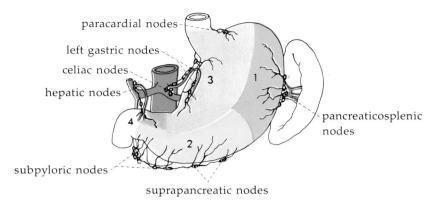

paracardial nodes

left gastric nodes

celiac nodes

hepatic nodes

pancreaticosplenic nodes

subpyloric nodes

suprapancreatic nodes

A. Schematic drawing of the lymph drainage of the stomach.

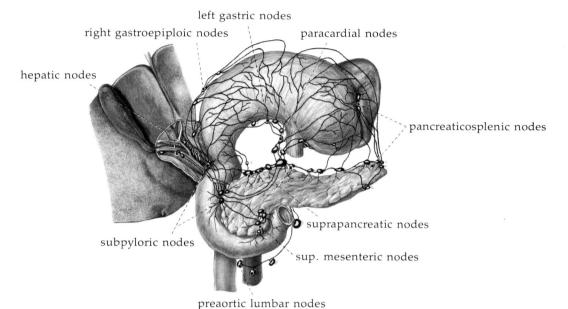

left gastric nodes

right gastroepiploic nodes

paracardial nodes

hepatic nodes

pancreaticosplenic nodes

suprapancreatic nodes

subpyloric nodes

sup. mesenteric nodes

preaortic lumbar nodes

B. Lymph drainage of the stomach.
The stomach has been reflected upward to show the relation to the spleen and pancreas.

Since carcinoma of the stomach is rather common, an understanding of the lymphatic drainage is desirable.

Four important areas should be considered (see *A*):

1. Lymph from the fundus and part of the greater curvature drains to the spleen. If a carcinoma is located in these areas the ligaments of the spleen are usually involved, and splenectomy has to be considered.

2. The subpyloric lymph nodes drain the remaining part of the greater curvature. This group, which drains into the liver, has to be carefully dissected when the stomach is removed. Sometimes pancreatic tissue also has to be removed.

When the cancer is located along the greater curvature, metastases can spread to the pancreaticosplenic group, the subpyloric group, and also to the greater omentum. In such cases the entire omentum is usually removed.

3. The lymph drainage of the lesser curvature and the area around the cardia is very extensive. The lymph enters the paracardial and left gastric nodes and passes subsequently to the celiac nodes.

4. A small but important lymph area is found in the upper portion of the pylorus. In this region carcinoma occurs frequently. The lymph vessels drain directly into the liver by way of the hepatoduodenal ligament.

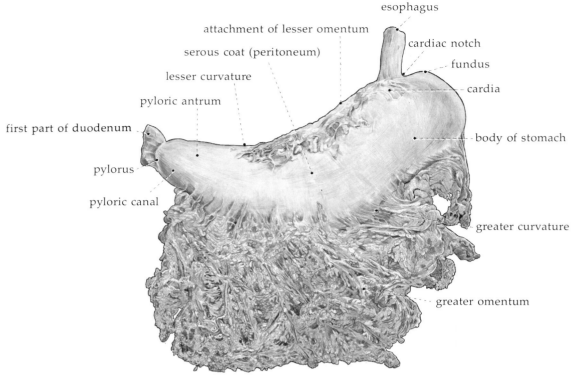

esophagus

attachment of lesser omentum

cardiac notch

serous coat (peritoneum)

fundus

lesser curvature

cardia

pyloric antrum

first part of duodenum

body of stomach

pylorus

pyloric canal

greater curvature

greater omentum

A.   Anterior view of the stomach and greater omentum.

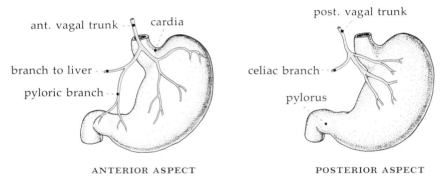

ant. vagal trunk

cardia

post. vagal trunk

branch to liver

celiac branch

pyloric branch

pylorus

ANTERIOR ASPECT

POSTERIOR ASPECT

B and C.   Schematic drawings of the nerve supply of the stomach.

¶   The *fundus*, located above the junction with the esophagus, usually contains a gas bubble. It bulges against the left cupola of the diaphragm up to the level of the fifth intercostal space. A full and distended stomach may cause accelerated respiration and possibly increased cardiac activity (see A34).

¶   The parasympathetic nerve supply to the stomach is provided by the vagus nerves (*B*). The *left* or *anterior* vagal trunk supplies the anterior wall. It also gives off a branch to the pylorus and antrum and a branch to the liver by way of the lesser omentum. The *right* or *posterior* vagal trunk gives branches to the posterior wall of the stomach, and also a few to the anterior surface. Its main branch extends to the celiac ganglion for distribution to the small intestine, the pancreas and the colon as far as the midtransverse colon. This branch is known as the celiac branch.

¶   The vagal trunks provide motor and secretory impulses to the stomach. Cutting the trunks abolishes gastric secretion but at the same time makes the stomach atonic; hence, it empties with great difficulty.

¶   The sympathetic nerve supply to the stomach arises from the celiac plexus, and reaches the stomach by way of the arteries. The greater splanchnic nerve, originating from the fifth to the tenth thoracic ganglia, passes through the diaphragm behind the suprarenal gland and terminates in the upper part of the celiac plexus; the lesser splanchnic nerve, arising from the ninth and tenth ganglia, reaches the lower end (see T63).

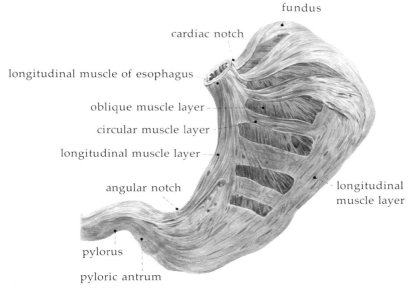

cardiac notch
fundus
longitudinal muscle of esophagus
oblique muscle layer
circular muscle layer
longitudinal muscle layer
angular notch
longitudinal muscle layer
pylorus
pyloric antrum

A. Muscle layers of the stomach.

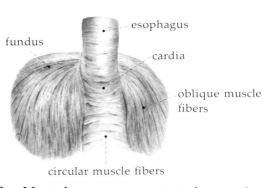

esophagus
fundus
cardia
oblique muscle fibers
circular muscle fibers

B. Muscular arrangement at the esophagogastric junction.
The longitudinal layer has been removed.

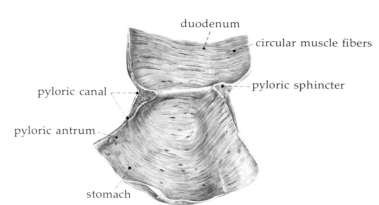

duodenum
circular muscle fibers
pyloric canal
pyloric sphincter
pyloric antrum
stomach

C. Circular muscular fibers in the pyloric region.

¶ The muscular coat consists of three layers:

1. A longitudinal coat, which is continuous with longitudinal fibers of the esophagus. It is found mainly along the curvatures (*A*).

2. A circular coat, which is particularly thick in the pyloric region (*C*). In infants the circular layer of the pylorus may be excessively thickened, a condition known as *congenital pyloric stenosis.*

3. Oblique fibers, which extend over the fundus and down on both surfaces of the stomach (*B*). They end proximal to the pyloric portion. Some longitudinal fibers interlace with the fibers of the pyloric sphincter.

¶ No special sphincter exists at the cardiac orifice. This opening is kept closed by the normal resting tone of the lowest circular fibers of the esophagus. The passage of food is permitted by a momentary relaxation in front of a peristaltic wave. The distal end then pouts temporarily into the stomach. Closure is assisted by the valvelike fold of the cardiac notch and possibly by the oblique muscular fibers of the stomach. Other factors which may help in the closing mechanism have been suggested: (a) mucosal folds at the esophagogastric junction act as a valve; (b) the intra-abdominal pressure compresses the walls of the intra-abdominal esophagus; (c) the acute angle of entry of the esophagus into the stomach produces a valvelike effect.

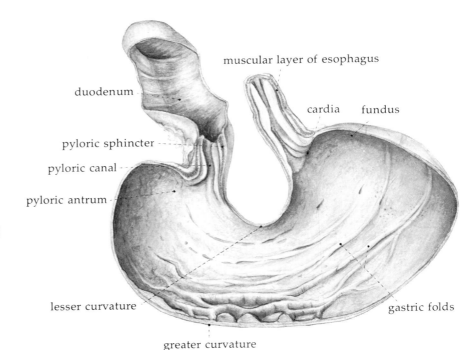

A. Mucosa of the stomach and pyloric region.

muscular layer of esophagus

duodenum

cardia   fundus

pyloric sphincter

pyloric canal

pyloric antrum

lesser curvature

gastric folds

greater curvature

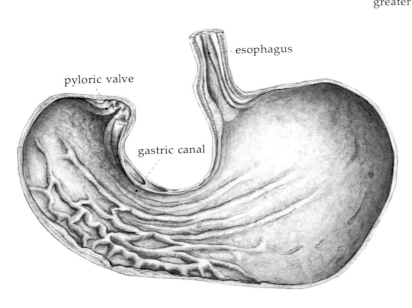

esophagus

pyloric valve

gastric canal

B. The stomach and its orifices.

¶ Gastric ulcers are most frequently seen along the lesser curvature of the stomach. When they perforate they penetrate through the mucosa, the submucosa, the muscular layers and the peritoneal layer covering the outside. They may break through anteriorly and also posteriorly, thereby releasing gastric fluid in the omental bursa (see A19).

¶ Sometimes a gastric ulcer or cancer erodes the pancreas, causing severe pain in the back. Ulceration occurs occasionally into the splenic artery, resulting in serious retroperitoneal hemorrhage (see A28).

¶ The stomach frequently adheres to the surrounding structures and organs as a result of chronic inflammation. In this manner it may be attached to the transverse mesocolon.

¶ The pyloric region consists of an antrum and a tubular canal, the *pyloric canal*. It is covered by the liver. Since most perforated peptic ulcers occur in this area, it is of great surgical importance. The circular musculature is thick and forms a ring around the pyloric orifice, the *pyloric sphincter*.

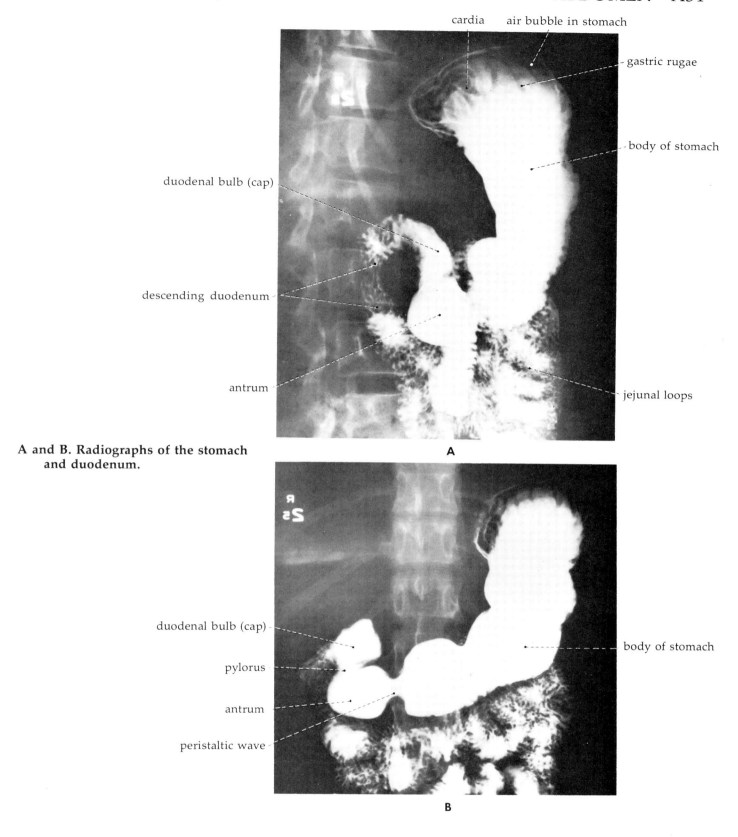

cardia   air bubble in stomach

gastric rugae

body of stomach

duodenal bulb (cap)

descending duodenum

antrum

jejunal loops

A

A and B. Radiographs of the stomach and duodenum.

duodenal bulb (cap)

body of stomach

pylorus

antrum

peristaltic wave

B

The great variability in the position, size and shape of the stomach is particularly striking in radiographs. Note the following features: (a) the air bubble in the fundus; (b) the esophagogastric region; (c) the rugae; (d) the pyloric antrum and sphincter; (e) the duodenal cap; and (f) the peristaltic waves.

By tipping the patient head-down, barium containing fluid can be directed so that it will impinge against the cardia. When the cardioesophageal sphincter is incompetent the radiopaque material flows into the esophagus.

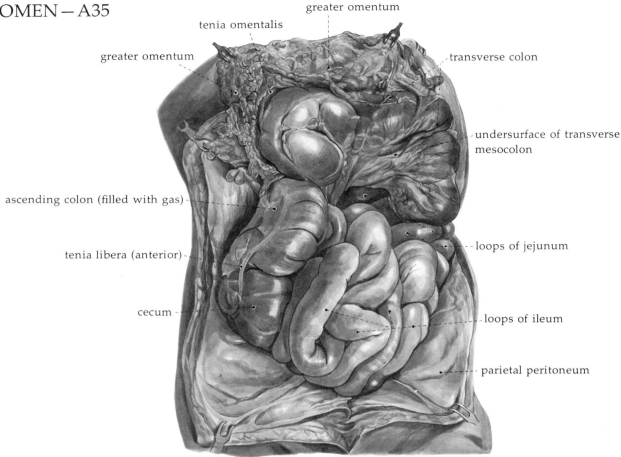

greater omentum

tenia omentalis

greater omentum

transverse colon

undersurface of transverse mesocolon

ascending colon (filled with gas)

loops of jejunum

tenia libera (anterior)

cecum

loops of ileum

parietal peritoneum

A.   Loops of the small and large intestines.

The greater omentum and transverse colon have been drawn upward to expose the transverse mesocolon.

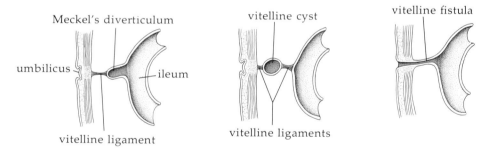

Meckel's diverticulum

vitelline cyst

vitelline fistula

umbilicus

ileum

vitelline ligament

vitelline ligaments

B, C and D.   Remnants of the vitelline duct.

(From Langman, J.: Radical Embryology, 3rd ed., Baltimore, The Williams & Wilkins Co., 1975.)

Normally the patent connection that exists between the gastrointestinal tract and the yolk sac during embryonic life disappears, but in 2 per cent of cases the vitelline duct persists (a) as a diverticulum attached to the ileum and known as Meckel's diverticulum (B). Its typical position is 2 feet from the ileocecal junction on the antimesenteric border of the ileum; (b) as a vitelline cyst between the umbilicus and small intestine, usually attached to both by fibrous cords (C); (c) as a narrow channel through which fecal discharge oozes to the surface at the umbilicus (D). It is important to know that Meckel's diverticulum may contain gastric tissue and even pancreatic tissue. On occasion a peptic ulcer may be found in the diverticulum.

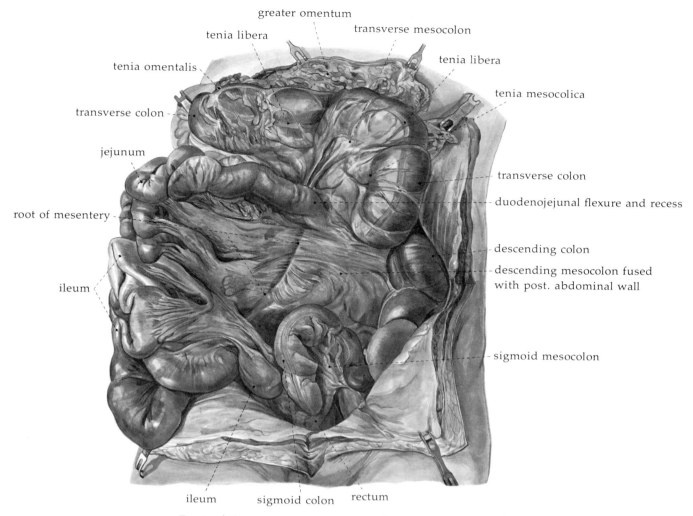

greater omentum

tenia libera

transverse mesocolon

tenia omentalis

tenia libera

transverse colon

tenia mesocolica

jejunum

transverse colon

duodenojejunal flexure and recess

root of mesentery

descending colon

descending mesocolon fused with post. abdominal wall

ileum

sigmoid mesocolon

ileum   sigmoid colon   rectum

Root of the mesentery proper and transverse mesocolon.
The loops of the small intestine have been drawn to the right and the transverse colon has been drawn upward.

Note the following important structures:

§ The transverse colon with the tenia libera, tenia omentalis and tenia mesocolica.

§ The transverse mesocolon.

§ The duodenojejunal flexure with the duodenojejunal recess.

§ The root of the mesentery. It is about 6 inches (17 cm.) in length and extends obliquely across the posterior abdominal wall from a point slightly to the left of the body of L2 to the right sacroiliac joint.

§ The descending mesocolon, fused with the posterior abdominal wall.

§ The sigmoid mesocolon which allows movement of the sigmoid colon (see A19 C).

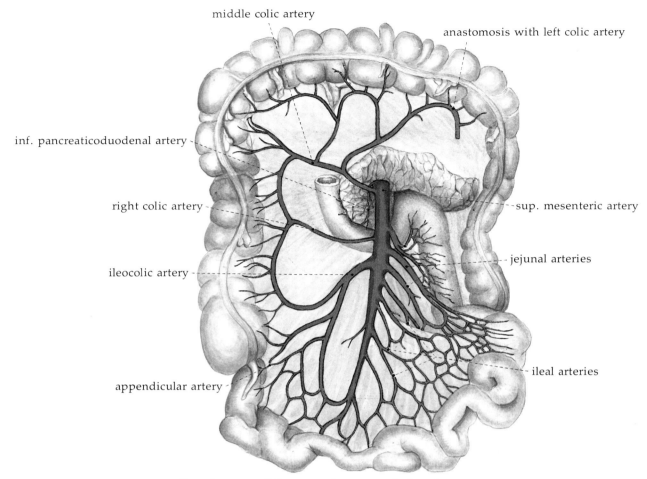

middle colic artery

anastomosis with left colic artery

inf. pancreaticoduodenal artery

sup. mesenteric artery

right colic artery

jejunal arteries

ileocolic artery

ileal arteries

appendicular artery

Supply area of the superior mesenteric artery.
The artery arises behind the neck of the pancreas and passes in front of the uncinate process and the horizontal part of the duodenum to enter the mesentery proper.

A number of important observations should be made:

¶ The inferior pancreaticoduodenal artery, supplying about two-thirds of the duodenum, is one of the first branches of the superior mesenteric. It courses along the medial wall of the duodenum and provides anterior and posterior branches.

¶ Note the intensive blood supply of the jejunum and the ileum. The branches form a network of arcades from which straight vessels move to the gut. These straight vessels (vasa recta) do not anastomose. Toward the ileum the arcades become larger and the vasa recta shorter and further apart.

¶ There is a series of large anastomosing loops along the colon that results in a continuous marginal artery along the wall of the gut. In case of embolus or occlusion an effective collateral circulation may develop. A dangerous point exists in the ileocecal area, where collateral formation is sometimes insufficient. Another weak point may be found at the left colic flexure where the supply areas of the superior and inferior mesenteric arteries sometimes fail to overlap (see also A43).

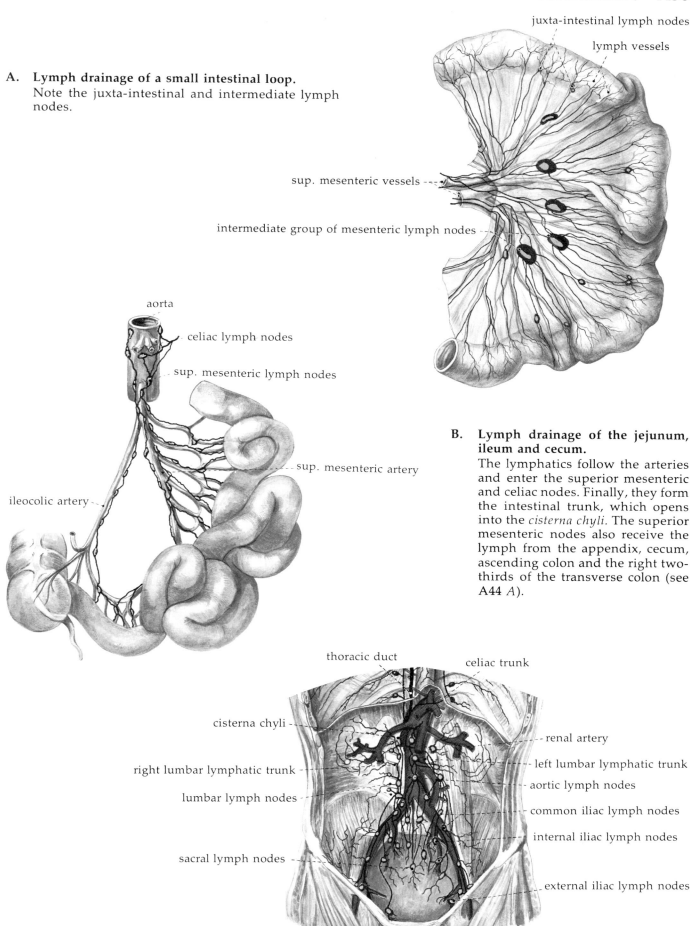

A. Lymph drainage of a small intestinal loop.
Note the juxta-intestinal and intermediate lymph nodes.

juxta-intestinal lymph nodes

lymph vessels

sup. mesenteric vessels

intermediate group of mesenteric lymph nodes

aorta

celiac lymph nodes

sup. mesenteric lymph nodes

sup. mesenteric artery

ileocolic artery

B. Lymph drainage of the jejunum, ileum and cecum.
The lymphatics follow the arteries and enter the superior mesenteric and celiac nodes. Finally, they form the intestinal trunk, which opens into the *cisterna chyli*. The superior mesenteric nodes also receive the lymph from the appendix, cecum, ascending colon and the right two-thirds of the transverse colon (see A44 *A*).

thoracic duct

celiac trunk

cisterna chyli

renal artery

right lumbar lymphatic trunk

left lumbar lymphatic trunk

lumbar lymph nodes

aortic lymph nodes

common iliac lymph nodes

internal iliac lymph nodes

sacral lymph nodes

external iliac lymph nodes

C. Cisterna chyli and abdominal lymph trunks.

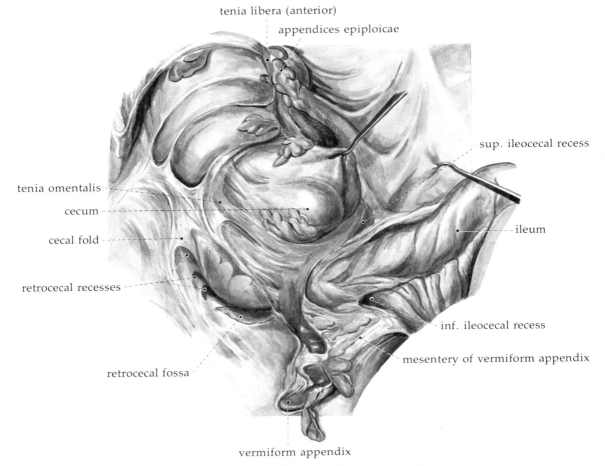

tenia libera (anterior)

appendices epiploicae

sup. ileocecal recess

tenia omentalis

cecum

cecal fold

ileum

retrocecal recesses

inf. ileocecal recess

mesentery of vermiform appendix

retrocecal fossa

vermiform appendix

Ileocecal region with vermiform appendix.
The cecum has been pulled to the left to expose the retrocecal recess.

Make the following observations:

❡ The vermiform appendix has its own mesentery, the *mesoappendix,* which has the shape of a triangular fold. It contains lymph vessels, lymph nodes, the appendicular artery and some fat lobules (see A40 *A*).

❡ The cecum has a complete peritoneal investment; from its anterior surface the peritoneum continues upward over the ascending colon, but from its posterior surface it is reflected backward and downward over the iliac muscle, thus forming a cul-de-sac behind the cecum. This retrocecal recess sometimes extends behind the ascending colon and frequently contains the vermiform appendix.

Occasionally the cecum and ascending colon retain a short mesentery. This permits mobility and makes it possible for the ileocecal segment to become twisted around its own mesentery. This situation is called volvulus, and since the blood vessels may be twisted, the blood supply may be insufficient, leading to ischemic necrosis.

❡ On the sides of the ileocecal junction are found the superior and inferior ileocecal recesses.

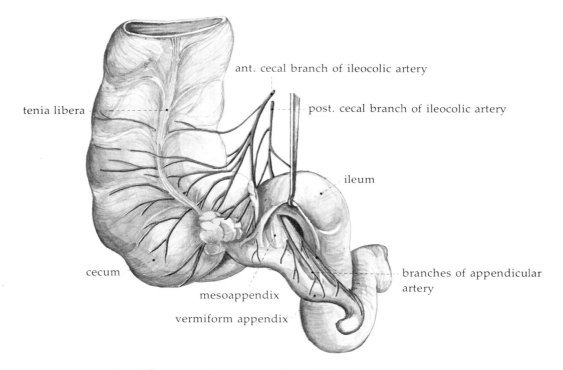

ant. cecal branch of ileocolic artery

tenia libera

post. cecal branch of ileocolic artery

ileum

cecum

branches of appendicular artery

mesoappendix

vermiform appendix

A. The vermiform appendix and the ileocecal region.

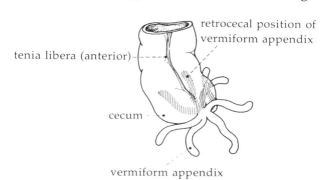

retrocecal position of vermiform appendix

tenia libera (anterior)

cecum

vermiform appendix

B. Various positions of the appendix.

Important clinical considerations:

¶ The appendix has a mesentery which is continuous with the left layer of the ileal mesentery; it reaches the appendix after passing behind the termination of the ileum. As a rule the mesentery does not extend to the tip of the appendix. In the mesentery lies the appendicular artery, a branch of the ileocolic. It passes behind the ileum.

¶ When an inflamed appendix is in the position shown in *A*, a point of tenderness is located at the junction of the middle and outer thirds of a line joining the umbilicus and the anterior superior iliac spine. This area of greatest tenderness is known as McBurney's point.

¶ In probably more than 50 per cent of cases the vermiform appendix is found in a retrocecal position (see A41 *A*). It may, however, also lie: (a) on the outside of the ascending colon, (b) toward the umbilicus, (c) over the promontory of the sacrum, (d) over the brim of the pelvis, and (e) in an inguinal position (see *B*).

¶ The symptoms of an inflamed vermiform appendix vary greatly depending on its position. An abscess behind the cecum may be intraperitoneal or retroperitoneal; in the latter case it may ascend to the perinephric or subphrenic regions. When located in the pelvis an abscess may cause vesical or rectal irritation.

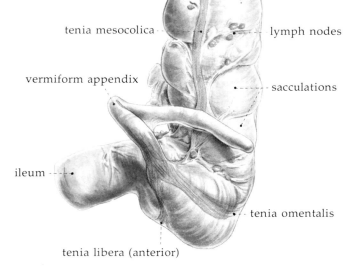

tenia mesocolica — lymph nodes

vermiform appendix

sacculations

ileum

tenia omentalis

tenia libera (anterior)

A. Ileocecal region with the appendix in a retro-cecal position.
The teniae of the colon converge toward the vermiform appendix. Small lymph nodes are present on the wall of the colon.

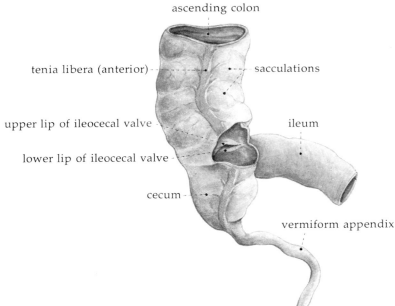

ascending colon

tenia libera (anterior) — sacculations

upper lip of ileocecal valve

ileum

lower lip of ileocecal valve

cecum

vermiform appendix

B. Ileocecal orifice.
The valves are formed by the circular muscle bundles of the ileum protruding into the cecum. It is important to realize that the valves do not prevent reflux from the cecum into the small intestine, as evidenced by the appearance of contrast fluid in the ileum after a rectal barium enema.

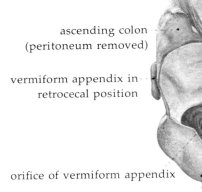

ascending colon with peritoneal covering

ascending colon (peritoneum removed)

vermiform appendix in retrocecal position

probe in ileocecal valve

ileum

orifice of vermiform appendix

cecum

C. Ileocecal valve and valve of the vermiform appendix.

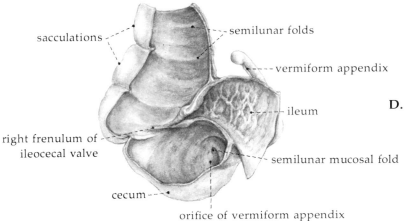

sacculations — semilunar folds

vermiform appendix

ileum

right frenulum of ileocecal valve

semilunar mucosal fold

cecum

orifice of vermiform appendix

D. Ileocecal junction.
Note: (a) the frenulum caused by merging of the upper and lower valves; (b) the difference in the mucosa between the ileum and the colon; (c) the opening into the vermiform appendix guarded by a semilunar mucosal fold.

A. Anterior view of the ascending colon.
The serosa has been partially removed to show a tenia.

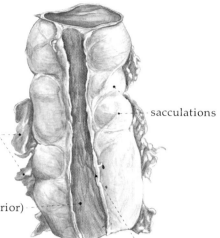

sacculations

appendices epiploicae

tenia libera (anterior)

serous coat (removed to show
muscle fibers of tenia)

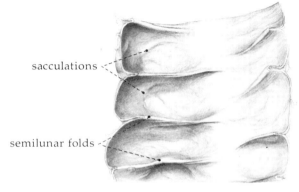

sacculations

semilunar folds

B. Interior view of the colon.

muscular fibers of tenia

serous coat

fatty tissue in serous coat

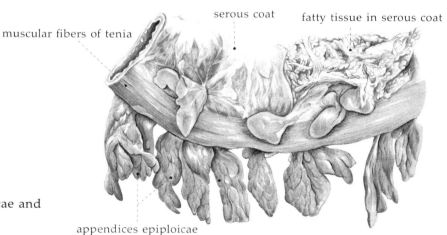

C. Ascending colon.
The serosa, the appendices epiploicae and
a muscular tenia are shown.

appendices epiploicae

¶ The colon has three typical characteristics:

1. *Teniae.* The outer longitudinal muscle coat is not complete but forms three bands, the *teniae coli.* They converge to the vermiform appendix where they form a continuous sheet of longitudinal muscle. Since the muscular bands are shorter than the gut itself the wall of the colon forms sacculations.

2. *Haustra.* Sacculations of the colon wall.

3. *Appendices epiploicae.* Fat lobules surrounded by peritoneum hang from the wall throughout the length of the colon. Usually they are located close to the anterior tenia. Those in the region of the appendix, the cecum and the rectum generally contain little fat or none.

¶ The transverse colon is completely invested by peritoneum and is attached to the posterior abdominal wall by its mesentery. The ascending and descending sections of the colon are usually surrounded on three sides but not on the posterior side. Sometimes they are completely surrounded by peritoneum but have no mesentery.

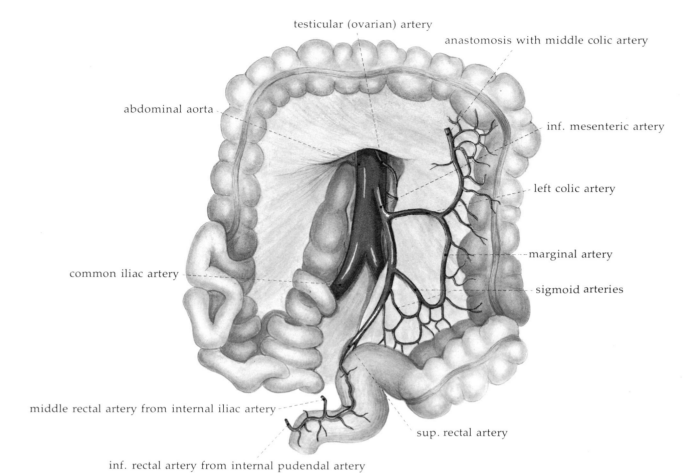

testicular (ovarian) artery

anastomosis with middle colic artery

abdominal aorta

inf. mesenteric artery

left colic artery

marginal artery

common iliac artery

sigmoid arteries

middle rectal artery from internal iliac artery

sup. rectal artery

inf. rectal artery from internal pudendal artery

Inferior mesenteric artery and its supply area.

ꟼ The inferior mesenteric artery forms anastomoses with the superior mesenteric artery at the left third of the transverse colon. Although in many cases the large marginal artery from the superior mesenteric continues into that of the inferior mesenteric, occasionally it does not. If occlusion of the artery in this region occurs, the left third of the transverse colon has little chance of collateral circulation.

ꟼ A second area with few anastomoses is located between the sigmoid and the rectum.

ꟼ The arterial supply to the rectum is provided by three vessels: (a) the superior rectal artery, a terminal branch from the inferior mesenteric; (b) the middle rectal, from the internal iliac artery; and (c) the inferior rectal, from the internal pudendal artery. The venous drainage of the rectum is particularly important, since the blood from the upper part will return to the inferior mesenteric vein and the portal vein, while blood from the lower part will drain by way of the inferior vena cava. (For a view of the porta-caval anastomoses, see A29.)

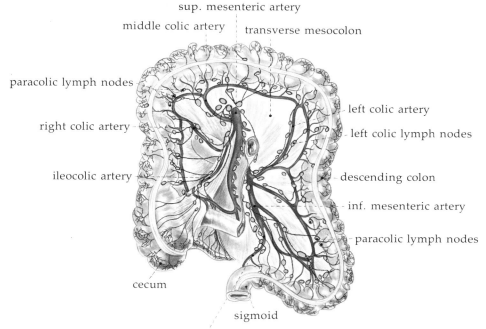

A. Lymph drainage of the large intestine.

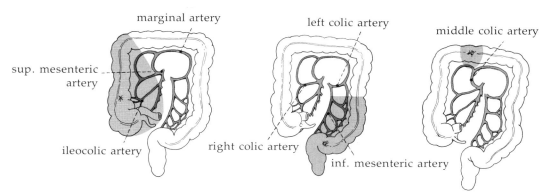

B, C and D. Practical application of the blood and lymph supply.

¶ As in the small intestine three groups of lymph nodes can be recognized: (a) the paracolic nodes along the marginal artery, (b) the intermediate nodes on the stems of the colic arteries, and (c) the main nodes near the roots of the arteries. The lymph vessels of the colon, between the appendix and the left colic flexure, join those of the small intestine and form the intestinal trunk toward the cisterna chyli (see A38). The lymph vessels from the left colic flexure to and including the upper part of the rectum follow the branches of the inferior mesenteric artery and end in the nodes of the left lumbar aortic chain.

¶ In patients with cancer of the colon the course of the lymph vessels is of utmost importance. Since the lymph vessels closely follow the arteries and veins, removal of the vessels is frequently a necessity. As removal of the arterial supply of a segment of bowel results in necrosis of that segment, a considerable length of colon has to be removed. For example, cancer of the cecum necessitates removal from the distal part of the ileum to the transverse colon up to the middle colic artery. Similarly, cancer of the upper part of the rectum requires removal of the sigmoid and part of the descending colon. Carcinoma of the middle of the transverse colon around the middle colic artery requires removal of the smallest section, namely, 7 to 10 cm on either side of the growth.

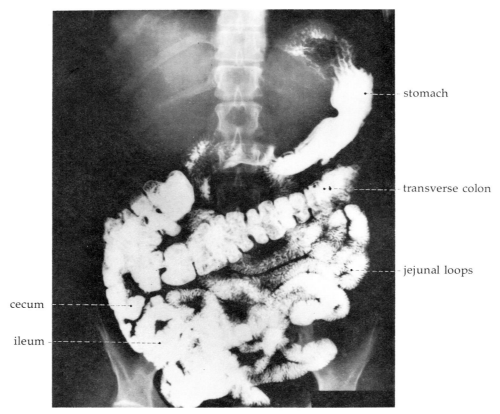

stomach

transverse colon

jejunal loops

cecum

ileum

A. Radiograph of the small intestinal loops.
Note the peristaltic contractions.

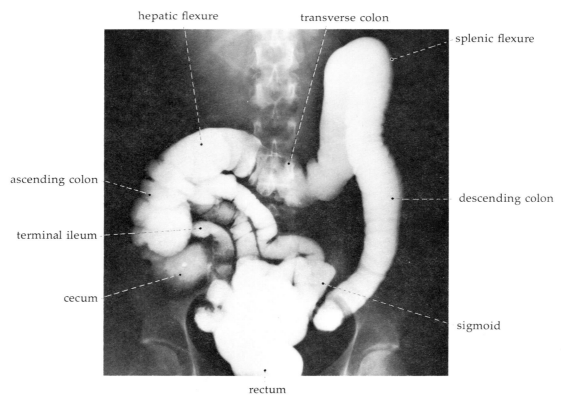

hepatic flexure

transverse colon

splenic flexure

ascending colon

descending colon

terminal ileum

cecum

sigmoid

rectum

B. Radiograph of the colon after a barium enema.
Note the reflux of barium into the ileum.

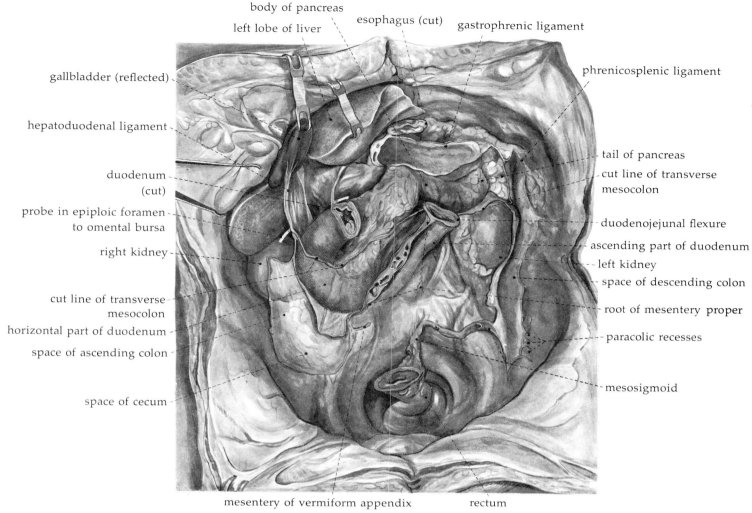

body of pancreas
left lobe of liver   esophagus (cut)   gastrophrenic ligament
gallbladder (reflected)
hepatoduodenal ligament
duodenum (cut)
probe in epiploic foramen to omental bursa
right kidney
cut line of transverse mesocolon
horizontal part of duodenum
space of ascending colon
space of cecum
phrenicosplenic ligament
tail of pancreas
cut line of transverse mesocolon
duodenojejunal flexure
ascending part of duodenum
left kidney
space of descending colon
root of mesentery proper
paracolic recesses
mesosigmoid
mesentery of vermiform appendix   rectum

Attachment of mesenteries.
The stomach, jejunum and ileum, and the colon and sigmoid have been removed, but the duodenum, pancreas and liver are left in position.

Note the following important landmarks:

1. Cut edge of the esophagus at its entrance into the stomach.

2. Cut edge of the duodenum close to the pylorus.

3. Cut edge of the jejunum at the duodenojejunal flexure.

4. Cut edge of the rectum.

5. Cut edge of the root of the small intestinal mesentery (mesentery proper) with the superior mesenteric vessels.

6. Cut edge of the mesentery of the vermiform appendix.

7. Cut edge of the mesentery of the transverse colon, passing over the duodenum and pancreas.

8. Cut edge of the sigmoid mesentery with branches of the inferior mesenteric vessels.

9. The "bed" of the cecum and ascending colon. On each side the covering peritoneum has been cut. Note its relation to the right kidney.

10. The "bed" of the descending colon. Note its relation to the left kidney.

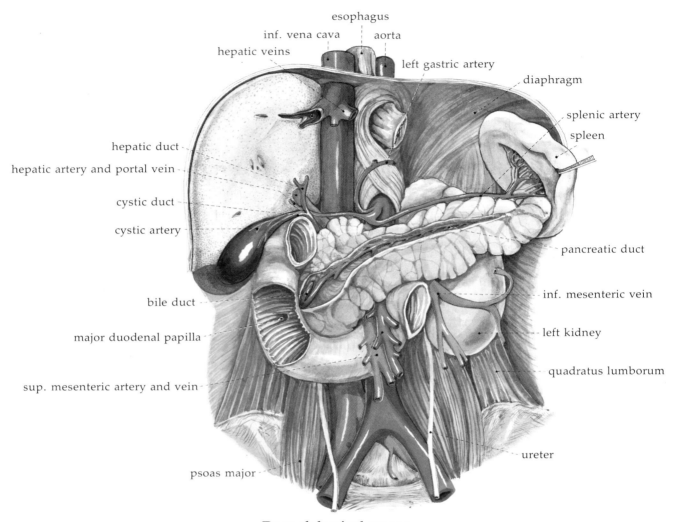

esophagus

inf. vena cava   aorta

hepatic veins

left gastric artery

diaphragm

splenic artery

spleen

hepatic duct

hepatic artery and portal vein

cystic duct

cystic artery

pancreatic duct

bile duct

inf. mesenteric vein

major duodenal papilla

left kidney

quadratus lumborum

sup. mesenteric artery and vein

ureter

psoas major

Deep abdominal organs.
The stomach, small intestinal loops, colon and part of the liver have been removed.

Make the following observations:

¶ The pancreas lies behind the peritoneum. The head of the pancreas fills the space between the extremities of the horseshoe-shaped duodenum; the body crosses over the
left kidney, and the tail reaches the intraperitoneally located spleen.

¶ The splenic artery passes to the left along the upper border of the body and tail of the
pancreas; the hepatic artery runs to the right along the upper border of the neck and the
head of the pancreas.

¶ The splenic vein runs parallel to the artery but lies behind the pancreas. Similarly, the
inferior and superior mesenteric veins pass behind the pancreas.

¶ The bile duct passes behind the first part of the duodenum and then through the head
of the pancreas. It joins the main pancreatic duct before entering the duodenum.

116

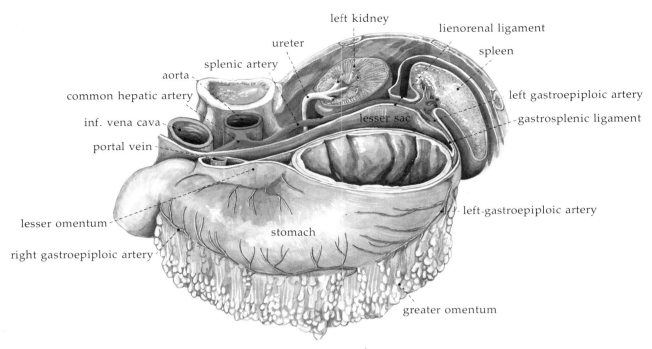

A. The spleen and its relation to the kidney and stomach.
Note the lienorenal and gastrosplenic ligaments.

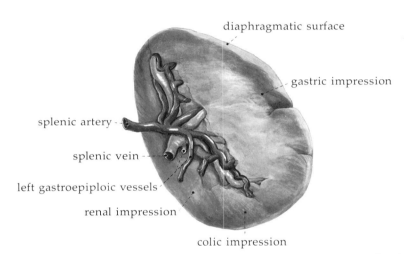

B. Medial view of the spleen showing the splenic artery and vein.
Note the left gastroepiploic vessels.

¶ The spleen is completely surrounded by peritoneum. At the hilus it is connected to the kidney and posterior abdominal wall by the lienorenal ligament. Through this ligament (a double fold of peritoneum) the splenic vessels enter the spleen. The left gastroepiploic vessels pass through the gastrosplenic ligament, which connects the greater curvature with the hilus. Note that the posterior wall of the omental bursa or lesser sac is formed by peritoneum which covers the posterior abdominal wall.

¶ Removal of the spleen in cases of rupture or extreme enlargement is relatively easy to accomplish since the organ is attached to its surroundings only by the lienorenal and gastrosplenic ligaments. By incising the left leaf of the lienorenal ligament and clamping the vessels at the hilus the blood supply to the stomach can be left uninterrupted.

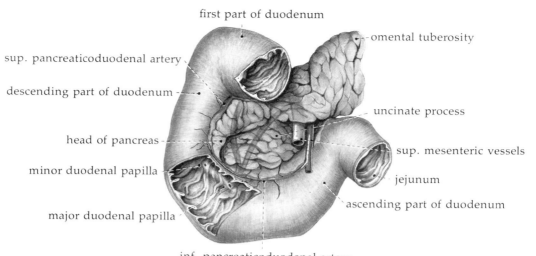

first part of duodenum

omental tuberosity

sup. pancreaticoduodenal artery

descending part of duodenum

uncinate process

head of pancreas

sup. mesenteric vessels

minor duodenal papilla

jejunum

ascending part of duodenum

major duodenal papilla

inf. pancreaticoduodenal artery

A. Head of the pancreas and the duodenum.

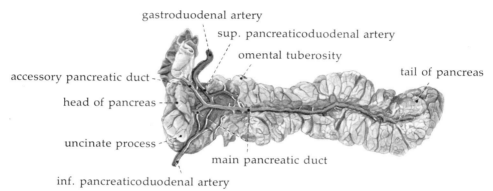

gastroduodenal artery

sup. pancreaticoduodenal artery

omental tuberosity

accessory pancreatic duct

tail of pancreas

head of pancreas

uncinate process

main pancreatic duct

inf. pancreaticoduodenal artery

B. Pancreatic ducts and blood supply of the head of the pancreas.

The head of the pancreas is an important area clinically since (a) the pancreatic ducts, the bile duct and the superior mesenteric vessels traverse it, and (b) carcinoma of the pancreas is usually located in the head region.

¶ When a carcinoma develops in the head of the pancreas it will slowly compress the surrounding organs and tissues. The first indication of the tumor may be caused by pressure on or obstruction of the bile duct, resulting in jaundice.

¶ Frequently the tumor compresses the duodenum; radiologic examination may reveal only a narrow passage through the duodenum.

¶ Since the superior mesenteric vein, the splenic vein, the inferior mesenteric vein and even the portal and inferior caval veins (see A47), are closely related to the head of the pancreas, the tumor may directly involve these veins and metastases may proceed along their walls.

¶ The lymphatics drain into the celiac glands around the root of the celiac artery. Metastases, however, may also proceed along the hepatoduodenal ligament into the liver.

¶ The *superior pancreaticoduodenal artery*, a branch of the gastroduodenal artery, and the *inferior pancreaticoduodenal*, a branch of the superior mesenteric, supply the duodenum and the head of the pancreas. Both arteries usually divide into two parallel vessels, one in front and one behind the head of the pancreas. In this manner the blood supply of the duodenum and head of the pancreas is very intensive.

¶ The body and tail of the pancreas are supplied by numerous branches of the splenic artery.

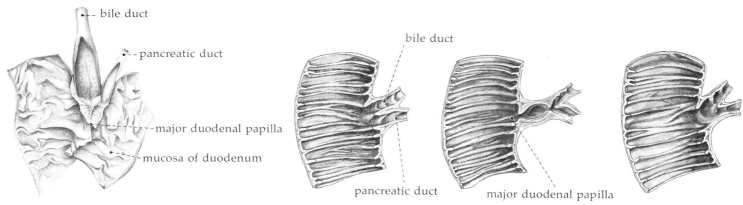

A. Major duodenal papilla.

B, C and D. Variation in the junction of the bile duct and the pancreatic duct.

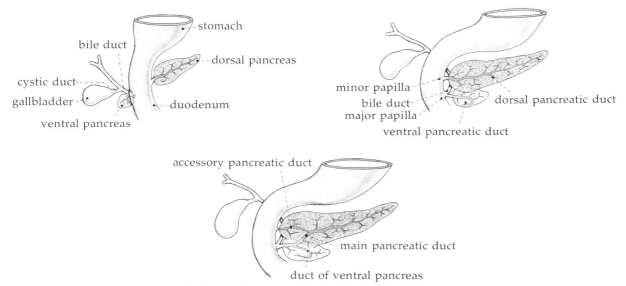

E, F and G. Development of the pancreas.

(From Langman, J.: Medical Embryology, 3rd ed. The Williams & Wilkins Co., Baltimore, 1975.)

¶ The bile duct widens considerably before entering the duodenum. In this widened area (the ampulla), small gallstones may be lodged. At the entrance into the duodenum the duct is surrounded by a circular muscle known as the sphincter of Oddi. The minor duodenal papilla is located about 2 cm above the major papilla.

¶ The bile duct and the main pancreatic duct join each other at a variable distance from the duodenum (B, C, D). They enter the duodenum at the major duodenal papilla. Sometimes the septum dividing the two ducts is visible in the duodenum, and sometimes the common duct is 1 cm long.

¶ When a gallstone is lodged in the ampulla, the consequences for the pancreas depend on the duct arrangement. When a large common duct exists, bile may flow into the pancreatic system; conversely, it is thought that pancreatic fluid may flow into the biliary system and cause formation of calculi in the gallbladder. If the common duct is very short, the pancreatic flow is usually not impeded or is channeled by way of the accessory duct.

¶ The main pancreatic duct is the result of a fusion between the duct in the tail and body of the pancreas with the duct of the original ventral pancreas. The accessory pancreatic duct, entering the duodenum at the minor duodenal papilla, is a part of the duct system of the original dorsal pancreas. In 10 per cent of persons, the dorsal and ventral pancreatic duct systems fail to fuse and the tail, body and major portion of the pancreatic head then drain at the minor papilla.

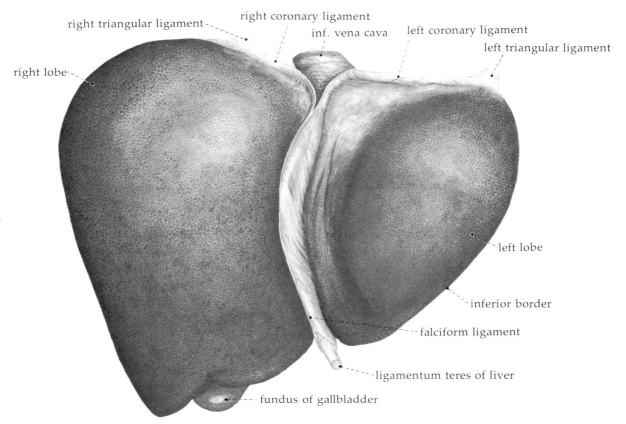

right triangular ligament

right coronary ligament

inf. vena cava

left coronary ligament

left triangular ligament

right lobe

left lobe

inferior border

falciform ligament

ligamentum teres of liver

fundus of gallbladder

Anterosuperior view of the liver.

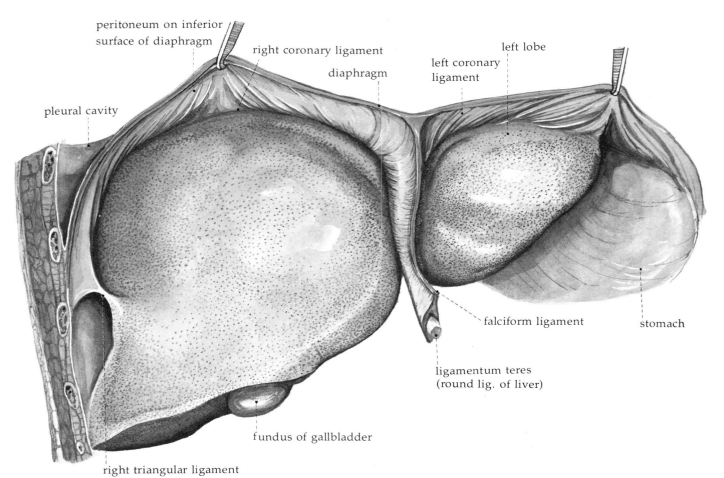

peritoneum on inferior
surface of diaphragm

right coronary ligament

diaphragm

left coronary
ligament

left lobe

pleural cavity

falciform ligament

stomach

ligamentum teres
(round lig. of liver)

fundus of gallbladder

right triangular ligament

Anterosuperior view of the liver.
Note the relation to the diaphragm and stomach.

If the fingers are passed upward over the right lobe of the liver, they are stopped by the upper layer of the right coronary ligament. From here the peritoneum of the right lobe is reflected onto the undersurface of the diaphragm. Similarly, on the left side the peritoneum is reflected onto the undersurface of the diaphragm at the left coronary ligament. The inferior vena cava is located at the site where the two leaves of the falciform ligament split into the upper layers of the right and left coronary ligaments(A51).

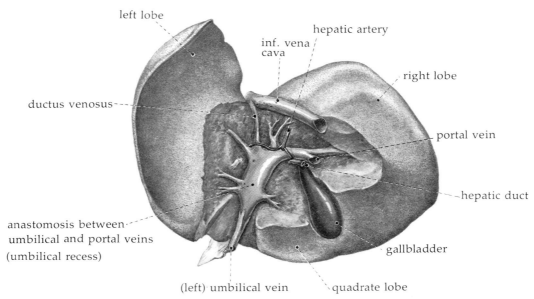

left lobe

inf. vena cava

hepatic artery

right lobe

ductus venosus

portal vein

hepatic duct

anastomosis between umbilical and portal veins (umbilical recess)

gallbladder

(left) umbilical vein

quadrate lobe

A. Inferior view of the liver of a fetus.

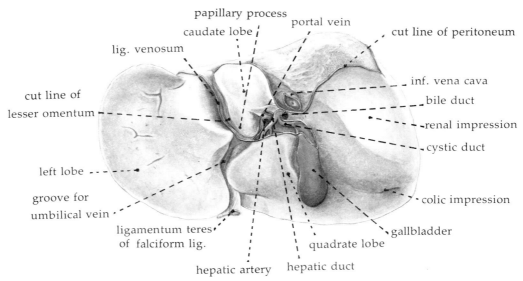

papillary process

caudate lobe

portal vein

cut line of peritoneum

lig. venosum

inf. vena cava

cut line of lesser omentum

bile duct

renal impression

cystic duct

left lobe

colic impression

groove for umbilical vein

ligamentum teres of falciform lig.

gallbladder

quadrate lobe

hepatic artery

hepatic duct

B. Inferior view of the liver at 9 months of age.

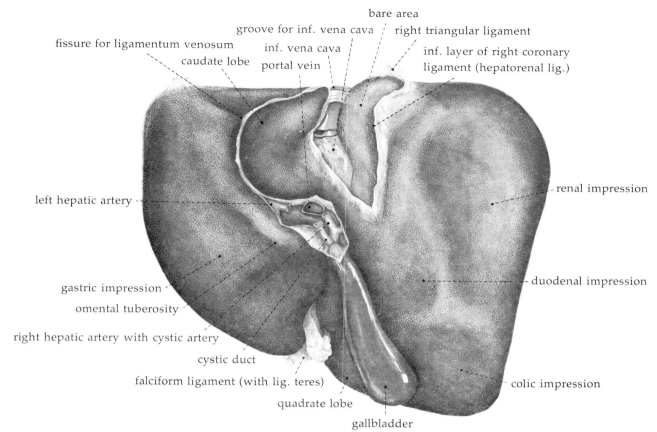

bare area
groove for inf. vena cava / right triangular ligament
fissure for ligamentum venosum   inf. vena cava
caudate lobe   portal vein   inf. layer of right coronary
                                     ligament (hepatorenal lig.)

left hepatic artery   renal impression

gastric impression
omental tuberosity
right hepatic artery with cystic artery   duodenal impression
cystic duct
falciform ligament (with lig. teres)   colic impression
quadrate lobe
gallbladder

Inferior view of the adult liver.
Note the attachment of the lesser omentum around the porta hepatis.

¶ In the fetus the left umbilical vein, which is located in the lower margin of the falciform ligament, passes from the umbilicus toward the liver. The oxygen-rich blood enters the umbilical recess and from there continues either into the liver or through the ductus venosus (ductus Arantii) directly into the inferior vena cava. The portal vein enters the liver through the lesser omentum, but during fetal life it carries little blood (see A53 *A*).

¶ After birth the umbilical vein forms the *round ligament of the liver* (ligamentum teres hepatis), which runs in the lower margin of the falciform ligament toward the liver (A53 *B*). The falciform ligament forms the dividing line between the right and left lobes of the liver.

¶ The ductus venosus is obliterated after birth and forms the ligamentum venosum; this creates a deep fissure known as the fissure for the ligamentum venosum.

¶ During fetal life the porta hepatis is occupied mainly by the umbilical recess, but after birth it becomes the port of entrance for the portal vein and hepatic artery and the port of exit for the hepatic duct.

¶ The lesser omentum connects the lesser curvature of the stomach and the first part of the duodenum with the inferior surface of the liver. Note that the attachment of the lesser omentum surrounds the porta hepatis and subsequently runs on each side of the ligamentum venosum.

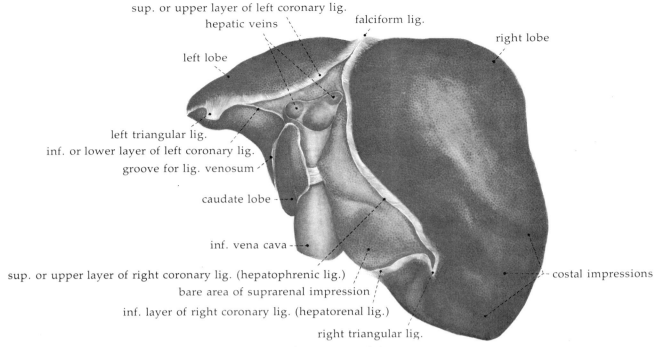

sup. or upper layer of left coronary lig.
hepatic veins
falciform lig.
right lobe
left lobe
left triangular lig.
inf. or lower layer of left coronary lig.
groove for lig. venosum
caudate lobe
inf. vena cava
sup. or upper layer of right coronary lig. (hepatophrenic lig.)
bare area of suprarenal impression
inf. layer of right coronary lig. (hepatorenal lig.)
right triangular lig.
costal impressions

A. Posterior aspect of the liver.

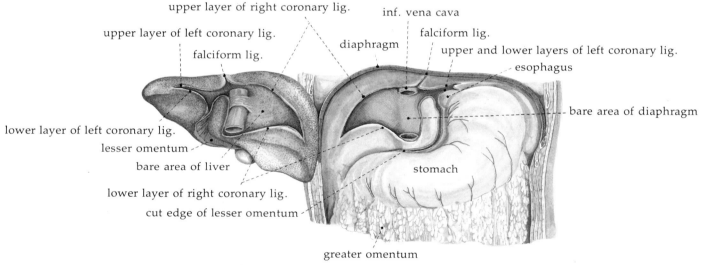

upper layer of right coronary lig.
inf. vena cava
upper layer of left coronary lig.
falciform lig.
diaphragm
falciform lig.
upper and lower layers of left coronary lig.
esophagus
lower layer of left coronary lig.
bare area of diaphragm
lesser omentum
bare area of liver
stomach
lower layer of right coronary lig.
cut edge of lesser omentum
greater omentum

B. The liver rotated 180 degrees out of its bed.

¶ The large bare area on the posterior aspect of the liver is located between the upper and lower layers of the right coronary ligament. The upper layer is called the hepatophrenic ligament, and the lower layer is known as the hepatorenal ligament. The right coronary ligament is reflected onto the right kidney, adrenal gland, and inferior vena cava. The bare area borders on the diaphragm, the inferior vena cava, and the upper part of the right suprarenal gland.

¶ The bare area between the upper and lower layers of the left coronary ligament is small. Both layers are reflected onto the diaphragm in the area of the central tendon.

¶ It is important to realize that the bare area of the liver on the right side is in contact with the muscular portion of the diaphragm. On the left side the bare area is in contact with the tendinous part of the diaphragm. This can be seen when the liver is lifted out of the peritoneal cavity, thereby exposing the undersurface of the diaphragm.

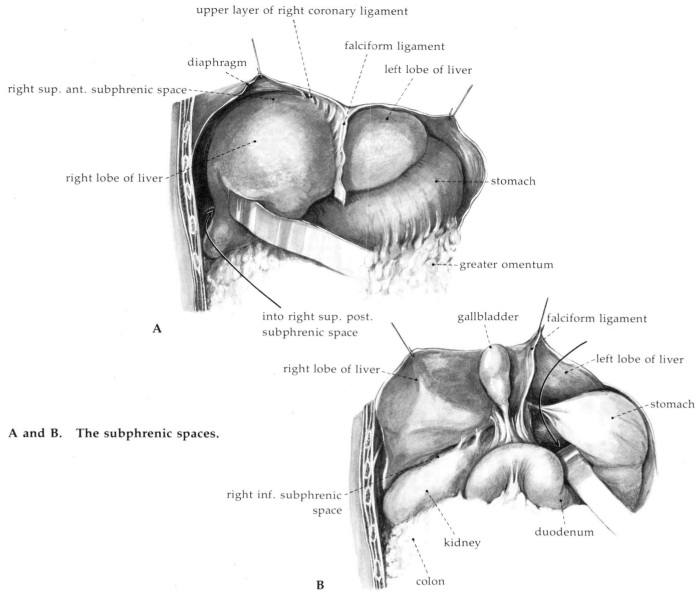

upper layer of right coronary ligament

falciform ligament

diaphragm

left lobe of liver

right sup. ant. subphrenic space

right lobe of liver

stomach

greater omentum

into right sup. post.
subphrenic space

A

gallbladder

falciform ligament

right lobe of liver

left lobe of liver

stomach

A and B.   The subphrenic spaces.

right inf. subphrenic
space

duodenum

kidney

colon

B

¶   The subphrenic spaces are clinically important because they are sites of predilection for abscesses. Although at least six subphrenic spaces have been defined, the following are of particular interest:

1.   *The right superior posterior subphrenic space* (see *A*) is bounded by the inferior or lower layer of the right coronary ligament, which forms its roof. Anteriorly is found the surface of the liver, and the posterior wall is formed by the parietal peritoneum covering the diaphragm. The space extends downward into the right inferior subphrenic space.

2.   *The right inferior subphrenic space (B)* is bounded above by the inferior surface of the liver and below by the transverse mesocolon and the colon. It extends over the right suprarenal gland and the right kidney. The space is also known as the hepatorenal pouch or recess.

3.   *The right superior anterior subphrenic space* is bounded by the right side of the falciform ligament, the upper layer of the right coronary ligament, the underside of the diaphragm and the superior surface of the liver (see *A*).

¶   When a patient lies in a supine position the lowest point of the peritoneal cavity is behind the liver, and fluid.and pus from the right side of the cavity will collect in the right subphrenic spaces. Most of the sources of peritoneal contamination are located on the right side (appendix, gallbladder and peptic ulcer), and consequently the right posterior and inferior subphrenic spaces are the most frequent sites of abscesses.

¶   Subphrenic abscesses, particularly in the posterior space, are often accompanied by infection of the adjoining pleural cavity. Localized empyema is sometimes found in a patient with a subphrenic abscess. The infection probably spreads from the peritoneum to the pleura through the diaphragmatic lymphatics.

¶   Patients with a subphrenic abscess frequently complain of pain over the right shoulder. The skin of the shoulder is supplied by the supraclavicular nerves originating from C3 and C4. These nerves have the same segmental origin as the phrenic nerve, which supplies not only the upper but also the undersurface of the diaphragm.

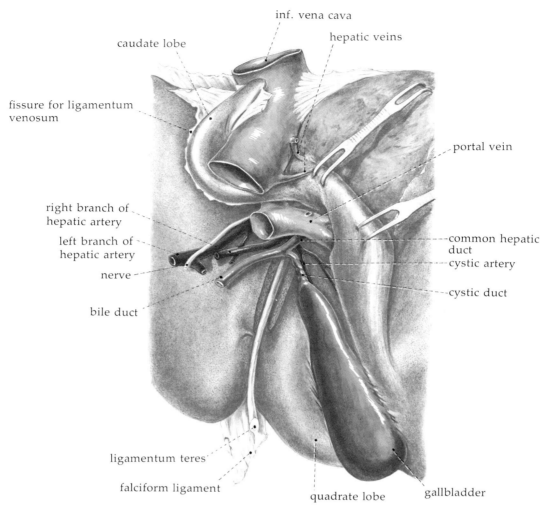

inf. vena cava

caudate lobe

hepatic veins

fissure for ligamentum venosum

portal vein

right branch of hepatic artery

left branch of hepatic artery

nerve

common hepatic duct

cystic artery

cystic duct

bile duct

ligamentum teres

falciform ligament

quadrate lobe

gallbladder

The porta hepatis.

The following structures are found in the porta hepatis:

§ The *hepatic arteries*. Great variation exists: sometimes one artery is present, but usually there are two. Their origin and course are variable. Note also the *cystic artery*.

§ The *portal vein* is the largest structure in the porta hepatis. It is formed by confluence of the splenic and mesenteric veins at the level of the head and neck of the pancreas. When the portal vein is obstructed by intrahepatic or extrahepatic causes, the blood is shunted to the systemic veins in the areas where the two systems meet (see A29).

§ The *hepatic* and *cystic ducts*.

§ The *nerves* of the liver are derived from the left vagal trunk and the sympathetic chain. They usually follow the arteries.

§ Most of the *lymph vessels* of the liver terminate in the lymph nodes in and around the porta hepatis. From there the lymph passes to the celiac lymph nodes. Some lymph vessels pass through the falciform ligament to the diaphragm and thus reach the mediastinal nodes. Others join the inferior vena cava and enter the thorax. Sometimes the lymph nodes in the porta hepatis compress the portal vein or the hepatic duct.

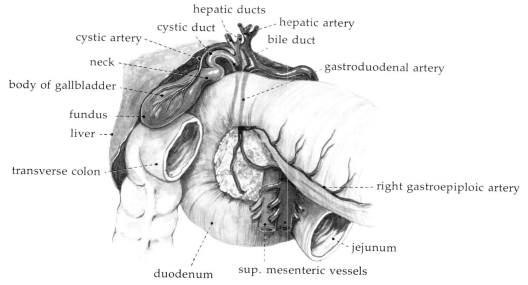

The gallbladder and its surroundings.

Important clinical considerations:

¶ When the fundus of the gallbladder protrudes beyond the anterior margin of the liver, it is frequently in contact with the anterior abdominal wall in the angle between the lateral border of the right rectus abdominis muscle and the costal margin (see A2).

¶ The body of the gallbladder, which is covered by the peritoneum at the sides and below (but usually not in the area where it contacts the liver), is in contact with the transverse colon or the right colic flexure and also with the second portion of the duodenum. Infections of the gallbladder thus may expand to the liver, duodenum, colon and the anterior abdominal wall and, of course, to the peritoneal cavity. Similarly, fistulas, that is, the development of open connections between the gallbladder and the duodenum and colon, may arise. Sometimes an anastomosis with the jejunum develops.

¶ The neck of the gallbladder is closely applied to the liver and, inferiorly, to the first part of the duodenum. The neck continues into the cystic duct, which is characterized by a spiral valve. This valve makes catheterization or probing of the duct difficult. The cystic duct, which is about 2½ cm long and has a tortuous course, extends to the porta hepatis where it joins the common hepatic duct to form the bile duct (ductus choledochus). Frequently the cystic duct passes downward with the common hepatic duct before joining it (see A59 *B*).

¶ The bile duct, an extremely important clinical feature, descends from the porta hepatis in the free margin of the lesser omentum. Here it can easily be palpated by putting one finger in the epiploic foramen (of Winslow) and another at the anterior surface of the lesser omentum. To the left is the hepatic artery; the portal vein lies posteriorly. The second or retroduodenal part of the bile duct runs parallel to the gastroduodenal artery, which lies on the left side of the duct. This part of the duct can easily be exposed. The next part of the duct passes through the pancreas in either a deep sulcus or a tunnel and is difficult to expose. It is closely related to the inferior vena cava, the portal vein and the gastroduodenal artery.

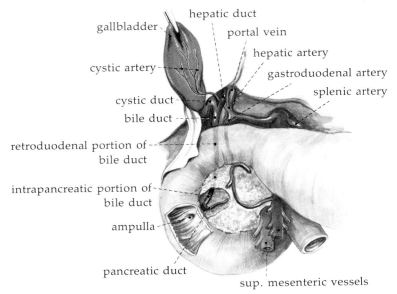

gallbladder
hepatic duct
portal vein
hepatic artery
cystic artery
gastroduodenal artery
splenic artery
cystic duct
bile duct
retroduodenal portion of bile duct
intrapancreatic portion of bile duct
ampulla
pancreatic duct
sup. mesenteric vessels

A. Gallbladder, extrahepatic biliary system and blood supply.

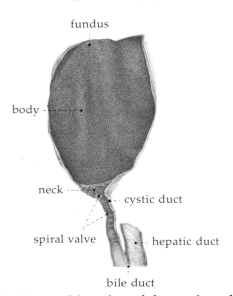

fundus
body
neck
cystic duct
spiral valve
hepatic duct
bile duct

B. Open gallbladder and junction of the cystic and hepatic ducts.

An understanding of the blood supply is very important in removing the gallbladder and in surgical procedures on the duct system.

¶ The cystic artery, one of the most variable structures in the body, arises in 60 per cent of cases from the right hepatic artery, passes behind the hepatic duct, and divides into a superficial branch to the peritoneal surface of the gallbladder and a deep branch to the nonperitoneal surface. The cystic artery usually does not follow the cystic duct. Frequently the cystic artery is duplicated or triplicated. When the gallbladder is removed, the arteries have to be carefully dissected; otherwise bleeding may easily develop.

¶ Many small veins in the wall of the gallbladder drain directly into the liver. Hence, removal of the gallbladder from its hepatic bed is sometimes followed by profuse bleeding from the liver.

¶ The greatest danger in removing calculi from the duct system is that surgical manipulation causes devascularization of the duct and subsequently necrosis. The small arteries supplying the bile duct arise from the cystic artery and the posterior branch of the superior pancreaticoduodenal artery (not from the hepatic artery). They approach the duct from its medial side; consequently, this side has to be handled carefully to avoid devascularization.

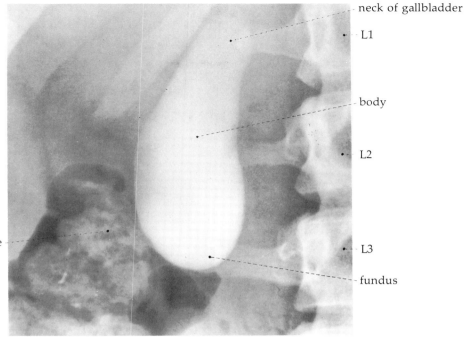

neck of gallbladder

L1

body

A. Cholecystogram.
Twelve hours after ingestion of contrast medium. Note the relation of the gallbladder to the vertebral bodies.

L2

right colic flexure

L3

fundus

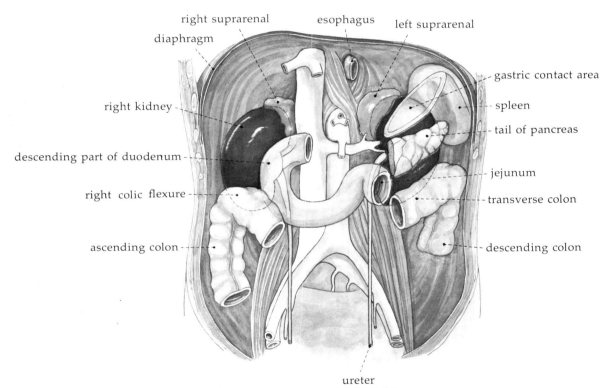

right suprarenal   esophagus   left suprarenal

diaphragm

gastric contact area

right kidney

spleen

tail of pancreas

descending part of duodenum

jejunum

right colic flexure

transverse colon

ascending colon

descending colon

ureter

B. Anterior relations of the kidney.
The liver is not shown.

The following points are clinically important:

¶ The kidneys are contiguous with many surrounding organs and structures, and infections of one organ may pass to another by direct contact. Both kidneys are capped by the suprarenal glands. Anteriorly the right kidney adjoins the liver, the right flexure of the colon and the descending duodenum. The left kidney borders anteriorly on the stomach, the spleen, the pancreas, the transverse colon and some coils of the jejunum. The pancreas and the duodenum are in so-called direct contact with the kidneys because there is no peritoneal covering between the apposing organs. The remaining organs have indirect contact with the kidneys.

¶ Keep in mind that posteriorly the kidney is separated from the pleura only by the diaphragm. No peritoneum exists between the two structures (see A61).

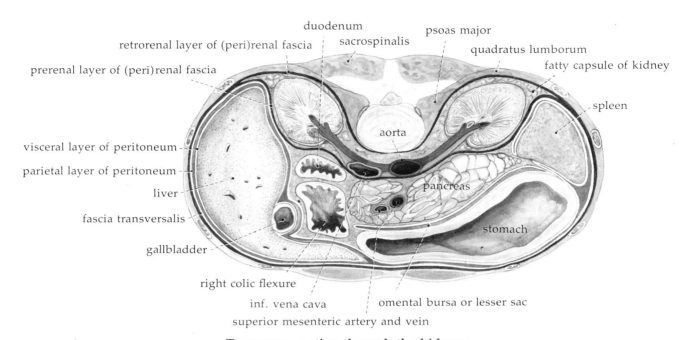

duodenum
psoas major
retrorenal layer of (peri)renal fascia
sacrospinalis
quadratus lumborum
prerenal layer of (peri)renal fascia
fatty capsule of kidney
spleen
aorta
visceral layer of peritoneum
parietal layer of peritoneum
liver
pancreas
fascia transversalis
gallbladder
stomach
right colic flexure
inf. vena cava
omental bursa or lesser sac
superior mesenteric artery and vein

Transverse section through the kidneys.
Note the fascia and the relationship of the kidneys to other abdominal organs.

Important clinical observations:

¶ At the lateral border of the kidney the fascia transversalis splits into a prerenal and a retrorenal layer to form the renal or perirenal fascia. The retrorenal layer blends with the fascia of the quadratus lumborum and psoas major muscles and with the vertebral column. The anterior layer extends medially in front of the renal vessels, the aorta and the inferior vena cava to blend with its partner from the opposite side. Some authors suggest that it also blends with the connective tissue around the aorta. Between the two layers and surrounding the kidney is the perirenal fat, which provides the kidney with a so-called "fatty capsule." Infections of the kidney, particularly perinephritic infections, may spread from right to left within the sheaths of the perirenal fascia.

¶ The kidney maintains its position by intra-abdominal pressure and by its fasciae. Because of the presence of the perirenal fat, slight mobility, for instance during respiration, is possible. During deep inspiration and in patients with a poorly developed abdominal musculature, the inferior pole of the left kidney can sometimes be palpated.

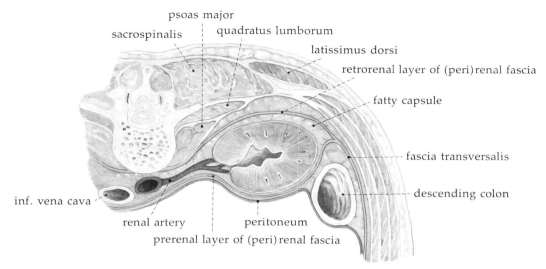

psoas major

sacrospinalis   quadratus lumborum

latissimus dorsi

retrorenal layer of (peri)renal fascia

fatty capsule

fascia transversalis

descending colon

inf. vena cava

renal artery   peritoneum

prerenal layer of (peri)renal fascia

A.   Transverse section through the region of the left kidney.
Note the peritoneum and the prerenal and retrorenal layer of the renal fascia.

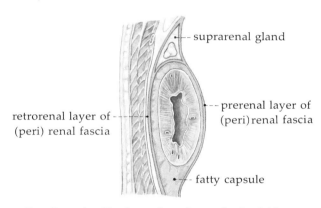

suprarenal gland

retrorenal layer of (peri) renal fascia

prerenal layer of (peri)renal fascia

fatty capsule

B.   Longitudinal section through the kidney.

The two layers of the renal fascia fuse at the upper pole of the kidney but remain separated at the lower pole. There are two important consequences of this arrangement: (a) When the amount of perirenal fat decreases, the mobility of the kidney increases; the kidney may move downward since the fascia layers are not fused at the lower pole. (b) The suprarenal gland does not move; it has its own fascial compartment. Sometimes the kidney descends to such an extent that the ureter develops a kink, thus producing symptoms of kidney obstruction. The kidney may be removed within its capsule, leaving the suprarenal gland undisturbed.

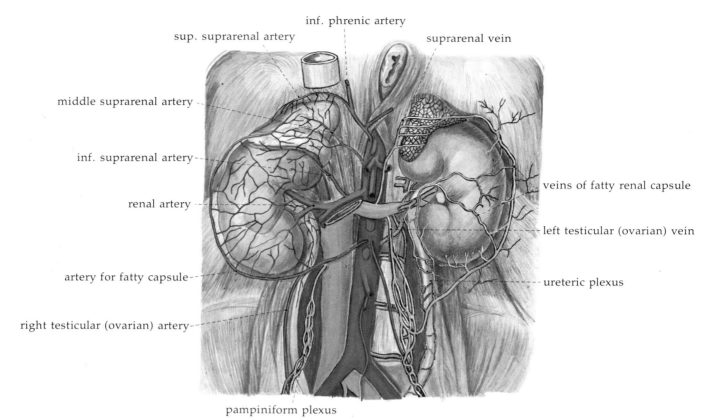

sup. suprarenal artery

inf. phrenic artery

suprarenal vein

middle suprarenal artery

inf. suprarenal artery

renal artery

veins of fatty renal capsule

left testicular (ovarian) vein

artery for fatty capsule

ureteric plexus

right testicular (ovarian) artery

pampiniform plexus

Arterial supply and venous drainage of the kidneys and suprarenal glands.

The arteries and veins present a number of interesting points:

¶ The renal artery may divide into two or more branches before entering the kidney. An important branch sometimes courses behind the ureter, thereby forming a vascular fork around the ureter. Occasionally this vascular fork causes constriction of the ureter and impedes its flow.

¶ Sometimes two or three renal arteries arise from the aorta. This arrangement probably results from the ascent of the kidney during its development. As it ascends to the lumbar level the kidney is supplied by new arteries at continuously higher levels. Hence, supernumerary arteries represent persistent fetal arteries.

¶ The testicular arteries usually arise from the aorta. In some cases, however, they originate from the renal artery or from the artery of the fatty capsule.

¶ The venous pattern is complex because of the confluence of veins from many surrounding structures. The drainage is particularly complicated on the left side since the veins from the suprarenal gland, the pampiniform plexus of the testis, and the fatty capsule, as well as the veins surrounding the ureter, make many anastomoses. Surgery is dangerous, as it permits the spread of infections or metastases. Malignant tumors of the kidney frequently spread along the renal vein. Since the left testicular vein drains into the left renal vein, its flow may be impeded, thus causing a left-sided varicocele in the scrotum.

¶ The blood supply to the suprarenal gland is intensive. Note: (a) the superior suprarenal artery, a branch of the inferior phrenic artery; (b) the middle suprarenal artery, originating directly from the aorta; and (c) the inferior suprarenal artery, a branch of the renal artery. Only one vein drains the gland.

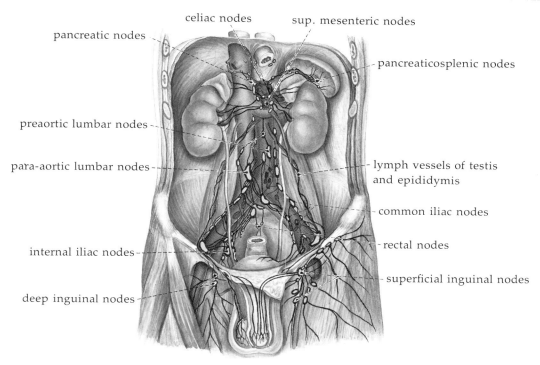

celiac nodes

sup. mesenteric nodes

pancreatic nodes

pancreaticosplenic nodes

preaortic lumbar nodes

lymph vessels of testis and epididymis

para-aortic lumbar nodes

common iliac nodes

rectal nodes

internal iliac nodes

superficial inguinal nodes

deep inguinal nodes

A. Lymph drainage of the kidney and testes.

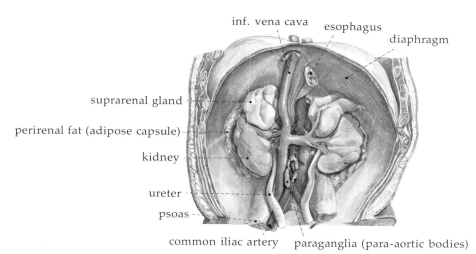

inf. vena cava   esophagus

diaphragm

suprarenal gland

perirenal fat (adipose capsule)

kidney

ureter

psoas

common iliac artery   paraganglia (para-aortic bodies)

B. Position of the kidneys and suprarenals in a newborn infant.
Note the paraganglia.

¶ The lymphatics of the kidney follow the course of the veins and drain into the lateral or para-aortic lymph nodes. Of particular interest are the lymphatics of the testes, which follow the testicular vein via the inguinal canal to end in the para-aortic nodes (the lymph vessels of the penis and scrotum drain into the inguinal nodes). Cancers of the testes usually metastasize early and are found in the region of the para-aortic nodes. Sometimes metastases are found before the cancer has caused any clinical symptoms.

¶ In the newborn infant note: (a) the large size of the suprarenal gland in comparison to the size of the kidney, (b) the lobulation of the kidney, (c) the large amount of perirenal fat surrounding the kidney, and (d) the paraganglia along the aorta.

¶ The paraganglia are large at birth but degenerate in childhood. They consist of chromaffin tissue (like that of the suprarenal gland) and are distributed along the sympathetic chain and near the sympathetic collateral ganglia. They are supplied by numerous preganglionic fibers.

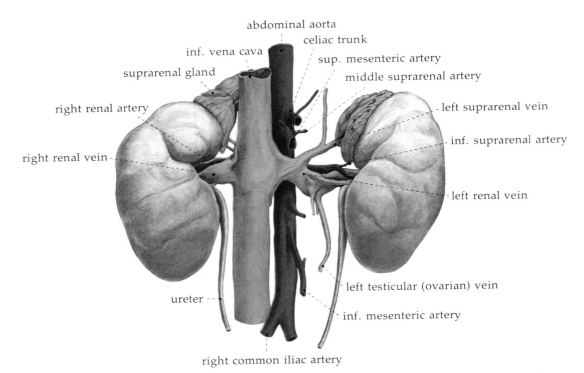

abdominal aorta
celiac trunk
inf. vena cava
sup. mesenteric artery
suprarenal gland
middle suprarenal artery
right renal artery
left suprarenal vein
right renal vein
inf. suprarenal artery
left renal vein
left testicular (ovarian) vein
ureter
inf. mesenteric artery
right common iliac artery

A. Anterior view of the kidneys and suprarenal glands and their vascular supply.
Note the complicated venous arrangement on the left.

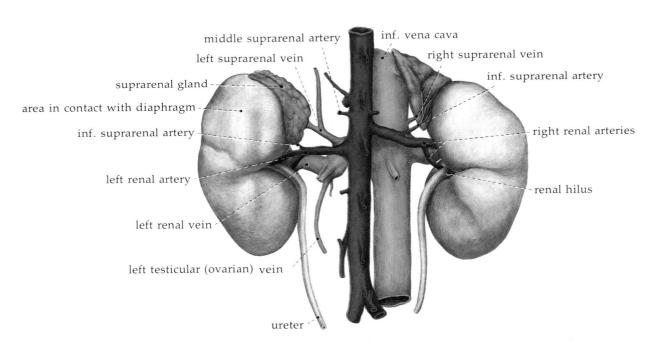

middle suprarenal artery
inf. vena cava
left suprarenal vein
right suprarenal vein
suprarenal gland
inf. suprarenal artery
area in contact with diaphragm
inf. suprarenal artery
right renal arteries
left renal artery
renal hilus
left renal vein
left testicular (ovarian) vein
ureter

B. Posterior view of the kidneys and suprarenal glands and their vascular supply.

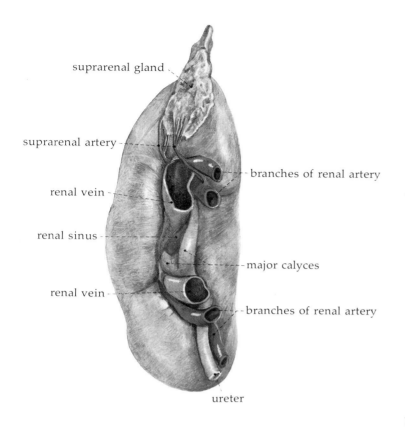

suprarenal gland

suprarenal artery

renal vein

renal sinus

branches of renal artery

renal vein

major calyces

branches of renal artery

ureter

A. **Medial view of the hilus of the right kidney.** Note the suprarenal branches from the renal artery.

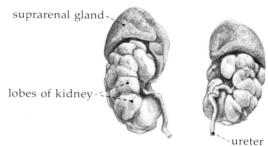

suprarenal gland

lobes of kidney

ureter

B. **The kidney and suprarenal gland in a fetus of 9 months.**

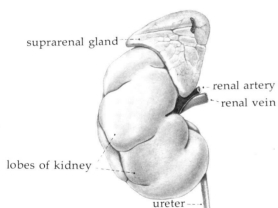

suprarenal gland

renal artery

renal vein

lobes of kidney

ureter

C. **Anterior view of the right kidney and suprarenal gland in a child.**

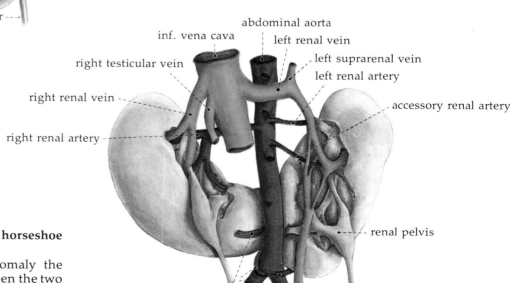

inf. vena cava

abdominal aorta

left renal vein

right testicular vein

left suprarenal vein

left renal artery

right renal vein

accessory renal artery

right renal artery

renal pelvis

accessory renal arteries

ureter

testicular vein

D. **Anterior view of a horseshoe kidney.**
Usually in such an anomaly the connecting bridge between the two lower poles is located in front of the aorta. Note also the many accessory arteries.

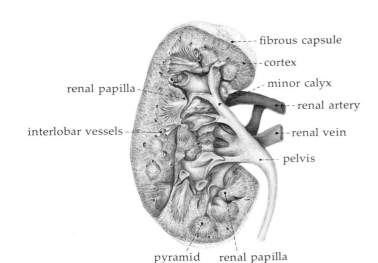

fibrous capsule
cortex
minor calyx
renal artery
renal vein
pelvis

renal papilla
interlobar vessels

pyramid   renal papilla

A. Posterior view of the pelvis and calyces.
Some calyces have been opened.

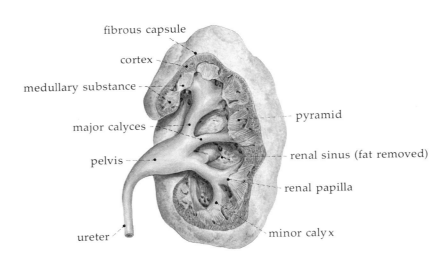

fibrous capsule
cortex
medullary substance
major calyces
pelvis
ureter

pyramid
renal sinus (fat removed)
renal papilla
minor calyx

B. Posterior view of the pelvis and calyces.
The vessels, fat and some of the kidney tissue have been removed.

C. Cast of the pelvis and calyces.

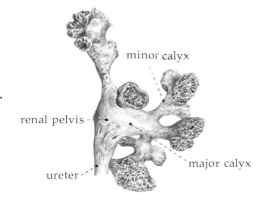

minor calyx
renal pelvis
ureter
major calyx

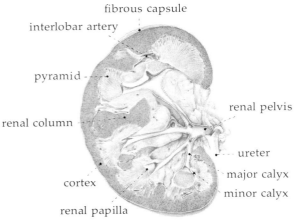

fibrous capsule
interlobar artery
pyramid
renal column
cortex
renal papilla
renal pelvis
ureter
major calyx
minor calyx

D. Longitudinal section through the kidney.

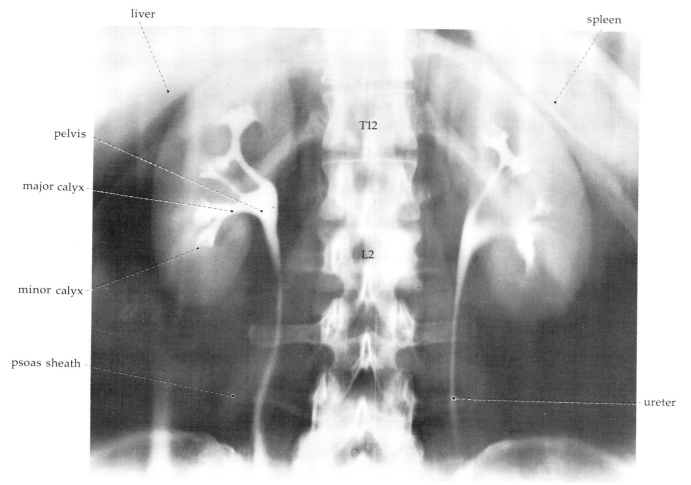

liver   spleen

T12

pelvis

major calyx

L2

minor calyx

psoas sheath   ureter

A.   Intravenous urogram showing the pelvic calyces and part of the ureter.

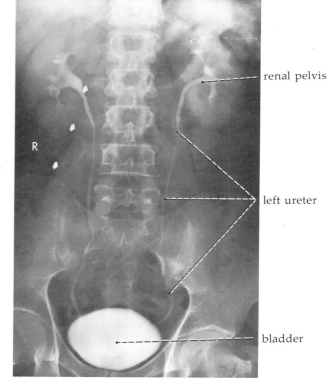

renal pelvis

R

left ureter

bladder

B.   **Intravenous urogram of the ureter.** (*A* and *B* from Meschan, I.: An Atlas of Anatomy Basic to Radiology. Philadelphia, W. B. Saunders Co., 1975.)

The ureter has a number of narrow areas. The uppermost constriction is at the junction of the ureter and the renal pelvis; the next is at the place where the ureter crosses the pelvic inlet, and the lowest one is at the entrance into the bladder. A renal or ureteral stone frequently stops at one of these constrictions as it passes down the ureter to the bladder.

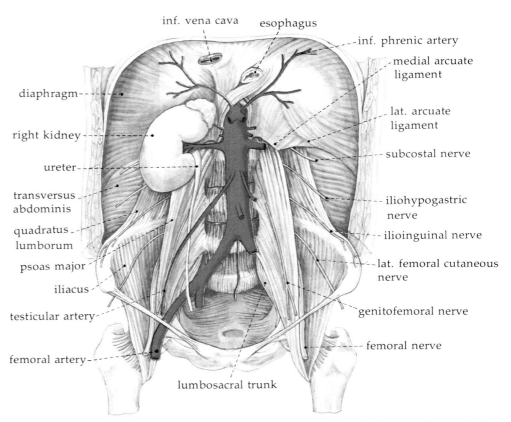

inf. vena cava
esophagus
inf. phrenic artery
medial arcuate ligament
diaphragm
lat. arcuate ligament
right kidney
ureter
subcostal nerve
transversus abdominis
iliohypogastric nerve
quadratus lumborum
ilioinguinal nerve
psoas major
lat. femoral cutaneous nerve
iliacus
genitofemoral nerve
testicular artery
femoral nerve
femoral artery
lumbosacral trunk

A. The kidney in its relation to the posterior abdominal wall.

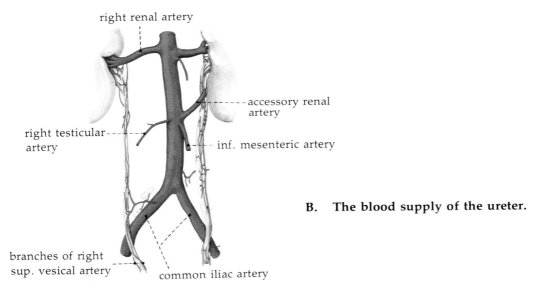

right renal artery

accessory renal artery

right testicular artery

inf. mesenteric artery

branches of right sup. vesical artery

common iliac artery

B. The blood supply of the ureter.

¶ The kidney rests in a retroperitoneal position on four muscles: the diaphragm, the transversus abdominis, the quadratus lumborum and the psoas major.

¶ The blood supply of the ureter is important since surgical manipulation of the ureter may interfere with its vascularization and thus cause necrosis. Usually, however, anastomoses are ample. The following arteries supply the ureter: (a) the renal artery, (b) the testicular or ovarian artery, (c) the common iliac artery, (d) the superior vesical artery, and sometimes (e) the middle rectal artery.

¶ The afferent nerve fibers of the pelvis of the kidney and of the ureter itself are connected to the spinal cord at segments T11, T12, L1 and L2. When a calculus passes along the ureter, strong peristaltic waves of the smooth muscles in the wall of the ureter try to move it to the bladder. The spasm of the muscle causes severe pain, which is referred to skin areas supplied by the nerves from T11 to L2. Sometimes the pain is referred to the testis or to the front of the thigh (genitofemoral nerve).

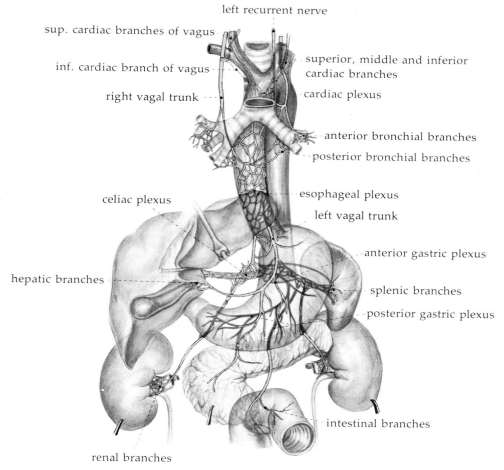

left recurrent nerve

sup. cardiac branches of vagus

inf. cardiac branch of vagus

right vagal trunk

superior, middle and inferior cardiac branches

cardiac plexus

anterior bronchial branches

posterior bronchial branches

celiac plexus

esophageal plexus

left vagal trunk

anterior gastric plexus

hepatic branches

splenic branches

posterior gastric plexus

intestinal branches

renal branches

Distribution of vagus trunks in the abdomen.

¶ In addition to innervating the stomach, the right (posterior) vagal trunk sends fibers to the celiac and renal plexuses of the autonomic nervous system. From the celiac plexus the vagal fibers are distributed along the visceral branches of the aorta to the intestinal tract as far as the transverse colon. Beyond the left colic flexure of the transverse colon the parasympathetic innervation comes from the sacral region.

¶ The left (anterior) vagal trunk sends fibers between the layers of the lesser omentum to the liver and biliary system and to the pylorus and first part of the duodenum.

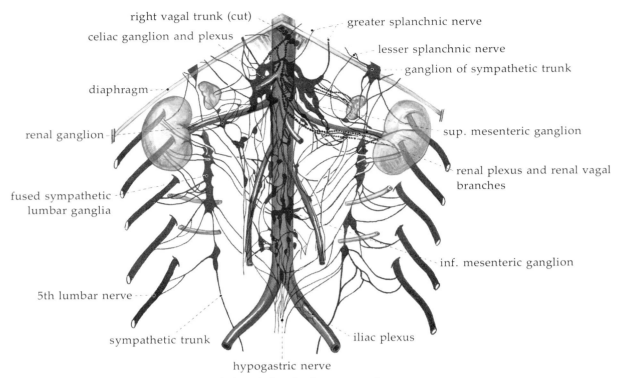

right vagal trunk (cut)

celiac ganglion and plexus

greater splanchnic nerve

lesser splanchnic nerve

ganglion of sympathetic trunk

diaphragm

renal ganglion

sup. mesenteric ganglion

renal plexus and renal vagal branches

fused sympathetic lumbar ganglia

inf. mesenteric ganglion

5th lumbar nerve

sympathetic trunk

iliac plexus

hypogastric nerve

Schematic drawing of the abdominal autonomic system.

¶ The sympathetic trunk of the thorax continues downward into the abdominal cavity and is represented by the lumbar ganglia. The right sympathetic trunk lies behind the inferior vena cava, and the left trunk lies behind the left border of the abdominal aorta. Four ganglia are present, but, as in the cervical region, fusion between the ganglia (L1 and L2) is not uncommon.

¶ Many branches of the sympathetic ganglia pass medially to the preaortic ganglia and plexuses. Preganglionic and postganglionic sympathetic fibers and preganglionic parasympathetic fibers of the vagus nerve form a plexus of nerves around the origin of the celiac, superior mesenteric, inferior mesenteric and renal arteries (the inferior mesenteric plexus also receives parasympathetic branches from the sacral parasympathetics).

¶ The celiac plexus consists of two large ganglia, the *celiac ganglia*, which receive preganglionic sympathetic fibers from the greater and lesser splanchnic nerves. The *renal* and *superior mesenteric ganglia* are much smaller than those of the celiac region.

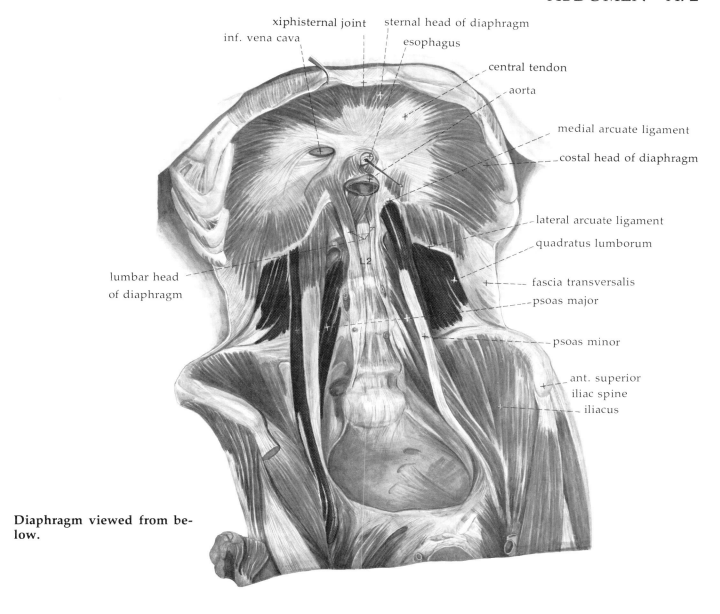

xiphisternal joint   sternal head of diaphragm

inf. vena cava

esophagus

central tendon

aorta

medial arcuate ligament

costal head of diaphragm

lateral arcuate ligament

quadratus lumborum

lumbar head
of diaphragm

fascia transversalis

psoas major

psoas minor

ant. superior
iliac spine

iliacus

L2

**Diaphragm viewed from be-
low.**

Important observations:

1. The right cupola of the diaphragm rises to the level of the fifth rib, just below the nipple; the left
    cupola rises to the fifth intercostal space about an inch below the nipple. The depressed median
    portion on which the heart lies rises to the level of the xiphisternal joint. The level of the dia-
    phragm varies with age and among individuals (see also T11 *D* and T66).

2. a. The *sternal head* attaches to the xiphoid process.
    b. The *costal head* attaches to the inner surfaces of the seventh to the twelfth costal cartilages.
    c. The *lumbar head* attaches to the vertebral column. On the right side it arises from the bodies
        and intervertebral discs of L1, L2, and L3; on the left it arises from the bodies of L1 and L2.
        Between the left and right crura is an opening for the aorta.

    Many fibers of the diaphragm arise from the medial and lateral arcuate ligaments. The *medial
    arcuate* ligament is formed by the thickened fascia of the psoas major muscle and runs from the
    body of L2 to the tip of the transverse process of L1. The *lateral arcuate ligament* extends from the
    tip of the transverse process of L1 to the lower border of the twelfth rib.

3. a. The *aortic opening*, located at the level of T12, transmits the aorta and the thoracic duct.
    b. The *esophageal opening* lies at the level of T10 and transmits the esophagus, the trunks of the
        vagus nerves and the branches of the left gastric vessels.
    c. The *inferior vena cava* passes through the diaphragm at the level of T8. It is accompanied by
        the right phrenic nerve (see also T66).

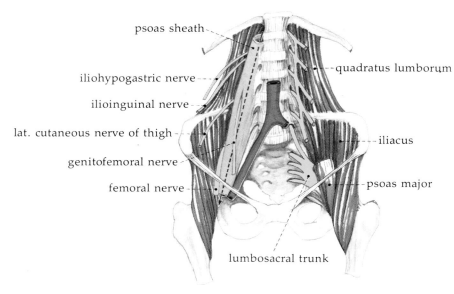

psoas sheath

iliohypogastric nerve

ilioinguinal nerve

lat. cutaneous nerve of thigh

genitofemoral nerve

femoral nerve

quadratus lumborum

iliacus

psoas major

lumbosacral trunk

A. **The psoas sheath and the lumbar plexus.**

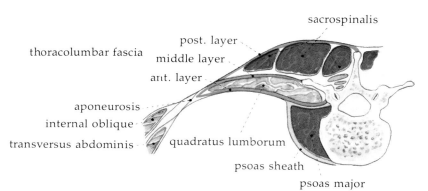

sacrospinalis

thoracolumbar fascia

post. layer

middle layer

ant. layer

aponeurosis

internal oblique

transversus abdominis

quadratus lumborum

psoas sheath

psoas major

B. **The psoas sheath and its relation to the thoracolumbar fascia.**

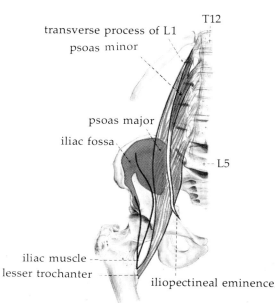

T12

transverse process of L1

psoas minor

psoas major

iliac fossa

L5

iliac muscle

lesser trochanter

iliopectineal eminence

C. **Schematic drawing of the psoas muscles.**

Psoas major
> *Origin*: Sides of the bodies and intervertebral discs of T12 and L1 to L5.
> *Insertion*: Lesser trochanter of the femur.

Psoas minor
> *Origin*: Ventral sides of the bodies of T12 and L1.
> *Insertion*: Iliopectineal eminence. (This muscle is present in 50 per cent of cases.)

The sheath of the psoas muscle is of clinical importance since infections from T12 may descend along the sheath to the hip joint. It is attached medially to the bodies of the lumbar vertebrae and blends laterally with the anterior layer of the thoracolumbar fascia. Superiorly the sheath is open (it attaches to the medial side of the body of L2 and the transverse process of L1 laterally). Pus from a tuberculous process of a thoracic vertebra may enter the sheath at its open end and descend to the hip joint or break through the sheath in the lumbar region.

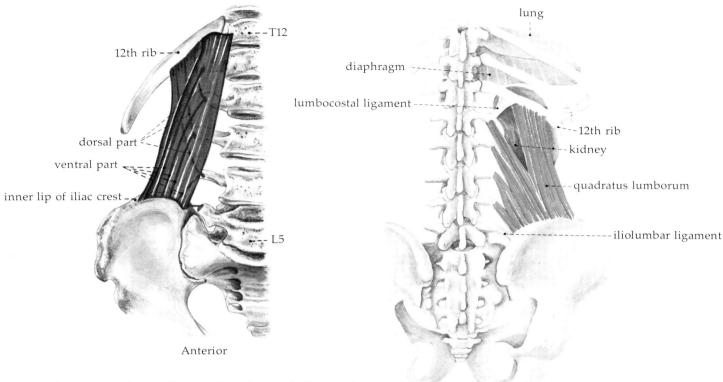

12th rib – –
dorsal part
ventral part
inner lip of iliac crest –

T12
L5

Anterior

lung
diaphragm
lumbocostal ligament
12th rib
kidney
quadratus lumborum
iliolumbar ligament

Posterior

A and B. Anterior and posterior views of the quadratus lumborum muscle.

Origin: Posterior part of inner lip of iliac crest; iliolumbar ligament; lumbar transverse processes.

Insertion: Medial 2 inches of twelfth rib; lumbar transverse processes. The fascial covering is slightly thickened above to form the lateral arcuate ligament, from which the diaphragm originates.

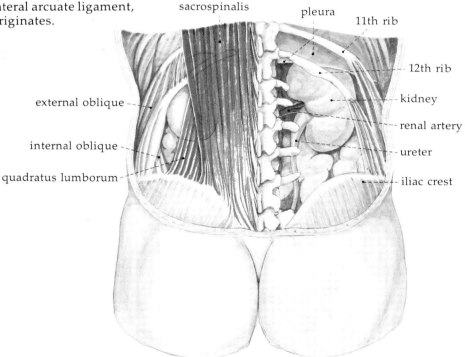

sacrospinalis
pleura
11th rib
12th rib
kidney
renal artery
ureter
iliac crest
external oblique
internal oblique
quadratus lumborum

C. Position of the kidneys seen from behind.

The deep musculature has been removed on the right side.

An important clinical landmark in the surgical approach to the kidney is provided by the twelfth rib, which crosses the kidney obliquely downward. The kidney is separated from the twelfth rib by fibers of the diaphragm and the pleura. The lower border of the pleura is horizontal; thus it crosses the twelfth rib. If the rib is short and the eleventh rib is mistaken for the twelfth, an incision may be placed too high and the pleural cavity may be opened. (Note that the right kidney lies lower than the left, owing to the bulk of the liver on the right side.)

PELVIS

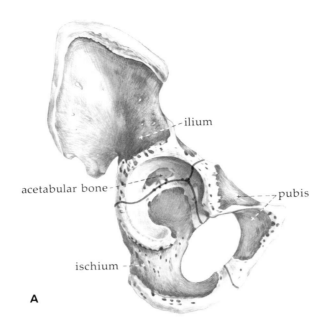

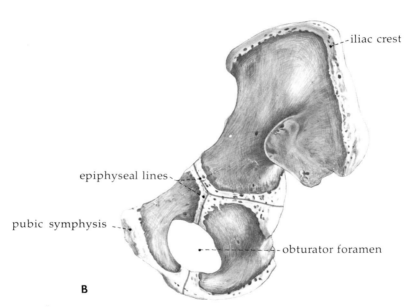

A and B.   Right hip bone of 6 year old boy in (A) lateral view and (B) medial view.

Two points of practical importance should be noted:

¶ The hip bone is formed by a fusion of three bones (the ilium, the ischium and the pubis). Each has its own ossification center. They meet each other in the acetabulum, making this the only part of the hip bone to which all three components contribute. Sometimes an additional little bone is found in the acetabulum (see *A*). This bone, the *acetabular bone,* complements the three main components. At a more advanced age an acetabular bone or part of it may become loose, causing considerable damage to the hip joint.

¶ Ossification of the hip bone is usually completed by early adult life. In a radiograph of the hip and acetabulum of a child an epiphyseal line should not be mistaken for a fracture line (see LL37).

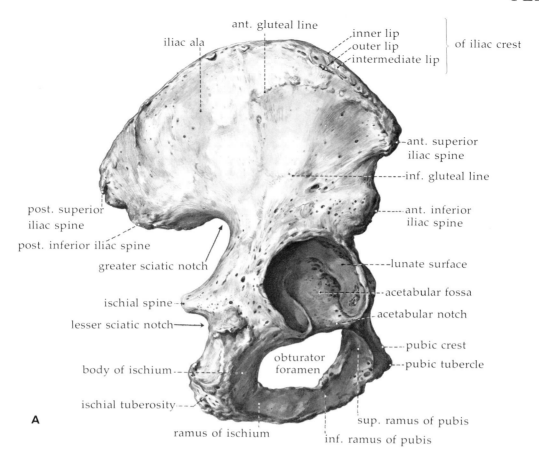

ant. gluteal line

iliac ala

inner lip
outer lip
intermediate lip

} of iliac crest

ant. superior
iliac spine

inf. gluteal line

ant. inferior
iliac spine

post. superior
iliac spine

post. inferior iliac spine

greater sciatic notch

lunate surface

acetabular fossa

acetabular notch

ischial spine

lesser sciatic notch →

pubic crest

pubic tubercle

body of ischium

obturator
foramen

ischial tuberosity

sup. ramus of pubis

A

ramus of ischium

inf. ramus of pubis

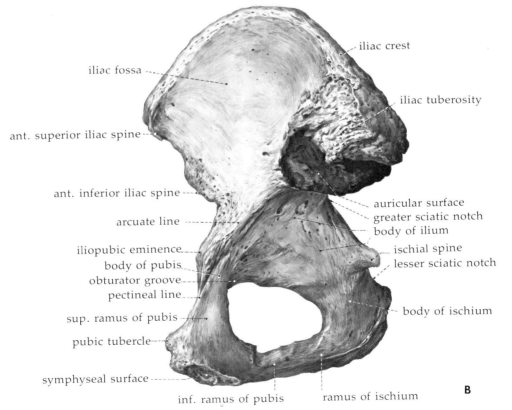

iliac crest

iliac fossa

iliac tuberosity

ant. superior iliac spine

ant. inferior iliac spine

arcuate line

auricular surface

greater sciatic notch

body of ilium

iliopubic eminence

body of pubis

obturator groove

pectineal line

ischial spine

lesser sciatic notch

sup. ramus of pubis

body of ischium

pubic tubercle

symphyseal surface

B

inf. ramus of pubis

ramus of ischium

A and B. Right hip bone of adult in (A) lateral view and (B) medial view.
Note the acetabulum with its joint surface for the femur and the rough auricular joint
surface for the sacrum.

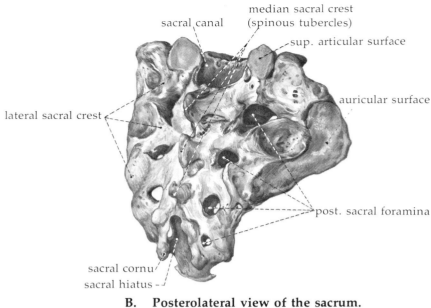

B. **Posterolateral view of the sacrum.**

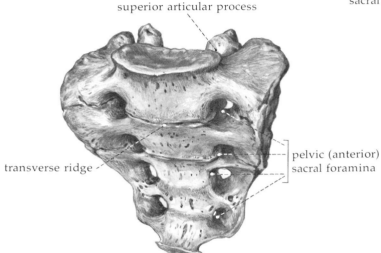

A. **Anterior aspect of the sacrum.**

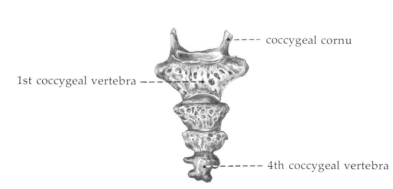

C. **Sacralization of the fifth lumbar vertebra.**

D. **Anterior surface of the coccyx.**

¶ Normally the five components of the sacrum are solidly fused and articulate with the fifth lumbar vertebra. Occasionally, however, L5 fuses entirely or partially with the sacrum. This process is known as the assimilation or sacralization of the lumbar vertebra with the sacrum.

¶ The first component of the coccyx is commonly fused with the sacrum. The joint between the first and second parts usually persists and may permit considerable movement, particularly in women who are nearing the end of pregnancy.

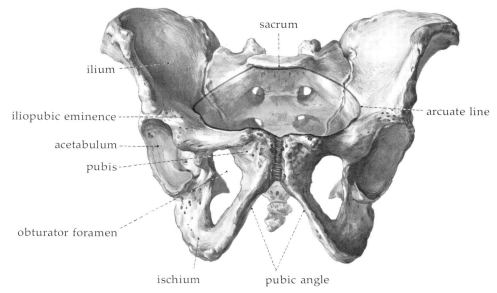

A. Anterior view of the male pelvis.

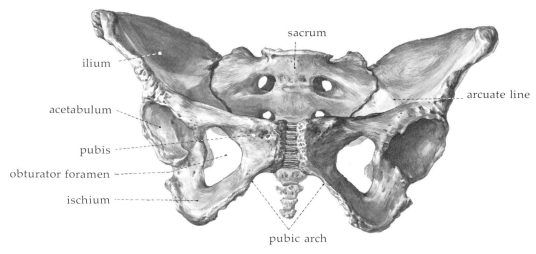

B. Anterior view of the female pelvis.

The bony pelvis consists of the two hip bones and the sacrum. They are joined by the pubic symphysis and the sacroiliac joints The pelvis is divided into two parts by the *pelvic brim* (see P5), which is formed by (a) the promontory of the sacrum, (b) the anterior border of the ala of the sacrum, (c) the arcuate line of the ilium, (d) the pectineal line of the pubic bone, (e) the pubic crest, and (f) the symphysis. Above the brim is the *false* or *greater pelvis*; below the brim is the *true* or *lesser pelvis.* In the practice of obstetrics the true pelvis is often referred to as "the pelvis."

The following differences are evident between the male and female pelves:

1. The male pelvis consists of heavy bones and is tall; the female pelvis consists of lighter bones and is broad and flat.

2. In the female the sacrum is shorter, wider and flatter than in the male.

3. The subpubic space between the ischiopubic rami forms a rather sharp angle in the male, but has the shape of an arch in the female.

4. The ischial spine is sharp and pointed in the male; in the female it is usually round.

5. The distance between the ischial spines is much shorter in the male than in the female.

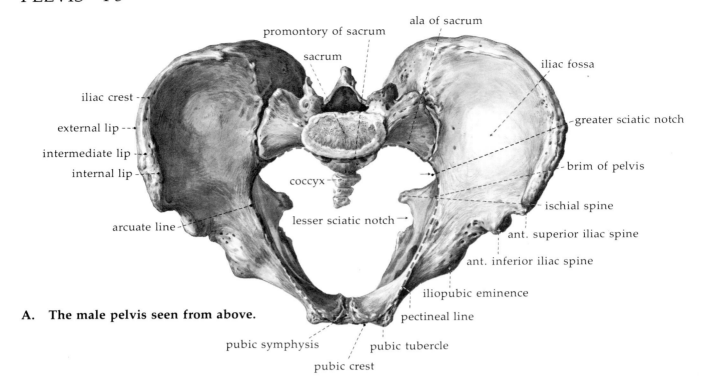

iliac crest
external lip
intermediate lip
internal lip

arcuate line

promontory of sacrum

ala of sacrum

sacrum

iliac fossa

greater sciatic notch

brim of pelvis

coccyx

ischial spine

lesser sciatic notch

ant. superior iliac spine

ant. inferior iliac spine

iliopubic eminence

pectineal line

pubic symphysis

pubic tubercle

pubic crest

A. The male pelvis seen from above.

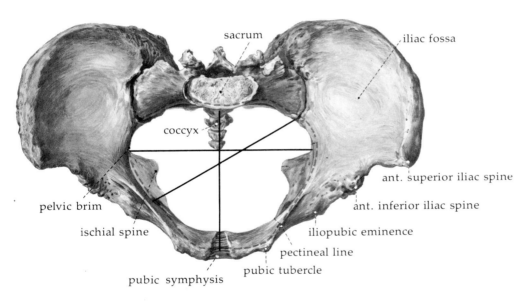

sacrum

iliac fossa

coccyx

pelvic brim

ischial spine

ant. superior iliac spine

ant. inferior iliac spine

iliopubic eminence

pectineal line

pubic tubercle

pubic symphysis

B. The female pelvis seen from above.

The inlet of the true pelvis is highly important, because it is the most narrow opening through which the child must pass during the birth process. It is also called the inlet to the birth canal.

¶ The plane of the pelvic inlet in the female is transversely oval, whereas in the male it is much more narrow and heart-shaped.

¶ The following diameters of the female pelvis should be remembered:

1. *The true conjugate* or *anteroposterior diameter* extends from the middle of the promontory of the sacrum to the upper edge of the pubic symphysis. It is about 10 to 11 cm and is the most narrow distance of the pelvic inlet (see P6).

2. *The transverse conjugate* or *diameter* extends from the left arcuate line to the right arcuate line. It is nearer to the promontory than to the symphysis and is the widest diameter of the pelvic inlet (about 13 cm).

3. *The oblique conjugate* or *diameter* extends from the sacroiliac joint on one side to the iliopubic eminence on the other. It is about 12 cm.

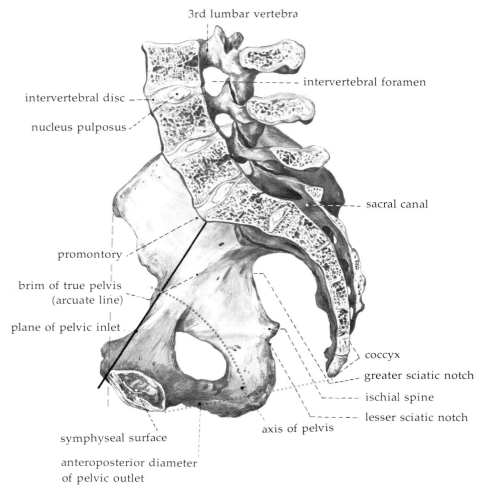

3rd lumbar vertebra

intervertebral foramen

intervertebral disc

nucleus pulposus

sacral canal

promontory

brim of true pelvis
(arcuate line)

plane of pelvic inlet

coccyx

greater sciatic notch

ischial spine

lesser sciatic notch

axis of pelvis

symphyseal surface

anteroposterior diameter
of pelvic outlet

Median section of the right half of the female pelvis.

Note the following important points:

§ In an individual in a standing position the anterior superior iliac spine and the upper rim of the symphysis are in a vertical plane (broken blue line). The ischial spine is then above the level of the symphysis.

§ The *plane of the pelvic inlet* forms an angle of about 60 degrees with the horizontal plane (solid black line).

§ The *plane of the pelvic outlet*, bounded in front by the lower rim of the symphysis, laterally by the ischial tuberosities and posteriorly by the tip of the coccyx, forms an angle of about 10 degrees with the horizontal plane. The anteroposterior diameter extends from the tip of the coccyx to the lower rim of the symphysis. It is about 13 cm (dotted blue line).

§ The pelvic cavity is the space between the pelvic inlet and pelvic outlet.

§ The *axis of the pelvis* is an imaginary line following the midway points of the anteroposterior diameters from the inlet to the outlet. It is the course taken by the baby's head as it descends through the pelvis (dotted red line).

§ The largest diameter of the baby's head is the anteroposterior measurement and the smallest is from side to side. Under normal conditions the anteroposterior diameter of the head enters the transverse or oblique diameter of the plane of the pelvic inlet. Once it has reached the pelvic cavity the head rotates so that the face is directed toward the hollow of the sacrum. At the plane of the pelvic outlet the anteroposterior diameter of the head is in the anteroposterior diameter of the outlet or is slightly oblique. The occipital bone is then found at the lower rim of the symphysis.

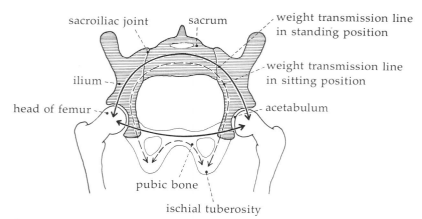

A. Schematic drawing showing the weight-transmitting function of the pelvis.

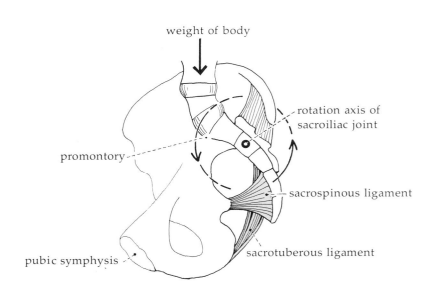

B. Schematic drawing indicating the function of the sacrotuberous and sacrospinous ligaments.

Note the following points:

¶ In addition to its function as a birth canal, the pelvis also has an important function of transmitting weight (*A*). The weight of the head, neck, thorax and abdomen is superimposed on the fifth lumbar vertebra, and from there it passes to the upper three segments of the sacrum. By way of the sacroiliac joints and the iliac bones the weight is then transmitted to the acetabula and, in a standing position, to the two femora. In a sitting position the weight is transmitted to the ischial tuberosities. Along the lines of weight transmission the bones of the pelvis are thick, as opposed to the alae of the iliac bones, which are usually very thin. The weight-transmission line forms an arch and the pubic bones, bound together by ligaments, act as struts to prevent the two ends of the arch from spreading.

¶ The weight of the body will tend to push the upper part of the sacrum forward into the pelvic cavity (see *B*). Since this movement involves rotation around the axis of the sacroiliac joint, the lower part of the sacrum and the coccyx will rotate backward. Forward movement of the sacrum into the pelvis results in a shortening of the anteroposterior diameter (promontory to upper rim of symphysis) of the pelvic inlet and has serious consequences, particularly in the female. The forward rotation, which is always accompanied by backward rotation of the posterior part of the sacrum, is strongly resisted by the sacrospinous and sacrotuberous ligaments. They are supported in this function by the posterior sacroiliac ligaments, the iliolumbar ligament and the interosseous sacroiliac ligaments (see P8).

¶ When the bones are soft, as in rickets, the sacrum will bend and the anterior portion will be pushed into the pelvis. Rickets was formerly one of the most common causes of narrowing of the plane of the pelvic inlet.

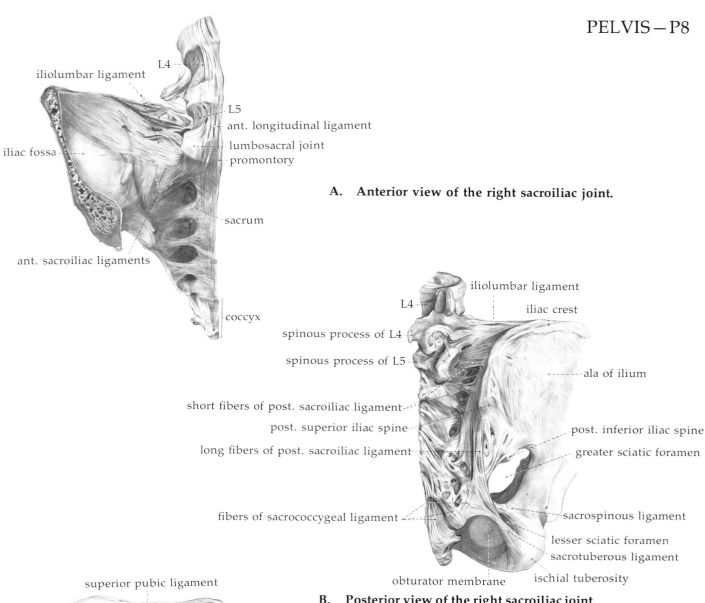

iliolumbar ligament
L4
iliac fossa
ant. sacroiliac ligaments
sacrum
L5
ant. longitudinal ligament
lumbosacral joint
promontory
coccyx

A. Anterior view of the right sacroiliac joint.

iliolumbar ligament
iliac crest
L4
spinous process of L4
spinous process of L5
ala of ilium
short fibers of post. sacroiliac ligament
post. superior iliac spine
post. inferior iliac spine
long fibers of post. sacroiliac ligament
greater sciatic foramen
fibers of sacrococcygeal ligament
sacrospinous ligament
lesser sciatic foramen
sacrotuberous ligament
obturator membrane
ischial tuberosity

B. Posterior view of the right sacroiliac joint.
Note also the sacrotuberous and sacrospinous ligaments.

superior pubic ligament
joint cavity
pubis
fibrocartilage in interpubic disc
arcuate pubic ligament

C. Frontal section through the pubic symphysis.

Note:

¶ The sacroiliac joints are synovial joints. Because of the strong ligaments surrounding the joints, only a limited amount of movement is possible. They act mainly as shock absorbers during walking and jumping.

¶ With advancing age the sacroiliac joints and the surrounding ligaments may ossify, thus eliminating the shock-absorbing ability of the joints.

¶ The opposing bony surfaces of the pubic bones (C) are coated with hyaline cartilage and united by fibrocartilage. In the fibrocartilage is a cleft which gives rise to a joint cavity, thus permitting some movement. The bones are united by dense anterior decussating fibers and the strong arcuate ligament.

¶ At the end of pregnancy both the sacroiliac joints and the symphysis permit greater movement than normal, owing to the hormone relaxin. As a result the birth canal becomes more flexible. Movement between the two pubic bones can sometimes be felt at this time.

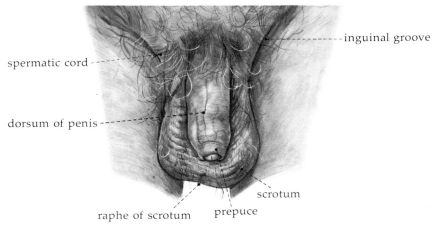

spermatic cord

inguinal groove

dorsum of penis

scrotum

raphe of scrotum   prepuce

A.   The male external genital organs.

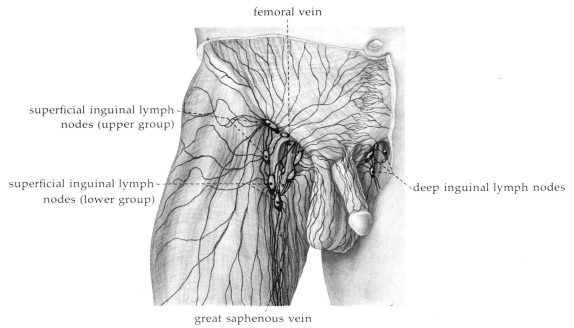

femoral vein

superficial inguinal lymph
nodes (upper group)

superficial inguinal lymph
nodes (lower group)

deep inguinal lymph nodes

great saphenous vein

B.   The superficial lymph vessels of the scrotum and penis.

Inspection and palpation of the penis and particularly of the scrotum are important.
Swellings of the scrotum, unilateral or bilateral, are frequently seen and are caused either
by the contents of the scrotum or by intestinal loops descending into the scrotum as an
inguinal hernia.

During palpation note:

1. *The superficial inguinal ring,* a triangular opening in the aponeurosis of the external
    oblique muscle. The ring is located slightly above and lateral to the pubic tubercle. The
    margins of the ring can be felt by invaginating the skin of the upper part of the scrotum
    with the index finger or little finger behind the spermatic cord (see A14).

2. *The spermatic cord,* which can be felt emerging from the superficial inguinal ring and
    can be followed as it descends into the scrotum over the pubic tubercle. In the
    upper part of the scrotum the cord can be palpated between the thumb and the index
    finger. The firm structure felt in the cord is the *ductus deferens.*

3. *The testis,* a firm ovoid body. It is mobile and is not attached to the skin and the sub-
    cutaneous tissue.

4. *The epididymis,* an elongated structure which is posterior to the testis and attached to
    it. Sometimes the enlarged upper end, the head, can be distinguished from the more
    narrow body and tail.

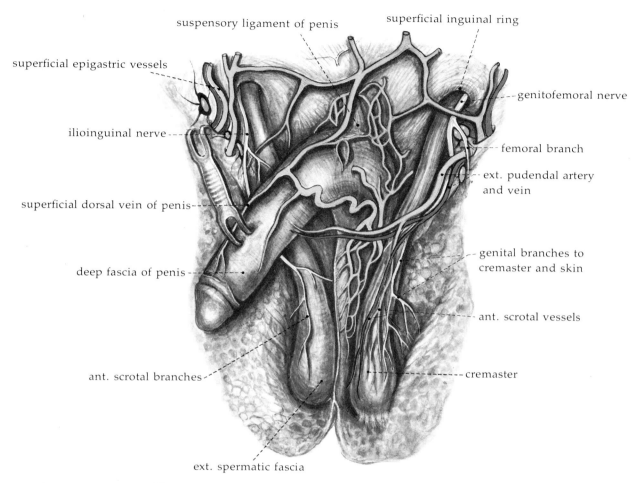

suspensory ligament of penis

superficial inguinal ring

superficial epigastric vessels

genitofemoral nerve

ilioinguinal nerve

femoral branch

ext. pudendal artery and vein

superficial dorsal vein of penis

genital branches to cremaster and skin

deep fascia of penis

ant. scrotal vessels

cremaster

ant. scrotal branches

ext. spermatic fascia

The external genital organs after removal of the skin.

Two nerves should be noticed:

¶ *The ilioinguinal nerve* (L1) passes into the inguinal canal and emerges through the superficial ring to supply the skin of the upper part of the scrotum (anterior scrotal branches), the root of the penis and the medial side of the thigh (see also A12 and A14).

¶ *The genital branch of the genitofemoral nerve* similarly passes through the inguinal canal to supply the cremaster muscle. The femoral branch supplies the skin of the medial side of the thigh. When the skin of the medial side of the thigh is scratched during physical examination, the testicle on the same side is drawn upward, a reaction known as the *cremasteric reflex*. The reflex involves the spinal cord segments of L1 and L2 (see A73).

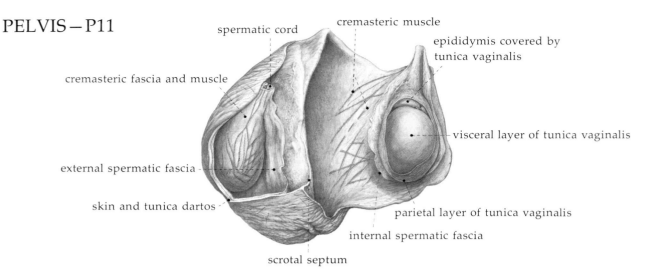

A. The testes and their surrounding layers.

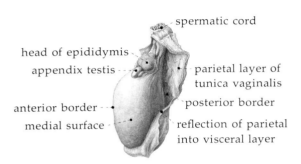

B. Medial aspect of the right testis.

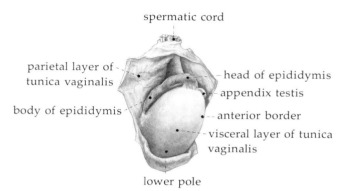

C. Lateral aspect of the right testis.

Note the following layers, beginning from the inside:

- ¶ The visceral layer of the tunica vaginalis, covering the testis and epididymis (see *A*).

- ¶ The parietal layer of the tunica vaginalis. The space between the two serous layers always contains some fluid.

- ¶ The internal spermatic fascia (a continuation of the fascia transversalis).

- ¶ The cremasteric fascia with some cremasteric muscle bundles (a continuation of the internal oblique muscle).

- ¶ The external spermatic fascia (a continuation of the external oblique muscle).

- ¶ Skin and tunica dartos, which on the inside is bordered by a membranous layer (Colles' fascia). (See A5 and P19.)

Note also:

- ¶ The *appendix testis* (B) is a remnant of the most cranial end of the paramesonephric duct. It is seen frequently and is located at the upper pole of the testis close to the head of the epididymis. Sometimes it is attached to the testis by a small stalk which may rotate, thereby closing off the blood supply and causing necrosis.

- ¶ The *appendix of the epididymis* is a remnant of the most cranial end of the mesonephric duct. In some cases both the appendix testis and the appendix of the epididymis are present (see P14).

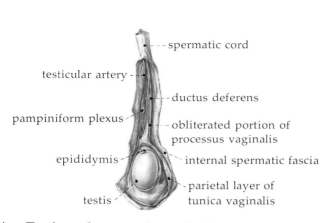

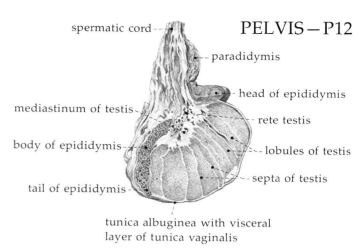

A. Testis and spermatic cord of a 1 year old boy.

B. Section through the testis and epididymis.

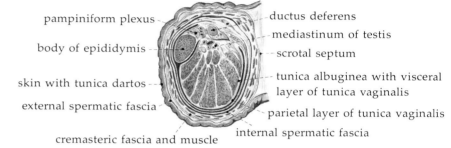

C. Horizontal section through the scrotum.

Note:

⁋ The tunica vaginalis surrounds the testis and the epididymis, with the exception of their posterior aspects. Here the parietal layer reflects into the visceral layer, which covers the testis and the epididymis. On the surface of the testis it is fused with the tunica albuginea, the true capsule of the testis.

⁋ The space between the parietal and visceral layers of the tunica vaginalis always contains some fluid. The most frequent swelling in the scrotum is caused by excessive fluid between the two layers of the tunica; this is the so-called *vaginal hydrocele*.

⁋ Other causes of swelling in the scrotum are cancers of the testis and inflammations of the epididymis.

⁋ The contents of the spermatic cord are:

1. The ductus deferens.

2. The deferential artery, a branch of the inferior vesical artery (see P14).

3. Sympathetic fibers around the ductus deferens from the lower thoracic and upper lumbar regions.

4. The testicular artery, arising from the abdominal aorta.

5. The pampiniform plexus, representing the veins from the testis and epididymis (see also P14). The veins in the pampiniform plexus number about one dozen. Approaching the inguinal canal they decrease in number but become larger. At the deep inguinal ring they form the testicular vein, which on the right enters the inferior vena cava but on the left enters the renal vein (see A63).

6. Lymph vessels of the epididymis and testis. The lymphatics follow the artery and veins and end in the lumbar nodes. This means that metastases from a cancer of the testis will go to the lumbar region, where they are difficult to detect (see A64).

7. The vaginal ligament, the obliterated part of the processus vaginalis (*A*). It is obliterated before birth or shortly thereafter. Its lower part remains patent and is invaginated by the testis and epididymis. Occasionally a middle portion of the vaginal ligament remains patent to form a cystlike structure in the upper part of the scrotum (see A18).

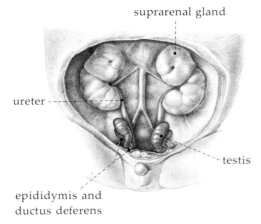

suprarenal gland

ureter

testis

epididymis and
ductus deferens

A.   Descent of the testis in a 5 month old fetus.
Note the large suprarenal gland, the lobulated
kidney and the course of the ductus deferens.

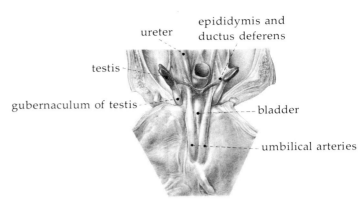

ureter

epididymis and
ductus deferens

testis

gubernaculum of testis

bladder

umbilical arteries

B.   Descent of the testis in a 6 month old fetus.
Note the large umbilical arteries on the anterior
abdominal wall, the gubernaculum of the testis
and the ductus deferens.

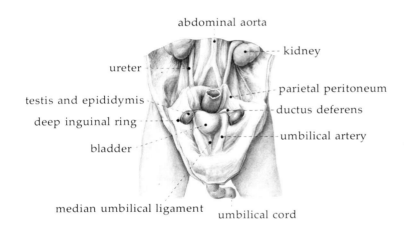

abdominal aorta

kidney

ureter

parietal peritoneum

testis and epididymis

ductus deferens

deep inguinal ring

umbilical artery

bladder

median umbilical ligament   umbilical cord

C.   Descent of the testis just before birth.
Note the relation of the ureter to the
ductus deferens, the umbilical arteries,
and the median umbilical ligament, a
remnant of the urachus.

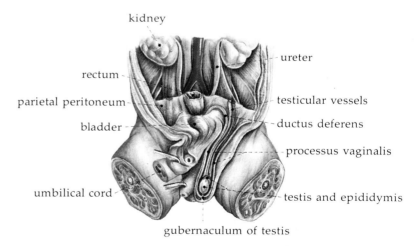

kidney

ureter

rectum

parietal peritoneum

testicular vessels

bladder

ductus deferens

processus vaginalis

umbilical cord

testis and epididymis

gubernaculum of testis

D.   Testis descended into the scrotum.
Note the ductus deferens and the testicular vessels.

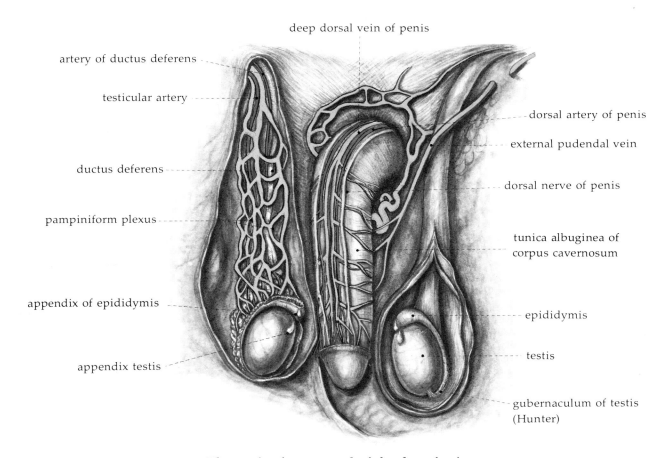

deep dorsal vein of penis

artery of ductus deferens

testicular artery

ductus deferens

pampiniform plexus

appendix of epididymis

appendix testis

dorsal artery of penis

external pudendal vein

dorsal nerve of penis

tunica albuginea of
corpus cavernosum

epididymis

testis

gubernaculum of testis
(Hunter)

The penis after removal of the deep fascia.
Note also the scrotum at various stages of dissection.

¶ The deep dorsal arteries and veins are the most important vessels of the corpora cavernosa and corpus spongiosum. They are located at the dorsal aspect of the penis under
the deep fascia. The veins are characterized by encircling branches. The deep dorsal
vein drains into the prostatic venous plexus and passes between the arcuate pubic
ligament and the urogenital diaphragm (see P23 A).

¶ The deep dorsal vein should not be confused with the superficial dorsal vein, which
lies in the superficial fascia and can be seen through the skin. This vein drains with
right and left branches into the external pudendal veins (see P10).

¶ The pampiniform venous plexus drains the testis and epididymis. The vessels form the
testicular vein or veins. On the left this vein drains into the left renal vein; on the right
it drains into the inferior vena cava. When the outflow of the plexus is impeded, the
veins of the pampiniform plexus may become varicose. On palpation of the scrotum
they give the impression of a bag of worms. The extension of the veins is known as
varicocele and is seen mainly on the left side.

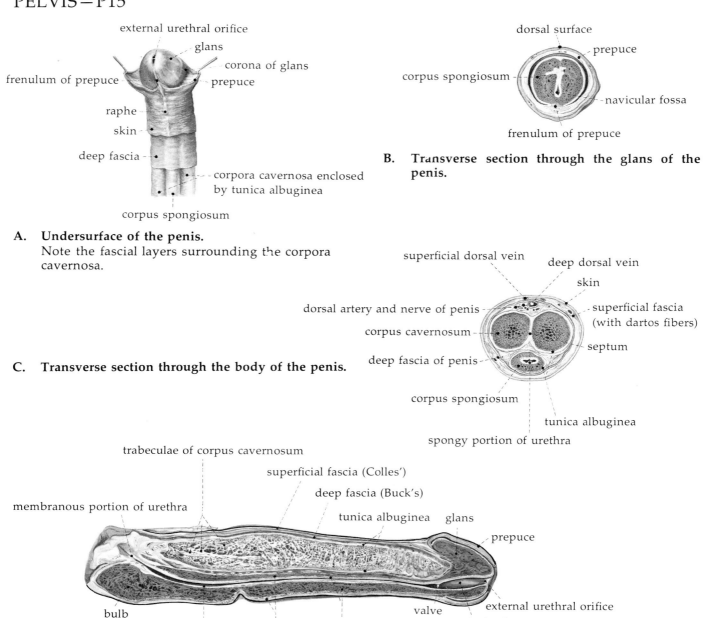

external urethral orifice
glans
corona of glans
frenulum of prepuce
prepuce
raphe
skin
deep fascia
corpora cavernosa enclosed
by tunica albuginea
corpus spongiosum

A. Undersurface of the penis.
Note the fascial layers surrounding the corpora cavernosa.

dorsal surface
prepuce
corpus spongiosum
navicular fossa
frenulum of prepuce

B. Transverse section through the glans of the penis.

superficial dorsal vein
deep dorsal vein
skin
dorsal artery and nerve of penis
corpus cavernosum
deep fascia of penis
corpus spongiosum
spongy portion of urethra
superficial fascia (with dartos fibers)
septum
tunica albuginea

C. Transverse section through the body of the penis.

trabeculae of corpus cavernosum
superficial fascia (Colles')
deep fascia (Buck's)
membranous portion of urethra
tunica albuginea
glans
prepuce
bulb
valve
external urethral orifice
navicular fossa
tunica albuginea
corpus spongiosum
spongy portion of urethra

D. Longitudinal section of the penis.

The fascial layers surrounding the penis are a continuation of those of the anterior abdominal wall (see A5 and P19).

¶ The superficial fascia of the abdomen consists of a fatty layer; and a membranous layer. Toward the penis the fatty layer disappears; in the scrotum it is represented by some subcutaneous smooth muscle fibers—the *dartos muscle*. The membranous layer is the superficial fascia of the penis.

¶ The deep fascia of the abdominal wall also forms the deep fascia of the penis. In front of the symphysis it forms the suspensory ligament of the penis (see P10).

¶ The tunica albuginea forms a dense fibrous sheath around the corpora cavernosa penis and around the corpus spongiosum penis. The septum separating the two corpora cavernosa is irregularly interrupted distally, thus permitting blood to flow from one to the other. The tunica around the corpus spongiosum, which contains the urethra, is not as dense as that around the corpora cavernosa.

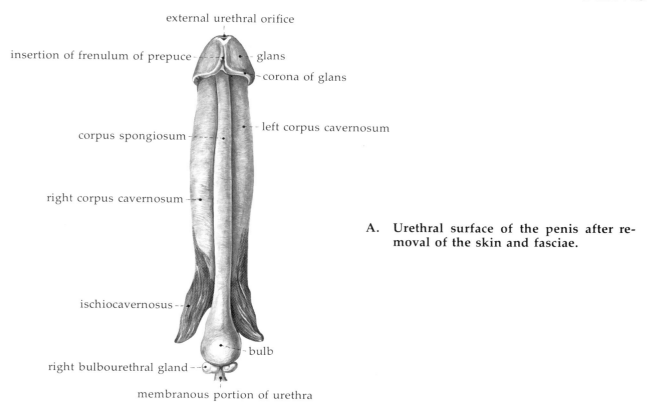

external urethral orifice

insertion of frenulum of prepuce — glans

corona of glans

left corpus cavernosum

corpus spongiosum

right corpus cavernosum

A. Urethral surface of the penis after removal of the skin and fasciae.

ischiocavernosus

bulb

right bulbourethral gland

membranous portion of urethra

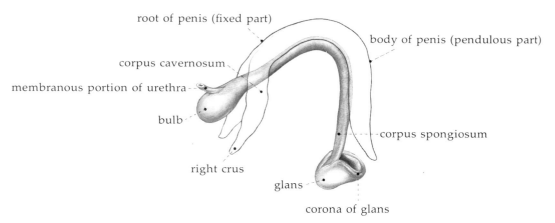

root of penis (fixed part)

body of penis (pendulous part)

corpus cavernosum

membranous portion of urethra

bulb

corpus spongiosum

right crus

glans

corona of glans

B. Drawing showing how the glans (the end of the corpus spongiosum) fits like a cone over the ends of the corpora cavernosa.

◖ During erection the cavernous spaces in the corpora cavernosa are filled with blood from the branches of the dorsal artery of the penis, a branch of the internal pudendal artery. As the cavernous spaces expand, the thin-walled venules are compressed. The subsequent swelling pushes the corpora against the tough tunica albuginea and the deep fascia of the penis. Consequently, many of the veins are compressed, thus further preventing the outflow of blood and promoting rigidity. Contractions of the ischiocavernosus muscle also help to close off the venous drainage. After orgasm the media in the wall of the arteries constrict and a gradual venous drainage begins.

◖ Vasodilation is under the influence of parasympathetic impulses. Postganglionic fibers join the internal pudendal arteries in the erectile tissue of the corpora cavernosa. During ejaculation the smooth muscle fibers of the duct of the epididymis, the ductus deferens, the seminal vesicles and the prostate contract. The spermatozoa together with secretions of the seminal vesicles and prostate are pushed into the prostatic urethra. Subsequent rhythmic contractions of the bulbospongiosus muscle move the semen along the urethra. At the same time the sphincter of the bladder contracts to prevent reflux of spermatozoa into the bladder.

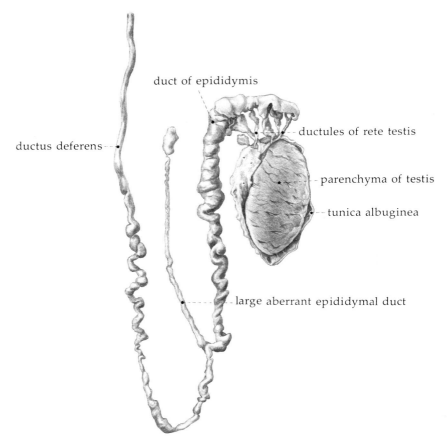

duct of epididymis

ductules of rete testis

ductus deferens

parenchyma of testis

tunica albuginea

large aberrant epididymal duct

A. **The testis, epididymis and ductus deferens after dissection.**
Note the ductules of the rete testis.

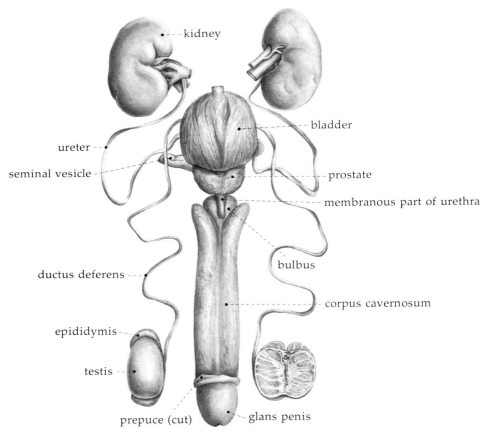

kidney

bladder

ureter

seminal vesicle

prostate

membranous part of urethra

bulbus

ductus deferens

corpus cavernosum

epididymis

testis

prepuce (cut)

glans penis

B. **The testis, epididymis and ductus deferens in relation to other male genitalia.**
Note the length of the ductus deferens.

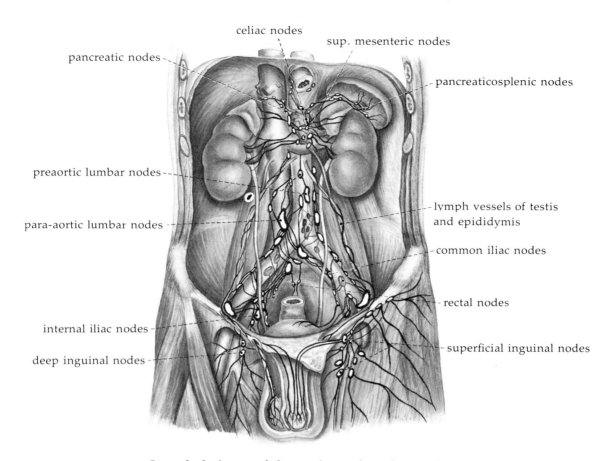

celiac nodes

sup. mesenteric nodes

pancreatic nodes

pancreaticosplenic nodes

preaortic lumbar nodes

lymph vessels of testis and epididymis

para-aortic lumbar nodes

common iliac nodes

rectal nodes

internal iliac nodes

superficial inguinal nodes

deep inguinal nodes

Lymph drainage of the penis, testis and scrotal wall.
The lymphatics of the external genitals are important because gonorrheal infections of the urethra and epididymis, as well as cancers of the testis, may spread by way of the lymph vessels.

With regard to the lymph drainage, note:

- The lymph vessels of the skin of the scrotum and of the penis and prepuce drain into the superficial inguinal lymph nodes (see P9).

- The glans, the corpora cavernosa and part of the urethra drain to the deep inguinal nodes on both sides. They follow the deep dorsal vein. Some lymph vessels pass directly to the external iliac lymph nodes. The lymph from the bulbar portion of the urethra follows the internal pudendal vessels to the internal iliac nodes.

- The lymphatics of the testis and the spermatic cord follow the testicular vessels through the inguinal canal. They do not follow the ductus deferens, but pass with the vessels toward the external iliac and lumbar nodes. Hence, metastases from cancers of the testis do not spread to the inguinal nodes but to the lumbar nodes, where they cannot be palpated.

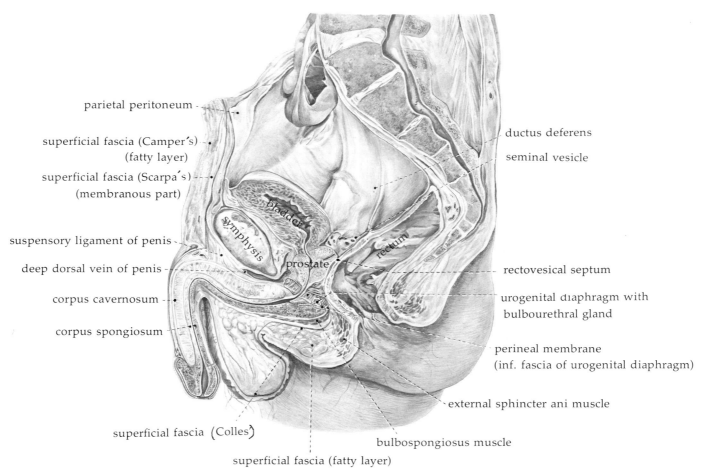

parietal peritoneum

ductus deferens

superficial fascia (Camper's)
(fatty layer)

seminal vesicle

superficial fascia (Scarpa's)
(membranous part)

bladder

symphysis

rectum

suspensory ligament of penis

deep dorsal vein of penis

prostate

rectovesical septum

corpus cavernosum

urogenital diaphragm with
bulbourethral gland

corpus spongiosum

perineal membrane
(inf. fascia of urogenital diaphragm)

external sphincter ani muscle

superficial fascia (Colles')

bulbospongiosus muscle

superficial fascia (fatty layer)

Median section through the penis, scrotum and perineum.
Note the fascial compartments and the pelvic organs.

Note:

¶ The *fatty layer* of the superficial fascia that is found on the anterior abdominal wall is absent on the penis and scrotum. In the urogenital triangle, however, it is present and extends into the region surrounding the rectum.

¶ The *membranous layer* of the superficial fascia continues over the penis and scrotum (*Colles' fascia*). In the region of the urogenital triangle it is clearly distinguishable. It is attached laterally to the pubic arch (P22 B) and fuses posteriorly with the *perineal membrane*, that is, the inferior fascia of the urogenital diaphragm.

¶ The urinary bladder rests on the pubis and, via the prostate, on the floor of the pelvis. As the bladder fills, it gradually rises above the pubic bones into the abdomen.

¶ Rectal examination may provide information about:

1. The sphincters and the mucous membrane of the anal canal and rectum.
2. Hemorrhoids, abscesses and cancers.
3. The entire posterior surface of the prostate.
4. Part of the seminal vesicles.
5. The surrounding bony points, which are particularly important in the female in obtaining some impression of the width of the birth canal.

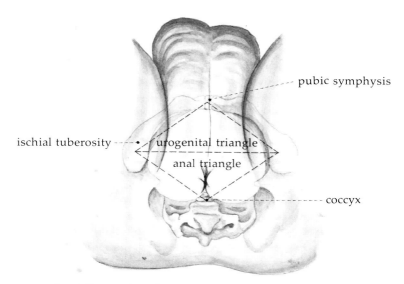

A. The anal and urogenital triangles in the male.

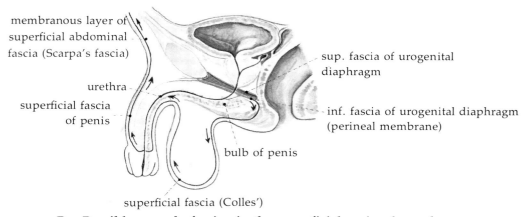

B. Possible spread of urine in the superficial perineal pouch.

¶ The main structure in the anal triangle is the anus, the terminal part of the anal canal. This canal extends from the upper aspect of the pelvic diaphragm to the anus. (In surgery the anal canal is considered to extend from the pectinate line to the anus, because this line forms the dividing line between the venous and lymphatic drainage of the upper and lower parts of the anal canal. (see P33.)

¶ The greater part of the corpora cavernosa and corpus spongiosum is found in the urogenital triangle under the urogenital diaphragm. The fascial relationship in this region is different from that in the penis and is significant in the spread of infections, urine and blood (see P22 A).

¶ The *superficial perineal pouch* (B) is inferiorly bordered by the membranous layer of the superficial fascia, and superiorly by the perineal membrane. When the urethra is ruptured beneath the perineal membrane, urine and blood will penetrate into the superficial perineal pouch. From the perineal region the extravasate may expand deep to the membranous layer into the scrotum, around the penis and on to the abdominal wall. (For deep perineal pouch see P22 B).

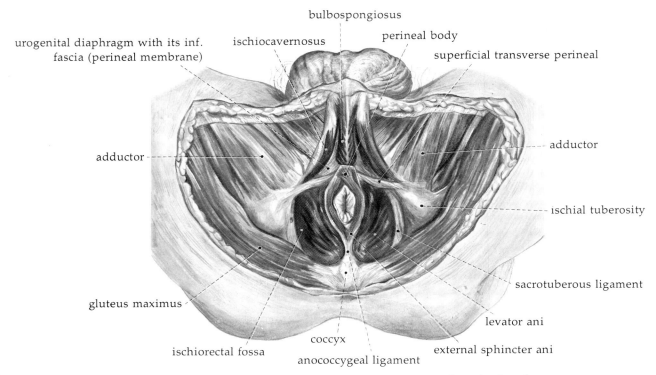

A. The muscles in the urogenital and anal triangles.

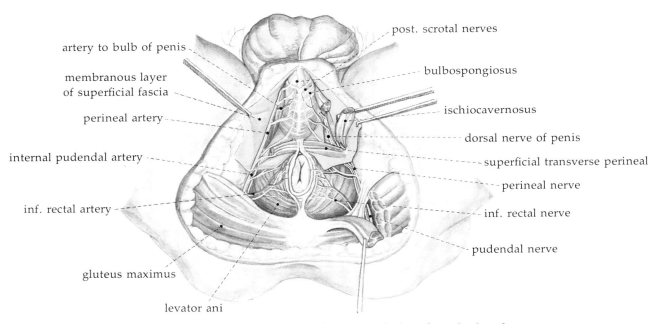

B. The nerves and vessels in the urogenital and anal triangles.

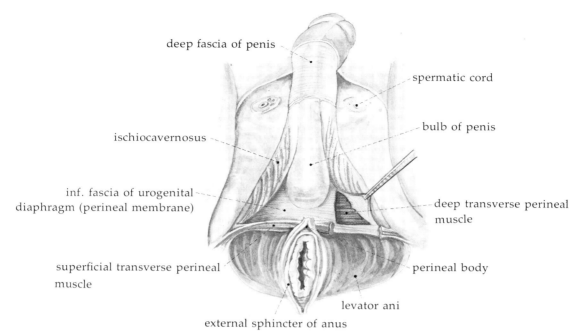

deep fascia of penis

spermatic cord

ischiocavernosus

bulb of penis

inf. fascia of urogenital
diaphragm (perineal membrane)

deep transverse perineal
muscle

superficial transverse perineal
muscle

perineal body

external sphincter of anus

levator ani

A. Relationship of the corpora cavernosa to the urogenital diaphragm.
The fatty layer and the membranous layer (Colles' fascia) of the superficial fascia have
been removed.

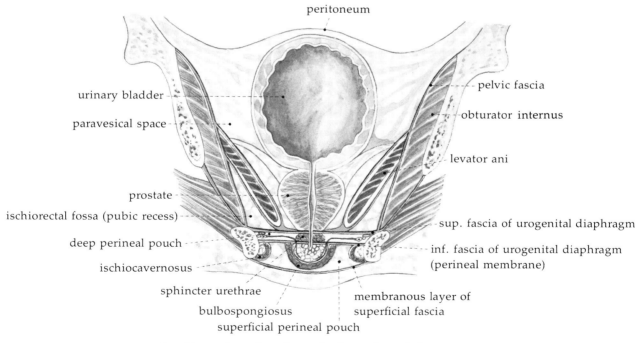

peritoneum

urinary bladder

pelvic fascia

paravesical space

obturator internus

levator ani

prostate

ischiorectal fossa (pubic recess)

sup. fascia of urogenital diaphragm

deep perineal pouch

inf. fascia of urogenital diaphragm
(perineal membrane)

ischiocavernosus

sphincter urethrae

membranous layer of
superficial fascia

bulbospongiosus

superficial perineal pouch

B. Frontal section through the male pelvis.
Note the superficial and deep perineal pouches.

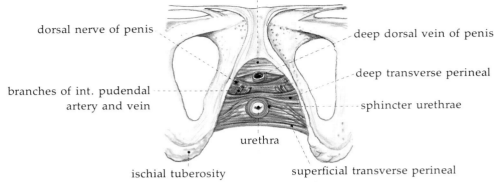

A.   Urogenital diaphragm after removal of the corpora cavernosa.

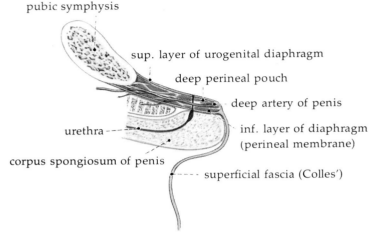

B.   Schematic drawing of the deep perineal pouch.

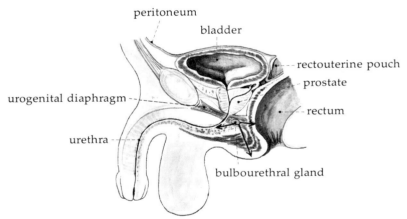

C.   The bulbourethral glands (Cowper's glands) in the deep pouch.

The *urogenital diaphragm* is a musculo-membranous diaphragm stretched across the pubic arch and attached to the ischio-pubic rami. It consists of two fascial layers with two muscles between them. The inferior fascial layer of the urogenital diaphragm (also called the perineal membrane) forms the lower or *perineal surface*. The superior layer is derived from the pelvic fascia and forms the upper or *pelvic surface*. Between the two fascial layers are found the *deep transverse perineal muscle* and the *sphincter urethrae*.

Clinically, the term *deep perineal pouch* is used to indicate the space between the two fasciae. The pouch contains (a) the sphincter urethrae and deep transverse perineal muscle, (b) the membranous part of the urethra, (c) the bulbourethral glands, (d) an important branch of the internal pudendal artery which supplies the bulb of the penis, and (e) the dorsal nerve to the penis.

The deep pouch has considerable clinical importance.

1.   The membranous portion of the urethra, about 1 cm long, is the narrowest part of the urethra. It is directed downward and slightly forward, in contrast to the spongy part of the urethra which curves upward and forward in the corpus spongiosum of the penis. When inserting a catheter into the bladder it may be difficult to proceed from the spongy part into the membranous part, and ruptures of the urethra in this region are not uncommon. If the rupture is below the membranous part, urine and blood will penetrate into the superficial perineal pouch (see P20 B). If the rupture occurs in the membranous portion, urine will enter the deep pouch. From here it may break either through the inferior fascia into the superficial pouch or through the superior fascia into the retropubic space between the bladder and symphysis. Subsequently, it may ascend between the peritoneum and the fascia transversalis.

2.   The *bulbourethral* glands (*C*), two pea-sized bodies, drain through 2 cm long ducts into the floor of the spongy portion of the urethra, thereby piercing the inferior fascia. Gonorrheal infections of the bulbourethral glands may cause abscesses. Such abscesses may break through into the rectum, the superficial perineal pouch or the urethra (see arrows in *C*).

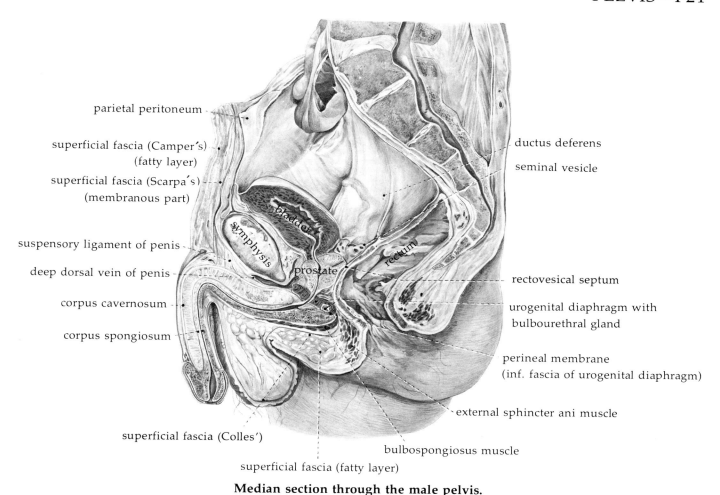

parietal peritoneum

superficial fascia (Camper's)
(fatty layer)

superficial fascia (Scarpa's)
(membranous part)

suspensory ligament of penis

deep dorsal vein of penis

corpus cavernosum

corpus spongiosum

ductus deferens

seminal vesicle

rectovesical septum

urogenital diaphragm with
bulbourethral gland

perineal membrane
(inf. fascia of urogenital diaphragm)

external sphincter ani muscle

superficial fascia (Colles')

bulbospongiosus muscle

superficial fascia (fatty layer)

Median section through the male pelvis.

Make the following observations:

¶ The peritoneum passes from the anterior abdominal wall to the upper surface of the bladder. From the bladder it continues over the tips of the seminal vesicles and then over the anterior part of the middle third of the rectum. The peritoneum covers the front as well as both sides of the upper third of the rectum (see P32).

¶ As the bladder fills, the superior wall rises above the symphysis and peels the peritoneum off the posterior surface of the anterior abdominal wall. When catheterization fails in cases of retention of urine, a needle may be inserted into the bladder by passing it through the abdominal wall above the symphysis without entering the peritoneal cavity. Similarly, in surgical operations involving the prostate a retropubic approach outside the peritoneum may be followed.

¶ The posterior surface of the prostate is closely related to the anterior surface of the rectal ampulla. The two surfaces are separated by the *rectovesical septum* (fascia of Denonvilliers). This septum is formed during fetal life by the fusion of the peritoneal leaves of the rectovesical pouch, which originally extended to the perineal body. The fascial plane thus formed can be used to approach the prostate through the perineum (see P28).

¶ The *prevesical* or *retropubic space* (space of Retzius) is filled with loose connective tissue and a large number of veins. Superiorly it extends into the space between the peritoneum and the fascia transversalis as far as the umbilical region. Bladder and prostate infections as well as urine and blood extravasates may enter and expand into the prevesical space.

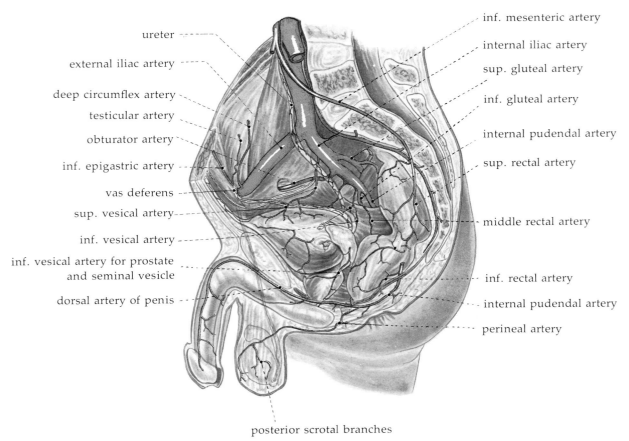

ureter

external iliac artery

deep circumflex artery

testicular artery

obturator artery

inf. epigastric artery

vas deferens

sup. vesical artery

inf. vesical artery

inf. vesical artery for prostate
and seminal vesicle

dorsal artery of penis

inf. mesenteric artery

internal iliac artery

sup. gluteal artery

inf. gluteal artery

internal pudendal artery

sup. rectal artery

middle rectal artery

inf. rectal artery

internal pudendal artery

perineal artery

posterior scrotal branches

The organs of the male pelvis and their blood supply.
The peritoneum has been removed.

¶ The blood supply of the organs of the pelvis derives mainly from the internal iliac artery; branches of the inferior mesenteric artery, however, also contribute to the supply of the rectum. The arterial supply of the rectum is threefold:

1. The *superior rectal artery*, a branch of the inferior mesenteric artery, supplies the upper third of the rectum. It is the main artery for the mucosa and may descend to the lower third (see also A43).

2. The *middle rectal artery*, a branch of the internal iliac artery, supplies mainly the muscular coat.

3. The *inferior rectal artery*, a branch of the internal pudendal artery, supplies the ano-rectal region. It anastomoses with the middle rectal artery at the anorectal junction.

¶ The arterial supply of the urinary bladder derives from: (a) the *superior vesical artery*, a branch of the internal iliac artery; and (b) the *inferior vesical artery*, which similarly originates from the internal iliac artery. The inferior vesical artery also supplies the prostate and seminal vesicles. (c) The *middle rectal artery* supplies part of the posterior surface of the bladder.

¶ Among the branches of the internal iliac artery, note (a) the superior vesical artery (originally this artery continues as the umbilical artery), (b) the obturator artery, (c) the small artery that supplies the ductus deferens, (d) the inferior vesical artery, (e) the middle rectal artery, (f) the internal pudendal artery, and (g) the inferior gluteal artery.

¶ Proceeding in a posterior direction the following branches are found: (a) the iliolumbar artery, (b) the lateral sacral artery, and (c) the superior gluteal artery (see P35).

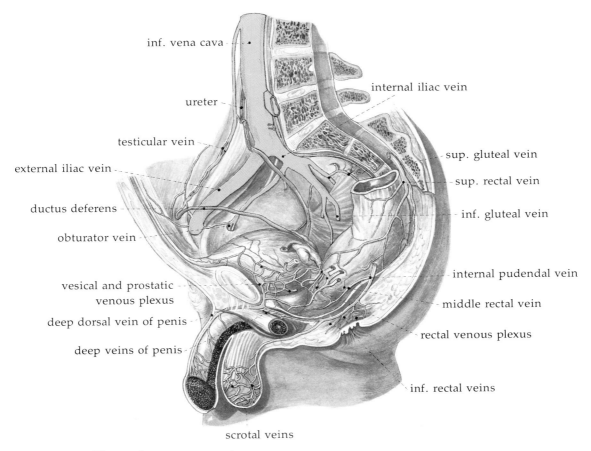

inf. vena cava

ureter

testicular vein

external iliac vein

ductus deferens

obturator vein

vesical and prostatic
venous plexus

deep dorsal vein of penis

deep veins of penis

scrotal veins

internal iliac vein

sup. gluteal vein

sup. rectal vein

inf. gluteal vein

internal pudendal vein

middle rectal vein

rectal venous plexus

inf. rectal veins

The main structures of the male pelvis and their venous drainage.

¶ The *venous drainage of the rectum* is important because of the large anastomoses between the portal and caval tributaries. The superior rectal vein drains into the inferior mesenteric vein and thus into the portal system; the middle and inferior rectal veins drain into the internal iliac and internal pudendal veins and thus into the caval system (see A29 and P33).

¶ The veins in the anal canal and rectum form a plexus within the wall. In the anal region the plexus is developed mainly in the submucosal position. It begins at the internal margin; somewhat higher it is found mainly among the anal columns. In the ampullary region the veins traverse the muscle layers and occupy a subperitoneal position; these veins have no valves and pass obliquely through the muscular wall. Any obstruction in the return flow toward the portal system causes the veins to become varicose (creating hemorrhoids). Internal hemorrhoids, mainly in the region of the middle and superior rectal veins, are covered with mucosa and are located above the pectinate line. External hemorrhoids are dilatations of the inferior rectal veins that are covered by skin (see P33).

¶ The *veins of the urinary bladder* form a large venous plexus into which blood flows from the penis and prostate. The plexus drains into the internal iliac vein (see also P31).

¶ Note the course of the ductus deferens. As soon as the duct has passed through the deep inguinal ring it leaves the testicular vein, which on the right side courses to the inferior vena cava and on the left to the renal vein.

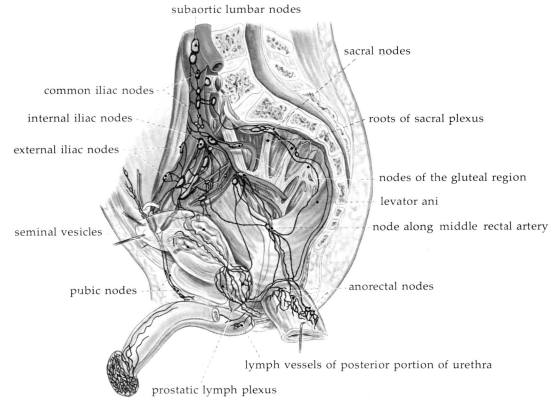

subaortic lumbar nodes

sacral nodes

common iliac nodes

internal iliac nodes

external iliac nodes

roots of sacral plexus

nodes of the gluteal region

levator ani

node along middle rectal artery

seminal vesicles

pubic nodes

anorectal nodes

lymph vessels of posterior portion of urethra

prostatic lymph plexus

Lymph drainage of the organs in the male pelvis.

Although the dissection of the lymph vessels and even of the lymph nodes is difficult, it is extremely important to understand the lymph drainage in this region. Cancers of the rectum and anal canal, the prostate and the bladder are common, and metastases frequently move along the lymph vessels to the nodes.

¶ *Lymph drainage of the rectum and anal canal.* The lymph vessels draining the upper part of the rectum follow the superior rectal artery to the inferior mesenteric nodes (see A44). Those of the middle portion follow the middle rectal artery to the internal iliac nodes. Lymph from the lower portion of the rectum and anal canal drains either in an upward direction, or downward to the medial group of the *superficial inguinal nodes* (see P9). The dividing line is formed by the pectinate line (see P33). A swelling of the inguinal nodes may be confused with an inguinal hernia. In any patient with a swelling in the inguinal region, the anal canal and rectum should be carefully examined.

¶ *Lymph drainage of the prostate.* The lymph vessels of the prostate course to the internal iliac lymph nodes. Cancers of the prostate also spread by way of the venous plexus, and metastases have a tendency to spread to the bones of the pelvis and vertebral column via the vertebral plexus (see P31).

¶ *Lymph drainage of the bladder.* The lymph vessels drain toward the internal and external iliac nodes.

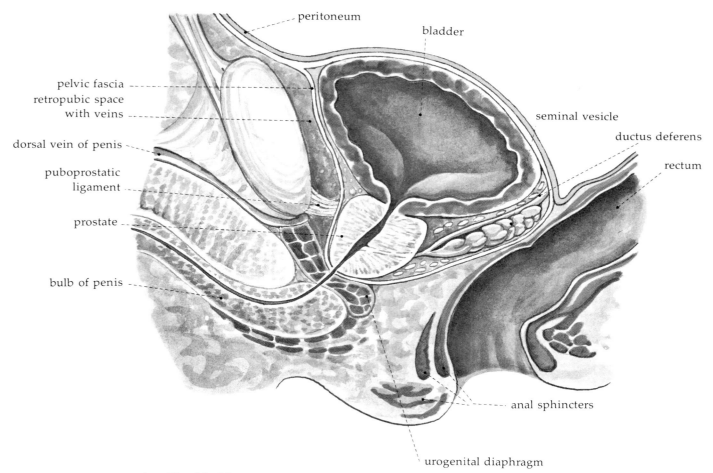

peritoneum

bladder

pelvic fascia

retropubic space
with veins

seminal vesicle

dorsal vein of penis

ductus deferens

rectum

puboprostatic
ligament

prostate

bulb of penis

anal sphincters

urogenital diaphragm

A. The bladder, prostate, seminal vesicle and urogenital diaphragm.

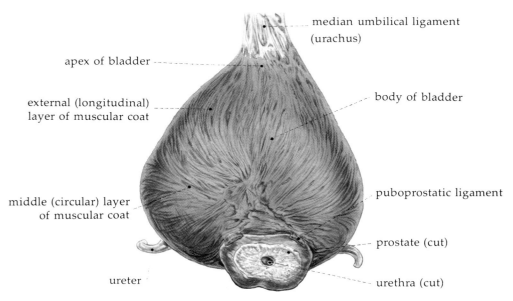

median umbilical ligament
(urachus)

apex of bladder

body of bladder

external (longitudinal)
layer of muscular coat

middle (circular) layer
of muscular coat

puboprostatic ligament

prostate (cut)

ureter

urethra (cut)

B. Anteroinferior surface of the urinary bladder.
The prostate and prostatic urethra have been cut
above the urogenital diaphragm.

Note:

¶ The bladder is anchored at its base by its continuity with the prostate and urethra,
which are in turn fixed to the urogenital diaphragm. In addition, the neck of the
bladder is fixed anteriorly by two ligamentous bands on each side of the median plane;
these bands are the puboprostatic ligaments. They extend from the back of the pubic
bone close to the middle of the symphysis, passing downward and medially to blend
with the upper part of the fascia of the prostate. In the female these bands are called
pubovesical ligaments.

173

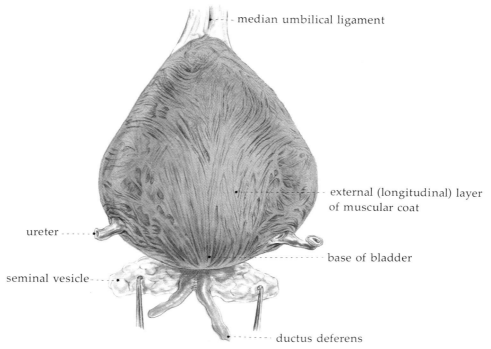

median umbilical ligament

external (longitudinal) layer
of muscular coat

ureter

base of bladder

seminal vesicle

ductus deferens

A. Posterosuperior surface of the urinary bladder.
The peritoneum has been removed and the
seminal vesicles pulled down.

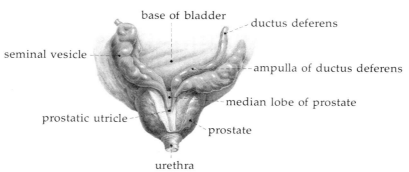

base of bladder

ductus deferens

seminal vesicle

ampulla of ductus deferens

median lobe of prostate

prostatic utricle

prostate

urethra

B. Posterior aspect of the urinary bladder.
Note the ductus deferens, seminal vesicles
and prostate.

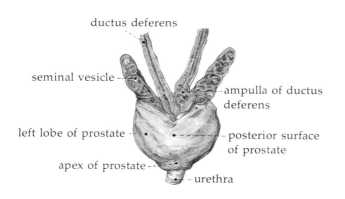

ductus deferens

seminal vesicle

ampulla of ductus
deferens

left lobe of prostate

posterior surface
of prostate

apex of prostate

urethra

**C. Section through the seminal vesicles and ampulla
of the ductus deferens.**

¶ The nonstriated muscular coat of the urinary bladder is arranged in three obliquely
encircling layers. At the neck of the bladder they form the *sphincter of the bladder* or
sphincter vesicae (see P30 *A*).

¶ As a result of the strong fixation of the prostate and the neck of the bladder, the urethra
between the prostate and the urogenital diaphragm is easily torn. This is likely to
result from severe trauma such as fractures of the pelvis in automobile accidents. Urine
and blood will then enter the prevesical space or retropubic space and may ascend between the peritoneum and fascia transversalis of the abdominal wall (see P28 *A*).

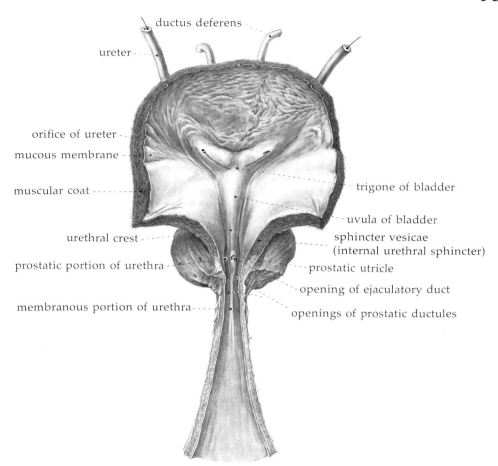

ductus deferens

ureter

orifice of ureter

mucous membrane

muscular coat

urethral crest

prostatic portion of urethra

membranous portion of urethra

trigone of bladder

uvula of bladder

sphincter vesicae
(internal urethral sphincter)

prostatic utricle

opening of ejaculatory duct

openings of prostatic ductules

**A. The trigone of the bladder and the floor of
the prostatic urethra.**

Make the following observations:

¶ The *trigone of the bladder* is a triangular area
of the posterior wall of the bladder. The apex is
formed by the internal urethral orifice, the
base by a line between the two ureteral orifices.
The latter two orifices appear as semilunar slits.
A probe passed through the openings takes an
oblique course through the bladder for about
1½ cm. This canal, surrounded on all sides by
muscle fibers, acts as a valve which allows
urine to pass into the bladder but prevents
regurgitation as the bladder fills. The trigone
remains smooth-walled even when the bladder is empty. On cystoscopic examination it
has a pink color.

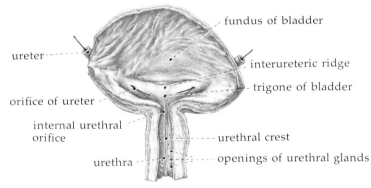

fundus of bladder

ureter

orifice of ureter

internal urethral
orifice

urethra

interureteric ridge

trigone of bladder

urethral crest

openings of urethral glands

**B. The trigone of the bladder and urethra in the
female.**

¶ The *internal urethral orifice* is at the apex of the
trigone. In the male the posterior margin protrudes slightly forward in the form of a fold.
This fold, the uvula, is caused by the middle lobe of the prostate. When the prostate
is hypertrophic, this lobe is enlarged and may block the internal urethral orifice
partially or completely.

¶ In addition to the pubovesical and puboprostatic ligaments, another important structure that supports the bladder is the levator ani muscle (see P54). In the female these
muscle fibers may be overstretched and damaged during a difficult delivery. As a
result, the angle between the neck of the bladder and the urethra may be changed,
leading to stress incontinence. This occurs particularly when the patient laughs or
strains excessively.

¶ The trigone of the bladder is a favorite site for ulcers and cancers of the bladder.

175

A. Coronal section through the prostate.

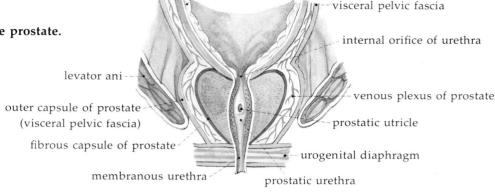

mucosa of urinary bladder
visceral pelvic fascia
internal orifice of urethra
levator ani
venous plexus of prostate
outer capsule of prostate
(visceral pelvic fascia)
prostatic utricle
fibrous capsule of prostate
urogenital diaphragm
membranous urethra
prostatic urethra

B. Sagittal section through the prostate.

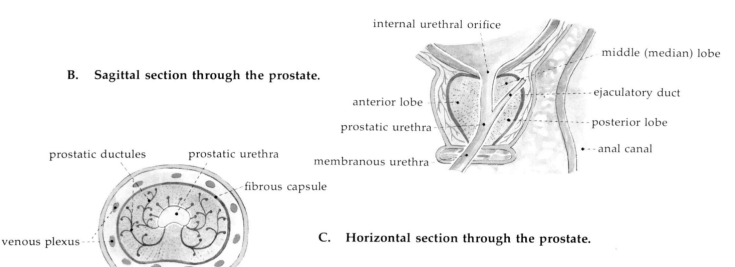

internal urethral orifice
middle (median) lobe
anterior lobe
ejaculatory duct
prostatic urethra
posterior lobe
membranous urethra
anal canal

prostatic ductules   prostatic urethra
fibrous capsule
venous plexus
fascial sheath

C. Horizontal section through the prostate.

The prostate gland is an extremely important organ because of its tendency toward inflammation, hypertrophy and cancers.

¶ Benign enlargement of the prostate occurs frequently. The median or middle lobe, located between the urethra and ejaculatory ducts, is usually most affected. It enlarges upward and pushes forward and upward into the posterior wall of the bladder. As a result the urethral crest begins to bulge forward into the bladder and may block the urethral outlet partially or completely. Since muscle fibers of the bladder continue in the prostate, particularly in the region of the sphincter vesicae, the sphincter action becomes impeded and urine leaks into the prostatic urethra (producing a desire to micturate). Further enlargement of the prostate causes compression of the prostatic urethra, so that the patient may have difficulty urinating. Back-pressure effects on the ureters and kidneys are a common complication.

¶ The prostate has two capsules: a fibrous capsule directly applied to the glandular tissue and an external capsule formed by the pelvic fascia, known as the fascia of the prostate. Between the two is an extremely rich venous plexus. During surgical procedures on the prostate extreme care must be taken with the venous plexus. The veins are thin and have no valves; they are drained by several trunks into the internal iliac veins (see P24 for surgical approach to prostate).

¶ The veins of the prostate not only drain into the internal iliac veins but also connect with the vertebral veins. These connections are thought to be the cause of the frequent occurrence of skeletal metastases in the lower vertebral column and pelvic bones in cancer of the prostate. It is thought that cancer cells may even enter the skull by way of the valveless veins of the vertebral column.

¶ Gonorrheal infections frequently cause abscesses in the prostate. When these abscesses expand and rupture, they may break through into the rectum, the bladder, the perineum, or the prevesical or retropubic space (see P23 and P28).

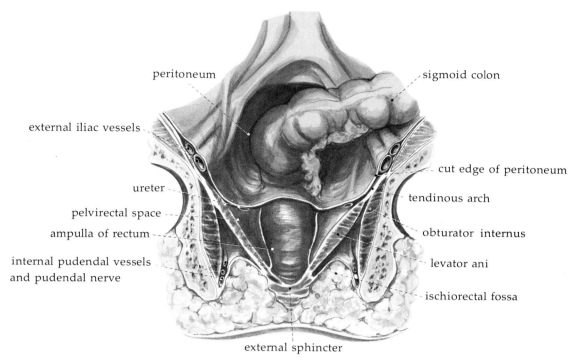

peritoneum

sigmoid colon

external iliac vessels

cut edge of peritoneum

ureter

tendinous arch

pelvirectal space

ampulla of rectum

obturator internus

internal pudendal vessels
and pudendal nerve

levator ani

ischiorectal fossa

external sphincter

Section through the pelvis with an anterior view of the rectum.
Note the relation of the rectum to the peritoneum, the levator ani and the ischiorectal fossa.

The space in the true pelvis is conveniently divided into three compartments:

1. *The peritoneal compartment.* In the male its lowest point is formed by the rectovesical pouch; in the female the low point is formed by the rectouterine pouch. The blood supply of that part of the rectum surrounded by the peritoneum comes from the superior rectal artery, a branch of the inferior mesenteric artery.

2. *The subperitoneal compartment.* This is the space found between the peritoneum and the diaphragm of the pelvis. It contains the urinary bladder, prostate, seminal vesicles, uterus and the middle part of the rectum. The blood supply of the organs in the subperitoneal compartment comes from the main branches of the internal iliac artery such as the vesical arteries, the uterine artery and the middle rectal artery.

3. *The subcutaneous compartment.* This is the space inferior to the diaphragm of the pelvis. The ischiorectal fossa is a part of the subcutaneous compartment. The tissues and organs in this compartment are all supplied by the internal pudendal artery.

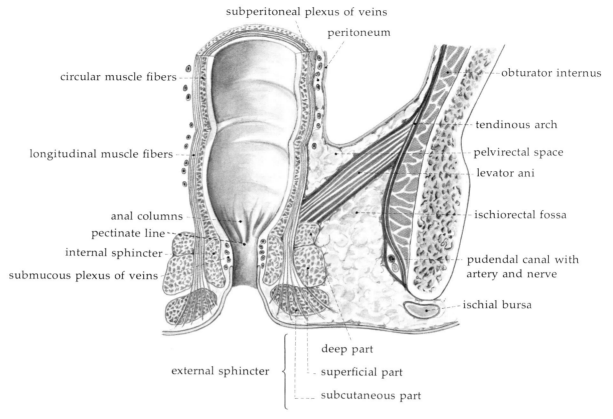

subperitoneal plexus of veins

peritoneum

circular muscle fibers

obturator internus

tendinous arch

longitudinal muscle fibers

pelvirectal space

levator ani

anal columns

ischiorectal fossa

pectinate line

internal sphincter

pudendal canal with artery and nerve

submucous plexus of veins

ischial bursa

deep part

external sphincter { superficial part

subcutaneous part

The ischiorectal fossa and the anal sphincters.
Note the position of the pudendal nerve.

¶ The ischiorectal fossa is part of the anal triangle and forms a prismatic space on each side of the anal canal. The lateral wall is formed by the lower part of the internal obturator muscle; the medial wall is formed by the levator ani and the sphincter musculature of the anal canal, and the floor by the skin. The fossa is filled with fat.

¶ The blood supply of the fatty tissue in the ischiorectal fossa is poor, and infections frequently develop into large abscesses. The fossa is a site of predilection for abscesses and infections due to its proximity to the anal canal. Infections of the anal canal and of the perianal sweat glands spread easily to the ischiorectal fossa. Abscesses usually open to the outside through the perianal region; only rarely do they break through the levator ani into the pelvirectal space.

¶ The sphincter ani surrounds the anal canal. This canal extends from the upper aspect of the pelvic diaphragm to the anus. The sphincter ani consists of an internal sphincter, a thickening of the circular muscle coat of the rectum, and an external sphincter. The latter muscle consists of (a) a subcutaneous part, (b) a superficial part which is attached to the coccyx and the perineal body, and (c) a deep part. In addition, fibers from the levator ani (the puborectal muscle) surround the canal like a sling and blend with the deep part of the external sphincter (see P55).

¶ Note the extensive venous network in the submucosal region. These veins are the source of external hemorrhoids.

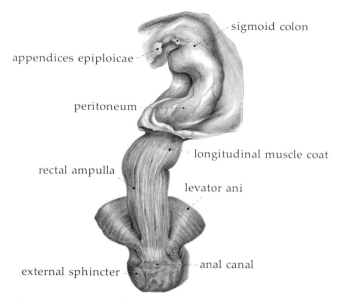

sigmoid colon

appendices epiploicae

peritoneum

rectal ampulla

longitudinal muscle coat

levator ani

external sphincter

anal canal

A. Anterior view of the rectum and its peritoneal covering.

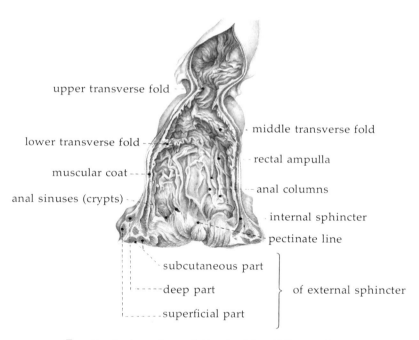

upper transverse fold

lower transverse fold

middle transverse fold

muscular coat

rectal ampulla

anal sinuses (crypts)

anal columns

internal sphincter

pectinate line

subcutaneous part

deep part   } of external sphincter

superficial part

B. Posterior view of the inside of the rectum.

¶ The crypts located between the anal columns are especially prone to infections, which gradually burrow themselves into the anal wall. Frequently they penetrate through the wall above, below or through the sphincter muscles, entering the ischiorectal fossa. Here they cause abscesses. These abscesses then may break through the skin around the anus, and a canal (fistula) from the anus toward the skin may develop.

¶ The rectum is involved in 50 per cent of all cases of cancer of the colon. In general, lymph from the lower part of the anal canal moves downward and forward across the perineum to the superficial inguinal lymph nodes (in cases of swelling of the inguinal lymph nodes, always examine the rectum!); from the upper part of the anal canal and rectum it moves to the inferior mesenteric nodes and the preaortic nodes (see A44). In surgery the dividing line between the lower and upper parts of the anal canal is considered to be the pectinate line. When rectal cancer occurs, it will be necessary to remove most of the pelvic colon, the mesocolon, the rectum, the anus, the surrounding skin, the fat in the ischiorectal fossa and the levator ani muscles.

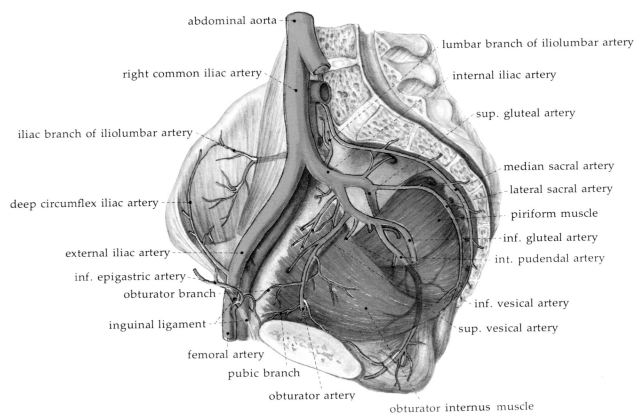

abdominal aorta

lumbar branch of iliolumbar artery

right common iliac artery

internal iliac artery

sup. gluteal artery

iliac branch of iliolumbar artery

median sacral artery

lateral sacral artery

deep circumflex iliac artery

piriform muscle

inf. gluteal artery

int. pudendal artery

external iliac artery

inf. epigastric artery

obturator branch

inf. vesical artery

inguinal ligament

sup. vesical artery

femoral artery

pubic branch

obturator artery

obturator internus muscle

The internal iliac artery and its branches.

Although many branches of the internal iliac artery have been encountered during the dissection of the bladder and rectum, their stems can be seen to best advantage after removal of the pelvic organs. Also, their relationships to the muscles and their exit foramina can now be explored.

¶ The superior gluteal artery leaves the pelvic cavity at the upper border of the piriform muscle and passes through the suprapiriform foramen to reach the lower extremity.

¶ The inferior gluteal artery, together with the internal pudendal artery, leaves the pelvis at the lower border of the piriform muscle, passing through the infrapiriform foramen. Whereas the inferior gluteal artery supplies the gluteal region, the internal pudendal artery returns to the perineal region through the lesser sciatic foramen.

¶ The obturator artery, which supplies mainly the medial region of the thigh, leaves the pelvis through the obturator foramen. Before entering the foramen, however, a pubic branch and an obturator branch are given off. The obturator branch communicates with the inferior epigastric artery, which originates from the external iliac artery.

¶ Note also the stems of the arteries for the bladder and rectum. (Dissection of the pelvic diaphragm is shown in P55.)

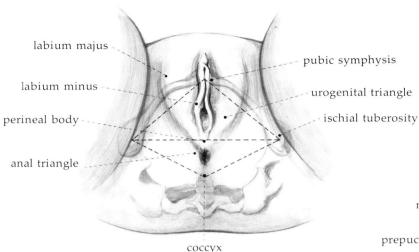

labium majus
labium minus
perineal body
anal triangle
pubic symphysis
urogenital triangle
ischial tuberosity
coccyx

A. **The female perineum, showing the anal and urogenital triangles.**

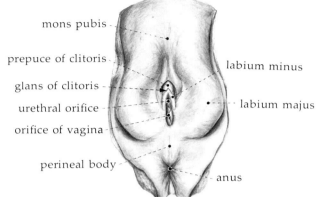

mons pubis
prepuce of clitoris
glans of clitoris
urethral orifice
orifice of vagina
perineal body
labium minus
labium majus
anus

B. **The external genitalia in a newborn girl.**

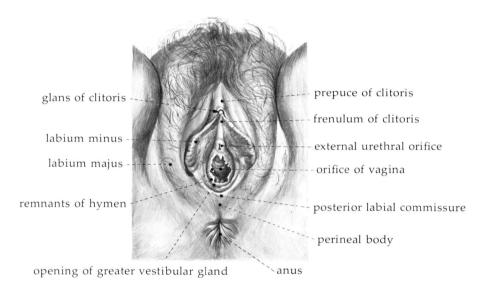

glans of clitoris
labium minus
labium majus
remnants of hymen
prepuce of clitoris
frenulum of clitoris
external urethral orifice
orifice of vagina
posterior labial commissure
perineal body
opening of greater vestibular gland
anus

C. **The external genitalia in an adult female.**
The labia have been pulled aside to show the entrance of the vagina and urethra.

Note the following points:

¶ The perineum is diamond-shaped. The boundaries are formed by the arcuate pubic ligament, the tip of the coccyx and the ischial tuberosities at each side. The pubic arch and the sacro-tuberous ligaments form the sides. A line drawn from one ischial tuberosity to the other lies in front of the anus and divides the perineum into the urogenital and anal triangles.

¶ The urethra and vagina enter the vestibule in close proximity to each other, so it is understandable that infections of the vagina easily spread to the urethra and bladder.

¶ The perineal body is a fibromuscular mass of tissue in the median plane extending from the posterior margin of the urogenital diaphragm to about 2 cm in front of the anal margin. A number of muscles converge and interlace in the perineal body. The most important of these are: (a) the external sphincter of the anus, (b) the bulbospongiosus, (c) the transverse perineal muscles, and (d) fibers of the levator ani see P38).

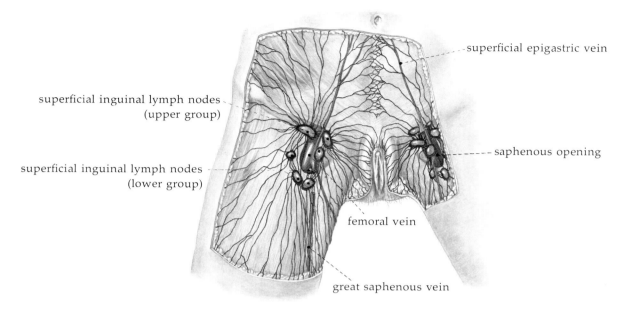

superficial epigastric vein

superficial inguinal lymph nodes
(upper group)

saphenous opening

superficial inguinal lymph nodes
(lower group)

femoral vein

great saphenous vein

A.   Lymphatic drainage of the labia and clitoris.

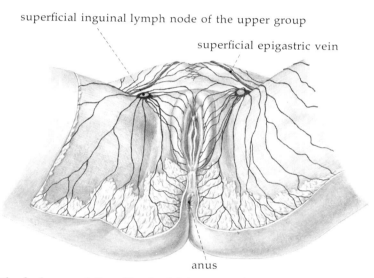

superficial inguinal lymph node of the upper group

superficial epigastric vein

anus

B.   Lymphatic drainage of the clitoris, labia, superficial perineal region and anus.

¶   Although the lymph vessels of the external genitalia and vagina are difficult to dissect, it is important to know that the labia majora, the labia minora and the lower third of the vagina drain to the superficial inguinal lymph nodes. The glans of the clitoris, however, drains to the deep inguinal nodes.

¶   When a swelling of the superficial inguinal nodes is observed, it should be remembered that the lower part of the anal canal also drains into the superficial nodes. Hence, careful examination of the anal canal is necessary in any patient with swellings of the inguinal lymph nodes.

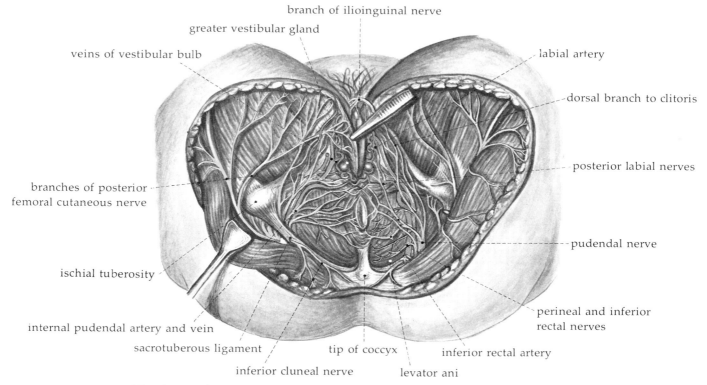

branch of ilioinguinal nerve
greater vestibular gland
veins of vestibular bulb
labial artery
dorsal branch to clitoris
posterior labial nerves
branches of posterior femoral cutaneous nerve
pudendal nerve
ischial tuberosity
perineal and inferior rectal nerves
internal pudendal artery and vein
sacrotuberous ligament
tip of coccyx
inferior rectal artery
inferior cluneal nerve
levator ani

The internal pudendal vessels and pudendal nerve with their branches.

⁋ The internal pudendal artery reaches the perineum by passing through the lesser sciatic foramen. It courses along the lateral wall of the ischiorectal fossa, accompanied by its vein and the pudendal nerve (see P33). Note the inferior rectal vessels supplying the anus and anal canal. The main artery continues into the urogenital triangle, where it supplies the labia and the clitoris (see also P35).

⁋ The pudendal nerve contains fibers from S2, S3 and S4. Some of its branches cross the ischiorectal fossa to supply the levator ani and the external sphincter muscle of the anus. In the urogenital area the branches of the pudendal nerve supply all the muscles and the skin over the labia. Some overlapping of the branches of the posterior femoral cutaneous nerve and the ilioinguinal nerve occurs in the sensory areas.

⁋ When the pudendal nerve enters the perineal region, the main stem courses through the pudendal canal beneath the fascia of the internal obturator muscle on the lateral wall of the ischiorectal fossa. In the area of the ischial tuberosity the nerve may be easily blocked by an anesthetic to produce analgesia of the perineum in patients who are experiencing difficulty in delivery.

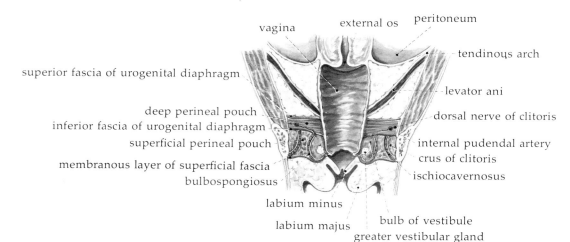

vagina
external os
peritoneum
tendinous arch
superior fascia of urogenital diaphragm
levator ani
deep perineal pouch
dorsal nerve of clitoris
inferior fascia of urogenital diaphragm
superficial perineal pouch
internal pudendal artery
crus of clitoris
membranous layer of superficial fascia
ischiocavernosus
bulbospongiosus
labium minus
labium majus
bulb of vestibule
greater vestibular gland

A. Schematic coronal section through the female external genitalia.
Note the urogenital diaphragm and the contents of the superficial pouch.

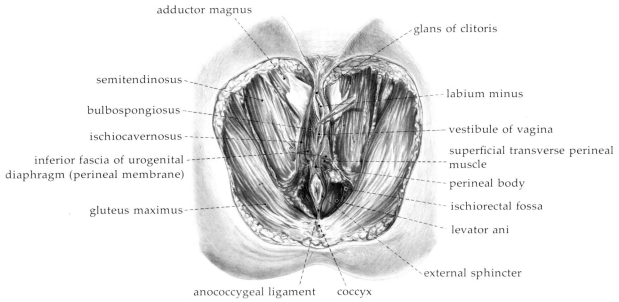

adductor magnus
glans of clitoris
semitendinosus
labium minus
bulbospongiosus
vestibule of vagina
ischiocavernosus
superficial transverse perineal muscle
inferior fascia of urogenital diaphragm (perineal membrane)
perineal body
ischiorectal fossa
gluteus maximus
levator ani
external sphincter
anococcygeal ligament
coccyx

B. The ischiocavernosus and bulbospongiosus muscles in the female.
The membranous layer of the superficial fascia has been removed, and the inferior fascia of the urogenital diaphragm (perineal membrane) is visible.

¶ The relationship of the fasciae in the urogenital region in the female is very similar to that seen in the anterior abdominal wall (A5). The fatty layer and the membranous layer of the superficial fascia are both present. However, the membranous layer (known as Scarpa's fascia on the abdominal wall) is now referred to as Colles' fascia. It is attached laterally to the pubic arch and fuses posteriorly with the perineal membrane (see also P20 and 22).

¶ The superficial pouch is bordered by the membranous layer of the superficial fascia inferiorly and by the inferior fascia of the urogenital diaphragm (perineal membrane) superiorly. The superficial pouch contains: (a) the *ischiocavernosus muscles* surrounding the crura of the clitoris; (b) the *bulbospongiosus muscles,* related to the vestibular bulbs; they act as constrictor muscles of the erectile tissue; and (c) the *greater vestibular glands* located on the side of the vagina under cover of the posterior part of the bulb. They secrete mucus into the vestibule. Gonococcal infections may cause swelling and cyst formation of the glands.

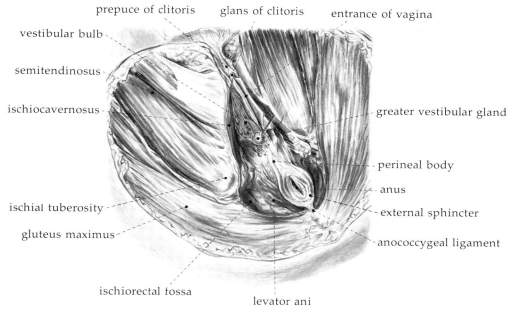

prepuce of clitoris   glans of clitoris   entrance of vagina
vestibular bulb
semitendinosus
ischiocavernosus   greater vestibular gland
                                                    perineal body
                                                    anus
                                                    external sphincter
ischial tuberosity   anococcygeal ligament
gluteus maximus
ischiorectal fossa
levator ani

A. The vestibular bulb and the greater vestibular gland.
The bulbospongiosus muscle and the superficial transverse perineal muscle have been removed.

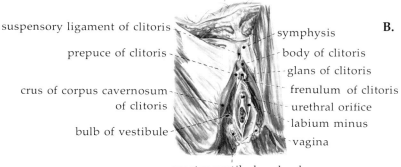

suspensory ligament of clitoris   symphysis
prepuce of clitoris   body of clitoris
                                               glans of clitoris
crus of corpus cavernosum   frenulum of clitoris
of clitoris   urethral orifice
                                               labium minus
bulb of vestibule   vagina
greater vestibular glands

B. The vestibular bulbs and the crura of the clitoris.
The bulbospongiosus and ischiocavernosus muscles have been removed.

C. The urogenital diaphragm seen from below.
The erectile tissue and related muscles have been removed.

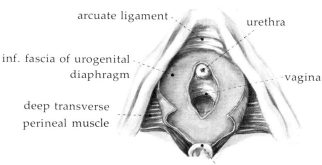

arcuate ligament   urethra
inf. fascia of urogenital
diaphragm   vagina
deep transverse
perineal muscle
perineal body

Note:

¶ The erectile tissue in the female is formed by the right and left crura (corpora cavernosa) of the clitoris and the bulbs of the vestibule. The vestibular bulbs correspond to the bulb of the penis. There are two of them because of the presence of the vagina. They unite to form the glans of the clitoris. The crura of the clitoris are comparable to the crura of the penis. The bulbs and the crura and their corresponding muscles are located in the superficial perineal pouch (see P39 *A*).

¶ After removal of the erectile tissue the inferior fascial layer (perineal membrane) of the urogenital diaphragm becomes visible. The urogenital diaphragm is a musculomembranous diaphragm, stretched across the pubic arch and attached to the ischiopubic rami. It consists of two layers of fascia with two muscles between them. The inferior fascial layer forms the lower or perineal surface, and the superior layer is derived from the pelvic fascia. The deep transverse perineal muscle, the sphincter urethrae and some muscular fibers around the vagina form the muscular component of the diaphragm. In addition, branches of the pudendal nerve and the internal pudendal artery and vein are found between the two fascial layers. In the female the diaphragm is much thinner than it is in the male. It is pierced by the urethra and the vagina.

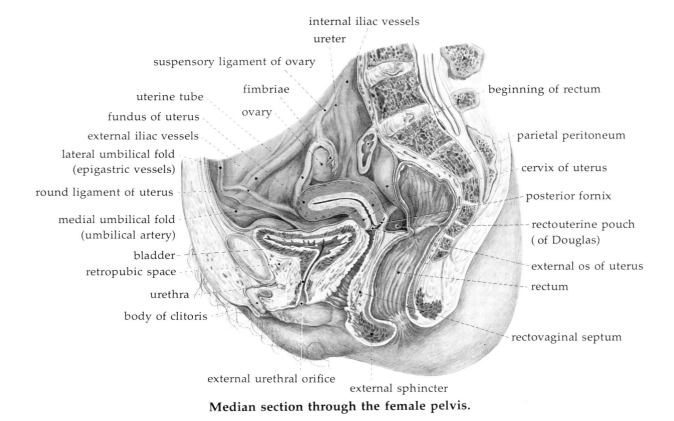

internal iliac vessels

ureter

suspensory ligament of ovary

fimbriae

uterine tube

ovary

fundus of uterus

external iliac vessels

lateral umbilical fold
(epigastric vessels)

round ligament of uterus

medial umbilical fold
(umbilical artery)

bladder

retropubic space

urethra

body of clitoris

external urethral orifice

external sphincter

beginning of rectum

parietal peritoneum

cervix of uterus

posterior fornix

rectouterine pouch
(of Douglas)

external os of uterus

rectum

rectovaginal septum

Median section through the female pelvis.

A number of important observations should be made.

¶ The peritoneum descends along the anterior abdominal wall and covers the superior surface of the bladder. Traced posteriorly it covers the anterior aspect of the body of the uterus but not the anterior aspects of the cervix and vagina. Hence, the anterior aspects of the cervix and vagina are in direct contact with the bladder. This is important because: (a) cancers of the cervix and vagina may penetrate directly into the wall of the bladder, and (b) the anterior aspect of the cervix can be reached without opening the peritoneum.

¶ The peritoneum covers entirely the fundus and posterior wall of the uterus and continues for a short distance on the posterior wall of the vagina. From there it passes onto the middle third of the rectum and covers its anterior wall. The deepest part of the peritoneal cavity is formed by the rectouterine pouch (or pouch of Douglas). Since it is in contact with the posterior fornix of the vagina, a needle can be passed through the posterior fornix into the pouch of Douglas to drain the peritoneal cavity.

¶ *Rectal examination.* If a finger is introduced through the anal canal into the rectum, the sphincters and the mucous membrane can be palpated. Anything in the lumen such as hemorrhoids, cancers or polyps can be felt. Posteriorly the pelvic surface of coccyx and the sacrum can be palpated; laterally the pelvic wall and the ischiorectal fossa may be examined for the presence of swollen lymph nodes. Anteriorly one can feel the posterior vaginal wall and the cervix. The rectouterine cavity or pouch of Douglas cannot be felt under normal conditions, but when fluid or metastases are present in the cavity they can be palpated.

¶ *Vaginal examination.* The walls of the vagina, the external orifice of the cervical part of the uterus and the fornices can be palpated. By placing the index and middle fingers of one hand in the vagina and the other hand on the abdominal wall above the symphysis and pushing downward on the uterus, an impression of the size of the uterus and ovaries can be gained. Usually the uterine tubes cannot be felt.

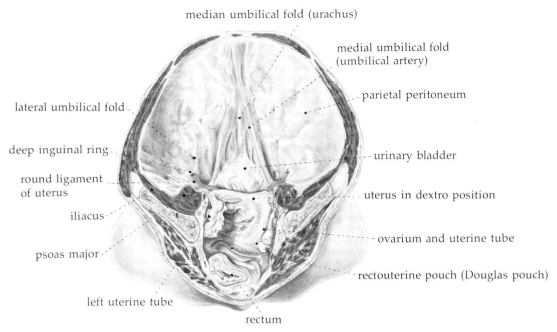

median umbilical fold (urachus)

medial umbilical fold
(umbilical artery)

parietal peritoneum

lateral umbilical fold

deep inguinal ring

urinary bladder

round ligament
of uterus

uterus in dextro position

iliacus

ovarium and uterine tube

psoas major

rectouterine pouch (Douglas pouch)

left uterine tube

rectum

Frontal section through the pelvis of a 2 month old girl.

On the posterior aspect of the anterior abdominal wall a number of folds can be seen:

¶ The *median umbilical fold* extending in the midline from the bladder to the umbilicus. This fold is caused by the remnants of the urachus, which obliterates after birth. Occasionally the connection between the bladder and the umbilicus remains open, an abnormality known as a *urachal fistula*. In such cases urine drips out of the umbilicus. If only a part of the urachus fails to obliterate, the result is a *urachal cyst* usually halfway between the bladder and the umbilicus.

¶ On each side of the bladder and coursing to the umbilicus are found the *medial umbilical folds*. They are caused by the ligamentous remnants of the umbilical arteries (see P13).

¶ An additional fold caused by the inferior epigastric vessels may be seen on each side. These folds, the *lateral umbilical ligaments*, begin on the medial side of the deep inguinal ring and course obliquely toward the rectus sheath (see A17).

¶ The *round ligaments of the uterus* also cause a fold that extends from the body of the uterus toward the deep inguinal ring. After passing through the inguinal canal, the ligaments terminate in the labia majora.

¶ Note the asymmetrical position of the uterus and the uterine tubes.

¶ After investing the posterior surface of the uterus the peritoneum passes to the middle third of the rectum, which it covers on its anterior aspect. The upper third is covered anteriorly and on both sides. At the level of S3, however, the peritoneum surrounds the rectum entirely (see P32).

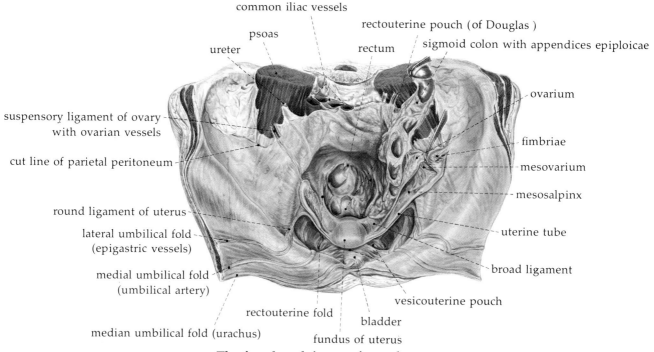

common iliac vessels

rectouterine pouch (of Douglas)

psoas

sigmoid colon with appendices epiploicae

ureter

rectum

suspensory ligament of ovary
with ovarian vessels

ovarium

cut line of parietal peritoneum

fimbriae

mesovarium

mesosalpinx

round ligament of uterus

uterine tube

lateral umbilical fold
(epigastric vessels)

broad ligament

medial umbilical fold
(umbilical artery)

vesicouterine pouch

rectouterine fold

bladder

median umbilical fold (urachus)

fundus of uterus

The female pelvis seen from above.

¶ The body and fundus of the uterus bend anteriorly and rest on the bladder. Hence, the peritoneal cavity between the bladder and the uterus, the vesicouterine pouch, cannot be seen.

¶ Note the deep rectouterine pouch (pouch of Douglas) between the posterior wall of the uterus and the rectum. Any fluid in the peritoneal cavity (blood, pus, transudate) will collect in the pouch of Douglas. Similarly, extrauterine pregnancies and metastases are often found in this space. They can be palpated through the anterior wall of the rectum.

¶ The sigmoid colon is completely surrounded by peritoneum. Note the appendices epiploicae.

¶ The ureters are found behind the peritoneum to which they are loosely attached. After coursing over the common iliac artery they enter the pelvis. Note particularly their relation to the cervix, from which they are separated by about 1.5 cm. In this area the uterine artery crosses the ureter anteriorly (see P44 B). The veins draining the bladder lie laterally and above the ureter as it reaches the bladder's posterior wall (see P45). Hence, in operating on the uterus and bladder great care must be taken to identify the ureters.

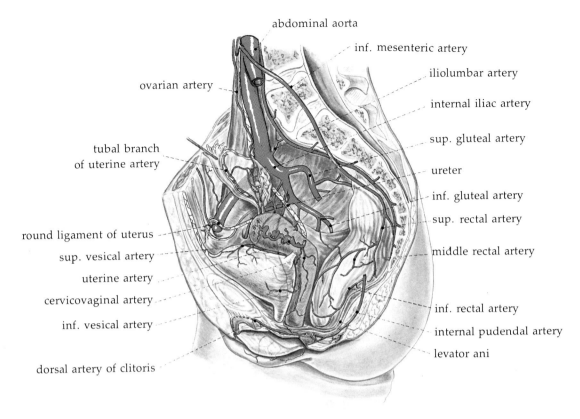

abdominal aorta

inf. mesenteric artery

iliolumbar artery

ovarian artery

internal iliac artery

sup. gluteal artery

tubal branch
of uterine artery

ureter

inf. gluteal artery

sup. rectal artery

round ligament of uterus

middle rectal artery

sup. vesical artery

uterine artery

cervicovaginal artery

inf. rectal artery

inf. vesical artery

internal pudendal artery

levator ani

dorsal artery of clitoris

A. The organs of the female pelvis and their arterial blood supply.
The peritoneum has been removed.

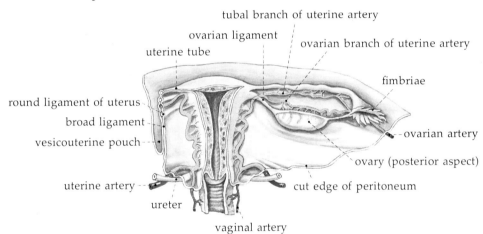

tubal branch of uterine artery

ovarian ligament

ovarian branch of uterine artery

uterine tube

fimbriae

round ligament of uterus

broad ligament

ovarian artery

vesicouterine pouch

ovary (posterior aspect)

uterine artery

cut edge of peritoneum

ureter

vaginal artery

B. The blood supply of the uterus, uterine tube and ovary (posterior view).

The branches of the internal iliac artery in the female are very similar to the branches in the male with the exception of:

¶ *The uterine artery.* It approaches the uterus from the lateral pelvic wall through the broad ligament. Just before reaching the uterus, the artery crosses the ureter near the level of the external os and about 1 or 2 cm lateral to it. Frequently the uterine artery provides a small branch to the ureter. Just after crossing anterior to the ureter it gives off the cervicovaginal artery, which supplies the posterior and anterior walls of the cervix and vagina. The main artery ascends, sending branches to the body, the fundus, the round ligament, the uterine tube and the ovary.

¶ *The ovarian artery.* This vessel, which is comparable to the testicular artery in the male, reaches the ovary by way of the suspensory ligament of the ovary. It courses subsequently between the two leaves of the mesovarium and enters the hilus of the ovary. In the mesovarium it forms anastomoses with the ovarian branch of the uterine artery.

¶ Note the close relationship between the ureter and the uterine artery.

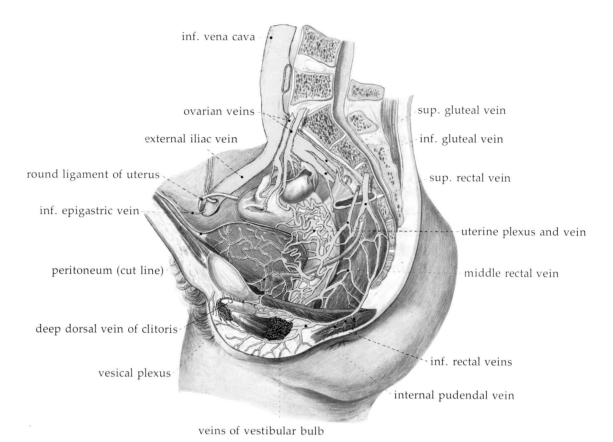

inf. vena cava

ovarian veins

external iliac vein

round ligament of uterus

inf. epigastric vein

peritoneum (cut line)

deep dorsal vein of clitoris

vesical plexus

sup. gluteal vein

inf. gluteal vein

sup. rectal vein

uterine plexus and vein

middle rectal vein

inf. rectal veins

internal pudendal vein

veins of vestibular bulb

The veins of the female pelvis.

Note:

¶ A dense venous plexus drains the uterus. Frequently the ureter is completely surrounded by veins. The uterine artery, usually single, always passes in front of and above the ureter.

¶ The ovarian veins do not enter the iliac veins but drain into the inferior vena cava on the right and the renal vein on the left, respectively.

¶ The round ligament of the uterus passes lateral to the inferior epigastric vessels at the deep inguinal ring.

¶ The venous blood from the external genital organs drains by two routes: (a) the dorsal vein of the clitoris, passing under the arcuate ligament to the vesical plexus, and (b) the internal pudendal vein.

¶ The rectal veins form a plexus within the wall of the rectum. (See the draining of the portal and caval systems in A29.)

A. Median section through the female pelvis.
Note the position of the uterus and its peritoneal covering.

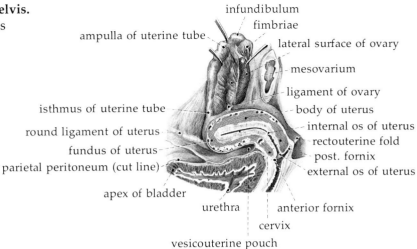

infundibulum
fimbriae
ampulla of uterine tube
lateral surface of ovary
mesovarium
ligament of ovary
isthmus of uterine tube
body of uterus
internal os of uterus
round ligament of uterus
rectouterine fold
fundus of uterus
post. fornix
parietal peritoneum (cut line)
external os of uterus
apex of bladder
urethra   anterior fornix
cervix
vesicouterine pouch

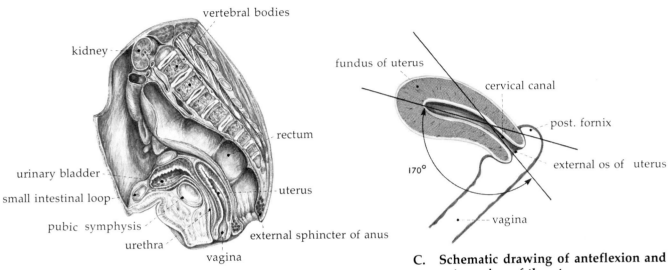

vertebral bodies
kidney
fundus of uterus
cervical canal
rectum
post. fornix
urinary bladder
170°   external os of uterus
small intestinal loop
uterus
pubic symphysis
vagina
urethra
external sphincter of anus
vagina

B. Position of the uterus in a neonate.

C. Schematic drawing of anteflexion and anteversion of the uterus.

- The position of the uterus is important and should be studied carefully. Normally the long axis of the body of the uterus is bent forward in relation to the long axis of the cervix at an angle of about 170 degrees. This position is called the *anteflexion of the uterus*. The long axis of the cervix forms an angle of about 90 degrees with the long axis of the vagina. This position is referred to as the *anteversion of the uterus.*

- In the *neonate* the positions of the bladder and the uterus are quite different. The bladder lies above the symphysis behind the anterior abdominal wall; the uterus is very immature and lies deep in the pelvis. It does not have the anteflexion and anteversion characteristic of the adult.

- The close relation between the anterior wall of the cervix and vagina and the posterior wall of the bladder is important. Cancers of the cervix frequently penetrate directly into the wall of the bladder.

- The body of the uterus is sometimes bent backward on the cervix (retroflexion) and the cervix on the vagina (retroversion). In extreme cases the fundus may lie in the rectouterine pouch. This position frequently causes a prolonged and painful menstrual bleeding and sometimes infertility.

- The proximity of the posterior fornix to the rectouterine pouch may be helpful in draining the peritoneal cavity. Sometimes, however, nonsterile instruments are inadvertently pushed through the wall of the posterior fornix into the peritoneal cavity instead of into the cervix. The result may be a fatal peritonitis.

- Cancers of the cervix may grow not only directly into the wall of the bladder but also into the anterior wall of the rectum. Similarly, fistulas between the cervix and vagina and between the bladder and rectum are not uncommon.

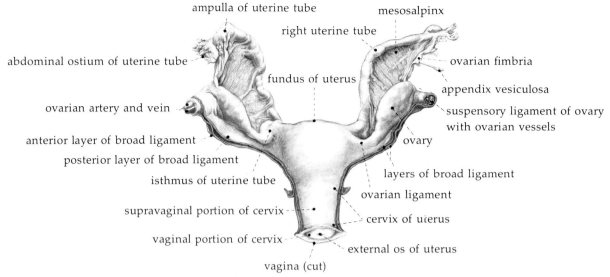

ampulla of uterine tube
mesosalpinx
right uterine tube
abdominal ostium of uterine tube
ovarian fimbria
fundus of uterus
appendix vesiculosa
ovarian artery and vein
suspensory ligament of ovary
with ovarian vessels
anterior layer of broad ligament
ovary
posterior layer of broad ligament
layers of broad ligament
isthmus of uterine tube
ovarian ligament
supravaginal portion of cervix
cervix of uterus
vaginal portion of cervix
external os of uterus
vagina (cut)

A. Posterior view of the female reproductive organs.

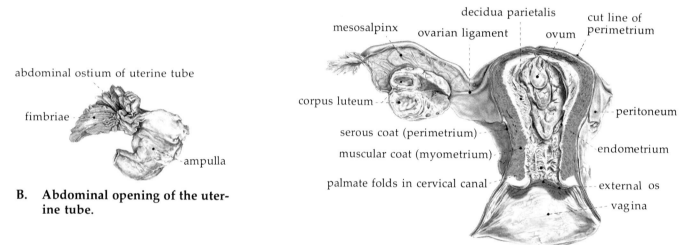

abdominal ostium of uterine tube

fimbriae

ampulla

B. Abdominal opening of the uterine tube.

decidua parietalis
cut line of
mesosalpinx   ovarian ligament   ovum   perimetrium

corpus luteum
peritoneum
serous coat (perimetrium)
muscular coat (myometrium)
endometrium
palmate folds in cervical canal
external os
vagina

C. Pregnant uterus after removal of the posterior wall.
The ovary has been cut to show the corpus luteum.

Note:

¶   The *broad ligament* of the uterus is the double layered fold of peritoneum extending
from the lateral margin of the uterus to the lateral pelvic wall. It hangs down from the
uterine tube as a double sheath of peritoneum. Inferiorly the two layers separate to
cover the pelvic floor. Two secondary ligaments are recognized: (a) the *mesosalpinx,*
the portion of the broad ligament that lies immediately below the uterine tube and
extends from the tube to the ovary, and (b) the *mesovarium,* which extends from the
ovary to the broad ligament.

¶   Between the two layers of the broad ligament are found: (a) the round ligament of
the uterus, (b) the ovarian ligament, (c) the uterine and ovarian vessels, (d) the lymph
nodes and (e) the epoophoron and paroophoron (see P48 *B*). Infections and cancers of
the uterus spread easily into the loose connective tissue of the broad ligament (see
P51 *A*).

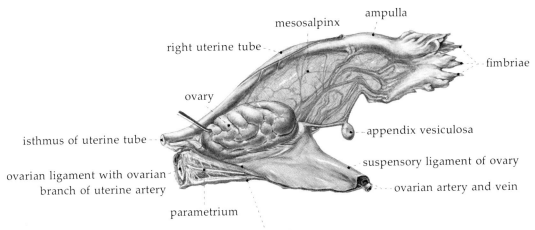

A. Posterior view of the right uterine tube and ovary.
Note the broad ligament.

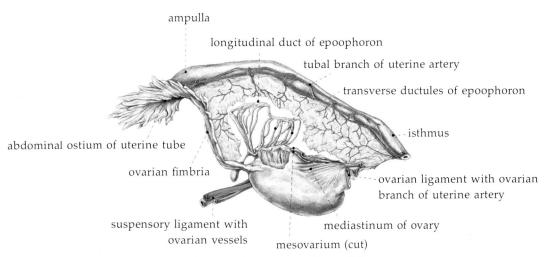

B. The left epoophoron and hilus of the ovary.

Note:

Small transverse ducts and a portion of a longitudinal duct are sometimes found between the two layers of the mesosalpinx. These structures are remnants of the excretory tubules of the mesonephros and of the original longitudinal mesonephric duct. It is not uncommon for these ductules to become cystic and cause complaints. The paroophoron and the appendix vesiculosa are similarly constituted. Sometimes remnants of the longitudinal duct are found along the lateral wall of the uterus and the vagina. These structures, known as Gärtner's cysts, may become large and carcinomatous.

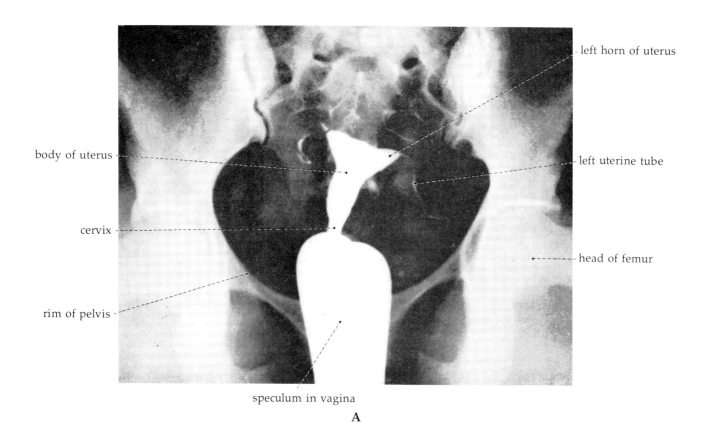

body of uterus

cervix

rim of pelvis

left horn of uterus

left uterine tube

head of femur

speculum in vagina

A

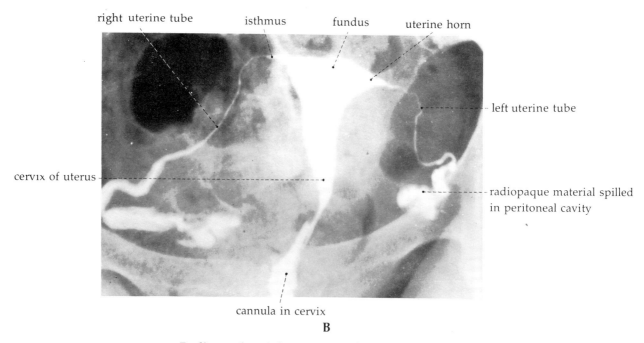

right uterine tube   isthmus   fundus   uterine horn

cervix of uterus

left uterine tube

radiopaque material spilled
in peritoneal cavity

cannula in cervix

B

Radiographs of the uterus and the uterine tubes.
(From Meschan, I.: An Atlas of Anatomy Basic to Radiology. Philadelphia, W. B. Saunders
Co., 1975.)

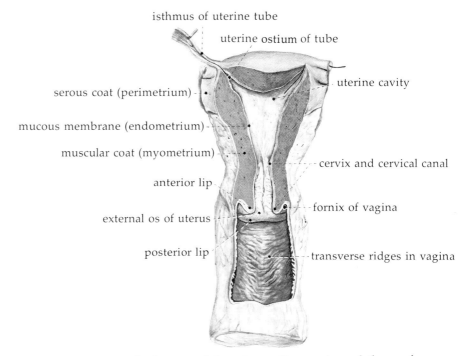

isthmus of uterine tube

uterine ostium of tube

uterine cavity

serous coat (perimetrium)

mucous membrane (endometrium)

muscular coat (myometrium)

cervix and cervical canal

anterior lip

external os of uterus

fornix of vagina

posterior lip

transverse ridges in vagina

A. The lumen of the uterus, the cervix and the vagina.

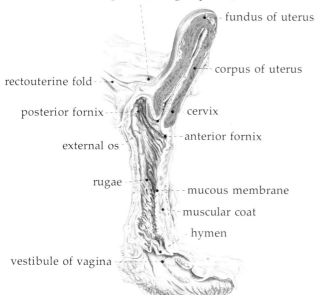

rectouterine pouch (Douglas pouch)

fundus of uterus

corpus of uterus

rectouterine fold

posterior fornix

cervix

external os

anterior fornix

rugae

mucous membrane

muscular coat

hymen

vestibule of vagina

B. Median section through the vagina and uterus.
Note the relation of the posterior fornix to the rectouterine pouch.

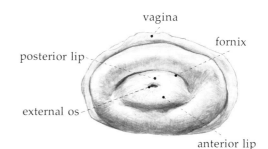

vagina

fornix

posterior lip

external os

anterior lip

C. The external os of the uterus in a nulliparous woman.

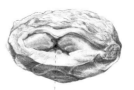

external os

D. The external os of the uterus in a multiparous woman.

Inspection and palpation of the external os are important.

¶ In a nulliparous woman the external os is round and smooth; in a multiparous woman it is usually highly irregular as a result of small ruptures that occur during childbirth.

¶ The external os of the uterus should be inspected regularly. It is a frequent site of ulcerations and cancers. Very early detection of a cancer at the external os of the uterus may save the patient's life.

¶ During pregnancy the external os of the uterus remains closed until the very end. Just before childbirth it begins to relax and opens slowly until it attains a diameter of about 10 cm. Progress in delivery can be easily judged by determining the speed at which the os opens.

¶ The external os usually contains a mucous plug. It is formed by secretions of the cervix and serves as a protective mechanism against uterine infections spreading from the vagina.

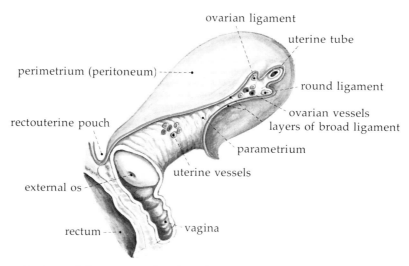

A. Lateral view of the uterus showing the attachment area of the broad ligament.

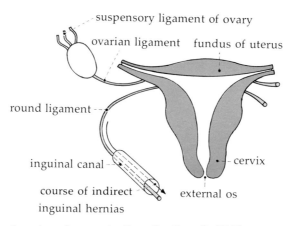

B. Schematic drawing demonstrating the "genital" ligaments of the uterus.

Note:

¶ The broad ligament is a double fold of peritoneum, extending from the lateral wall of the uterus to the lateral wall of the pelvis. Between the two leaves is found loose connective tissue through which the arteries, veins, lymph vessels and ligaments course to and from the uterus. When the uterus is removed surgically great care should be taken to ligate the vessels, particularly since the venous plexus may be dense (remember the ureter!).

¶ Three ligaments are found in the connective tissue of the broad ligament: (a) the suspensory ligament of the ovary, (b) the ovarian ligament, and (c) the round ligament of the uterus. Together they can be classified as the "genital" ligaments. The suspensory ligament of the ovary is formed from the embryologic superior genital ligament, and the other two arise from the embryologic inferior genital ligament. The ovarian ligament and the round ligament of the uterus are comparable to the gubernaculum testis (Hunter) in the male.

¶ The round ligament passes from the superolateral angle of the uterus to the deep inguinal ring and subsequently through the inguinal canal, terminating in the labia majora as fibrous strands. It contains smooth muscle fibers. During pregnancy it may become as thick as the little finger, and at the end of pregnancy it can sometimes be felt through the abdominal wall. The ligament is thought to play a role in keeping the uterus in its anteflexed position.

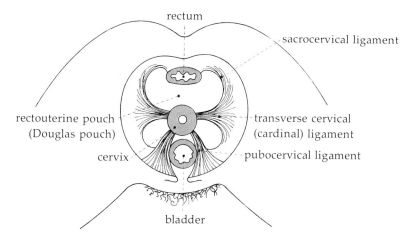

A. The cervical ligaments seen from above.

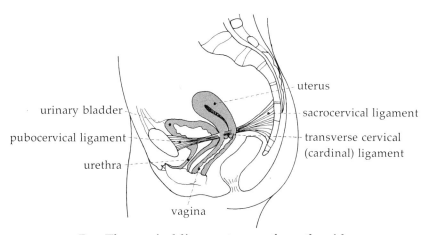

B. The cervical ligaments seen from the side.

The pubocervical, sacrocervical and particularly the transverse cervical (cardinal) ligaments are the most important ligaments in keeping the uterus in position and preventing the prolapse of the uterus and vagina.

⁋ The *lateral cervical (cardinal) ligament* forms the base of the parametrium and is a condensation of the connective tissue. It also strengthens the pelvic fascia of the levator ani muscle. The ligaments attach on each side to the cervix and upper part of the vagina and radiate to the lateral pelvic wall. They are considered the most important ligaments in preventing prolapse of the uterus.

⁋ The *sacrocervical ligaments*, two firm fibromuscular bands, pass from the lower part of the sacrum to the sides of the cervix and vagina. They course immediately under the peritoneum and form two folds, the rectouterine folds, one on each side of the rectouterine pouch. The sacrocervical ligaments keep the cervix up and back; if they fail to function, the cervix is displaced downward and forward. This permits a displacement of the body of the uterus so that the axes of the uterus and the vagina coincide. Intra-abdominal pressure then forces the cervix and the uterus into the vagina.

⁋ The *pubocervical ligaments* attach to the anterior aspect of the cervix and pass on each side of the neck of the bladder toward the posterior surface of the pubic bone.

During childbirth the ligaments are frequently damaged. Prolapse of the uterus may occur as a result. Since the vagina is supported by the same structures, prolapse of the uterus is usually accompanied by prolapse of the vagina.

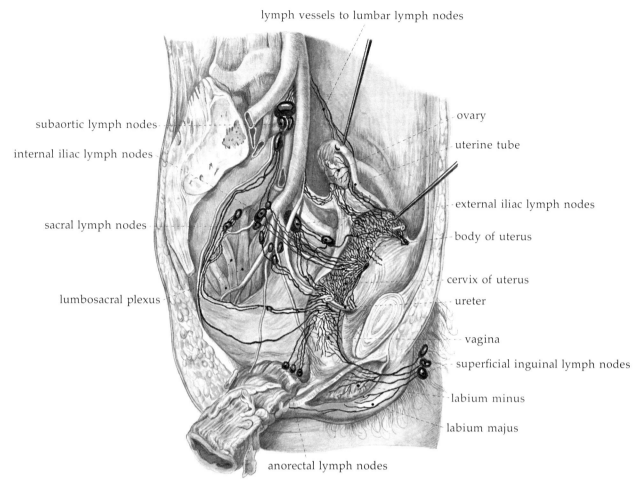

lymph vessels to lumbar lymph nodes

subaortic lymph nodes

internal iliac lymph nodes

sacral lymph nodes

lumbosacral plexus

ovary

uterine tube

external iliac lymph nodes

body of uterus

cervix of uterus

ureter

vagina

superficial inguinal lymph nodes

labium minus

labium majus

anorectal lymph nodes

Lymphatic drainage of the female reproductive system.

The lymph drainage of the female reproductive organs is very important because cancers of the uterus metastasize by way of the lymph vessels.

¶ The lymph vessels of the *cervix*, the most frequently affected part of the uterus, drain into the internal and external iliac lymph nodes. They pass from the lateral aspect of the uterus through the parametrium. Therefore, in patients with cancer of the cervix (and also cancer of the body of the uterus) the parametrium must be removed as far laterally as possible (posing a great danger to the ureter).

¶ The lymph from the *body of the uterus* follows the same routes as that from the cervix. Some lymph channels follow the round ligament through the inguinal canal and drain into the superficial inguinal lymph nodes.

¶ The lymph vessels from the *fundus*, the *uterine tube* and the *ovary* follow the ovarian vein and drain into the para-aortic nodes at the level of the first lumbar vertebra.

¶ Lymph from the *vagina* drains in two directions: (a) that from the lower portion and the tissues of the vulva drains into the superficial inguinal lymph nodes; (b) lymph from the middle and upper portions drains into the sacral, internal and external iliac lymph nodes.

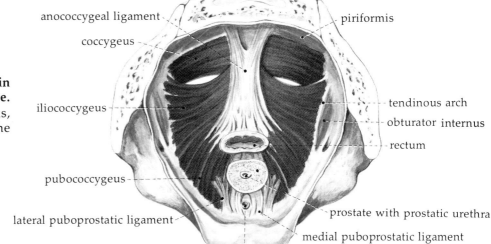

anococcygeal ligament
coccygeus
piriformis

A. The pelvic diaphragm in the male seen from above.
Note the pubococcygeus, the iliococcygeus and the coccygeus muscles.

iliococcygeus
tendinous arch
obturator internus
rectum

pubococcygeus
lateral puboprostatic ligament
prostate with prostatic urethra
medial puboprostatic ligament

deep dorsal vein of penis

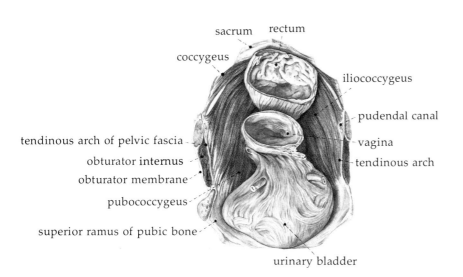

sacrum   rectum
coccygeus
iliococcygeus
pudendal canal
tendinous arch of pelvic fascia
obturator internus
vagina
obturator membrane
tendinous arch
pubococcygeus
superior ramus of pubic bone

B. The pelvic diaphragm in the female seen from above.
The rectum and vagina have been cut, the bladder has been left intact.

urinary bladder

The pelvic diaphragm is a fibromuscular sheet which forms the floor of the pelvis. It supports the pelvic viscera and prevents the prolapse of the pelvic organs that might result from the downward thrust of the intra-abdominal pressure. The diaphragm consists on each side of two muscles: the levator ani and the coccygeus.

¶ The *levator ani*. This muscle has two parts: the *pubococcygeus* and the *iliococcygeus*. The pubococcygeus, the more important of the two, arises from the back of the pubic bone just lateral of the symphysis and from the anterior part of the tendinous arch of the pelvic fascia. The fibers run on each side of the anal canal and meet each other behind the canal. These fibers form the *puborectalis* muscle and are part of the sphincter mechanism of the anus. The most anterior fibers of the pubococcygeus in the male course backward across the side of the prostate to end in the perineal body. They constitute the *levator of the prostate*. In the female similar fibers course on each side of the vagina, thus forming an additional *sphincter of the vagina.*

The iliococcygeus arises from the ischial spine and the posterior part of the tendinous arch of the pelvic fascia. The fibers are attached to the coccyx and the median raphe. Its fibers have no relation to the organs.

¶ The *coccygeus*. This muscle fills the space between the ischial spine and the coccyx. It helps to complete the pelvic diaphragm posteriorly.

Anteriorly the space between the prostate and the bladder is filled by the puboprostatic (*A*) and pubovesical ligaments (not shown).

199

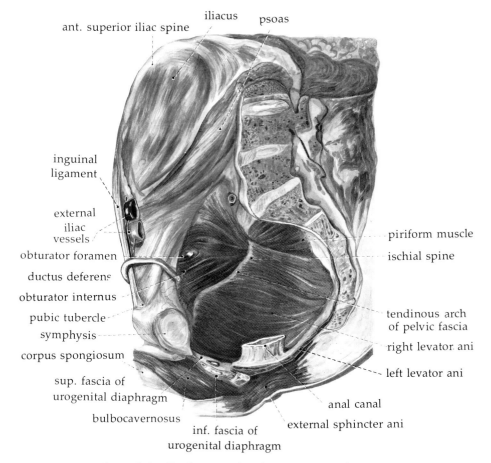

ant. superior iliac spine

iliacus

psoas

inguinal ligament

external iliac vessels

obturator foramen

ductus deferens

obturator internus

pubic tubercle

symphysis

corpus spongiosum

sup. fascia of urogenital diaphragm

bulbocavernosus

inf. fascia of urogenital diaphragm

piriform muscle

ischial spine

tendinous arch of pelvic fascia

right levator ani

left levator ani

anal canal

external sphincter ani

A.   The pelvic diaphragm after hemisection of the pelvis.

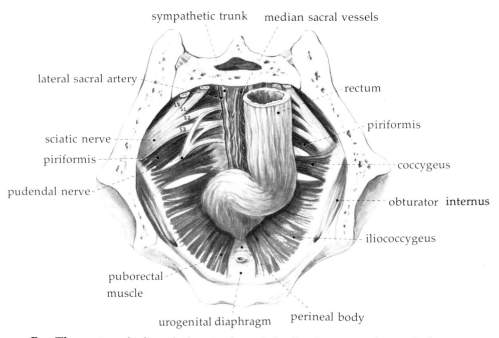

sympathetic trunk

median sacral vessels

lateral sacral artery

sciatic nerve

piriformis

pudendal nerve

puborectal muscle

urogenital diaphragm

perineal body

rectum

piriformis

coccygeus

obturator internus

iliococcygeus

B.   The rectum in its relation to the pelvic diaphragm and sacral plexus.

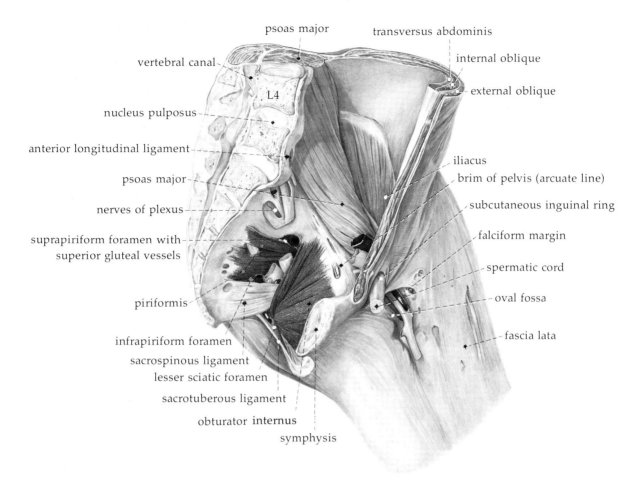

psoas major

transversus abdominis

vertebral canal

internal oblique

external oblique

L4

iliacus

nucleus pulposus

brim of pelvis (arcuate line)

anterior longitudinal ligament

subcutaneous inguinal ring

psoas major

nerves of plexus

falciform margin

suprapiriform foramen with
superior gluteal vessels

spermatic cord

oval fossa

piriformis

fascia lata

infrapiriform foramen

sacrospinous ligament

lesser sciatic foramen

sacrotuberous ligament

obturator internus

symphysis

Hemisection of the pelvis after removal of the pelvic diaphragm.
Note the piriform and internal obturator muscles.

Note the following:

❡ The piriform muscle leaves the pelvis through the greater sciatic foramen; the obturator internus leaves through the lesser sciatic foramen.

❡ Through the suprapiriform foramen pass the superior gluteal artery, vein and nerve. Through the infrapiriform foramen pass (a) the inferior gluteal artery, vein and nerve; (b) the internal pudendal artery and vein; (c) the pudendal nerve; (d) the sciatic nerve; (e) the posterior cutaneous femoral nerve.

❡ The pudendal nerve and internal pudendal artery and vein loop around the sciatic spine and then pass into the perineal region through the lesser sciatic foramen.

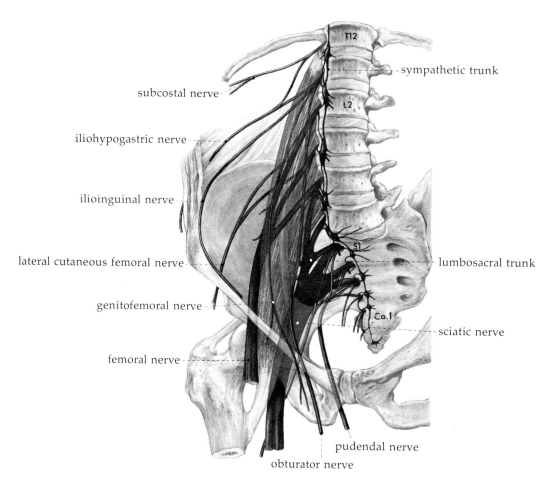

subcostal nerve

iliohypogastric nerve

ilioinguinal nerve

lateral cutaneous femoral nerve

genitofemoral nerve

femoral nerve

T12

L2

S1

Co.1

sympathetic trunk

lumbosacral trunk

sciatic nerve

pudendal nerve

obturator nerve

The lumbosacral plexus and its relation to the psoas major.
Note the sympathetic trunk; it is frequently highly irregular.

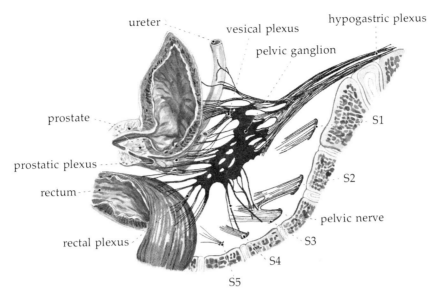

A. The innervation of the bladder and rectum in the male.

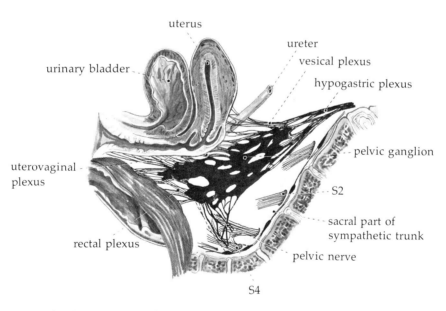

B. The innervation of the bladder, uterus and rectum in the female.

¶ The parasympathetic innervation of the pelvic organs is formed by the preganglionic fibers of S2, S3 and S4. They form the splanchnic pelvic nerves, which reach the pelvic plexuses and are subsequently distributed to the pelvic viscera. Some of the fibers supply the colon from the left colic flexure to the upper half of the anal canal. The preganglionic fibers synapse with postganglionic neurons located in the pelvic plexuses or in the walls of the organs.

¶ The pelvic part of the sympathetic trunk forms the hypogastric plexus. This plexus lies in the retroperitoneal tissue in front of the promontory and between the common iliac arteries. As the branches of the hypogastric plexus enter the pelvis, they form the right and left pelvic plexuses. Branches from these plexuses extend to the pelvic organs.

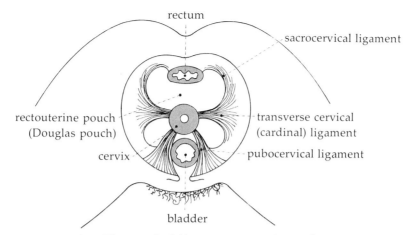

rectum

sacrocervical ligament

rectouterine pouch (Douglas pouch)

transverse cervical (cardinal) ligament

cervix

pubocervical ligament

bladder

A. The cervical ligaments seen from above.

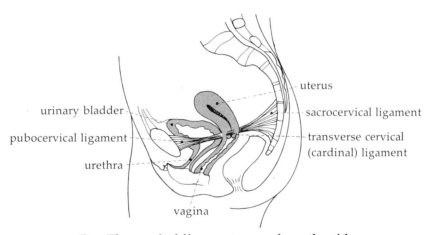

uterus

urinary bladder

sacrocervical ligament

pubocervical ligament

transverse cervical (cardinal) ligament

urethra

vagina

B. The cervical ligaments seen from the side.

The pubocervical, sacrocervical and particularly the transverse cervical (cardinal) ligaments are the most important ligaments in keeping the uterus in position and preventing the prolapse of the uterus and vagina.

¶   The *lateral cervical (cardinal) ligament* forms the base of the parametrium and is a condensation of the connective tissue. It also strengthens the pelvic fascia of the levator ani muscle. The ligaments attach on each side to the cervix and upper part of the vagina and radiate to the lateral pelvic wall. They are considered the most important ligaments in preventing prolapse of the uterus.

¶   The *sacrocervical ligaments*, two firm fibromuscular bands, pass from the lower part of the sacrum to the sides of the cervix and vagina. They course immediately under the peritoneum and form two folds, the rectouterine folds, one on each side of the rectouterine pouch. The sacrocervical ligaments keep the cervix up and back; if they fail to function, the cervix is displaced downward and forward. This permits a displacement of the body of the uterus so that the axes of the uterus and the vagina coincide. Intra-abdominal pressure then forces the cervix and the uterus into the vagina.

¶   The *pubocervical ligaments* attach to the anterior aspect of the cervix and pass on each side of the neck of the bladder toward the posterior surface of the pubic bone.

During childbirth the ligaments are frequently damaged. Prolapse of the uterus may occur as a result. Since the vagina is supported by the same structures, prolapse of the uterus is usually accompanied by prolapse of the vagina.

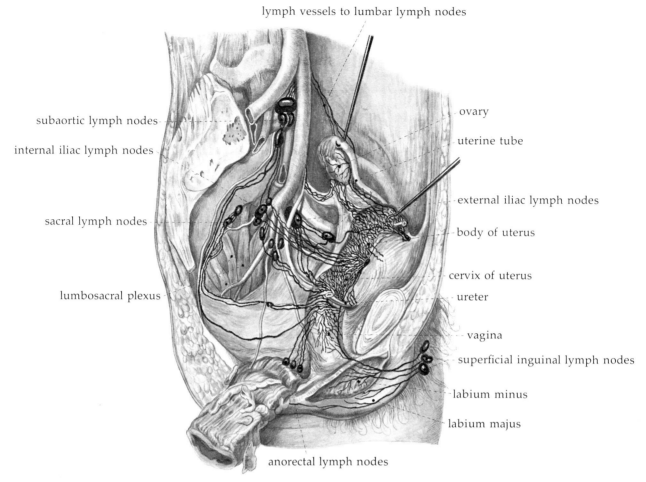

lymph vessels to lumbar lymph nodes

subaortic lymph nodes

internal iliac lymph nodes

sacral lymph nodes

lumbosacral plexus

ovary

uterine tube

external iliac lymph nodes

body of uterus

cervix of uterus

ureter

vagina

superficial inguinal lymph nodes

labium minus

labium majus

anorectal lymph nodes

Lymphatic drainage of the female reproductive system.

The lymph drainage of the female reproductive organs is very important because cancers of the uterus metastasize by way of the lymph vessels.

¶ The lymph vessels of the *cervix*, the most frequently affected part of the uterus, drain into the internal and external iliac lymph nodes. They pass from the lateral aspect of the uterus through the parametrium. Therefore, in patients with cancer of the cervix (and also cancer of the body of the uterus) the parametrium must be removed as far laterally as possible (posing a great danger to the ureter).

¶ The lymph from the *body of the uterus* follows the same routes as that from the cervix. Some lymph channels follow the round ligament through the inguinal canal and drain into the superficial inguinal lymph nodes.

¶ The lymph vessels from the *fundus*, the *uterine tube* and the *ovary* follow the ovarian vein and drain into the para-aortic nodes at the level of the first lumbar vertebra.

¶ Lymph from the *vagina* drains in two directions: (a) that from the lower portion and the tissues of the vulva drains into the superficial inguinal lymph nodes; (b) lymph from the middle and upper portions drains into the sacral, internal and external iliac lymph nodes.

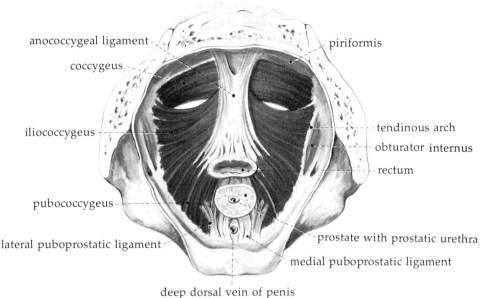

anococcygeal ligament

coccygeus

piriformis

A. The pelvic diaphragm in the male seen from above.
Note the pubococcygeus, the iliococcygeus and the coccygeus muscles.

iliococcygeus

tendinous arch

obturator internus

rectum

pubococcygeus

lateral puboprostatic ligament

prostate with prostatic urethra

medial puboprostatic ligament

deep dorsal vein of penis

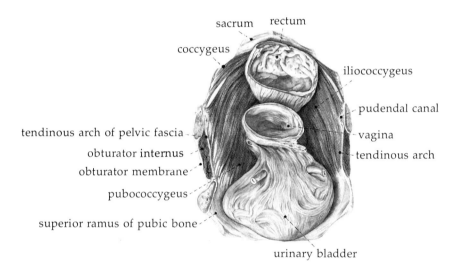

sacrum   rectum

coccygeus

iliococcygeus

pudendal canal

tendinous arch of pelvic fascia

obturator internus

vagina

obturator membrane

tendinous arch

pubococcygeus

superior ramus of pubic bone

urinary bladder

B. The pelvic diaphragm in the female seen from above.
The rectum and vagina have been cut, the bladder has been left intact.

The pelvic diaphragm is a fibromuscular sheet which forms the floor of the pelvis. It supports the pelvic viscera and prevents the prolapse of the pelvic organs that might result from the downward thrust of the intra-abdominal pressure. The diaphragm consists on each side of two muscles: the levator ani and the coccygeus.

¶ The *levator ani.* This muscle has two parts: the *pubococcygeus* and the *iliococcygeus.* The pubococcygeus, the more important of the two, arises from the back of the pubic bone just lateral of the symphysis and from the anterior part of the tendinous arch of the pelvic fascia. The fibers run on each side of the anal canal and meet each other behind the canal. These fibers form the *puborectalis* muscle and are part of the sphincter mechanism of the anus. The most anterior fibers of the pubococcygeus in the male course backward across the side of the prostate to end in the perineal body. They constitute the *levator of the prostate.* In the female similar fibers course on each side of the vagina, thus forming an additional *sphincter of the vagina.*

The iliococcygeus arises from the ischial spine and the posterior part of the tendinous arch of the pelvic fascia. The fibers are attached to the coccyx and the median raphe. Its fibers have no relation to the organs.

¶ The *coccygeus.* This muscle fills the space between the ischial spine and the coccyx. It helps to complete the pelvic diaphragm posteriorly.

Anteriorly the space between the prostate and the bladder is filled by the puboprostatic (*A*) and pubovesical ligaments (not shown).

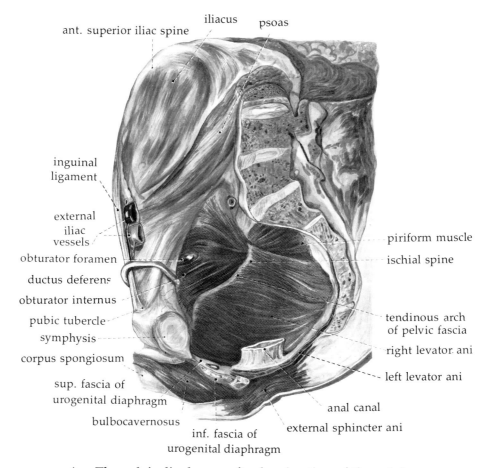

ant. superior iliac spine
iliacus
psoas

inguinal ligament

external iliac vessels

obturator foramen

ductus deferens

obturator internus

pubic tubercle

symphysis

corpus spongiosum

sup. fascia of urogenital diaphragm

bulbocavernosus

inf. fascia of urogenital diaphragm

piriform muscle

ischial spine

tendinous arch of pelvic fascia

right levator ani

left levator ani

anal canal

external sphincter ani

A. The pelvic diaphragm after hemisection of the pelvis.

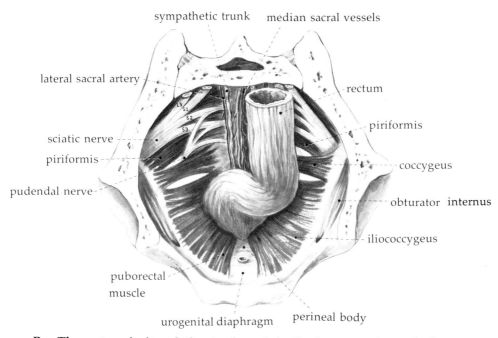

sympathetic trunk
median sacral vessels

lateral sacral artery

sciatic nerve

piriformis

pudendal nerve

puborectal muscle

urogenital diaphragm

perineal body

rectum

piriformis

coccygeus

obturator internus

iliococcygeus

B. The rectum in its relation to the pelvic diaphragm and sacral plexus.

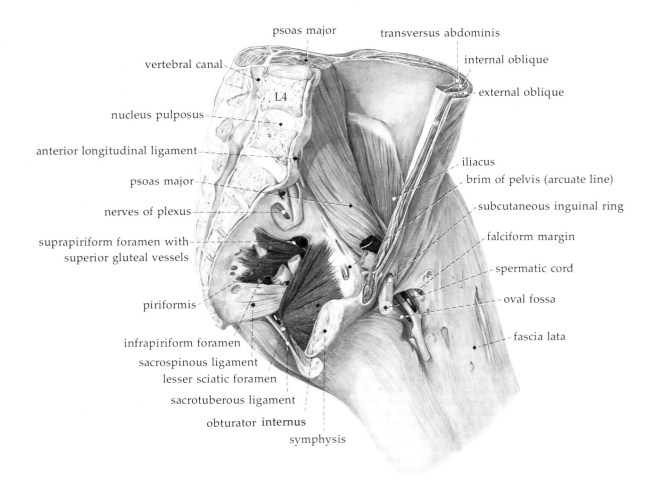

psoas major

transversus abdominis

vertebral canal

internal oblique

L4

external oblique

nucleus pulposus

iliacus

anterior longitudinal ligament

brim of pelvis (arcuate line)

psoas major

subcutaneous inguinal ring

nerves of plexus

falciform margin

suprapiriform foramen with
superior gluteal vessels

spermatic cord

oval fossa

piriformis

fascia lata

infrapiriform foramen

sacrospinous ligament

lesser sciatic foramen

sacrotuberous ligament

obturator internus

symphysis

Hemisection of the pelvis after removal of the pelvic diaphragm.
Note the piriform and internal obturator muscles.

Note the following:

⁋ The piriform muscle leaves the pelvis through the greater sciatic foramen; the obturator internus leaves through the lesser sciatic foramen.

⁋ Through the suprapiriform foramen pass the superior gluteal artery, vein and nerve. Through the infrapiriform foramen pass (a) the inferior gluteal artery, vein and nerve; (b) the internal pudendal artery and vein; (c) the pudendal nerve; (d) the sciatic nerve; (e) the posterior cutaneous femoral nerve.

⁋ The pudendal nerve and internal pudendal artery and vein loop around the sciatic spine and then pass into the perineal region through the lesser sciatic foramen.

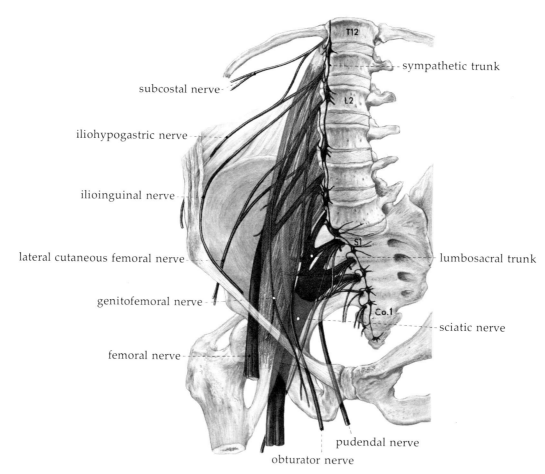

subcostal nerve

iliohypogastric nerve

ilioinguinal nerve

lateral cutaneous femoral nerve

genitofemoral nerve

femoral nerve

obturator nerve

pudendal nerve

sympathetic trunk

T12

L2

S1

Co.1

lumbosacral trunk

sciatic nerve

The lumbosacral plexus and its relation to the psoas major.
Note the sympathetic trunk; it is frequently highly irregular.

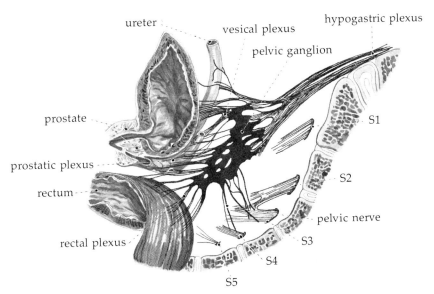

A. The innervation of the bladder and rectum in the male.

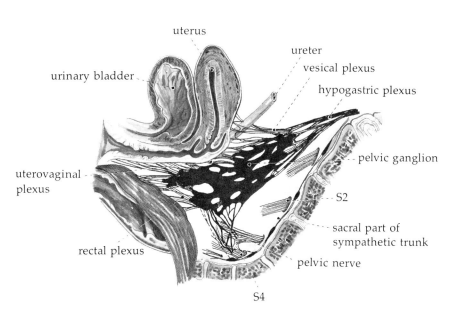

B. The innervation of the bladder, uterus and rectum in the female.

¶ The parasympathetic innervation of the pelvic organs is formed by the preganglionic fibers of S2, S3 and S4. They form the splanchnic pelvic nerves, which reach the pelvic plexuses and are subsequently distributed to the pelvic viscera. Some of the fibers supply the colon from the left colic flexure to the upper half of the anal canal. The preganglionic fibers synapse with postganglionic neurons located in the pelvic plexuses or in the walls of the organs.

¶ The pelvic part of the sympathetic trunk forms the hypogastric plexus. This plexus lies in the retroperitoneal tissue in front of the promontory and between the common iliac arteries. As the branches of the hypogastric plexus enter the pelvis, they form the right and left pelvic plexuses. Branches from these plexuses extend to the pelvic organs.

UPPER LIMB

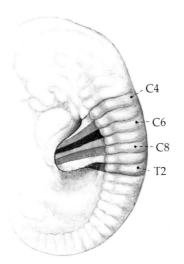

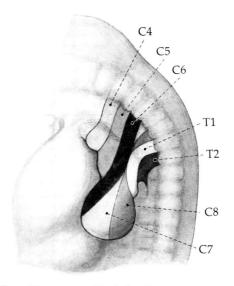

A. The upper limb bud at 5 weeks.   **B. The upper limb bud at 6 weeks.**

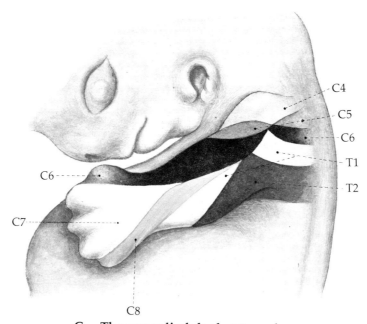

C. The upper limb bud at 7 weeks.

At the beginning of the fifth week of development, the upper limb buds appear as flattened paddles. They lie opposite the lower five cervical and the upper two thoracic segments. It is important to remember this because the nerves innervating the muscles and skin initially have a segmental character.

The segmentally organized spinal nerves penetrate into the limbs as soon as the buds are formed. At first they enter with isolated dorsal and ventral branches. Soon, however, the branches unite to form large dorsal and ventral nerves. Similarly, the muscle components fuse, and most muscles in the arm are derived from several segments. Although the original segmental pattern changes with growth of the limbs, an orderly sequence can still be recognized in the adult, particularly in the sensory innervation (see UL2 *B* and *C*).

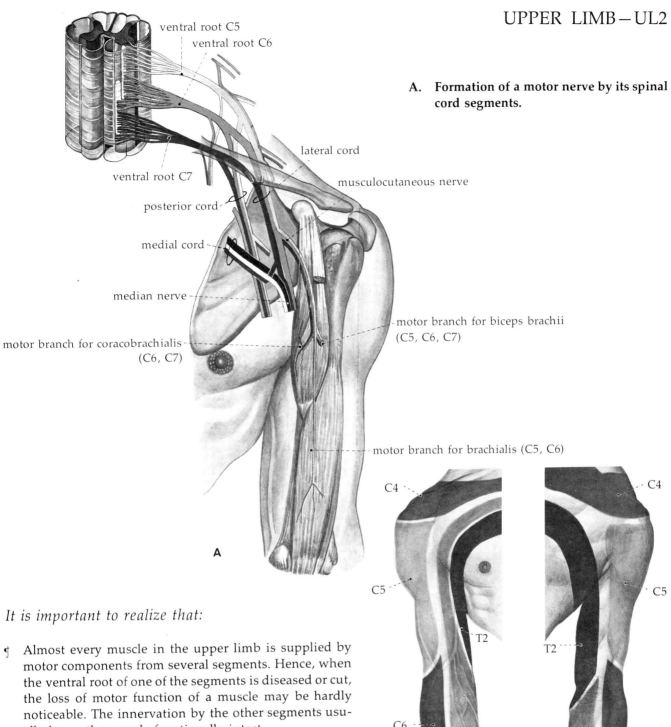

ventral root C5
ventral root C6
ventral root C7
lateral cord
musculocutaneous nerve
posterior cord
medial cord
median nerve
motor branch for coracobrachialis (C6, C7)
motor branch for biceps brachii (C5, C6, C7)
motor branch for brachialis (C5, C6)

A

A. Formation of a motor nerve by its spinal cord segments.

It is important to realize that:

❡ Almost every muscle in the upper limb is supplied by motor components from several segments. Hence, when the ventral root of one of the segments is diseased or cut, the loss of motor function of a muscle may be hardly noticeable. The innervation by the other segments usually keeps the muscle functionally intact.

❡ If the dorsal sensory root of one of the segments is diseased or cut, a large area of skin will be affected. In some areas of the body considerable overlapping of segmentally innervated areas exists, but in the upper limb the overlapping of the dermatomes (segmentally innervated areas) is small. Hence, if the dorsal root of one of the segments is damaged, a distinct area of skin loses its sensory innervation.

❡ In diseases that affect the motor roots (poliomyelitis) or the sensory roots (syphilis), paralysis of the muscles and and sensory deprivation usually extend over large areas. Gunshot wounds or fractures of a vertebra are more likely to be the cause of restricted segmental lesions.

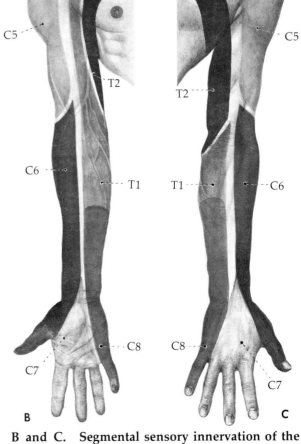

B and C. Segmental sensory innervation of the right upper limb.

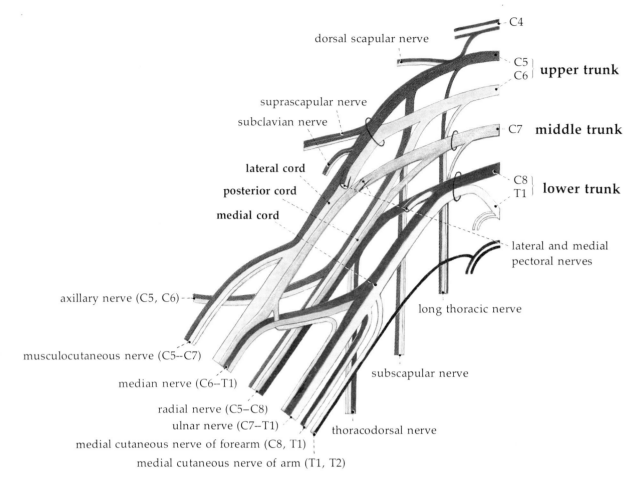

Schematic drawing of the right brachial plexus.

Before starting the dissection it is useful to study the origin and composition of the brachial plexus. The main nerve components of the upper limb arise from four cervical (C5 to C8) and one thoracic segment (T1). The contributions from C4 and T2 are variable. The ventral rami of these segments form the brachial plexus; the dorsal rami are small and innervate the skin and small muscles of the back.

The segmental character of the ventral rami is lost by fusion, intermingling and subdivision.

¶ The ventral rami of C5 and C6 unite to form the *upper trunk*; the ventral ramus of C7 forms the *middle trunk*; those of C8 and T1 form the *lower trunk*. The trunks are found in the neck above the clavicle.

¶ Each trunk divides into anterior and posterior divisions. The posterior divisions of all three trunks form the *posterior cord*. The anterior divisions of the upper and middle trunks form the *lateral cord*; those of the lower trunk form the *medial cord*.

¶ In the axillary region, the posterior cord forms two important nerves: the *radial nerve* and the *axillary (circumflex) nerve*. After further intermingling the lateral cord gives rise to: the *musculocutaneous nerve* and the *median nerve*. From the medial cord arise: the *ulnar nerve* and the *medial cutaneous nerves of the arm and forearm*.

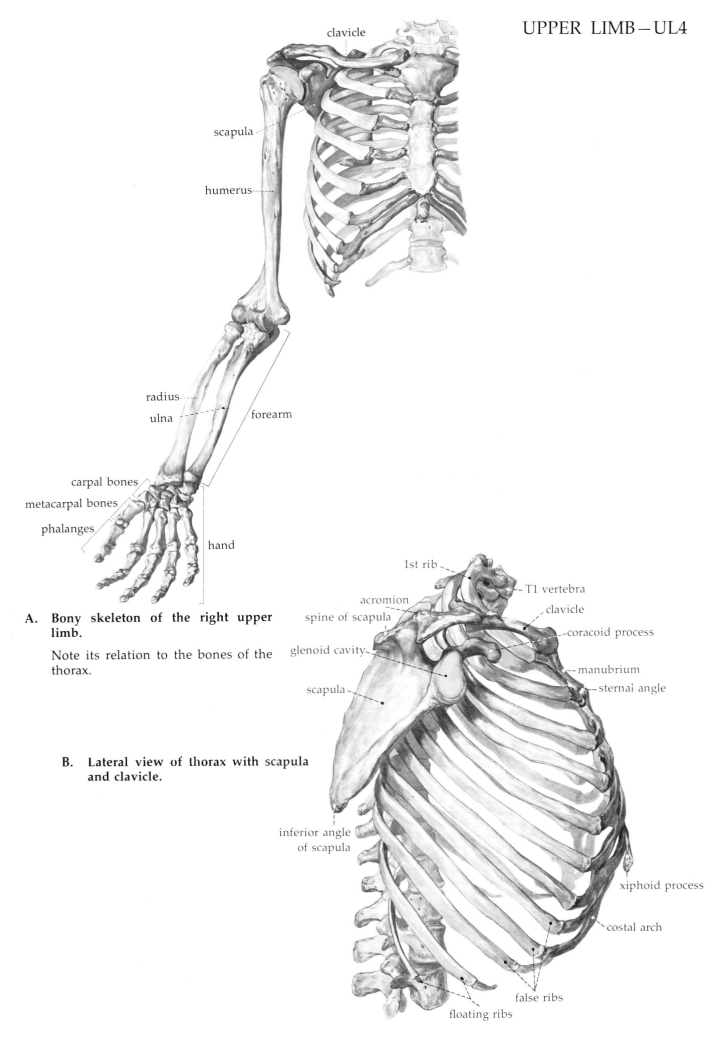

clavicle

scapula

humerus

radius

ulna

forearm

carpal bones

metacarpal bones

phalanges

hand

A. Bony skeleton of the right upper limb.

Note its relation to the bones of the thorax.

1st rib

acromion

spine of scapula

glenoid cavity

scapula

T1 vertebra

clavicle

coracoid process

manubrium

sternal angle

B. Lateral view of thorax with scapula and clavicle.

inferior angle of scapula

xiphoid process

costal arch

false ribs

floating ribs

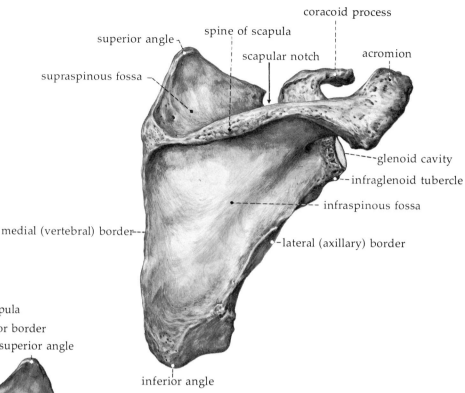

A. Posterior view of the right scapula.

coracoid process
spine of scapula
superior angle
scapular notch
acromion
supraspinous fossa
glenoid cavity
infraglenoid tubercle
infraspinous fossa
medial (vertebral) border
lateral (axillary) border
inferior angle

B. Anterior view of the right scapula.

scapular notch
articular surface for clavicle
spine of scapula
superior border
superior angle
acromion
coracoid process
neck of scapula
glenoid cavity
infraglenoid tubercle
ridges for muscle attachment
subscapular fossa
inferior angle

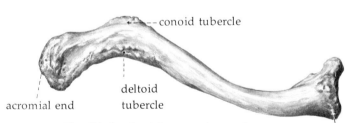

conoid tubercle
deltoid tubercle
acromial end
C. Right clavicle seen from above.
sternal end

acromial end
subclavian groove
tuberosity for costoclavicular ligament
conoid tubercle
sternal end

D. Right clavicle seen from below.
Note the conoid tubercle for attachment of the coracoclavicular ligament.

It is important to know that:

§ The clavicle is fractured more frequently than any other bone. Usually the fracture occurs at the junction of the outer (acromial) and middle thirds of the bone. The medial fragment is pulled upward by the pull of the sternocleidomastoid muscle, and the lateral third is pulled downward by the weight of the arm. Sometimes the fractured ends may severely damage the underlying vessels and nerves (see UL7, UL13 and UL14).

§ The clavicle has two centers of membranous ossification: one in the outer third and one more medially. They are separated by a cartilaginous growth zone. The location of so many fractures at the outer (acromial) third of the clavicle is probably related to the fact that this is where the two ossification centers meet.

§ The clavicle is the first bone in the body in which ossification begins. This occurs at the fifth week of development.

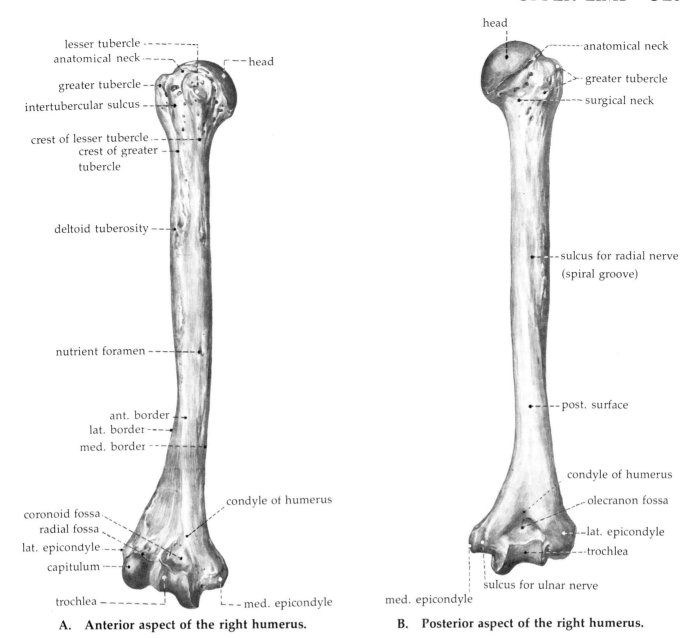

lesser tubercle
anatomical neck
head
greater tubercle
intertubercular sulcus
crest of lesser tubercle
crest of greater tubercle
deltoid tuberosity
nutrient foramen
ant. border
lat. border
med. border
condyle of humerus
coronoid fossa
radial fossa
lat. epicondyle
capitulum
trochlea
med. epicondyle

A. Anterior aspect of the right humerus.

head
anatomical neck
greater tubercle
surgical neck
sulcus for radial nerve (spiral groove)
post. surface
condyle of humerus
olecranon fossa
lat. epicondyle
trochlea
sulcus for ulnar nerve
med. epicondyle

B. Posterior aspect of the right humerus.

Note the following details:

1. The anatomical neck forms a constriction immediately adjacent to the head of the humerus. The surgical neck, found between the shaft of the bone and the head, is a common site for fractures. Since the axillary nerve and the posterior circumflex artery lie in direct contact with the surgical neck, fractures of the bone in this area may cause paralysis and severe bleeding (see UL13 and UL20).

2. On the posterior side of the humerus is an ill-defined groove. In this groove lies the radial nerve and the profunda brachii artery. As the shaft of the humerus frequently is fractured at the level of the groove, severe damage to the radial nerve may result.

3. The posterior aspect of the medial epicondyle is characterized by a rather deep groove for the ulnar nerve. The nerve can easily be felt and rolled against the bone. Whenever the medial epicondyle is fractured, the ulnar nerve is usually damaged (see UL45 and UL61).

4. The medial epicondyle gives origin to the flexor muscles of the forearm; the lateral epicondyle to the supinator and extensor muscles of the forearm and to the anconeus.

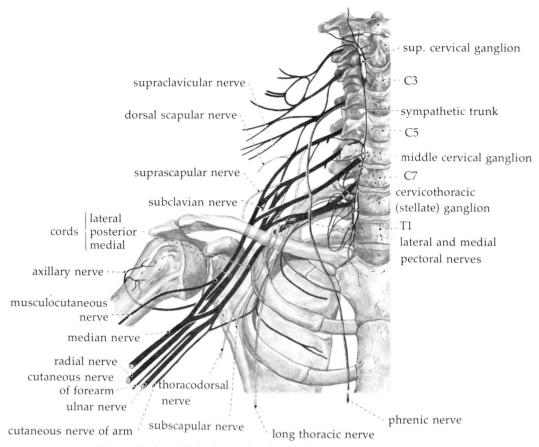

supraclavicular nerve

dorsal scapular nerve

suprascapular nerve

subclavian nerve

cords { lateral / posterior / medial

axillary nerve

musculocutaneous nerve

median nerve

radial nerve

cutaneous nerve of forearm

ulnar nerve

cutaneous nerve of arm

subscapular nerve

thoracodorsal nerve

long thoracic nerve

sup. cervical ganglion

C3

sympathetic trunk

C5

middle cervical ganglion

C7

cervicothoracic (stellate) ganglion

T1

lateral and medial pectoral nerves

phrenic nerve

The right brachial plexus in the neck and axillary region.
Note the relation of the plexus to the first rib and the clavicle.

Before entering the axillary region the nerve components of the plexus give off a number of branches in the neck. Some of these arise directly from the ventral rami, some arise after formation of the trunks, and others originate from the cords. It is of interest to know that:

⁋ The *phrenic nerve* is derived from C4 but occasionally receives a contribution from C3 and C5. The nerve supplies the motor and sensory innervation to the diaphragm. Since the supraclavicular nerves originate from the same segments, pain impulses from the diaphragm and related organs are sometimes carried over to the supraclavicular nerves, causing pain in the shoulder region (referred pain).

⁋ Since the anterior rami of C5 to C8 and T1 send no cutaneous branches to the pectoral region, the supraclavicular branches of C3 and C4 descend over the clavicle to the level of the second thoracic segment.

⁋ The following nerves arise from the plexus before entering the axillary region (segments of chief origin are indicated in bold type):
1. The *dorsal scapular nerve* (**C5**) to the levator scapulae and rhomboids.
2. The *suprascapular nerve* (**C5, C6**) to the supraspinatus and infraspinatus (see UL20).
3. The *subclavian nerve* (**C5, C6**) to the subclavius.
4. The *long thoracic nerve* (**C5, C6, C7**) to the serratus anterior (see UL11 *A*).
5. The *medial pectoral nerve* from the lower trunk and the *lateral pectoral nerve* from the upper and middle trunks. They supply the pectoralis major and minor.
6. The *thoracodorsal nerve* (C6, **C7, C8**) to the latissimus dorsi.
7. The *subscapular nerve* (**C5, C6**, C7) to the subscapularis and teres major.

212

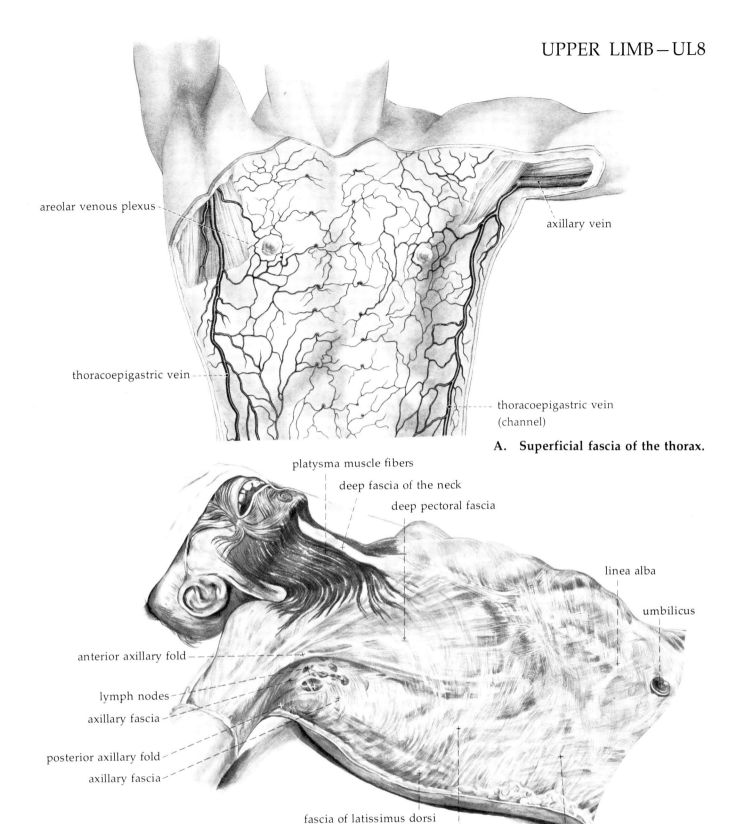

areolar venous plexus

axillary vein

thoracoepigastric vein

thoracoepigastric vein
(channel)

A. Superficial fascia of the thorax.

platysma muscle fibers

deep fascia of the neck

deep pectoral fascia

linea alba

umbilicus

anterior axillary fold

lymph nodes

axillary fascia

posterior axillary fold

axillary fascia

fascia of latissimus dorsi

fascia of serratus anterior

abdominal fascia

B. Deep fascia of the thorax.

Make the following observations:

¶ The *superficial fascia* is formed by the subcutaneous tissue immediately under the skin. With a few exceptions, such as in the palm of the hand, the superficial fascia contains much fat, a large number of veins and small branches of the nerves and arteries on their way to the skin. The superficial fascia is loosely attached to the skin and to the underlying deep fascia, which invests the muscles. When tumors are found in the superficial fascia, it is important to determine whether they are connected to the skin or deep fascia, and whether they are movable or fixed to the overlying and underlying layers.

¶ The *deep fascia* is whitish and fibrous. It is the investing layer of all muscles. In the living, it is slippery and smooth, thus allowing for movement of the muscles.

¶ In the neck region, small thin muscular fibers belonging to the platysma are found in the superficial fascia. These superficial muscles, also found in the region of the face, are attached to the skin and can move the skin.

213

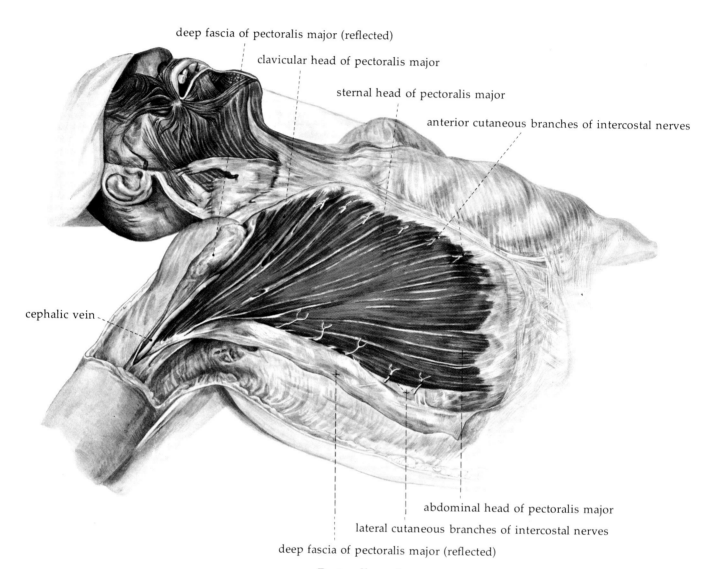

deep fascia of pectoralis major (reflected)

clavicular head of pectoralis major

sternal head of pectoralis major

anterior cutaneous branches of intercostal nerves

cephalic vein

abdominal head of pectoralis major

lateral cutaneous branches of intercostal nerves

deep fascia of pectoralis major (reflected)

Pectoralis major.
Note the anterior and lateral cutaneous branches of the intercostal nerves.

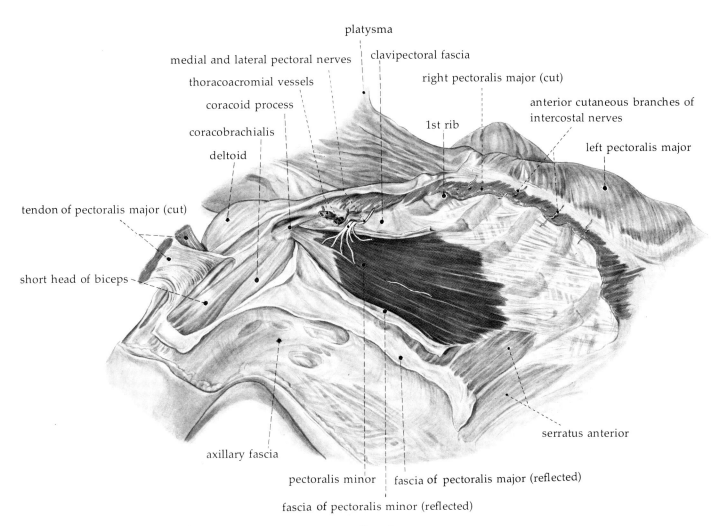

platysma

medial and lateral pectoral nerves

clavipectoral fascia

thoracoacromial vessels

right pectoralis major (cut)

coracoid process

anterior cutaneous branches of
intercostal nerves

coracobrachialis

1st rib

left pectoralis major

deltoid

tendon of pectoralis major (cut)

short head of biceps

serratus anterior

axillary fascia

pectoralis minor

fascia of pectoralis major (reflected)

fascia of pectoralis minor (reflected)

Pectoralis minor.

When the pectoralis major is reflected toward the arm, the medial and lateral pectoral nerves become visible. Also note the clavipectoral fascia, which is pierced by branches of the thoracoacromial artery, the cephalic vein and the lateral pectoral nerve (see T15 *B*). Removal of the pectoralis major exposes the axilla, since the muscle forms its anterior wall. Note also the coracobrachialis and the short head of the biceps. The pectoralis minor is an important landmark in locating the underlying plexus and vessels (see UL13 and UL15).

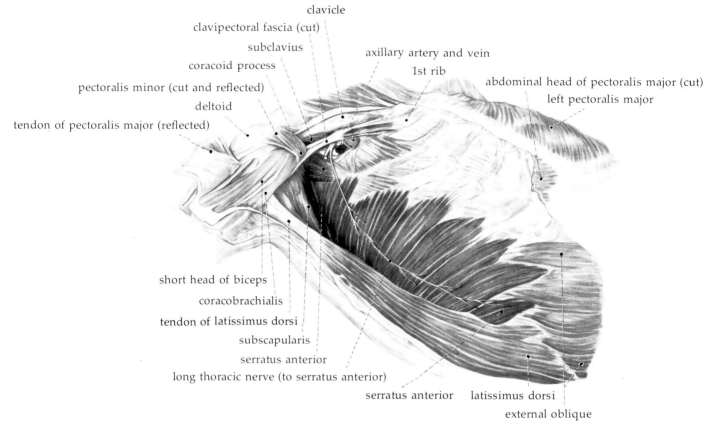

clavicle

clavipectoral fascia (cut)

subclavius

coracoid process

axillary artery and vein

1st rib

pectoralis minor (cut and reflected)

abdominal head of pectoralis major (cut)

left pectoralis major

deltoid

tendon of pectoralis major (reflected)

short head of biceps

coracobrachialis

tendon of latissimus dorsi

subscapularis

serratus anterior

long thoracic nerve (to serratus anterior)

serratus anterior   latissimus dorsi

external oblique

A.   Serratus anterior and latissimus dorsi.

The upper limb is extended in the shoulder joint; the neurovascular bundle is cut.

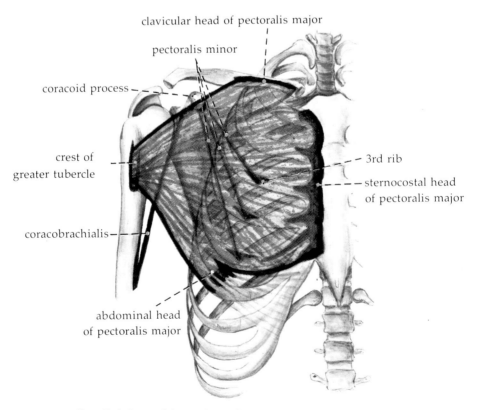

clavicular head of pectoralis major

pectoralis minor

coracoid process

crest of
greater tubercle

3rd rib

sternocostal head
of pectoralis major

coracobrachialis

abdominal head
of pectoralis major

B.   Origin and insertion of pectoralis minor and major.

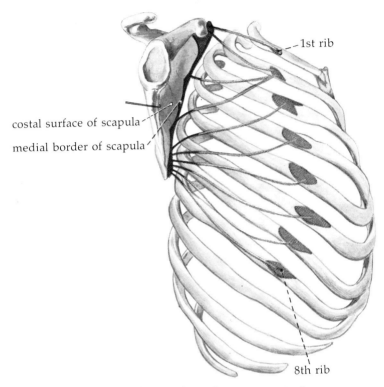

costal surface of scapula

medial border of scapula

1st rib

8th rib

Origin and insertion of serratus anterior.

Pectoralis major

Origin:

1. Clavicular part: anterior aspect of medial half of clavicle.
2. Sternocostal part: anterior surface of sternum and adjacent upper six costal cartilages.
3. Abdominal part: Aponeurosis of external oblique.

Insertion: Crest of greater tubercle of humerus.

Function: Adduction and medial rotation of the arm; also flexion of the arm in the shoulder joint.

Pectoralis minor

Origin: Third, fourth and fifth ribs near costal cartilages.

Insertion: Coracoid process of scapula.
Function: Depresses the point of the shoulder.

Serratus anterior

Origin: Outer surfaces of upper eight ribs.

Insertion: Costal aspect of medial border of scapula, mainly the area of the inferior angle.

Function: Pulls scapula forward and rotates it in an upward direction. When paralyzed the arm cannot be raised forward and abducted more than 90 degrees. Winged scapula.

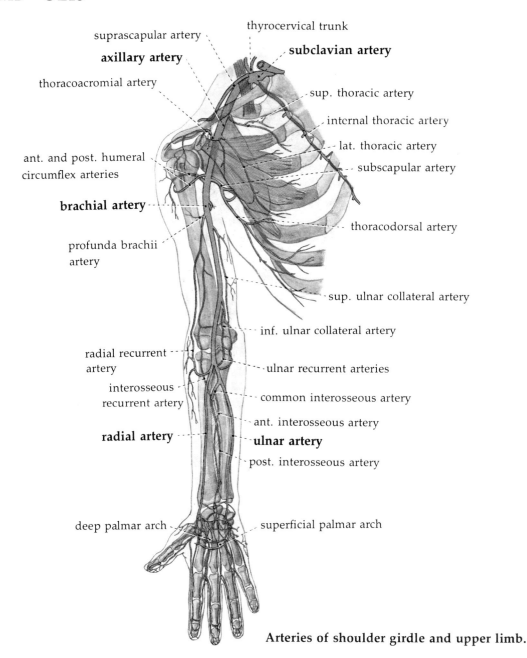

thyrocervical trunk

suprascapular artery

axillary artery

subclavian artery

thoracoacromial artery

sup. thoracic artery

internal thoracic artery

lat. thoracic artery

subscapular artery

ant. and post. humeral
circumflex arteries

brachial artery

thoracodorsal artery

profunda brachii
artery

sup. ulnar collateral artery

inf. ulnar collateral artery

radial recurrent
artery

ulnar recurrent arteries

interosseous
recurrent artery

common interosseous artery

ant. interosseous artery

radial artery

ulnar artery

post. interosseous artery

deep palmar arch

superficial palmar arch

Arteries of shoulder girdle and upper limb.

Before starting the dissection of the neurovascular bundle it is useful to study the general vascular pattern of the upper limb.

¶ As soon as the *subclavian artery* passes beneath the clavicle and crosses the lower border of the first rib, it is referred to as the *axillary artery*. At the level of the lower margin of the teres major it becomes the *brachial artery* (see UL20).

¶ The axillary artery passes behind the pectoralis minor, which divides it into three parts: (a) a first part from which arises the superior thoracic artery; (b) a second part behind the muscle from which arise the lateral thoracic and thoracoacromial arteries; and (c) a third part from which originate the subscapular and the anterior and posterior humeral circumflex arteries.

¶ Clinically important are the many anastomoses around the scapula (see UL20), in the region of the elbow (see UL27) and in the region of the wrist (see UL43). These anastomoses are important when a large artery must be ligated.

¶ Since the subclavian artery passes over the first rib, it can be compressed against the rib when severe arterial bleeding in the upper limb makes this necessary. Compression in the angle between the clavicle and the posterior margin of the sternocleidomastoid is most effective. A simple way to compress the artery is to push the arm backward, thus narrowing the space between the clavicle and the first rib.

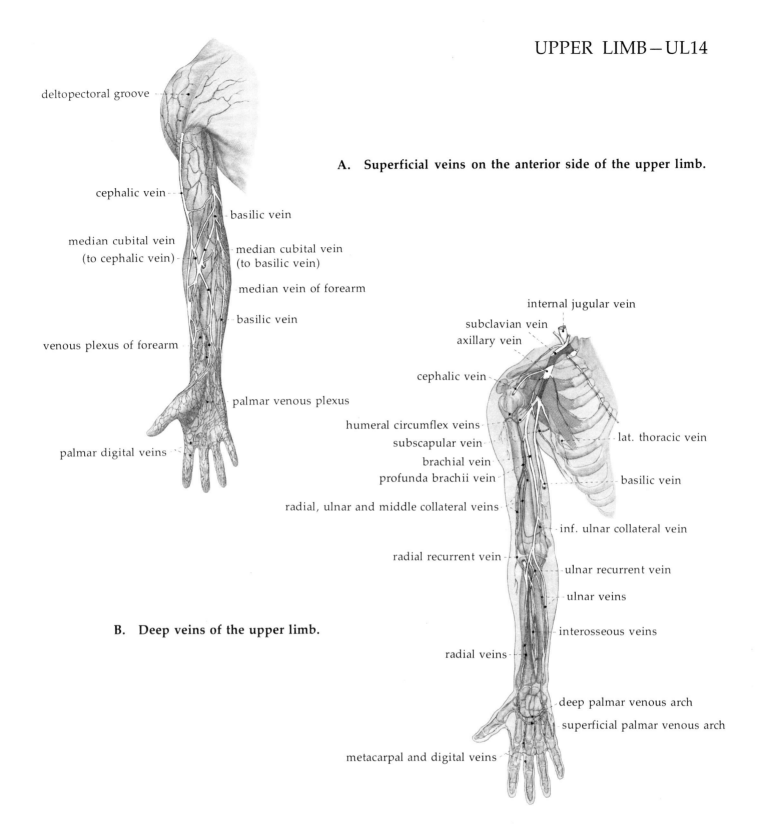

deltopectoral groove

A. Superficial veins on the anterior side of the upper limb.

cephalic vein

basilic vein

median cubital vein
(to cephalic vein)

median cubital vein
(to basilic vein)

median vein of forearm

basilic vein

internal jugular vein

subclavian vein

axillary vein

cephalic vein

venous plexus of forearm

humeral circumflex veins

lat. thoracic vein

subscapular vein

brachial vein

palmar venous plexus

profunda brachii vein

basilic vein

radial, ulnar and middle collateral veins

inf. ulnar collateral vein

palmar digital veins

radial recurrent vein

ulnar recurrent vein

ulnar veins

interosseous veins

B. Deep veins of the upper limb.

radial veins

deep palmar venous arch

superficial palmar venous arch

metacarpal and digital veins

¶ The deep veins of the upper limb form extensive venous networks in the scapular region, around the elbow and in the carpal–metacarpal region. In addition, the deep and superficial veins are connected to each other by many perforating branches. Hence, the venous system, even more than the arterial system, is characterized by many anastomoses; ligation of a vein therefore does not usually interfere with the drainage of the upper limb.

¶ Note the cephalic vein. In modern surgery the cephalic vein is frequently used in passing thin catheters into the heart. The catheter is pushed through the cephalic, axillary and subclavian veins and then by way of the superior vena cava into the heart.

¶ The median cubital vein is often used for venipuncture (e.g., blood sampling, transfusions, intravenous injections). It lies on the bicipital aponeurosis. It is important to be careful because the brachial artery and median nerve lie directly beneath the aponeurosis.

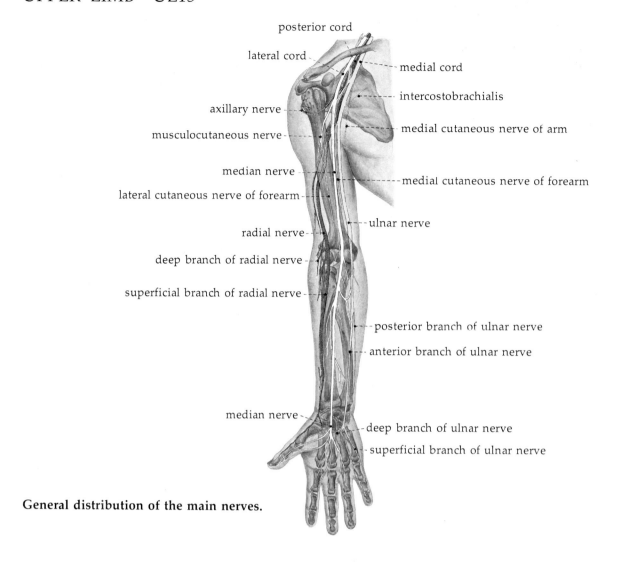

posterior cord

lateral cord

medial cord

intercostobrachialis

axillary nerve

musculocutaneous nerve

medial cutaneous nerve of arm

median nerve

medial cutaneous nerve of forearm

lateral cutaneous nerve of forearm

ulnar nerve

radial nerve

deep branch of radial nerve

superficial branch of radial nerve

posterior branch of ulnar nerve

anterior branch of ulnar nerve

median nerve

deep branch of ulnar nerve

superficial branch of ulnar nerve

General distribution of the main nerves.

With regard to the distribution of the major nerves, in general terms it may be stated that:

¶ The main nerves of the *posterior cord* (radial and axillary) supply the muscles and the skin on the posterior aspect of the limb.

¶ The main branches of the *lateral cord* (musculocutaneous and median nerves) supply the flexor muscles of the shoulder, elbow and most of the muscles on the anterolateral side of the forearm and thenar eminence. Similarly, most of the skin on the anterolateral side of the arm, forearm and hand is supplied by the lateral cord.

¶ The main branches of the *medial cord* (ulnar nerve and cutaneous nerves of arm and forearm) supply some deep muscles on the medial side of the forearm, most of the muscles of the hand and the skin of the medial aspect of the arm, forearm and hand.

Two lesions of the cords are known:

1. When the cords are damaged by a blow on the neck or when the arm is pulled downward and the head drawn away from the shoulder, the components of C5 and C6 are seriously injured. When this "upper" type of injury occurs during birth (the arm of the baby is pulled downward and the head moves in the opposite direction), it is referred to as "birth palsy." Since elements of C5 and C6 participate in the formation of the lateral cord and to a lesser extent in that of the posterior cord, the damage may be extensive. The motor and sensory components of all nerves which have contributions from C5 and C6 are affected (musculocutaneous, axillary, median and radial nerves). (For details see UL3.)

2. When the first rib is pulled upward or when a cervical rib is present, the nerve component of T1 may become stretched ("lower" type lesion). Since the T1 segment participates in the medial cord (ulnar nerve), the main result of such a lesion is paralysis of the small muscles of the hand, which assumes a clawlike shape (for more details see UL45).

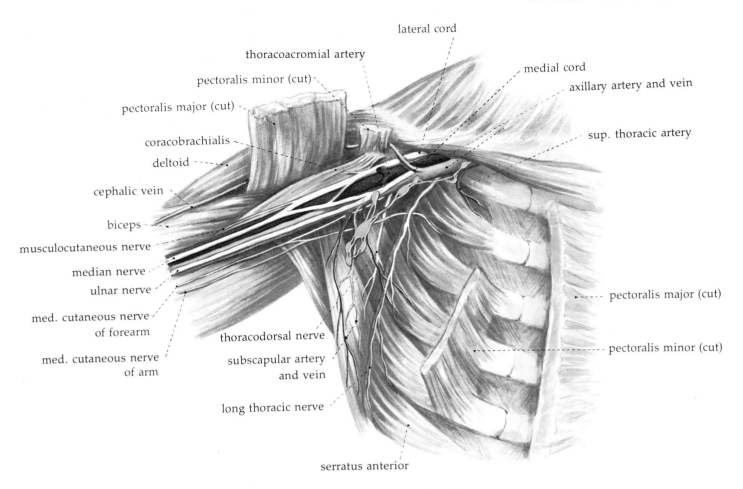

lateral cord

thoracoacromial artery

medial cord

pectoralis minor (cut)

axillary artery and vein

pectoralis major (cut)

coracobrachialis

sup. thoracic artery

deltoid

cephalic vein

biceps

musculocutaneous nerve

median nerve

ulnar nerve

pectoralis major (cut)

med. cutaneous nerve
of forearm

med. cutaneous nerve
of arm

pectoralis minor (cut)

thoracodorsal nerve

subscapular artery
and vein

long thoracic nerve

serratus anterior

The right neurovascular bundle.
The pectoral muscles have been removed and the clavicle has been cut to
show the nerves and their relation to the vessels.

Large groups of lymph nodes are found in the axillary region, and in every routine examination the nodes should be palpated. They are particularly important in relation to the
lymph drainage of the mammary gland, but it should be kept in mind that all lymph
from the upper limb also drains into the axillary region. Many infections of the upper
limb cause swelling of the nodes in the axillary region. For details of the different groups
of nodes see T6.

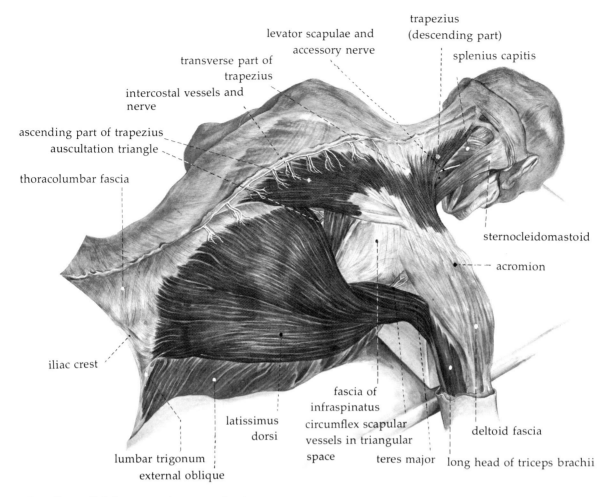

levator scapulae and
accessory nerve

trapezius
(descending part)

splenius capitis

transverse part of
trapezius

intercostal vessels and
nerve

ascending part of trapezius
auscultation triangle

thoracolumbar fascia

sternocleidomastoid

acromion

iliac crest

fascia of
infraspinatus
circumflex scapular
vessels in triangular
space

latissimus
dorsi

deltoid fascia

teres major

long head of triceps brachii

lumbar trigonum
external oblique

A. **Superficial musculature of the back.**
Note the accessory nerve to the sternocleidomastoid and trapezius.

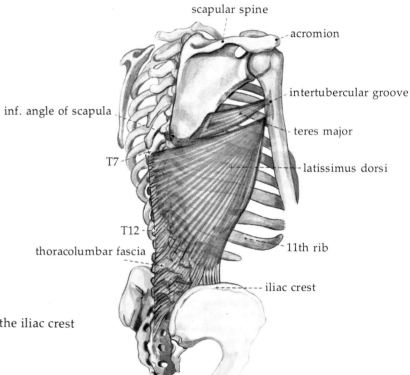

scapular spine

acromion

inf. angle of scapula

intertubercular groove

teres major

T7

latissimus dorsi

T12

11th rib

thoracolumbar fascia

iliac crest

B. **Schematic drawing of latissimus dorsi and teres major.**

Latissimus dorsi
Origin:
1. Spines of T7 to T12.
2. By way of the thoracolumbar fascia from the iliac crest and lumbar and sacral spines.
3. Lower three or four ribs.
Insertion: Floor of the intertubercular groove.
Function: Adduction and extension of arm; medial rotator.

Teres major
Origin: Inferior angle and dorsal surface of scapula.
Insertion: Crest of lesser tubercle of humerus.
Function: Adduction of arm; medial rotator.

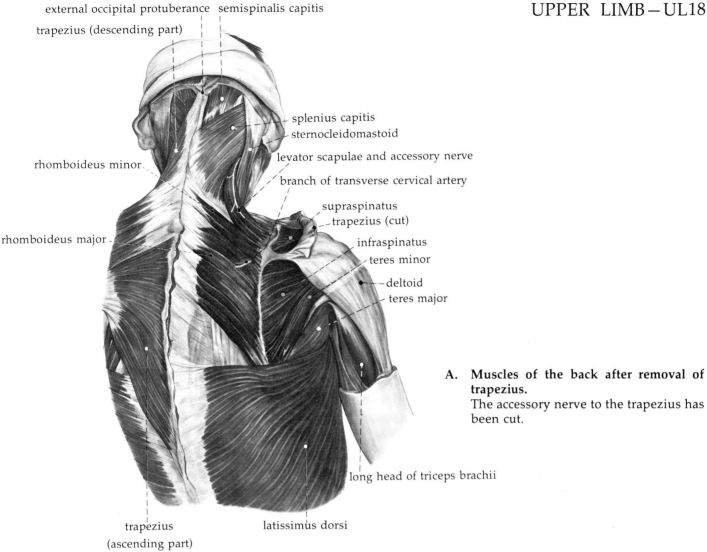

external occipital protuberance semispinalis capitis

trapezius (descending part)

splenius capitis

sternocleidomastoid

levator scapulae and accessory nerve

branch of transverse cervical artery

rhomboideus minor

supraspinatus

trapezius (cut)

rhomboideus major

infraspinatus

teres minor

deltoid

teres major

long head of triceps brachii

trapezius (ascending part)

latissimus dorsi

A. Muscles of the back after removal of trapezius.
The accessory nerve to the trapezius has been cut.

transverse process of C1 (atlas)

transverse process of C4

C6

levator scapulae

rhomboideus minor

medial border of scapula

B. Schematic drawing of the rhomboids and levator scapulae.

T4

rhomboideus major

medial border of scapula

Rhomboideus minor
Origin: Spines of C6 to T1; nuchal ligament.
Insertion: Medial border of scapula at root of scapular spine.

Rhomboideus major
Origin: Spines of T2 to T5; supraspinous ligaments.
Insertion: Medial border of scapula below the scapular spine.
Function of rhomboids: Retract and hold scapula to vertebral column.

Levator scapulae
Origin: Posterior tubercles of transverse processes of C1 to C4.
Insertion: Medial border of scapula above the scapular spine.
Function: Elevates scapula.

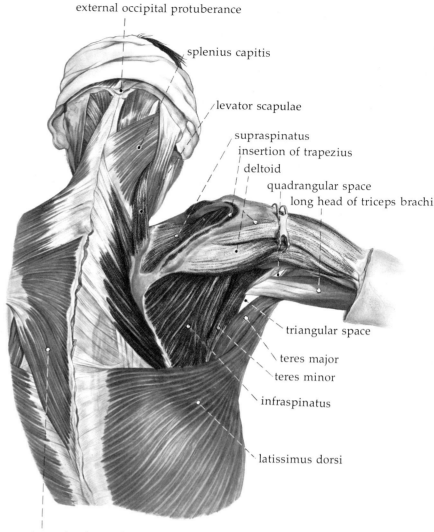

external occipital protuberance

splenius capitis

levator scapulae

supraspinatus
insertion of trapezius
deltoid
quadrangular space
long head of triceps brachi

triangular space

teres major

teres minor

infraspinatus

latissimus dorsi

trapezius (ascending part)

A. Muscles on the posterior aspect of the scapula.

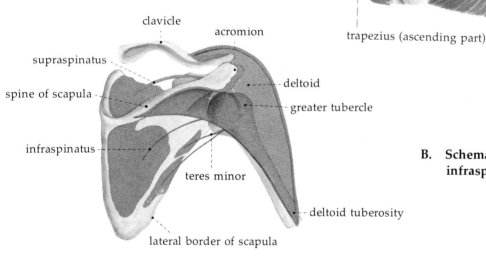

clavicle

acromion

supraspinatus

spine of scapula

infraspinatus

deltoid

greater tubercle

teres minor

deltoid tuberosity

lateral border of scapula

B. Schematic drawing of the supraspinatus, infraspinatus, teres minor and deltoid.

Supraspinatus

Origin: Medial two thirds of supraspinous fossa.

Insertion: Capsule of shoulder joint; greater tubercle of humerus.

Function: Abduction of arm.

Deltoid

Origin: Lateral third of clavicle; acromion; spine of scapula.

Insertion: Deltoid tuberosity.

Function: Abduction of arm; medial rotation of arm; lateral rotation of arm.

Infraspinatus

Origin: Medial two thirds of infraspinous fossa.

Insertion: Capsule of shoulder joint; greater tubercle of humerus.

Function: Lateral rotation of arm.

Teres minor

Origin: Lateral margin of infraspinous fossa.

Insertion: Capsule of shoulder joint; greater tubercle of humerus.

Function: Lateral rotation of arm.

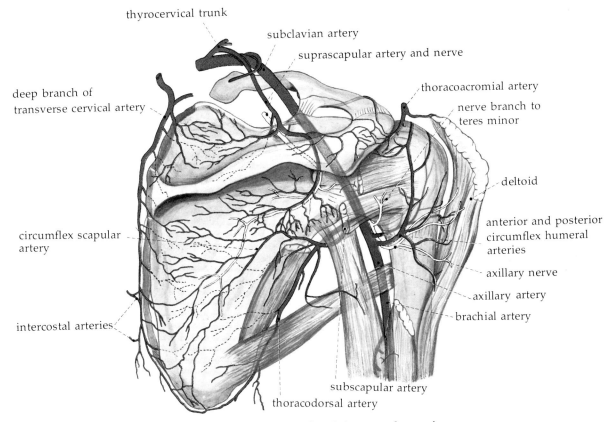

thyrocervical trunk

subclavian artery

suprascapular artery and nerve

deep branch of
transverse cervical artery

thoracoacromial artery

nerve branch to
teres minor

deltoid

circumflex scapular
artery

anterior and posterior
circumflex humeral
arteries

axillary nerve

axillary artery

brachial artery

intercostal arteries

subscapular artery

thoracodorsal artery

Nerves and vessels in the right scapular region.

Note:

⁋ The *triangular space,* bordered by the long head of the triceps, teres minor and teres major, allows the circumflex scapular artery to reach the posterior aspect of the scapula.

⁋ The *quadrangular space* is bordered by the long head of the triceps, teres minor, teres major and the medial aspect of the humerus. Through this space pass the posterior circumflex humeral artery and the axillary nerve.

Several observations of clinical importance should be made:

⁋ The subclavian or axillary artery can be ligated between the origins of the thyrocervical trunk and the subscapular artery. This is possible because the suprascapular artery (a branch from the thyrocervical trunk) has many anastomoses with the circumflex scapular artery, a branch from the subscapular artery. The latter in turn originates directly from the axillary artery. When the subclavian artery is ligated above the subscapular artery, the flow of blood is reversed and blood enters the axillary artery from the circumflex scapular. Other important anastomoses of the subclavian artery are formed by the transverse cervical, intercostal and thoracodorsal arteries. The axillary artery cannot be ligated below the origin of the subscapular artery, since no collateral circulation exists to supply the upper limb.

⁋ The axillary nerve and the posterior circumflex humeral artery pass through the quadrangular space, where the axillary nerve lies in close contact with the capsule of the shoulder joint. When the humerus dislocates in a downward direction, the nerve may be damaged if it is caught between the head of the humerus and the lateral margin of the scapula. Paralysis of the deltoid and teres minor results, and the patient has difficulty in abducting the arm (see UL29 and UL33).

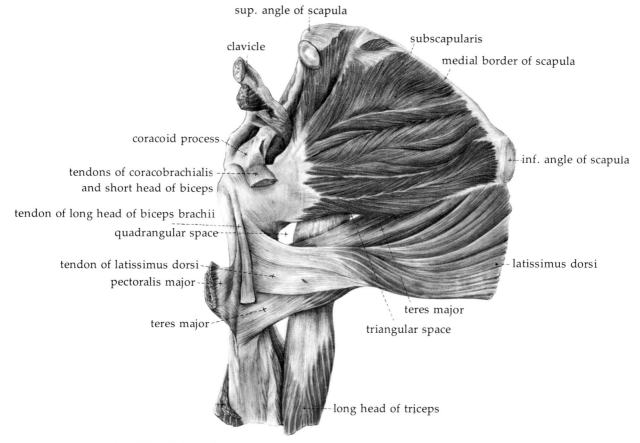

sup. angle of scapula

clavicle

subscapularis

medial border of scapula

coracoid process

tendons of coracobrachialis
and short head of biceps

tendon of long head of biceps brachii

quadrangular space

tendon of latissimus dorsi

pectoralis major

teres major

inf. angle of scapula

latissimus dorsi

teres major

triangular space

long head of triceps

A. The right subscapular muscle and its relation to the shoulder joint.

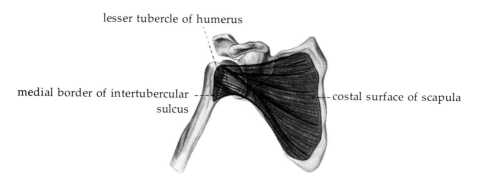

lesser tubercle of humerus

medial border of intertubercular
sulcus

costal surface of scapula

B. Schematic drawing of subscapular muscle.

The tendinous part of the subscapularis is closely related to the anterior aspect of the shoulder capsule and in this way enforces the capsule. Under the tendon is a large bursa, which usually communicates with the cavity of the shoulder joint and thus forms a protrusion of the joint cavity.

Subscapularis

Origin: Subscapular fossa.

Insertion: Capsule of shoulder joint; lesser tubercle and its crest.

Function: Medial rotation of humerus.

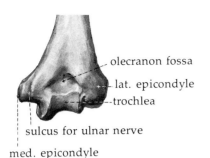

A. **Posterior view of the distal part (condyle) of the right humerus.**

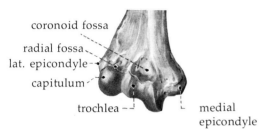

B. **Anterior aspect of the distal part (condyle) of the right humerus.**

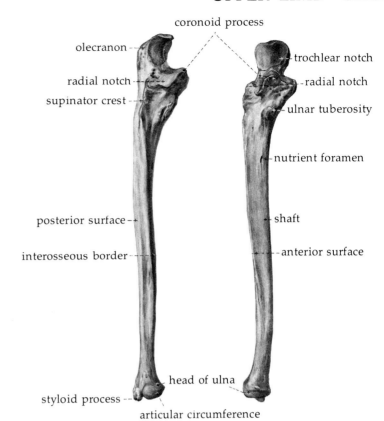

C. **Anteromedial view of the right ulna.**

D. **Anterior aspect of the right ulna.**

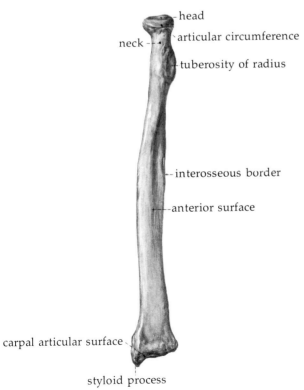

E. **Anterior aspect of the right radius.**

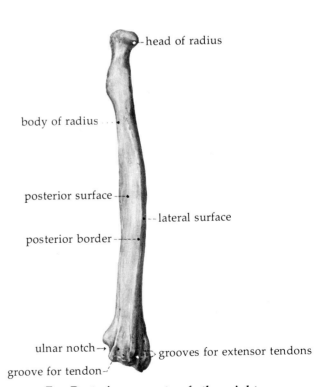

F. **Posterior aspect of the right radius.**

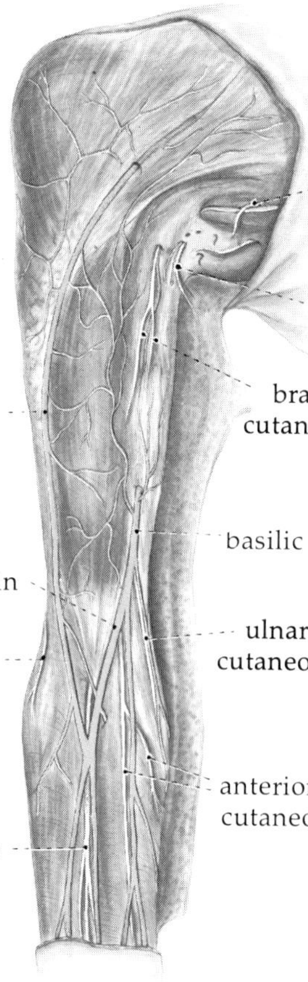

supraclavicular
cutaneous nerves
(C3, C4)

intercostalbrachial
nerve (T2)

branches of medial
cutaneous nerve of arm
(C8, T1, T2)

cephalic vein

basilic vein

median cubital vein

ulnar branch of medial
cutaneous nerve of forearm
(C8, T1)

post. cutaneous nerve
of forearm

anterior branches of medial
cutaneous nerve of forearm

lateral cutaneous nerve
of forearm (branch of
musculocutaneous n.)

A. Veins and nerves in the superficial fascia of the right arm.
The veins serve as landmarks for the cutaneous nerves, which run parallel and deep to them. In transverse cuts of the forearm, the nerves are often damaged.

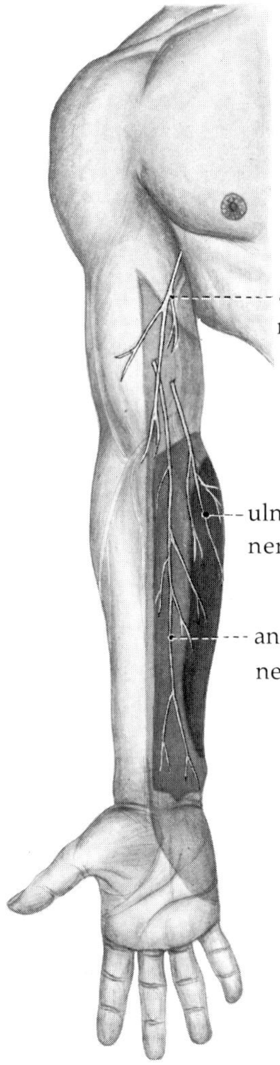

ant. branch of medial cutaneous
nerve of arm

ulnar branch of medial cutaneous
nerve of forearm

ant. branch of medial cutaneous
nerve of forearm

B. Skin area supplied by the medial cutaneous nerves of the right arm and forearm.

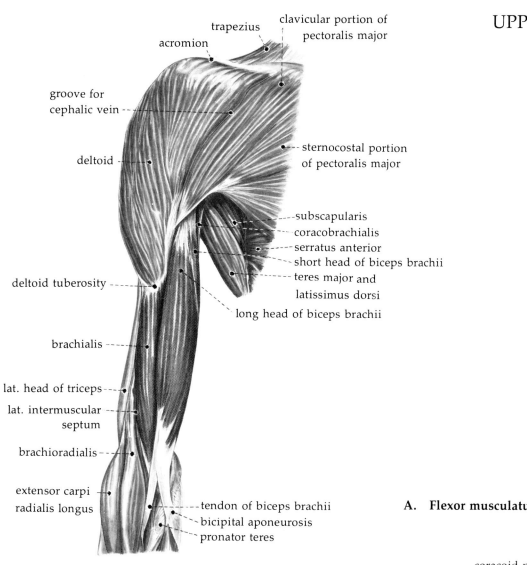

trapezius
acromion
clavicular portion of
pectoralis major

groove for
cephalic vein

deltoid

sternocostal portion
of pectoralis major

subscapularis
coracobrachialis
serratus anterior
short head of biceps brachii
teres major and
latissimus dorsi
long head of biceps brachii

deltoid tuberosity

brachialis

lat. head of triceps
lat. intermuscular
septum

brachioradialis

extensor carpi
radialis longus

tendon of biceps brachii
bicipital aponeurosis
pronator teres

A. Flexor musculature of the right arm.

B. Origin and insertion of the flexor musculature of the right arm.

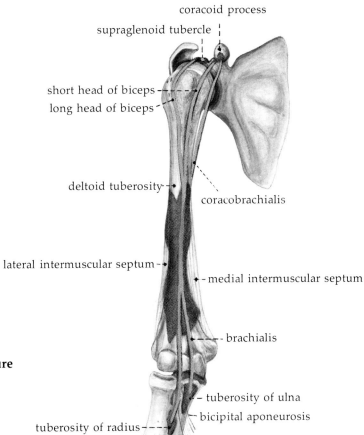

coracoid process
supraglenoid tubercle

short head of biceps
long head of biceps

deltoid tuberosity

coracobrachialis

lateral intermuscular septum

medial intermuscular septum

brachialis

tuberosity of ulna
bicipital aponeurosis
tuberosity of radius

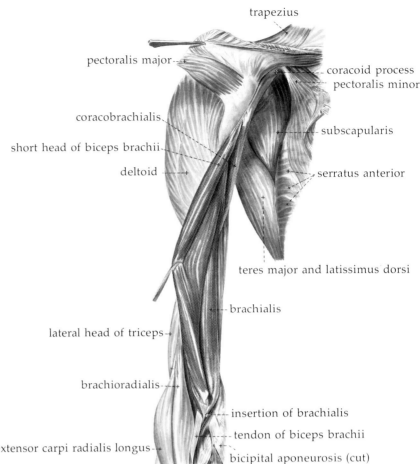

trapezius

pectoralis major

coracoid process

pectoralis minor

coracobrachialis

subscapularis

short head of biceps brachii

deltoid

serratus anterior

teres major and latissimus dorsi

brachialis

lateral head of triceps

brachioradialis

insertion of brachialis

tendon of biceps brachii

extensor carpi radialis longus

bicipital aponeurosis (cut)

A. Flexor musculature of the right arm.
The biceps has been pulled aside to show the coracobrachialis.

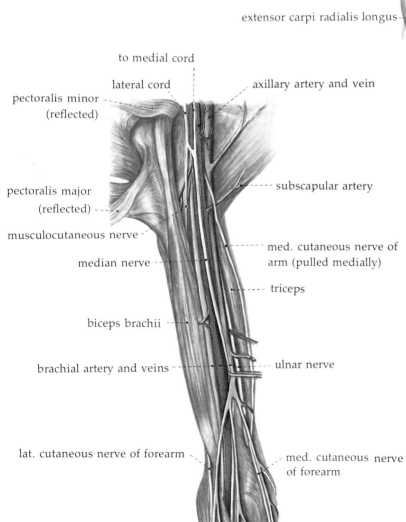

to medial cord

lateral cord

axillary artery and vein

pectoralis minor (reflected)

pectoralis major (reflected)

subscapular artery

musculocutaneous nerve

median nerve

med. cutaneous nerve of arm (pulled medially)

triceps

biceps brachii

brachial artery and veins

ulnar nerve

lat. cutaneous nerve of forearm

med. cutaneous nerve of forearm

brachioradialis

B. Anterior view of the vessels and nerves of the right arm.

230

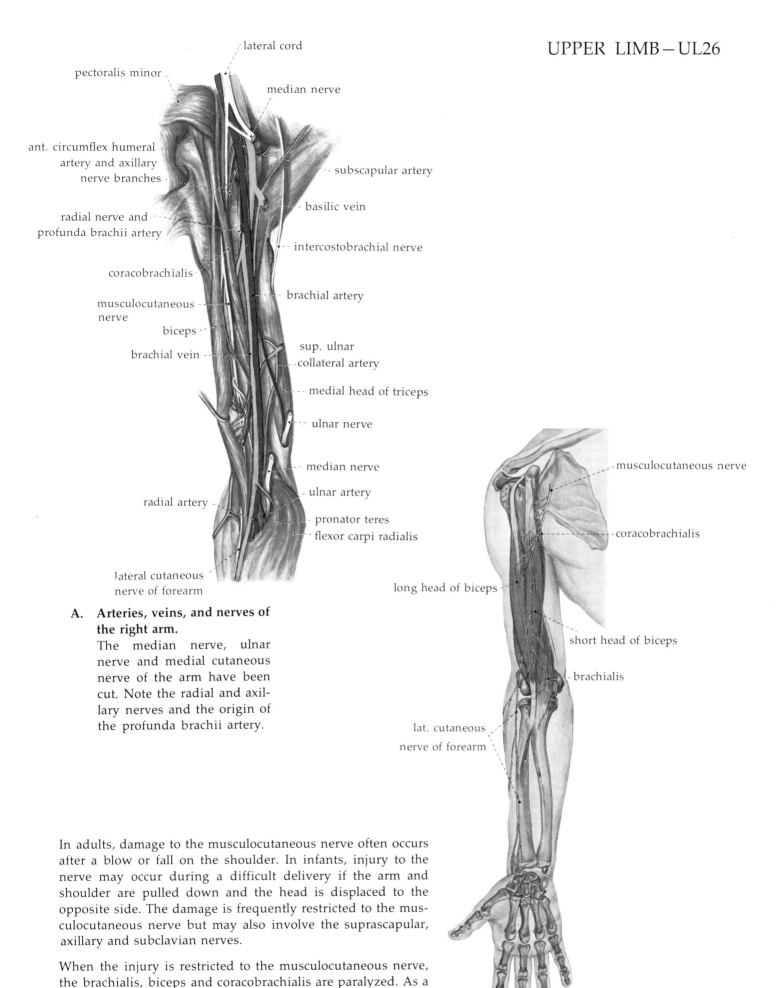

lateral cord

pectoralis minor

median nerve

ant. circumflex humeral artery and axillary nerve branches

subscapular artery

basilic vein

radial nerve and profunda brachii artery

intercostobrachial nerve

coracobrachialis

brachial artery

musculocutaneous nerve

biceps

sup. ulnar collateral artery

brachial vein

medial head of triceps

ulnar nerve

median nerve

ulnar artery

radial artery

pronator teres
flexor carpi radialis

lateral cutaneous nerve of forearm

A. Arteries, veins, and nerves of the right arm.
The median nerve, ulnar nerve and medial cutaneous nerve of the arm have been cut. Note the radial and axillary nerves and the origin of the profunda brachii artery.

musculocutaneous nerve

coracobrachialis

long head of biceps

short head of biceps

brachialis

lat. cutaneous nerve of forearm

In adults, damage to the musculocutaneous nerve often occurs after a blow or fall on the shoulder. In infants, injury to the nerve may occur during a difficult delivery if the arm and shoulder are pulled down and the head is displaced to the opposite side. The damage is frequently restricted to the musculocutaneous nerve but may also involve the suprascapular, axillary and subclavian nerves.

When the injury is restricted to the musculocutaneous nerve, the brachialis, biceps and coracobrachialis are paralyzed. As a result, the patient will have great difficulty with flexion of the arm in the shoulder and elbow joints. The forearm will be somewhat pronated owing to the loss of the strong supinating function of the biceps. Sensory loss will be restricted to the lateral aspect of the forearm but will not involve the hand.

B. Musculocutaneous nerve with motor and sensory innervation.

231

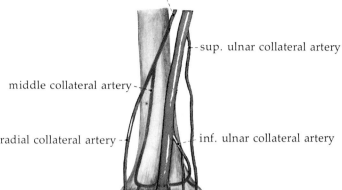

A. Anterior view of collateral circulation at the right elbow.

profunda brachii artery

sup. ulnar collateral artery

middle collateral artery

radial collateral artery

inf. ulnar collateral artery

radial recurrent artery

ulnar recurrent arteries

interosseous recurrent artery

ant. interosseous artery

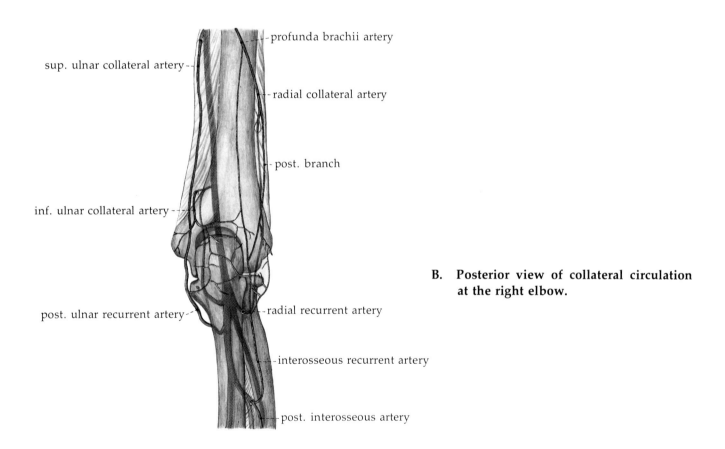

profunda brachii artery

sup. ulnar collateral artery

radial collateral artery

post. branch

inf. ulnar collateral artery

B. Posterior view of collateral circulation at the right elbow.

post. ulnar recurrent artery

radial recurrent artery

interosseous recurrent artery

post. interosseous artery

The rich collateral circulation in the elbow region is important. In patients with severe wounds of the arm, the brachial artery can be ligated below the inferior ulnar collateral artery. The many recurrent and collateral arteries will be able to supply the elbow joint and the remaining part of the forearm and hand.

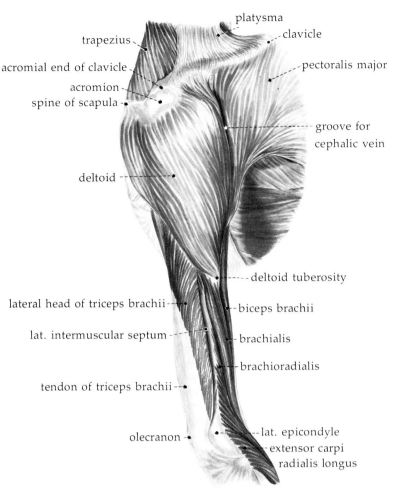

platysma
clavicle
trapezius
acromial end of clavicle
pectoralis major
acromion
spine of scapula
groove for
cephalic vein
deltoid

deltoid tuberosity
lateral head of triceps brachii
biceps brachii
lat. intermuscular septum
brachialis
brachioradialis
tendon of triceps brachii
lat. epicondyle
olecranon
extensor carpi
radialis longus

A. Lateral view of the muscles of the right arm.
Note that the brachioradialis and the extensor carpi radialis longus are anterior to the lateral intermuscular septum and the triceps brachii behind it.

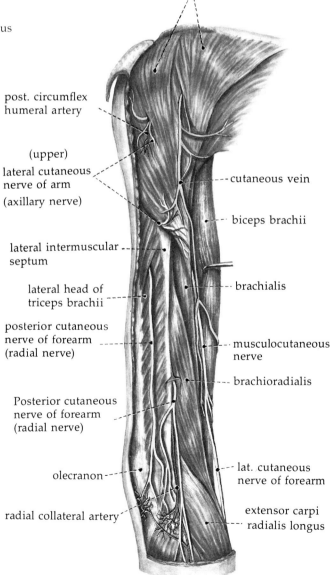

deltoideus

post. circumflex
humeral artery

(upper)
lateral cutaneous
nerve of arm
(axillary nerve)

cutaneous vein

biceps brachii

lateral intermuscular
septum

brachialis

lateral head of
triceps brachii

posterior cutaneous
nerve of forearm
(radial nerve)

musculocutaneous
nerve

brachioradialis

Posterior cutaneous
nerve of forearm
(radial nerve)

lat. cutaneous
nerve of forearm

olecranon

extensor carpi
radialis longus

radial collateral artery

B. Superficial nerves and arteries on the lateral side of the right arm.
Note the cutaneous branches of the axillary and radial nerves.

233

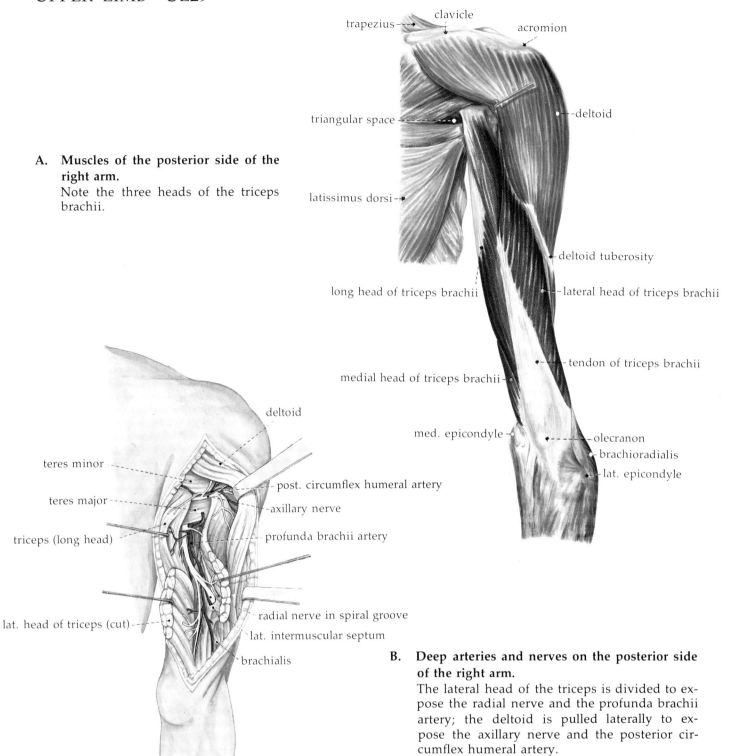

A. Muscles of the posterior side of the right arm.
Note the three heads of the triceps brachii.

B. Deep arteries and nerves on the posterior side of the right arm.
The lateral head of the triceps is divided to expose the radial nerve and the profunda brachii artery; the deltoid is pulled laterally to expose the axillary nerve and the posterior circumflex humeral artery.

After the radial nerve has left the axilla, it passes between the long and medial heads of the triceps. When the lateral head of the triceps is cut, the nerve can be seen to lie in the spiral groove on the posterior aspect of the humerus. In the groove the nerve is accompanied by the profunda brachii artery and is in direct contact with the bone. This particular course has some clinical implications:

1. In patients with fractures of the humerus, particularly fractures of the lower part of the bone, or in subsequent formation of callus, the radial nerve may be damaged. Since in the lower part of the arm the cutaneous and motor branches to the posterior aspect of the arm and the triceps have already left the main stem of the nerve, the motor damage is restricted to the extensors of the forearm. The main symptom is wrist drop and inability to extend the wrist and fingers. Sensory loss is restricted to a small area over the root of the thumb (see UL41 C).

2. Temporary damage to the radial nerve may occur after prolonged application of a tourniquet or when a patient lies with the back of the arm over the rim of a table. The latter injury sometimes occurs after a prolonged operation.

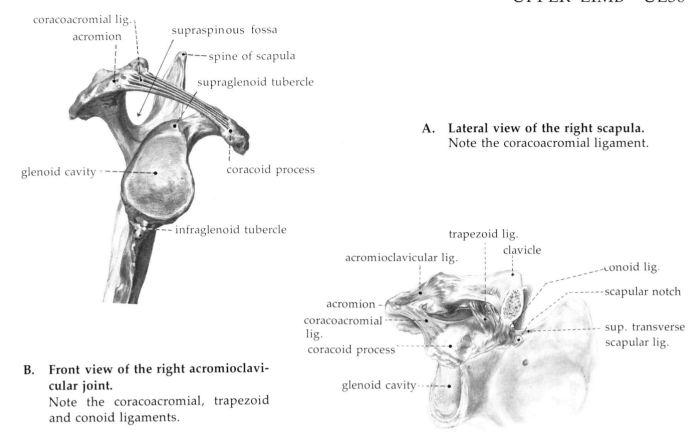

coracoacromial lig.
acromion
supraspinous fossa
spine of scapula
supraglenoid tubercle

glenoid cavity
coracoid process

infraglenoid tubercle

A. Lateral view of the right scapula.
Note the coracoacromial ligament.

trapezoid lig.
clavicle
acromioclavicular lig.
conoid lig.
scapular notch
acromion
coracoacromial lig.
sup. transverse scapular lig.
coracoid process
glenoid cavity

B. Front view of the right acromioclavicular joint.
Note the coracoacromial, trapezoid and conoid ligaments.

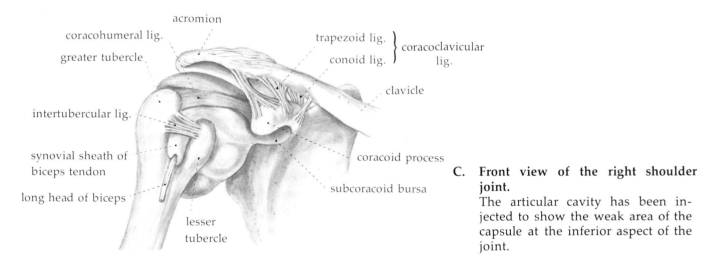

acromion
coracohumeral lig.
greater tubercle
trapezoid lig.
conoid lig.
} coracoclavicular lig.
clavicle
intertubercular lig.
synovial sheath of biceps tendon
coracoid process
long head of biceps
subcoracoid bursa
lesser tubercle

C. Front view of the right shoulder joint.
The articular cavity has been injected to show the weak area of the capsule at the inferior aspect of the joint.

Note the following points:

¶ The acromion and coracoid process are connected by the coracoacromial ligament. Together these three components form a bony ligamentous roof over the glenoid cavity and thus over the shoulder joint. When the humerus is thrust upward, this roof prevents the bone from dislocating in the shoulder joint.

¶ The outer end of the clavicle is sometimes dislocated by a fall on the point of the shoulder. The conoid (coracoclavicular) ligament is then usually torn and the acromion pushed under the lateral end of the clavicle. The dislocated end can easily be brought into position, but there is a strong possibility that redislocation will occur.

¶ When heavy loads are carried, the weight of the arm is transmitted to the scapula mainly by the coracohumeral ligament and to a lesser extent through the coracobrachialis and the short head of the biceps. Hence, the coracoid process is the central point in weight transmission. The coracoid process in turn is connected to the clavicle through the strong trapezoid and conoid ligaments. In this manner the weight of the upper limb is transmitted to the shoulder girdle.

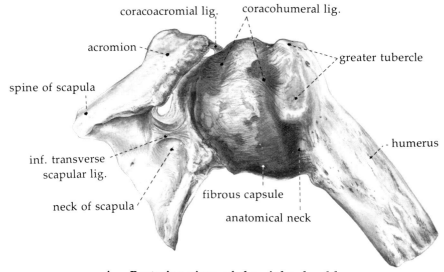

coracoacromial lig.

coracohumeral lig.

acromion

greater tubercle

spine of scapula

humerus

inf. transverse
scapular lig.

neck of scapula

fibrous capsule

anatomical neck

A. Posterior view of the right shoulder joint.
The joint cavity has been injected.

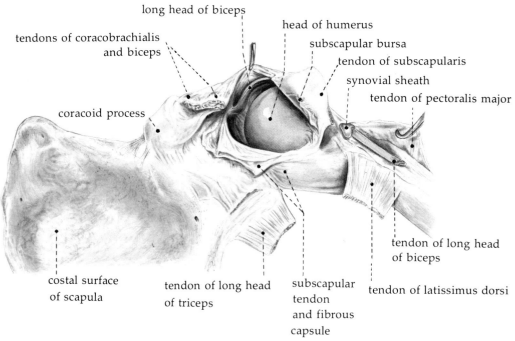

long head of biceps

head of humerus

tendons of coracobrachialis
and biceps

subscapular bursa

tendon of subscapularis

synovial sheath

tendon of pectoralis major

coracoid process

costal surface
of scapula

tendon of long head
of triceps

subscapular
tendon
and fibrous
capsule

tendon of long head
of biceps

tendon of latissimus dorsi

B. Anterior view of the opened left shoulder joint.
Note the long head of the biceps inside the joint cavity.

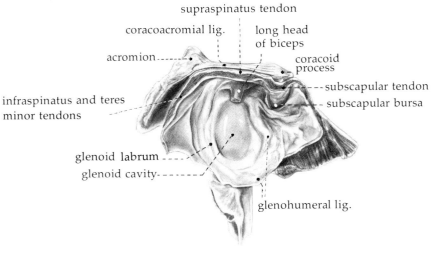

supraspinatus tendon
coracoacromial lig.
long head of biceps
acromion
coracoid process
subscapular tendon
subscapular bursa
infraspinatus and teres minor tendons
glenoid labrum
glenoid cavity
glenohumeral lig.

A. Lateral view of the right glenoid cavity.
The joint capsule and surrounding muscles have been cut.

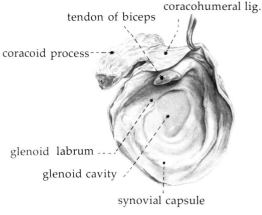

coracohumeral lig.
tendon of biceps
coracoid process
glenoid labrum
glenoid cavity
synovial capsule

B. Lateral view of the left glenoid cavity.
The muscle tendons surrounding the joint have been removed.

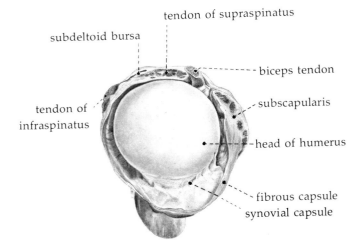

tendon of supraspinatus
subdeltoid bursa
biceps tendon
subscapularis
tendon of infraspinatus
head of humerus
fibrous capsule
synovial capsule

C. View of the head of the left humerus.
The joint capsule and surrounding tendons have been cut.

The shoulder region is characterized by two types of medical problems: dislocations of the shoulder joint and inflammations of the "rotator cuff."

¶ The shallowness of the glenoid cavity and the laxness of the fibrous capsule allow great movement of the arm. This freedom of movement, however, promotes dislocation. The dislocation is almost always in an inferior direction because: (a) the superior part of the capsule is strengthened by the broad tendon of the supraspinatus and the bony ligamentous roof formed by the acromion, the coracoid process and the coracoacromial ligament (see UL30); (b) the anterior part of the capsule is enforced by the tendon of the subscapularis and to a lesser extent by the glenohumeral ligament; and (c) the posterior part of the capsule is enforced by the tendons of the infraspinatus and teres minor.

¶ The inferior part of the capsule is weak, and hence the head of the humerus easily escapes in an inferior direction. From this position the head usually moves anteriorly to a subcoracoid position. Sometimes the head of the humerus moves in a posterior direction into the quadrangular space; if so, the axillary nerve may be damaged. The result is paralysis of the deltoid and teres minor muscles and loss of feeling over the lower portion of the deltoid (see UL33).

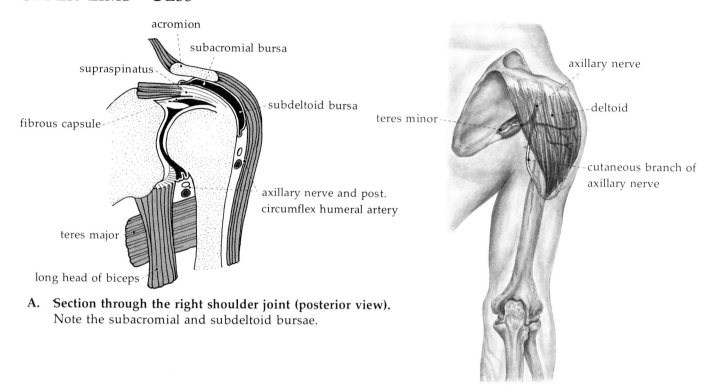

acromion

subacromial bursa

supraspinatus

subdeltoid bursa

fibrous capsule

axillary nerve and post.
circumflex humeral artery

teres major

long head of biceps

A. Section through the right shoulder joint (posterior view).
Note the subacromial and subdeltoid bursae.

axillary nerve

teres minor

deltoid

cutaneous branch of
axillary nerve

B. Motor innervation of the right axillary nerve.

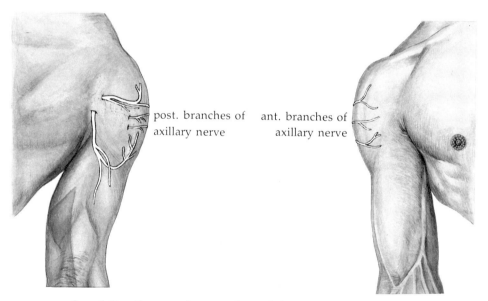

post. branches of   ant. branches of
axillary nerve   axillary nerve

C and D. Sensory innervation of the right axillary nerve.

A good understanding of the structures surrounding the shoulder joint is important:

¶ Lesions of the "rotator cuff" are the most common cause of pain in the shoulder region. The rotator cuff consists of the tendons of the subscapularis, supraspinatus, infraspinatus and teres minor. The tendon of the supraspinatus is most important, since it is frequently affected by early degenerative changes and inflammations. These pathologic processes probably are the result of friction between the head of the humerus and the bony ligamentous roof. The degenerative changes and inflammatory reactions often spread to the subacromial bursa and subsequently to the subdeltoid bursa. As a result of the swelling of the bursa, abduction and medial rotation in the shoulder become extremely painful.

¶ Occasionally the degenerative changes and inflammations proceed to the capsule of the joint, and perforations may occur. It is not uncommon that the synovial sheath of the long head of the biceps is also affected, and sometimes this tendon ruptures.

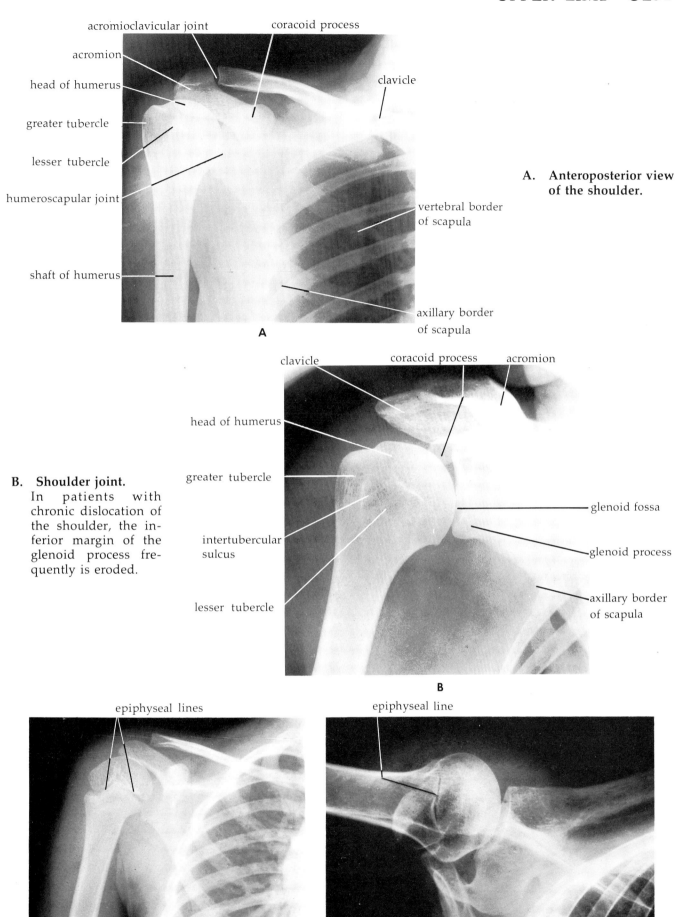

acromioclavicular joint

coracoid process

acromion

head of humerus

greater tubercle

lesser tubercle

humeroscapular joint

shaft of humerus

clavicle

vertebral border of scapula

axillary border of scapula

A.   Anteroposterior view of the shoulder.

A

B.   Shoulder joint.
In patients with chronic dislocation of the shoulder, the inferior margin of the glenoid process frequently is eroded.

clavicle

coracoid process

acromion

head of humerus

greater tubercle

intertubercular sulcus

lesser tubercle

glenoid fossa

glenoid process

axillary border of scapula

B

epiphyseal lines

epiphyseal line

C

D

C and D.   Shoulder region in an adolescent child.
Note the epiphyseal lines. Care must be taken not to confuse the epiphyseal lines with fracture lines. (*A* to *D* from Meschan, I.: *An Atlas of Anatomy Basic to Radiology*. Philadelphia, W. B. Saunders Co., 1975.)

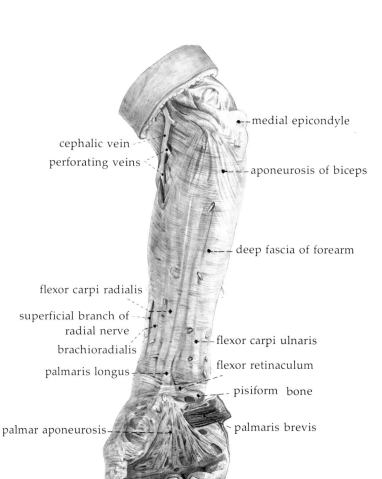

cephalic vein

perforating veins

medial epicondyle

aponeurosis of biceps

deep fascia of forearm

flexor carpi radialis

superficial branch of radial nerve

brachioradialis

palmaris longus

flexor carpi ulnaris

flexor retinaculum

pisiform bone

palmar aponeurosis

palmaris brevis

A. The deep fascia of the right forearm.
Most of the veins and sensory nerves in the superficial fascia have been removed.

lat. cutaneous nerve of forearm

ant. and med. branches of medial cutaneous nerve of forearm

brachioradialis

palmaris longus

superficial branch of radial nerve

flexor carpi ulnaris

radial artery with venae comitantes

flexor carpi radialis

ulnar artery and nerve

tendon of palmaris longus

median nerve

B. The superficial vessels and nerves of the right forearm.
The muscles lateral to the radial artery receive their motor innervation from the radial nerve, but those on the medial side are innervated by the median and ulnar nerves.

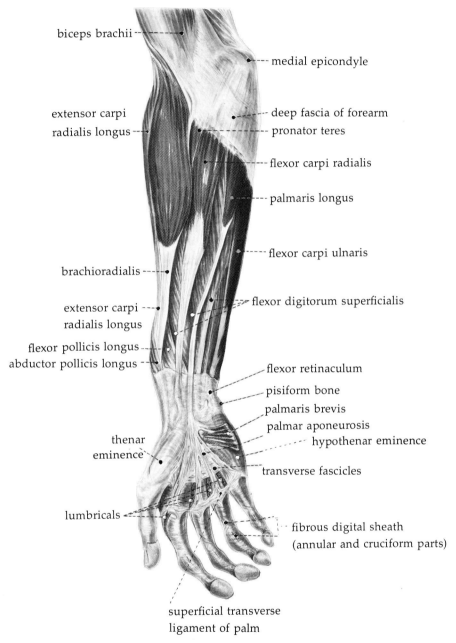

biceps brachii

medial epicondyle

extensor carpi
radialis longus

deep fascia of forearm

pronator teres

flexor carpi radialis

palmaris longus

flexor carpi ulnaris

brachioradialis

extensor carpi
radialis longus

flexor digitorum superficialis

flexor pollicis longus
abductor pollicis longus

flexor retinaculum

pisiform bone

palmaris brevis

palmar aponeurosis

thenar
eminence

hypothenar eminence

transverse fascicles

lumbricals

fibrous digital sheath
(annular and cruciform parts)

superficial transverse
ligament of palm

Superficial muscles on the anterior side of the right forearm.
The superficial flexor group consists of: (1) the pronator teres, (2) the flexor carpi radialis, (3) the palmaris longus, and (4) the flexor carpi ulnaris. The brachioradialis belongs to the lateral muscle group and, unlike the other muscles, is innervated by the radial nerve.

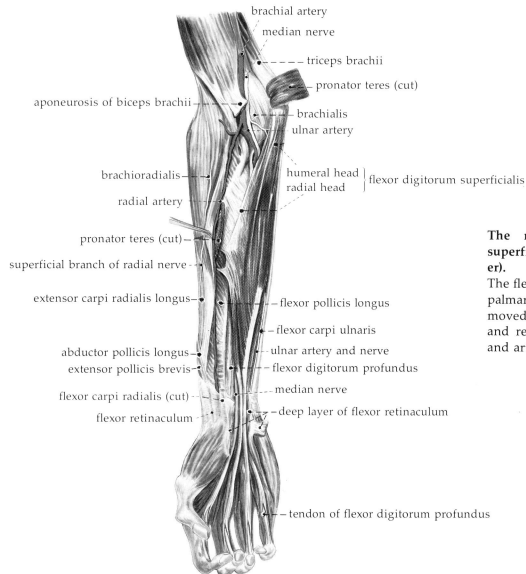

brachial artery

median nerve

triceps brachii

pronator teres (cut)

aponeurosis of biceps brachii

brachialis

ulnar artery

brachioradialis

humeral head
radial head } flexor digitorum superficialis

radial artery

pronator teres (cut)

superficial branch of radial nerve

extensor carpi radialis longus

flexor pollicis longus

flexor carpi ulnaris

abductor pollicis longus

ulnar artery and nerve

extensor pollicis brevis

flexor digitorum profundus

flexor carpi radialis (cut)

median nerve

flexor retinaculum

deep layer of flexor retinaculum

tendon of flexor digitorum profundus

The right flexor digitorum superficialis (second flexor layer).
The flexor carpi radialis and the palmaris longus have been removed; the pronator teres is cut and reflected. Note the nerves and arteries.

The median nerve is sometimes injured in the region of the elbow by supracondylar fractures of the humerus. As a result the following symptoms occur:

1. All the flexors of the forearm, with the exception of the flexor carpi ulnaris and the medial half of the flexor digitorum profundus, are paralyzed. The forearm is kept in a supine position (the biceps is not paralyzed), and flexion of the wrist is weak and is accompanied by adduction due to the function of the flexor carpi ulnaris (see UL51 and UL61).

2. Flexion of the interphalangeal joints of the index and middle fingers is impossible. When the patient makes a fist, the index and middle fingers remain straight.

3. The muscles of the thenar eminence are paralyzed, with the exception of the adductor pollicis (see UL50 and UL51).

4. For sensory loss see UL41.

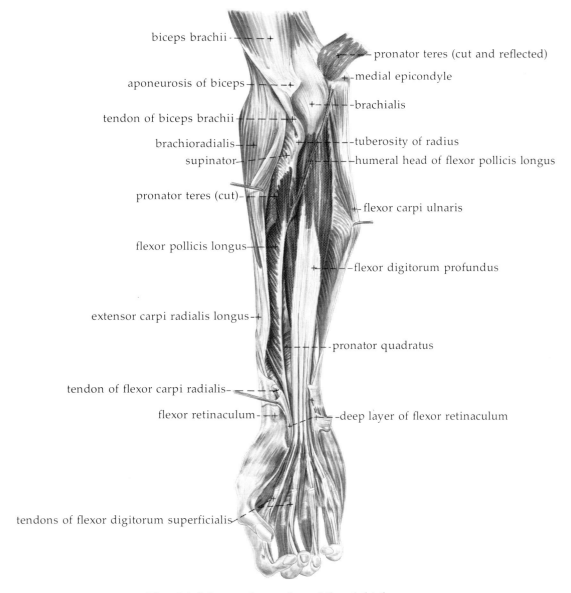

biceps brachii

pronator teres (cut and reflected)

aponeurosis of biceps

medial epicondyle

tendon of biceps brachii

brachialis

brachioradialis

tuberosity of radius

supinator

humeral head of flexor pollicis longus

pronator teres (cut)

flexor carpi ulnaris

flexor pollicis longus

flexor digitorum profundus

extensor carpi radialis longus

pronator quadratus

tendon of flexor carpi radialis

flexor retinaculum

deep layer of flexor retinaculum

tendons of flexor digitorum superficialis

The third layer of muscles of the right forearm.
The third flexor layer consists of the flexor pollicis longus and the flexor digitorum
profundus. The brachioradialis and flexor carpi ulnaris have been pulled to the side.

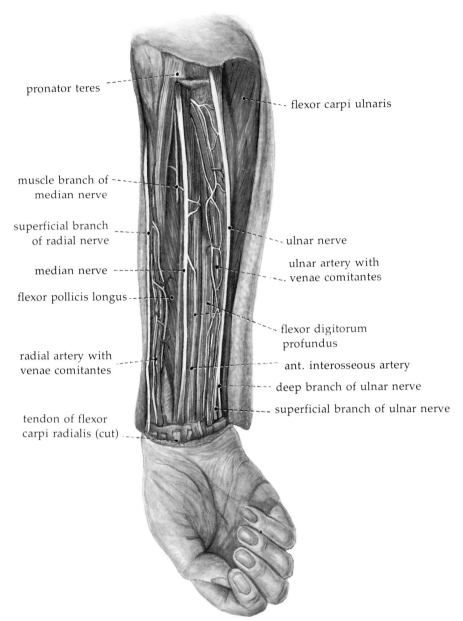

pronator teres

flexor carpi ulnaris

muscle branch of
median nerve

superficial branch
of radial nerve

ulnar nerve

ulnar artery with
venae comitantes

median nerve

flexor pollicis longus

flexor digitorum
profundus

radial artery with
venae comitantes

ant. interosseous artery

deep branch of ulnar nerve

superficial branch of ulnar nerve

tendon of flexor
carpi radialis (cut)

The arteries and nerves of the right forearm.
The flexor digitorum superficialis has been removed.

The most common injuries to the median nerve occur just above the flexor retinaculum.
In this area, the nerve is superficial between the tendons of the flexor carpi radialis and
the palmaris longus (see UL35 B and UL37).

When the nerve is injured at the wrist the following results occur:

1. The patient cannot oppose the thumb to the other fingers (paralysis of opponens
    pollicis).

2. Part of the thumb, index finger and middle finger and part of the fourth finger have
    lost their sensory innervation (see UL41).

3. The muscles of the thenar are paralyzed, and the thumb is in an adducted position.
    (The adductor pollicis is innervated by the ulnar nerve—see UL45 and UL51).

4. The first two lumbricals are paralyzed, and the index and middle fingers tend to stay
    behind the ring and little fingers in flexion of the fingers (see also UL50).

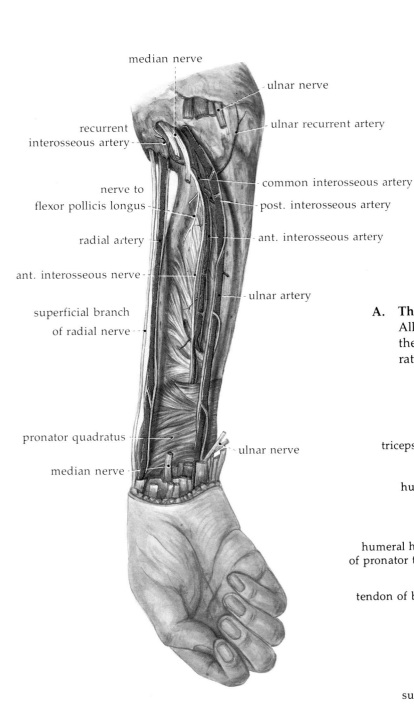

median nerve

ulnar nerve

recurrent interosseous artery

ulnar recurrent artery

nerve to flexor pollicis longus

common interosseous artery

post. interosseous artery

radial artery

ant. interosseous artery

ant. interosseous nerve

ulnar artery

superficial branch of radial nerve

pronator quadratus

ulnar nerve

median nerve

A. The arteries of the right forearm
All muscles have been removed with the exception of the pronator quadratus.

triceps brachii

humerus

medial epicondyle

humeral head of pronator teres

tendon of biceps

supinator

ulna

B. The right pronator and supinator muscles.
The main pronators of the forearm are: the pronator teres and the pronator quadratus. The main supinators are: the biceps femoris (see UL38) and the supinator.

interosseous membrane

radius

tendon of brachioradialis

pronator quadratus

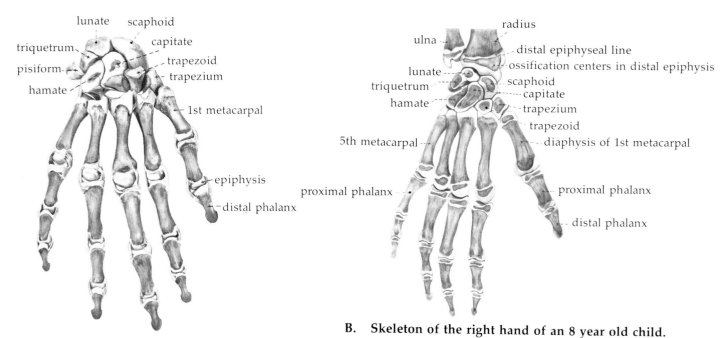

A. **Skeleton of the right hand of a 3 year old child.**

B. **Skeleton of the right hand of an 8 year old child.**

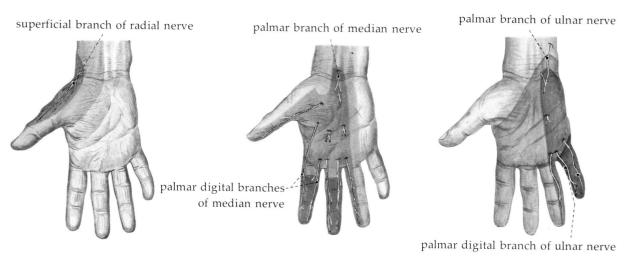

C. **Sensory innervation of the palm of the right hand.**

Knowledge of the time of ossification of the carpal bones is sometimes used to determine growth retardation in a child. At birth none of the carpal bones shows an ossification center. The capitate, however, starts to ossify soon after birth, followed by the hamate; ossification of the triquetrum starts at 2½ years of age; that of the lunate at 3½ years. Between the ages of 5 and 6 the scaphoid, trapezium and trapezoid show ossification centers. The pisiform is the last of all carpal bones to ossify at the age of 10.

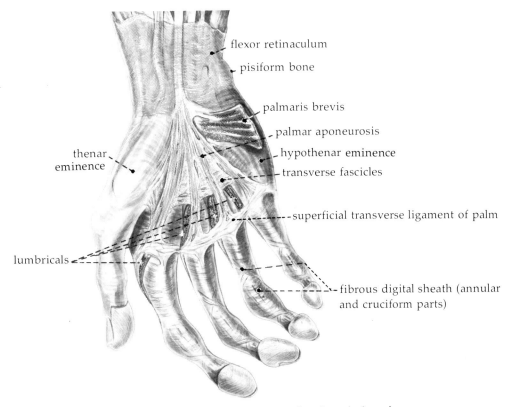

flexor retinaculum

pisiform bone

palmaris brevis

palmar aponeurosis

thenar eminence

hypothenar eminence

transverse fascicles

superficial transverse ligament of palm

lumbricals

fibrous digital sheath (annular and cruciform parts)

Right palmar aponeurosis and palmaris brevis.

The palmar aponeurosis is firmly attached to the skin of the palm. Toward the fingers it divides into four tendinous components, one for each finger. Each of these splits into two parts, which are inserted at the base of the proximal phalanges and the flexor sheaths. The palmar aponeurosis and the fascial spaces of the hand are clinically important:

¶ From the medial border of the palmar aponeurosis a fibrous septum passes deep to the anterior border of the fifth metacarpal bone; from the lateral border a septum passes deep to the anterior border of the third metacarpal bone. Hence, the septa divide the palm of the hand into: (a) the thenar space, (b) the midpalmar space, and (c) the hypothenar space. Proximally these spaces are closed by the walls of the carpal tunnel (see UL44). It is important to know these fascial compartments, since they limit the spread of infections in the hand.

¶ Frequently the palmar aponeurosis becomes thickened and contracted. This contracture, known as Dupuytren's contracture, begins usually at the ring finger. The result is flexion in the metacarpophalangeal joint, which draws the finger into the palm. Later the little finger becomes involved in a similar manner, thereby making the hand almost useless. In chronic cases all fingers become involved, and most of the fingers then also become flexed in the proximal interphalangeal joints.

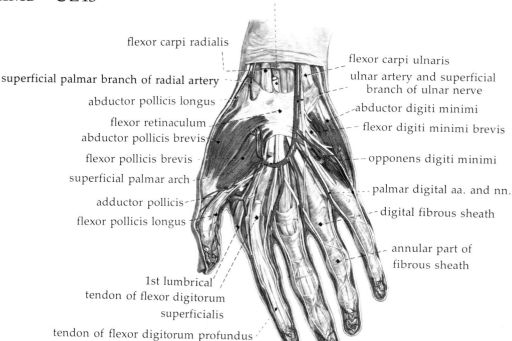

median nerve

flexor carpi radialis

superficial palmar branch of radial artery

abductor pollicis longus

flexor retinaculum

abductor pollicis brevis

flexor pollicis brevis

superficial palmar arch

adductor pollicis

flexor pollicis longus

flexor carpi ulnaris

ulnar artery and superficial branch of ulnar nerve

abductor digiti minimi

flexor digiti minimi brevis

opponens digiti minimi

palmar digital aa. and nn.

digital fibrous sheath

annular part of fibrous sheath

1st lumbrical

tendon of flexor digitorum superficialis

tendon of flexor digitorum profundus

A. Superficial arteries and nerves in the palm of the right hand.

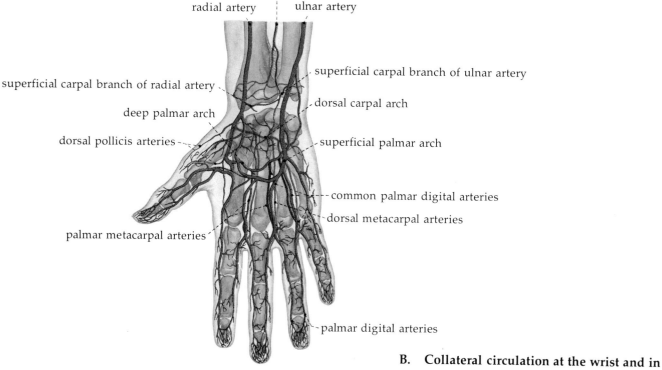

ant. interosseous artery

radial artery

ulnar artery

superficial carpal branch of radial artery

deep palmar arch

dorsal pollicis arteries

palmar metacarpal arteries

superficial carpal branch of ulnar artery

dorsal carpal arch

superficial palmar arch

common palmar digital arteries

dorsal metacarpal arteries

palmar digital arteries

B. Collateral circulation at the wrist and in the palm of the right hand.

Make the following observations:

¶ The superficial position of the ulnar nerve and artery at the wrist makes them vulnerable to injuries. Such injuries are particularly dangerous since both nerve and artery pass into the palm in front of the flexor retinaculum. The superficial branch of the ulnar nerve supplies the medial side of the palm, the palmaris brevis and the palmar surface of the medial one and a half fingers. Hence, injury to the nerve results mainly in sensory loss (see UL41 C).

¶ The ulnar or radial artery can be ligated safely since each is united by many anastomoses in the form of two palmar arches and two carpal arches. The superficial palmar arch lies under the skin and palmar aponeurosis; the deep palmar arch and the carpal connections lie in contact with the skeletal elements. The interosseous arteries also play a role in the communicating network.

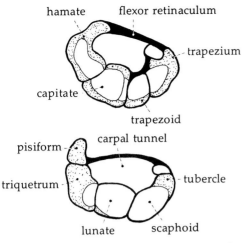

A. The carpal tunnel (transverse sections).

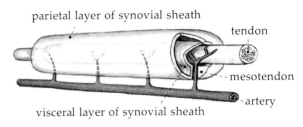

B. Schematic drawing of synovial sheath and blood supply of the tendon.

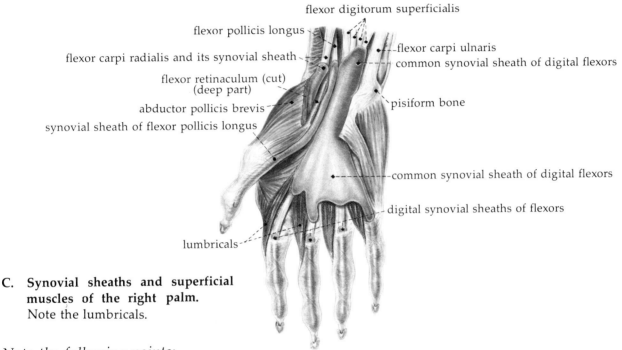

C. Synovial sheaths and superficial muscles of the right palm.
Note the lumbricals.

Note the following points:

¶ The carpal tunnel is formed by the flexor retinaculum and the palmar surface of the carpal bones. Through the tunnel pass the median nerve and the long flexor tendons with their sheaths. The tunnel is narrow, and the median nerve may be compressed if the synovial sheaths are swollen or if arthritic changes occur in the intercarpal joint. The result is a tingling sensation and loss of feeling in the lateral three and a half fingers and weakness in the thenar muscles. A longitudinal incision through the retinaculum usually makes the symptoms disappear rapidly.

¶ The synovial sheaths are lubricating sleeves through which the flexor tendons move smoothly under the flexor retinaculum and in the fascial coverings of the fingers. Since the synovial sheaths are closed at both ends, the blood supply passes through small mesotendons. The relation of the sheaths toward each other is very important. Those of the second, third, and fourth fingers do not communicate with the common sheath surrounding the tendons of the flexor digitorum superficialis and profundus. The sheath of the little finger almost always communicates with the common sheath.

¶ Small wounds penetrating the sheath are dangerous, particularly if infection occurs. Infections spread rapidly along the sheath. In the thumb, infections may expand into the common sheath at the wrist and subsequently descend to the little finger. The finger becomes swollen and is held in a semiflexed position to relieve the tension.

¶ If infections of the sheaths are neglected, pus may burst through the proximal parts. Infections of the little finger may spread into the subthenar fascial space, and those of the thumb into the thenar fascial space. Infections of the middle finger expand into the midpalmar space, and those of the index finger may expand either into the thenar space or into the midpalmar space.

¶ The synovial sheath of the flexor pollicis longus is also referred to as the *radial bursa*. Similarly, that of the little finger is referred to as the *ulnar bursa*. Infections of these bursae may expand into the fascial space of the forearm between the flexor digitorum profundus and the pronator quadratus. This space is known clinically as the *space of Parona*.

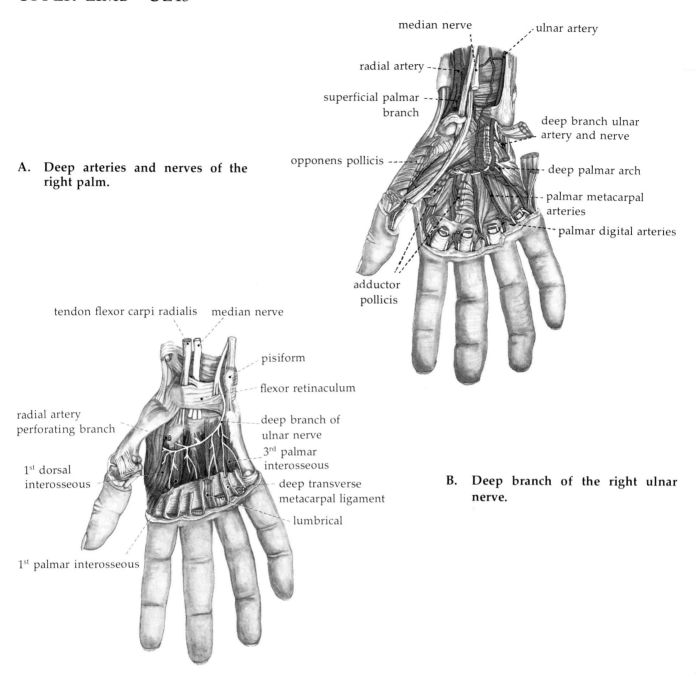

A. Deep arteries and nerves of the right palm.

median nerve

ulnar artery

radial artery

superficial palmar branch

deep branch ulnar artery and nerve

opponens pollicis

deep palmar arch

palmar metacarpal arteries

palmar digital arteries

adductor pollicis

tendon flexor carpi radialis   median nerve

pisiform

flexor retinaculum

radial artery perforating branch

deep branch of ulnar nerve

3rd palmar interosseous

1st dorsal interosseous

deep transverse metacarpal ligament

lumbrical

B. Deep branch of the right ulnar nerve.

1st palmar interosseous

The course and function of the deep branch of the ulnar nerve are important:

The deep branch supplies all the hypothenar muscles, all interossei, the two medial lumbricals and both heads of the adductor of the thumb. When the nerve is cut all small muscles of the hand are paralyzed, with the exception of those of the thenar and the first two lumbricals (supplied by the median nerve). Since all interossei are paralyzed, the fingers cannot be adducted and abducted, and the patient is unable to hold a sheet of paper between the fingers.

The interphalangeal joints are flexed owing to paralysis of the lumbricals and interossei, which under normal conditions extend these joints. The metacarpophalangeal joints are hyperextended—hence, the hand forms a claw. In time the muscles become atrophic, and a flattening of the hypothenar and interdigital spaces becomes evident. Sensory deprivation is restricted to the medial part of the hand; the patient is still able to oppose the thumb and index fingers (pincer action).

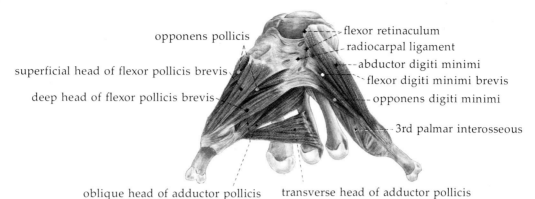

opponens pollicis

superficial head of flexor pollicis brevis

deep head of flexor pollicis brevis

flexor retinaculum

radiocarpal ligament

abductor digiti minimi

flexor digiti minimi brevis

opponens digiti minimi

3rd palmar interosseous

oblique head of adductor pollicis

transverse head of adductor pollicis

A. Muscles of the thenar and hypothenar of the right hand.
Note the heads of the adductor pollicis.

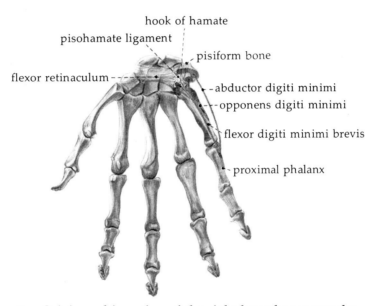

hook of hamate

pisohamate ligament

pisiform bone

flexor retinaculum

abductor digiti minimi

opponens digiti minimi

flexor digiti minimi brevis

proximal phalanx

B. Origin and insertion of the right hypothenar muscles.

The thenar and hypothenar eminences are each formed by three muscles: (a) an abductor near the border of the hand, (b) a flexor near the palm of the hand, and (c) an opponens deep to the other two.

Abductor digiti minimi (ulnar nerve)

Origin: Pisiform bone; adjacent proximal part of flexor retinaculum; tendon of flexor carpi ulnaris.

Insertion: Ulnar aspect of proximal phalanx.

Flexor digiti minimi (ulnar nerve)

Origin: Hook of hamate; adjacent distal part of flexor retinaculum.

Insertion: Ulnar aspect of proximal phalax.

Opponens digiti minimi (ulnar nerve)

Origin: Hook of hamate; distal part of flexor retinaculum.

Insertion: Shaft of fifth metacarpal bone.

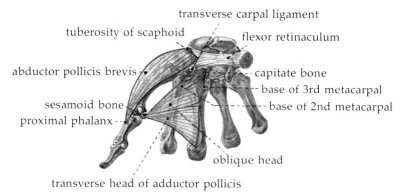

A. Origin and insertion of the right abductor pollicis brevis and adductor pollicis.

Abductor pollicis brevis (median nerve)

Origin: Scaphoid; trapezium; adjacent proximal part of flexor retinaculum.

Insertion: Radial aspect of proximal phalanx.

Adductor pollicis (ulnar nerve)

Origin: Oblique head: bases of second and third metacarpals and adjacent carpal bones. *Transverse head:* anterior surface of the shaft of the third metacarpal bone.

Insertion: Medial side of the base of the proximal phalanx of the thumb. Usually a sesamoid bone is present.

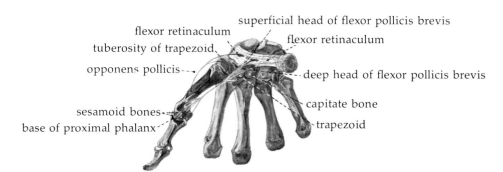

B. Origin and insertion of the right opponens pollicis and flexor pollicis brevis.

Flexor pollicis brevis (median nerve)

Origin: Ridge of trapezium; adjacent distal part of flexor retinaculum.

Insertion: Base of proximal phalanx.

Opponens pollicis (median nerve)

Origin: Distal part of flexor retinaculum.

Insertion: Shaft of first metacarpal bone.

252

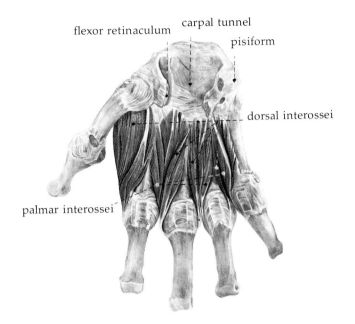

A. Right interosseous muscles seen from the palmar side.
Note the floor of the carpal tunnel.

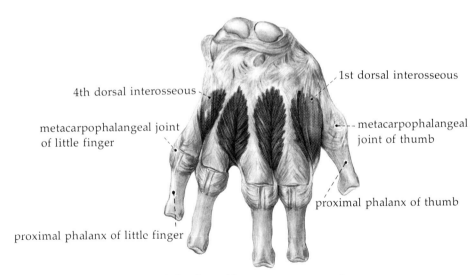

B. Right dorsal interosseous muscles.

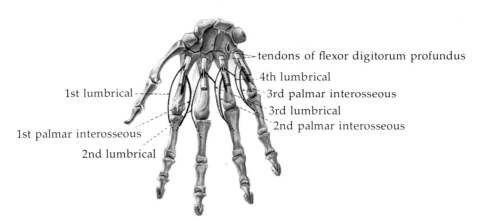

1st lumbrical

1st palmar interosseous

2nd lumbrical

tendons of flexor digitorum profundus

4th lumbrical

3rd palmar interosseous

3rd lumbrical

2nd palmar interosseous

A. Schematic drawing of the right lumbricals and palmar interosseous muscles.

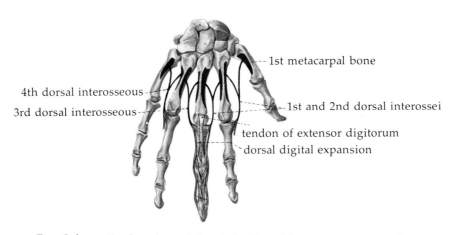

4th dorsal interosseous

3rd dorsal interosseous

1st metacarpal bone

1st and 2nd dorsal interossei

tendon of extensor digitorum

dorsal digital expansion

B. Schematic drawing of the right dorsal interosseous muscles.

Lumbricals

Origin: Tendons of flexor digitorum profundus.

Insertion: Lateral side of corresponding extensor expansion.

Function: Flexion of metacarpophalangeal joints.

Dorsal interossei

Origin: Contiguous sides of metacarpal bones.

Insertion: First and second dorsal interossei insert on lateral side of base of proximal phalanx of index and middle fingers. Third and fourth dorsal interossei insert on medial side of middle and ring fingers.

In addition, all these muscles insert into the extensor expansion of the digit on which they act.

Function: Abduction away from middle finger; flexion of metacarpophalangeal joints; extension of interphalangeal joints.

Palmar interossei

Origin: Shafts of second, fourth and fifth metacarpal bones.

Insertion: Medial side of base of proximal phalanx of index finger. Lateral side of base of proximal phalanx of ring and little fingers.

In addition, all are inserted into the extensor expansion of the digit on which they act.

Function: Adduction toward middle finger; flexion of metacarpophalangeal joints; extension of interphalangeal joints.

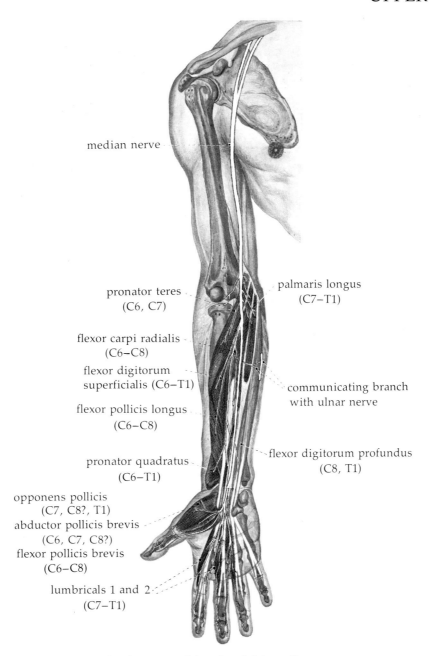

median nerve

pronator teres
(C6, C7)

palmaris longus
(C7–T1)

flexor carpi radialis
(C6–C8)

flexor digitorum
superficialis (C6–T1)

communicating branch
with ulnar nerve

flexor pollicis longus
(C6–C8)

flexor digitorum profundus
(C8, T1)

pronator quadratus
(C6–T1)

opponens pollicis
(C7, C8?, T1)
abductor pollicis brevis
(C6, C7, C8?)
flexor pollicis brevis
(C6–C8)

lumbricals 1 and 2
(C7–T1)

Muscles innervated by the right median nerve.

When reviewing the median nerve note:

¶ There are no sensory or motor branches in the axilla or arm.

¶ In the forearm the median nerve supplies all the anterior muscles except the flexor carpi ulnaris and the medial part of the flexor digitorum profundus.

¶ In the hand it supplies the muscles of the thenar eminence (except the adductor pollicis) and two lateral lumbricals.

¶ The nerve is most frequently injured: (a) in the elbow region by supracondylar fractures of the humerus; (b) just proximal to the flexor retinaculum by cuts at the wrist; (c) by dislocation of the lunate bone in a palmar direction. For results of lesions see UL37 and UL39.

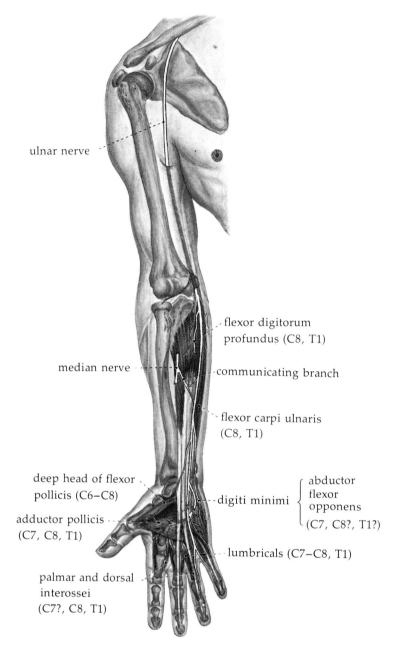

ulnar nerve

flexor digitorum
profundus (C8, T1)

median nerve

communicating branch

flexor carpi ulnaris
(C8, T1)

deep head of flexor
pollicis (C6–C8)

adductor pollicis
(C7, C8, T1)

digiti minimi
$\begin{cases} \text{abductor} \\ \text{flexor} \\ \text{opponens} \\ \text{(C7, C8?, T1?)} \end{cases}$

lumbricals (C7–C8, T1)

palmar and dorsal
interossei
(C7?, C8, T1)

Muscles innervated by the right ulnar nerve.

When reviewing the ulnar nerve note:

¶ There are no cutaneous or motor branches in the axilla or arm.

¶ In the forearm the ulnar nerve supplies only the flexor carpi ulnaris and the medial part of the flexor digitorum profundus.

¶ In the hand it supplies the hypothenar muscles, the two medial lumbricals, the palmar and dorsal interossei and the adductor pollicis.

¶ The nerve is most frequently injured: (a) at the elbow, where it lies behind the medial epicondyle; (b) at the wrist, where it lies in front of the flexor retinaculum. For results of lesions see UL45 and UL61.

anconeus

brachioradialis

extensor carpi radialis longus

extensor carpi ulnaris

extensor digitorum

extensor carpi radialis brevis

medial cutaneous nerve of forearm (ulnar)

extensor digiti minimi

abductor pollicis longus

post. cutaneous nerve of forearm (radial)

lat. cutaneous nerve of forearm (musculocutaneous)

extensor pollicis brevis

dorsal cutaneous branch of ulnar nerve

dorsal carpal branch of radial artery

dorsal carpal branch of ulnar artery

superficial branch of radial nerve

A. Superficial nerves and vessels of the right posterior forearm.

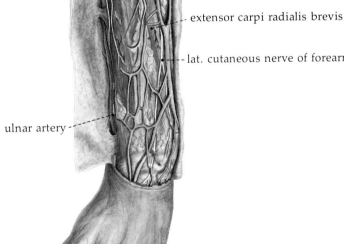

post. cutaneous nerve of forearm

lat. cutaneous nerve of forearm

brachioradialis

extensor digitorum

extensor carpi radialis longus

medial cutaneous nerve of forearm (ulnar branches)

extensor carpi radialis brevis

lat. cutaneous nerve of forearm

ulnar artery

The radial nerve gives off its sensory branches considerably proximal to the part innervated:

¶ The posterior cutaneous nerve of the arm, which innervates the back of the arm to the elbow joint, arises in the axilla.

¶ The posterior cutaneous nerve of the forearm arises in the spiral groove and innervates the posterior side of the forearm as far as the wrist.

¶ The superficial branch of the radial nerve arises in the elbow region and courses on the lateral side of the radial artery on the anterior side of the forearm. It leaves the artery in the lower part of the forearm to reach the posterior surface of the wrist and supplies the skin on the lateral two-thirds of the dorsal surface of the hand. Hence, lesions to this nerve are usually found at a much higher level than the affected sensory area.

B. Superficial nerves and vessels on the posterior side of the forearm.
Note the various cutaneous nerves.

257

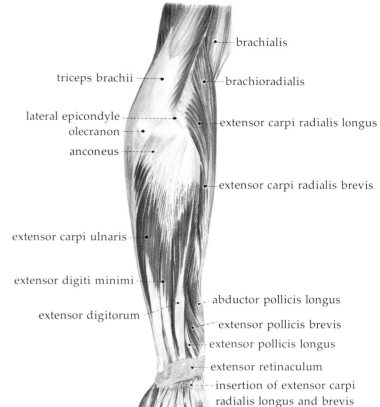

brachialis
triceps brachii
brachioradialis
lateral epicondyle
olecranon
anconeus
extensor carpi radialis longus
extensor carpi radialis brevis
extensor carpi ulnaris
extensor digiti minimi
extensor digitorum
abductor pollicis longus
extensor pollicis brevis
extensor pollicis longus
extensor retinaculum
insertion of extensor carpi radialis longus and brevis
tendon of extensor digiti minimi
tendons of extensor digitorum

A. Muscles of the extensor region of the right forearm.

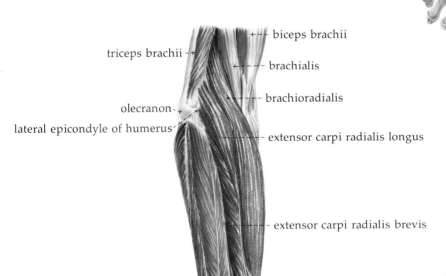

biceps brachii
triceps brachii
brachialis
brachioradialis
olecranon
lateral epicondyle of humerus
extensor carpi radialis longus
extensor carpi radialis brevis
extensor digitorum
extensor digiti minimi
abductor pollicis longus
extensor carpi ulnaris
extensor pollicis brevis
head of ulna
tendons of extensor carpi radialis longus and brevis
styloid process of radius

B. Muscles on the posterolateral side of the right forearm.

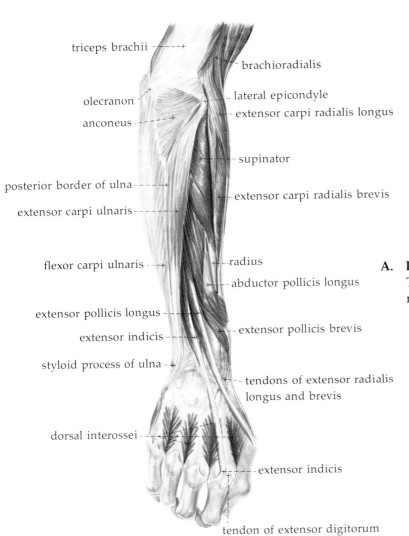

triceps brachii

brachioradialis

olecranon

lateral epicondyle

anconeus

extensor carpi radialis longus

supinator

posterior border of ulna

extensor carpi radialis brevis

extensor carpi ulnaris

flexor carpi ulnaris

radius

abductor pollicis longus

extensor pollicis longus

extensor pollicis brevis

extensor indicis

styloid process of ulna

tendons of extensor radialis longus and brevis

dorsal interossei

extensor indicis

tendon of extensor digitorum

A. Deep extensor muscles of the right forearm.
The extensor digitorum and extensor digiti minimi have been removed.

Unlike the ulnar nerve which passes behind the medial epicondyle, the radial nerve passes in front of the lateral epicondyle. After its course through the spiral groove, the nerve pierces the lateral intermuscular septum and lies between the brachialis medially and the brachioradialis laterally and superior to the extensor carpi radialis longus. The nerve then splits into the superficial branch and the deep branch, which pierces the supinator muscle.

During surgical procedures on the head of the radius, the deep branch of the radial nerve may be damaged, paralyzing all extensor muscles of the forearm. There is no sensory loss, since the nerve provides motor innervation exclusively. Surprisingly, the effect of paralysis is not too serious, since many other muscles can take over the function of the paralyzed ones. For example, the extensor carpi radialis longus is not affected and will be able to extend the wrist joint. Wrist drop does not occur.

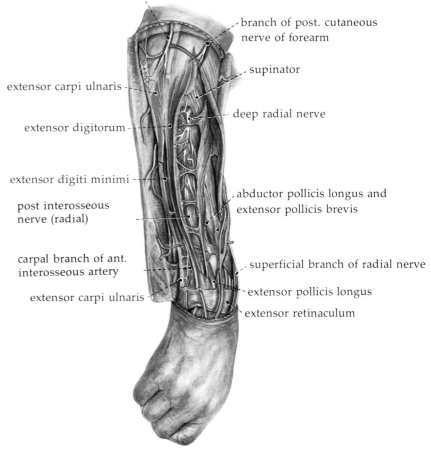

branch of post. cutaneous nerve of arm

branch of post. cutaneous nerve of forearm

extensor carpi ulnaris

supinator

extensor digitorum

deep radial nerve

extensor digiti minimi

post interosseous nerve (radial)

abductor pollicis longus and extensor pollicis brevis

carpal branch of ant. interosseous artery

superficial branch of radial nerve

extensor carpi ulnaris

extensor pollicis longus

extensor retinaculum

B. Deep branch of the right radial nerve.
The extensor digitorum has been split and pulled aside.

259

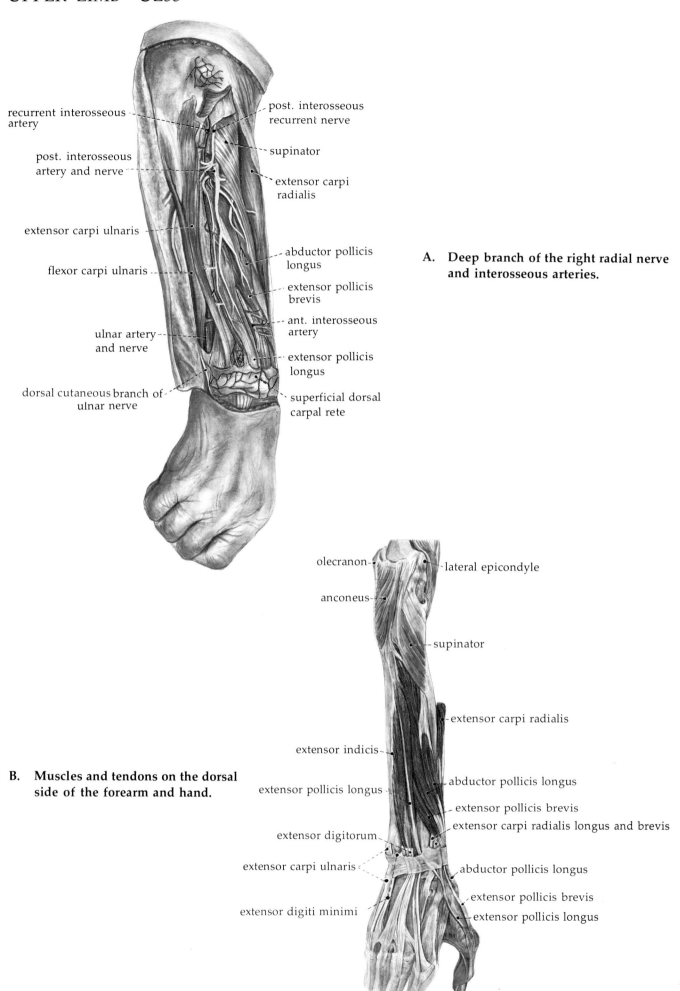

recurrent interosseous artery

post. interosseous artery and nerve

extensor carpi ulnaris

flexor carpi ulnaris

ulnar artery and nerve

dorsal cutaneous branch of ulnar nerve

post. interosseous recurrent nerve

supinator

extensor carpi radialis

abductor pollicis longus

extensor pollicis brevis

ant. interosseous artery

extensor pollicis longus

superficial dorsal carpal rete

A. Deep branch of the right radial nerve and interosseous arteries.

olecranon

anconeus

lateral epicondyle

supinator

extensor carpi radialis

extensor indicis

extensor pollicis longus

extensor digitorum

extensor carpi ulnaris

extensor digiti minimi

abductor pollicis longus

extensor pollicis brevis

extensor carpi radialis longus and brevis

abductor pollicis longus

extensor pollicis brevis

extensor pollicis longus

B. Muscles and tendons on the dorsal side of the forearm and hand.

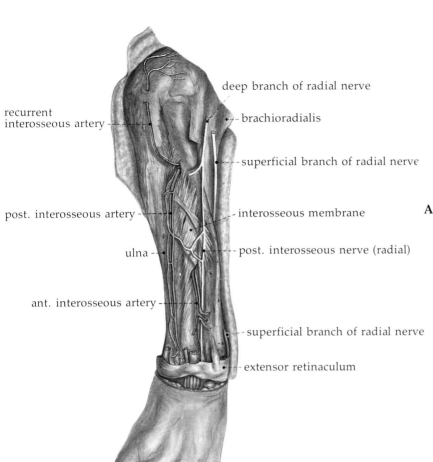

recurrent interosseous artery

deep branch of radial nerve

brachioradialis

superficial branch of radial nerve

post. interosseous artery

interosseous membrane

ulna

post. interosseous nerve (radial)

ant. interosseous artery

superficial branch of radial nerve

extensor retinaculum

A. Deep dissection of the posterior side of the right forearm.
Note the branch of the anterior interosseous artery piercing the interosseous membrane.

abductor pollicis longus
extensor pollicis brevis

extensor carpi radialis longus
extensor carpi radialis brevis

extensor retinaculum

extensor pollicis longus

extensor carpi ulnaris

extensor digitorum

extensor digiti minimi

B. Synovial sheaths on the dorsum of the right wrist.

¶ Fibrous septa pass from the extensor retinaculum (B) to the underlying radius and ulna, thus forming six compartments containing the tendons of the extensor muscles. To avoid friction, each compartment is provided with a synovial sheath, which extends above and below the retinaculum. Although infections of the synovial sheaths occur, they are rare in comparison with those on the palmar side of the wrist.

¶ Remember that the superficial branch of the radial nerve and the dorsal cutaneous branch of the ulnar nerve as well as the cephalic and basilic veins pass superficially over the extensor retinaculum (see UL52 A).

261

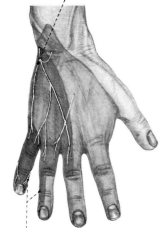
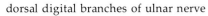
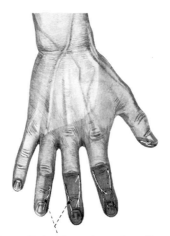
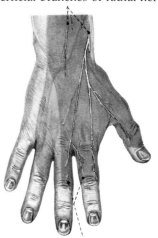

dorsal branch of ulnar nerve

superficial branches of radial nerve

dorsal digital branches of ulnar nerve

palmar digital branches of median nerve

dorsal digital branches of radial nerve

A.   Sensory innervation of the dorsum of the right hand.

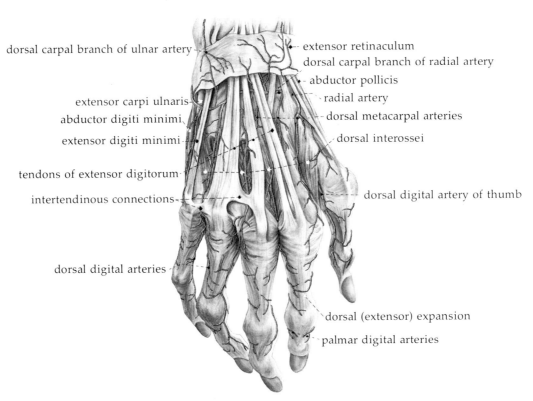

dorsal carpal branch of ulnar artery

extensor retinaculum

dorsal carpal branch of radial artery

abductor pollicis

radial artery

extensor carpi ulnaris

abductor digiti minimi

dorsal metacarpal arteries

extensor digiti minimi

dorsal interossei

tendons of extensor digitorum

intertendinous connections

dorsal digital artery of thumb

dorsal digital arteries

dorsal (extensor) expansion

palmar digital arteries

B.   Arteries of the dorsum of the right hand.

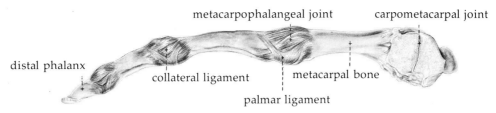

A. Joints of the middle finger.

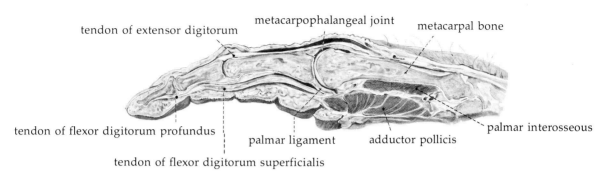

B. Longitudinal section through the index finger.

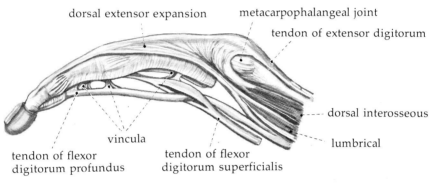

C. Muscles acting on the index finger.

In flexion movements of the fingers it is important to keep in mind:

❡ The distal phalanx is flexed by the flexor digitorum profundus.

❡ The middle phalanx is flexed by the flexor digitorum superficialis.

❡ The proximal phalanx is flexed by the interosseous and lumbrical muscles.

In extension of the fingers:

❡ The distal and middle phalanges are extended by the lumbrical and interosseous muscles.

❡ The proximal phalanx is extended by the extensor digitorum and extensor muscles of the index and little finger.

❡ For abduction and adduction movements see UL49.

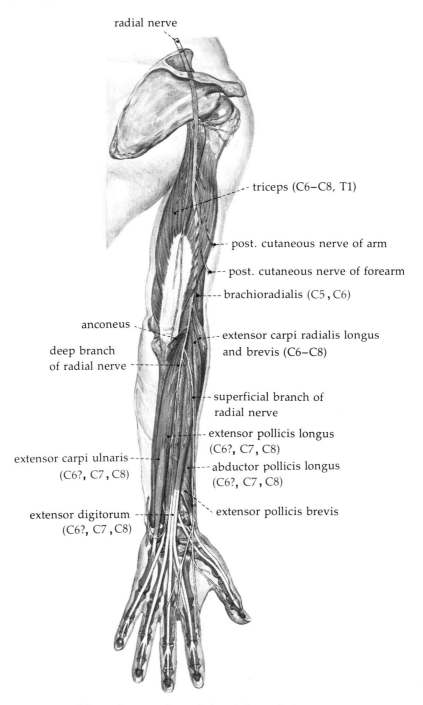

radial nerve

triceps (C6–C8, T1)

post. cutaneous nerve of arm

post. cutaneous nerve of forearm

brachioradialis (C5, C6)

anconeus

extensor carpi radialis longus
and brevis (C6–C8)

deep branch
of radial nerve

superficial branch of
radial nerve

extensor pollicis longus
(C6?, C7, C8)

extensor carpi ulnaris
(C6?, C7, C8)

abductor pollicis longus
(C6?, C7, C8)

extensor digitorum
(C6?, C7, C8)

extensor pollicis brevis

Motor innervation of the right radial nerve.

The radial nerve in the axilla may be damaged by fractures of the upper end of the humerus or dislocations with strong downward displacement of the humerus. In such cases the nerve may be stretched excessively. Continuous pressure in the axilla by a crutch may also damage the nerve.

When the nerve is injured in the axilla all extensors will be affected. The patient is unable to extend the elbow joint, the wrist joint and the fingers. Since the flexor muscles are unopposed, the arm will be flexed in the elbow, wrist drop will occur and gripping will be difficult because the patient is unable to fully extend his fingers. The middle and distal phalanges can be extended through the lumbricals and interossei. Although the brachioradialis and supinator are paralyzed, supination is still possible by the biceps brachii.

Lesions high in the radial nerve will produce complete loss of sensation. (For nerve injuries in the spiral groove and in the elbow region see UL29 and UL54.)

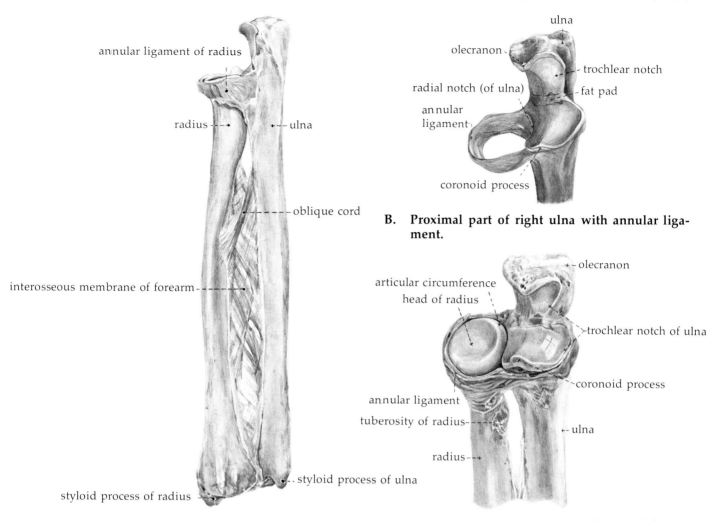

A. **Right interosseous membrane and annular ligament.**

B. **Proximal part of right ulna with annular ligament.**

C. **Right proximal radioulnar joint.**

The annular ligament is attached to the anterior and posterior margins of the radial notch of the ulna. It forms a collar around the head of the radius but is not attached to the radius. The annular ligament is of considerable importance:

¶ In young children the head of the radius is small and can easily be pulled out of its "buttonhole." This happens frequently when parents pull the child along by the hand or lift the child unexpectedly off the ground by one arm.

¶ In some cases the head of the radius may be fractured, and the ligament may be torn. During surgery on the head of the radius, the deep branch of the radial nerve has to be kept in mind. The nerve winds around the neck of the radius between the layers of the supinator muscle. When it is injured the brachioradialis and extensor carpi radialis remain unaffected, since they are innervated by branches of the radial nerve that originate at a higher level.

¶ Keep in mind that the proximal radioulnar joint is in open connection with the elbow joint, and any infection of the elbow joint will involve the proximal radioulnar joint. The distal radioulnar joint does not communicate with the wrist joint.

medial border of humerus

medial epicondyle

annular ligament

sacciform recess

radius

olecranon

post. portion
oblique portion } ulnar collateral ligament
ant. portion

oblique cord

ulna

A. Medial aspect of the right elbow joint.

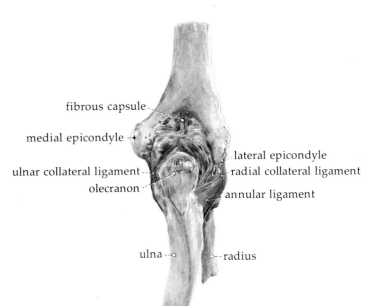

fibrous capsule

medial epicondyle

lateral epicondyle

ant. part of ulnar collateral ligament

radial collateral ligament

annular ligament

sacciform recess

tuberosity of radius

oblique cord

ulna

B. Anterior aspect of the right elbow joint.

lateral border of humerus

lateral epicondyle

olecranon

annular ligament

sacciform recess

radius

radial collateral ligament

ulna

C. Lateral aspect of the right elbow joint.

fibrous capsule

medial epicondyle

lateral epicondyle

ulnar collateral ligament

radial collateral ligament

olecranon

annular ligament

ulna

radius

D. Posterior aspect of the right elbow joint.

Note the following points:

¶ Inflammations of the joint cause the anterior and posterior aspects to become swollen and distended by fluid. The lateral and medial sides do not bulge. Aspiration of fluid is performed preferably on the radial side of the olecranon. It is too dangerous to approach the anterior aspect of the capsule because of the brachial artery and the median nerve, and the medial side is unapproachable because of the ulnar nerve.

¶ The sacciform recess is located below the annular ligament and forms an extension of the capsule. Its fibrous wall is relatively thin, so fluid and pus easily collect in this recess when the joint is inflamed.

¶ In dislocations of the ulna or fractures of the medial epicondyle the ulnar nerve may easily be damaged or overstretched. When the ulnar nerve is damaged, the flexor carpi ulnaris and the medial half of the flexor digitorum profundus are paralyzed, and flexion of the wrist joint results in abduction. The terminal phalanges of the ring and little fingers are not capable of flexion. Similarly, all small muscles of the hand will be paralyzed, except the three thenar muscles and the first two lumbricals.

266

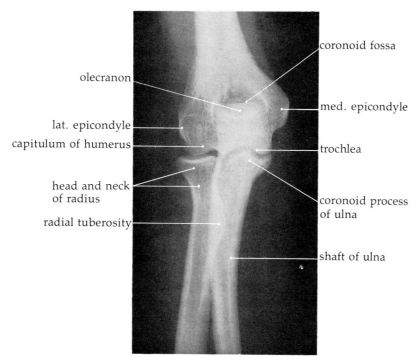

olecranon

coronoid fossa

lat. epicondyle

med. epicondyle

capitulum of humerus

trochlea

head and neck
of radius

coronoid process
of ulna

radial tuberosity

shaft of ulna

A. Right elbow joint, anteroposterior view.

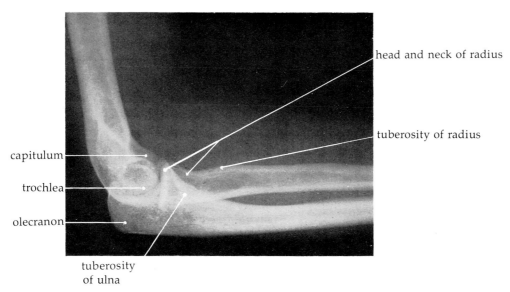

head and neck of radius

tuberosity of radius

capitulum

trochlea

olecranon

tuberosity
of ulna

B. **Right elbow joint, lateral view.**
Fractures of the head and neck of the radius are sometimes missed in radiographic examination of the joint. (*A* and *B* from Meschan, I.: *An Atlas of Anatomy Basic to Radiology*. Philadelphia, W. B. Saunders Co., 1975.)

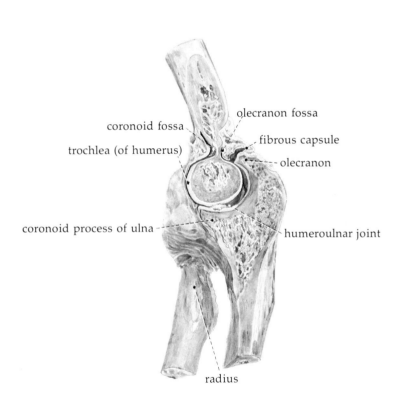

A. Sagittal section through the right humeroradial joint.
Note the sacciform recess.

capitulum (of humerus)
olecranon
articular cartilage
humeroulnar joint
fibrous capsule
annular ligament
fatty tissue
sacciform recess
proximal radioulnar joint
humeroradial joint

coronoid fossa
olecranon fossa
trochlea (of humerus)
fibrous capsule
olecranon
coronoid process of ulna
humeroulnar joint
radius

B. Sagittal section through the right humeroulnar joint.

Make the following observations:

¶ The bony plate between the coronoid fossa and the olecranon fossa at the distal end of the humerus is very thin. Occasionally it disappears entirely, and a periosteal membrane then fills the space between the two fossae. In such cases the arm can be considerably overextended in the elbow joint.

¶ Posterior dislocations of the ulna are common in children because the bones are not fully developed. The coronoid process is then found in the olecranon fossa, and the posterior aspect of the capsule is usually ruptured. Similarly, the tendon of the brachialis is usually ruptured, since it attaches to the coronoid process.

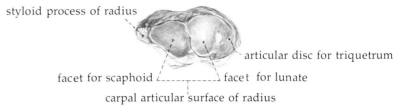

styloid process of radius

articular disc for triquetrum

facet for scaphoid

facet for lunate

carpal articular surface of radius

A. Articular surface of right radius and ulna for carpal bones.

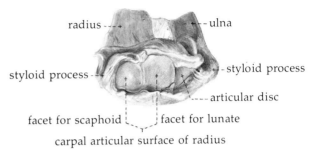

radius

ulna

styloid process

styloid process

articular disc

facet for scaphoid

facet for lunate

carpal articular surface of radius

B. Proximal articular surface of right radius and ulna for carpal bones.

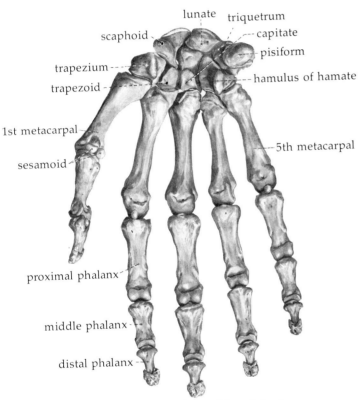

lunate   triquetrum

scaphoid

capitate

trapezium

pisiform

trapezoid

hamulus of hamate

1st metacarpal

sesamoid

5th metacarpal

proximal phalanx

middle phalanx

distal phalanx

C. Bones of the right wrist and hand (palmar aspect).

The carpal bones are arranged in a proximal and a distal row, each consisting of four bones. Only two are of clinical importance:

1. The *scaphoid bone.* In young adults the scaphoid is frequently fractured in falls on the outstretched hand, with the hand in radial abduction. The blood vessels entering the scaphoid at its proximal and distal ends (frequently only the distal end) are usually torn. As a result, the proximal fragment of the bone loses its arterial supply and undergoes necrosis. In other cases the two parts do not unite, causing weakness in the joint and osteoarthritis at a later age.

2. The *lunate bone.* This is the carpal bone most frequently dislocated. Because of its form the dislocation almost always occurs in a palmar direction. In this event the median nerve, which passes directly over the bone, may be damaged, and paralysis and sensory deprivation of the hand follows (see UL39 and UL41).

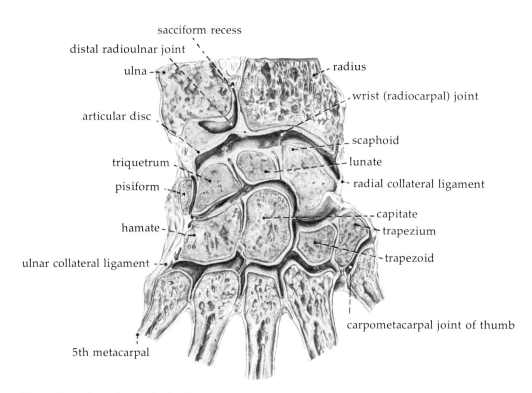

Frontal section through the left radiocarpal, intercarpal and carpometacarpal joints.

Make the following observations:

¶ The proximal part of the radiocarpal or wrist joint is formed by the concave lower articular surface of the radius and the articular disc. Hence, the ulna is not in direct contact with the carpal bones. In addition, because the articular disc closes off the distal radioulnar joint, this joint cavity is not in open communication with the wrist joint.

¶ The distal part of the wrist joint is formed by the scaphoid and lunate bones (which articulate with the radius) and the triquetrum (which articulates with the articular disc).

¶ The intercarpal joints are formed by the transverse carpal joint and the small pisiform joint. The transverse joint is formed by the three bones of the proximal row and the four of the distal row. The pisiform joint is independent, and its cavity is shut off from the other cavities.

¶ Of the five carpometacarpal joints, the joint of the thumb is entirely separated from the other four, which are in communication with each other.

¶ In a fall on the outstretched hand, the force is directed from the third metacarpal to the capitate and then (depending on whether the hand is in a radial or an ulnar position) to the scaphoid or lunate, respectively. Such a fall may cause a fracture of the scaphoid or a dislocation of the lunate.

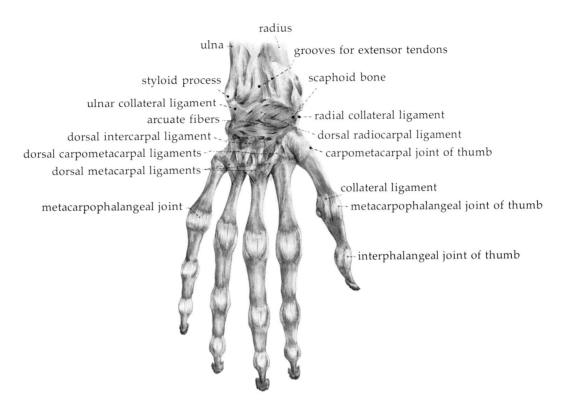

radius

ulna

grooves for extensor tendons

styloid process

scaphoid bone

ulnar collateral ligament

arcuate fibers

radial collateral ligament

dorsal intercarpal ligament

dorsal radiocarpal ligament

dorsal carpometacarpal ligaments

carpometacarpal joint of thumb

dorsal metacarpal ligaments

collateral ligament

metacarpophalangeal joint

metacarpophalangeal joint of thumb

interphalangeal joint of thumb

A. Ligaments on the dorsal side of the right wrist and hand.

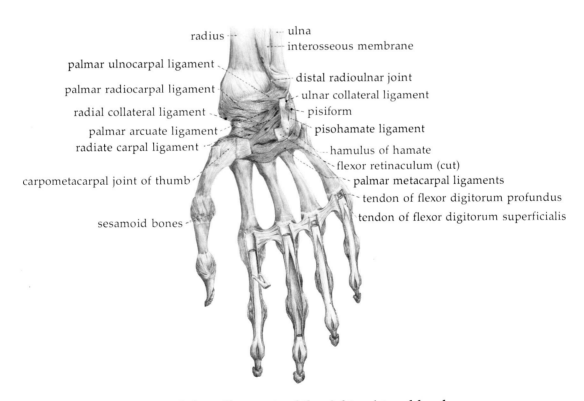

radius

ulna

interosseous membrane

palmar ulnocarpal ligament

distal radioulnar joint

palmar radiocarpal ligament

ulnar collateral ligament

radial collateral ligament

pisiform

palmar arcuate ligament

pisohamate ligament

radiate carpal ligament

hamulus of hamate

flexor retinaculum (cut)

carpometacarpal joint of thumb

palmar metacarpal ligaments

tendon of flexor digitorum profundus

sesamoid bones

tendon of flexor digitorum superficialis

B. Palmar ligaments of the right wrist and hand.

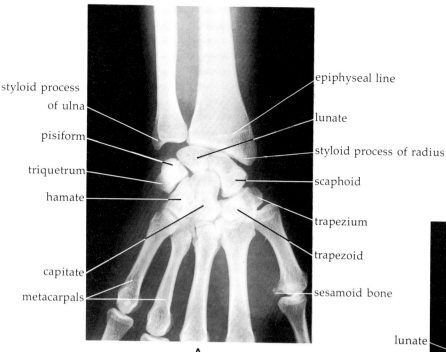

styloid process of ulna
pisiform
triquetrum
hamate
capitate
metacarpals

epiphyseal line
lunate
styloid process of radius
scaphoid
trapezium
trapezoid
sesamoid bone

A

A. Posteroanterior view of the wrist.

B. Oblique view of the wrist.
This view is particularly suitable for examination of the joint between the trapezium and the first metacarpal bone; it also gives a good view of the scaphoid, which is most likely to be fractured in a fall on the hand.

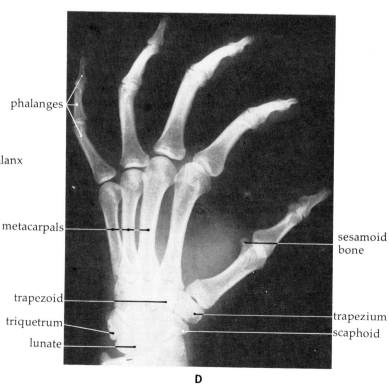

lunate
triquetrum
capitate
hamate
trapezoid

styloid process of radius
scaphoid
trapezium
1st metacarpal

B

C. Posteroanterior view of the hand.
Pathological processes such as tuberculosis may cause minute but important changes in the metacarpals and phalanges. Note also the tufted ends of the distal phalanges.

lunate
triquetrum
metacarpals
proximal phalanx
middle phalanx

scaphoid
1st metacarpal
sesamoid bone
tufted distal phalanx

C

D. Oblique view of the hand.
The various metacarpal bones do not overlap as much in this view as in a lateral view, and displacement of the metacarpals and phalanges in an anterior or posterior direction can be seen. (*A* to *D* from Meschan, I.: *An Atlas of Anatomy Basic to Radiology.* Philadelphia, W. B. Saunders Co., 1975.)

phalanges
metacarpals
trapezoid
triquetrum
lunate

sesamoid bone
trapezium
scaphoid

D

LOWER LIMB

A. Lower limb bud at 6 weeks.
Part of the bud has been cut
away to show its core.

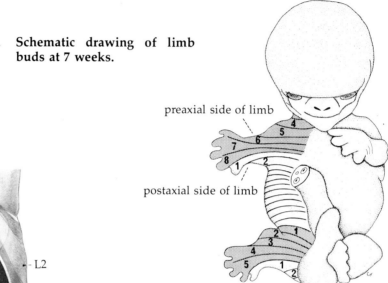

**B. Schematic drawing of limb
buds at 7 weeks.**

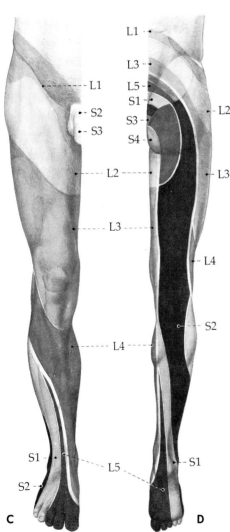

**C. Segmental innervation of anterior
aspect of lower limb.**

**D. Segmental innervation of posterior
aspect of lower limb.**

The buds of the lower limbs are always somewhat behind in development when compared with those of the upper limbs, but basically their developmental pattern is similar. They lie opposite the lumbar and upper two sacral segments, and the ventral rami of these segments enter the buds initially with isolated ventral and dorsal branches. Soon, however, the branches unite to form large dorsal and ventral nerves, and the segmental pattern largely disappears. In the adult the original segmental organization of the limbs can be recognized only in the sensory innervation of the skin, the so-called *dermatomes.* In patients with isolated lesions of the dorsal roots a thorough knowledge of the dermatomes is helpful and important. Note that (a) most of the anterior aspect of the lower limb is supplied by the lumbar segments; (b) most of the posterior aspect is supplied by the sacral segments; (c) the anal, perineal and genital regions are supplied by the sacral segments; (d) L5 supplies the first toe; and (e) S1 supplies the fifth toe.

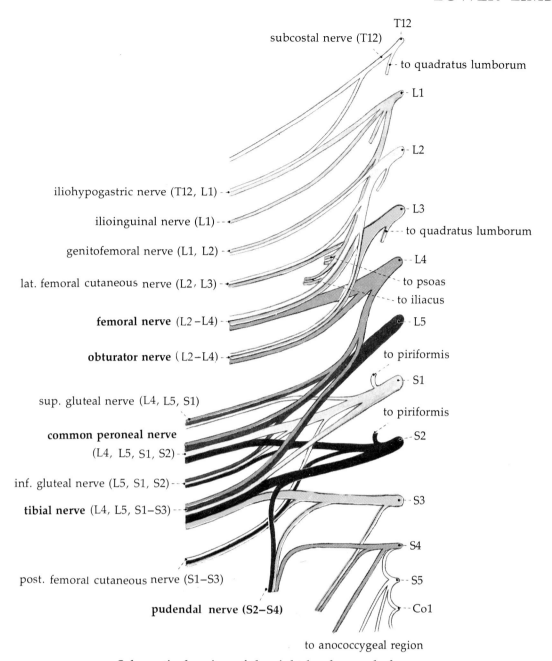

T12

subcostal nerve (T12)

to quadratus lumborum

L1

L2

iliohypogastric nerve (T12, L1)

ilioinguinal nerve (L1)

L3

genitofemoral nerve (L1, L2)

to quadratus lumborum

lat. femoral cutaneous nerve (L2, L3)

L4

to psoas

to iliacus

femoral nerve (L2–L4)

L5

obturator nerve (L2–L4)

to piriformis

S1

sup. gluteal nerve (L4, L5, S1)

to piriformis

common peroneal nerve
(L4, L5, S1, S2)

S2

inf. gluteal nerve (L5, S1, S2)

tibial nerve (L4, L5, S1–S3)

S3

S4

S5

post. femoral cutaneous nerve (S1–S3)

Co1

pudendal nerve (S2–S4)

to anococcygeal region

Schematic drawing of the right lumbosacral plexus.

The lumbosacral plexus consists of two components:

¶ The *lumbar plexus*, formed by the ventral rami of the first three lumbar nerves and the greater part of the fourth. T12 usually contributes a small twig to the first lumbar nerve. The two main nerves are the *femoral nerve* (L2–L4) and the *obturator nerve* (L2–L4).

¶ The *sacral plexus*, formed by the ventral rami of L5, S1, S2, or S3 and part of L4. The rami of L4 and L5 unite before joining those of the other segments; together they are known as the *lumbosacral trunk*. The two main nerves of the plexus are the *common peroneal nerve* (L4–S2) and the *tibial nerve* (L4–S3). These two are usually combined into one large nerve, the *sciatic nerve*. A third important nerve of the sacral plexus is the *pudendal nerve* (S2–S4). This nerve does not supply muscles of the lower limb but innervates those of the perineal region.

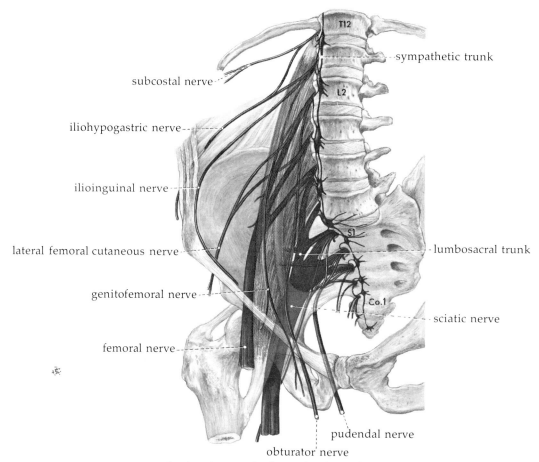

The lumbosacral plexus in the pelvis.
Note its relation to the psoas major and sympathetic trunk.

The nerves formed by the lumbosacral plexus are not restricted to the femoral, obturator and sciatic (common peroneal and tibial) nerves but include a number of smaller groups:

¶ On the abdominal wall and scrotum are found: (a) the subcostal nerve (T12), (b) the iliohypogastric nerve (T12, L1), (c) the ilioinguinal nerve (L1) and (d) the genitofemoral nerve (L1, L2).

¶ In the pelvis are found small motor nerves to: (a) the quadratus lumborum, (b) the psoas major and minor, (c) the iliacus and (d) the piriformis.

¶ Coursing from the pelvis to the lower limb are: (a) the lateral femoral cutaneous nerve (L2, L3), (b) the superior gluteal nerve (L4, L5, S1) (providing motor innervation to the gluteus medius, gluteus minimus and tensor fasciae latae), (c) the inferior gluteal nerve (L5, S1, S2) (motor innervation to the gluteus maximus) and (d) the posterior femoral cutaneous nerve (S1–S3).

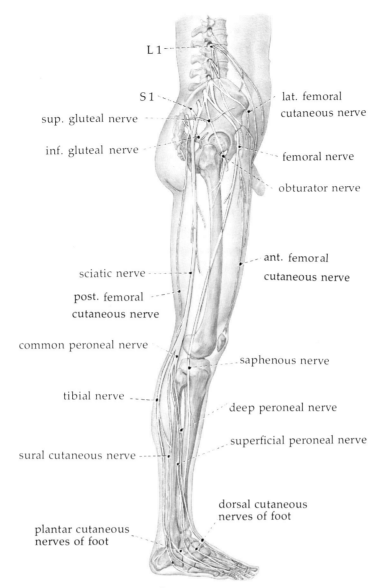

L 1

S 1

sup. gluteal nerve

inf. gluteal nerve

lat. femoral
cutaneous nerve

femoral nerve

obturator nerve

ant. femoral
cutaneous nerve

sciatic nerve

post. femoral
cutaneous nerve

common peroneal nerve

saphenous nerve

tibial nerve

deep peroneal nerve

superficial peroneal nerve

sural cutaneous nerve

dorsal cutaneous
nerves of foot

plantar cutaneous
nerves of foot

Major nerves of the lower limb.

Note:

¶ The *femoral nerve* innervates the musculature on the anterior side of the thigh and the skin over the muscles. Its terminal branch — the saphenous nerve — supplies the skin on the medial side of the leg and foot. (For details see LL20 *A* and *B*.)

¶ The *obturator nerve* innervates the musculature on the medial side of the thigh (the adductor group) and a small cutaneous area over the muscle group. (For details see LL20 *C*.)

¶ The *sciatic nerve*, which divides into the common peroneal and tibial nerves, innervates the musculature on the posterior side of the thigh and all the muscles of the leg and foot. It also innervates the skin of the leg as well as that of the dorsal and plantar sides of the foot. (For details see LL29 *A* and LL66.)

¶ The *superior and inferior gluteal nerves* innervate the gluteal muscles and the tensor fasciae latae (see LL22 *B* and LL29 *B*).

¶ The *lateral and posterior femoral cutaneous nerves* (see LL9 *B* and LL21 *B*).

277

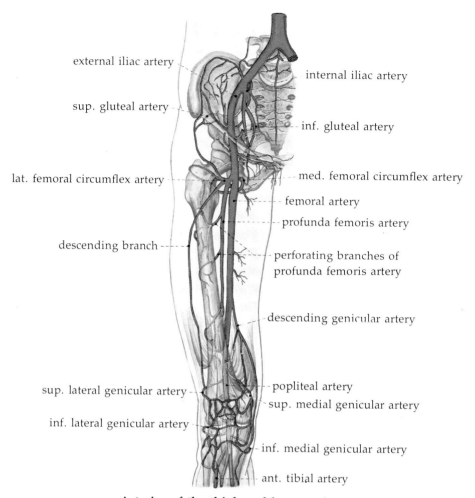

external iliac artery

internal iliac artery

sup. gluteal artery

inf. gluteal artery

lat. femoral circumflex artery

med. femoral circumflex artery

femoral artery

profunda femoris artery

descending branch

perforating branches of profunda femoris artery

descending genicular artery

sup. lateral genicular artery

popliteal artery

sup. medial genicular artery

inf. lateral genicular artery

inf. medial genicular artery

ant. tibial artery

Arteries of the thigh and knee regions.

The following points are important when studying the femoral artery and its branches:

¶ The femoral artery can easily be palpated midway between the anterior superior iliac spine and the pubic symphysis. At this point it passes over the superior ramus of the pubis. In emergencies the artery can be compressed against this bony point.

¶ The popliteal artery lies under the taut popliteal fascia and can be palpated only when the knee is flexed and all the muscles are relaxed (see also LL22 *A*).

¶ Gradual occlusion of the femoral artery due to arteriosclerosis may be followed by development of a collateral circulation. When occlusion occurs in the proximal part of the femoral artery the collateral circulation is established through the medial and lateral femoral circumflex arteries, and through the inferior and superior gluteal arteries. When the lower part of the femoral artery is occluded, collaterals are established between the perforating branches of the profunda femoris artery and the muscular and articular branches of the femoral artery. The descending branch of the lateral femoral circumflex artery plays an important role in establishing a collateral circulation when the proximal as well as the distal part of the femoral artery is occluded.

¶ Intermittent claudication is a condition caused by occlusive arterial disease of the leg. Obstruction of the femoral artery causes an insufficiency of the blood supply to the calf muscles. This results in intense pain in the leg during walking. When the patient stops walking, the oxygen supply improves and walking is again possible.

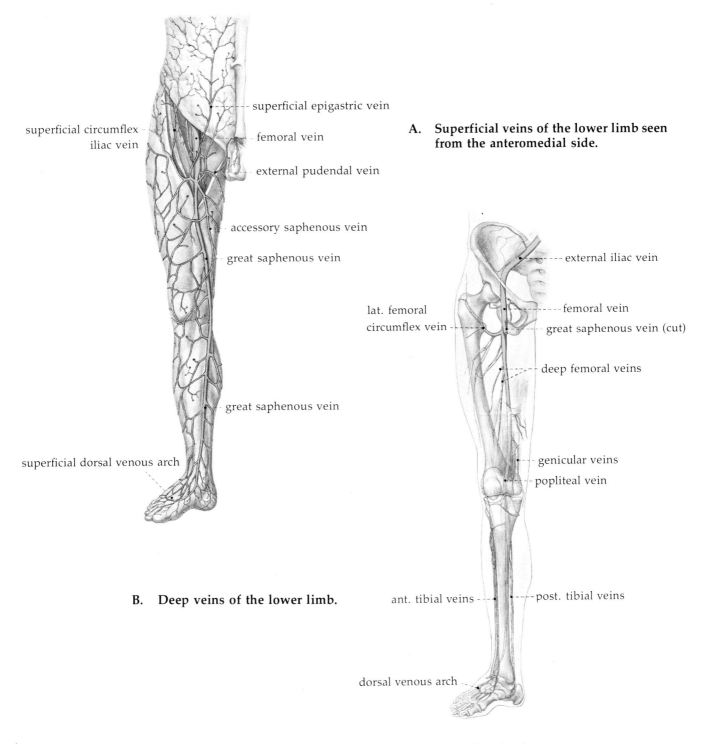

superficial epigastric vein

superficial circumflex iliac vein

femoral vein

external pudendal vein

accessory saphenous vein

great saphenous vein

great saphenous vein

superficial dorsal venous arch

A. Superficial veins of the lower limb seen from the anteromedial side.

external iliac vein

lat. femoral circumflex vein

femoral vein

great saphenous vein (cut)

deep femoral veins

genicular veins

popliteal vein

ant. tibial veins

post. tibial veins

B. Deep veins of the lower limb.

dorsal venous arch

The superficial veins are located in the superficial fascia and are connected to the deep veins by communicating perforating veins. The perforating veins possess valves that prevent the return flow of blood from the deep to the superficial veins. The venous networks in the lower limb are important for the following reasons:

¶ The superficial veins are frequently varicose—that is, the diameter is larger than normal and the course is tortuous. The most frequent cause of varicose veins is an elevated intra-abdominal pressure resulting from pregnancy or tumors. Varicose veins, however, may also develop in people who stand for prolonged periods of time and also when the valves of the perforating veins are incompetent.

¶ The deep veins are under pressure from contraction of the muscles and pulsations of the adjacent arteries. These forces compress the veins and force the blood upwards. When the valves of the perforating veins are incompetent, blood will be pressed into the superficial network.

¶ Remember that the great saphenous vein passes just in front of the medial malleolus. Sometimes blood transfusions are given at this location.

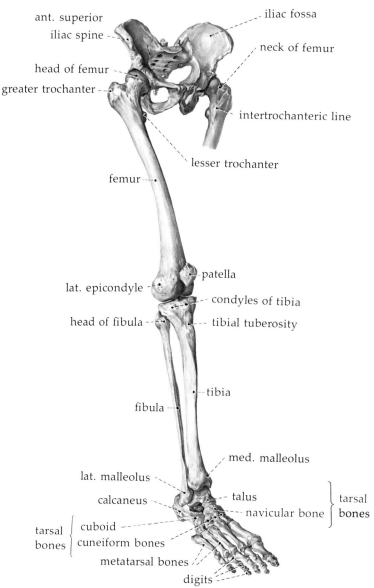

ant. superior
iliac spine

iliac fossa

head of femur

neck of femur

greater trochanter

intertrochanteric line

lesser trochanter

femur

patella

lat. epicondyle

condyles of tibia

head of fibula

tibial tuberosity

tibia

fibula

med. malleolus

lat. malleolus

calcaneus

talus

navicular bone

tarsal
bones

tarsal
bones

cuboid

cuneiform bones

metatarsal bones

digits

Bony skeleton of the right lower limb.
Note the important bones and landmarks.

Note:

¶ The bones of the lower limb are connected to the trunk by the pelvic girdle, which is formed by the two hip bones and the sacrum. The pelvic girdle transmits the weight of the body toward the lower limbs (see LL32 C).

¶ Since the main function of the bones of the lower limb is to support the weight of the body, they are thicker and stronger than those of the upper limb.

¶ Three segments are recognized in the lower limb: (a) the thigh with the femur as its bony component (see LL30); (b) the leg with the tibia and fibula as the bony components (see LL53); and (c) the foot with the tarsal, metatarsal and digital bones (see LL69).

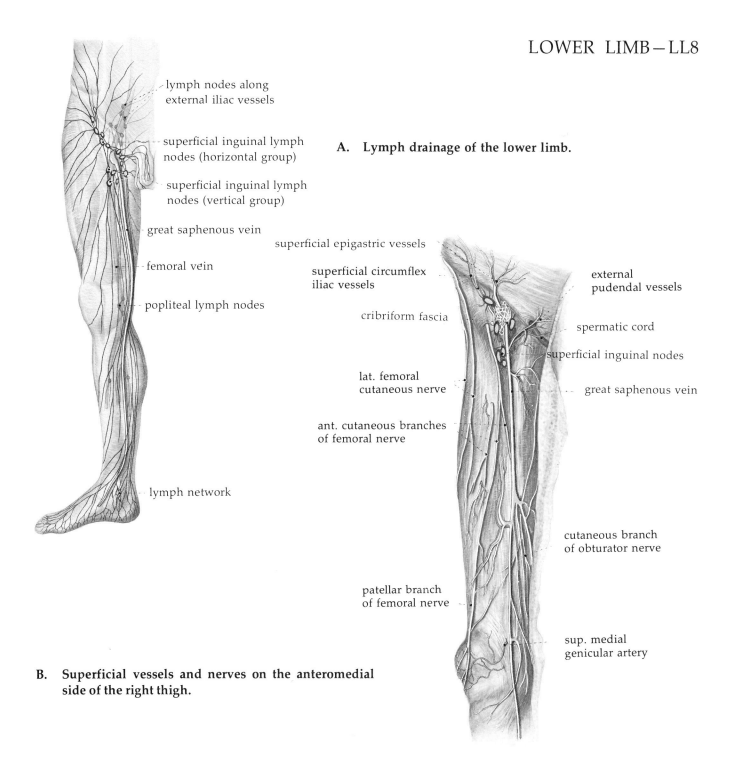

lymph nodes along
external iliac vessels

superficial inguinal lymph
nodes (horizontal group)

A. Lymph drainage of the lower limb.

superficial inguinal lymph
nodes (vertical group)

great saphenous vein

superficial epigastric vessels

superficial circumflex
iliac vessels

external
pudendal vessels

femoral vein

cribriform fascia

spermatic cord

popliteal lymph nodes

superficial inguinal nodes

lat. femoral
cutaneous nerve

great saphenous vein

ant. cutaneous branches
of femoral nerve

lymph network

cutaneous branch
of obturator nerve

patellar branch
of femoral nerve

sup. medial
genicular artery

**B. Superficial vessels and nerves on the anteromedial
side of the right thigh.**

Note:

¶ The superficial inguinal lymph nodes consist of a horizontal group of nodes just below and parallel to the inguinal ligament and a vertical group parallel to the terminal
part of the great saphenous vein. When swollen lymph nodes are found in the inguinal
region, remember that the vertical group receives lymph mainly from the lower limb as
far as the toes but that the horizontal group receives lymph from: (a) the anterior abdominal wall below the umbilicus; (b) the posterior abdominal wall below the iliac
crest; (c) the perineum; (d) the external genitalia in both sexes (not the testes); (e) part
of the urethra; and (f) the anal canal below the pectinate line.

¶ The deep inguinal nodes lie along the femoral vein. They receive lymph from the superficial nodes through the saphenous opening.

¶ The great saphenous vein as well as the other superficial veins passes through a gap in
the fascia lata (the deep fascia of the thigh) to join the femoral vein. This gap, the saphenous opening, is ill-defined because of the presence of the superficial inguinal lymph
nodes, the lymph vessels, the veins and loose connective tissue. The loose connective
tissue that fills the saphenous opening is known as the cribriform fascia (see *B*).

281

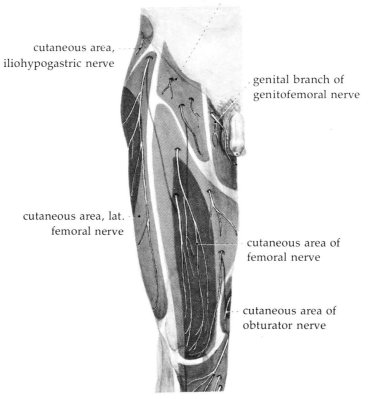

femoral branch of genitofemoral nerve

cutaneous area,
iliohypogastric nerve

genital branch of
genitofemoral nerve

cutaneous area, lat.
femoral nerve

cutaneous area of
femoral nerve

cutaneous area of
obturator nerve

A. Sensory innervation of the anterior aspect of the thigh.

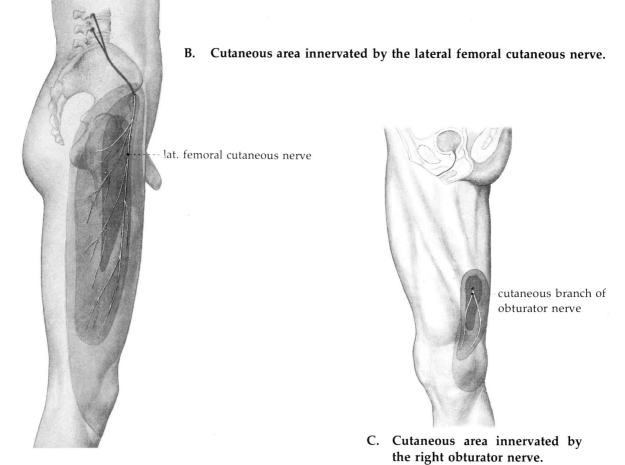

B. Cutaneous area innervated by the lateral femoral cutaneous nerve.

lat. femoral cutaneous nerve

cutaneous branch of
obturator nerve

**C. Cutaneous area innervated by
the right obturator nerve.**

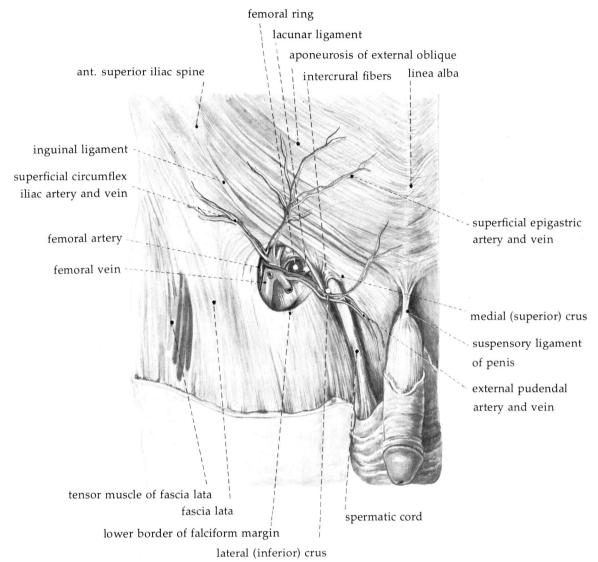

femoral ring

lacunar ligament

aponeurosis of external oblique

ant. superior iliac spine

intercrural fibers

linea alba

inguinal ligament

superficial circumflex
iliac artery and vein

femoral artery

femoral vein

superficial epigastric
artery and vein

medial (superior) crus

suspensory ligament
of penis

external pudendal
artery and vein

tensor muscle of fascia lata

fascia lata

lower border of falciform margin

spermatic cord

lateral (inferior) crus

Right saphenous opening.
The lymph nodes and cribriform
fascia have been removed.

¶ The saphenous opening is a gap in the fascia lata through which pass: (a) the great saphenous vein; (b) the superficial epigastric vein; (c) the superficial external pudendal vein; (d) the superficial circumflex iliac vein; (e) an accessory lateral saphenous vein; (f) numerous lymph vessels; and (g) the arteries accompanying some of the veins.

¶ The fascia lata is fused with the inguinal ligament from the anterior superior iliac spine to the pubic tubercle. From the pubic tubercle the fascia is reflected downward and laterally, thus forming the lower border of the falciform margin. The fascia then turns cranially, forming the upper border (superior corner) of the falciform margin.

¶ Note the boundaries and location of the femoral ring (see also LL12 A).

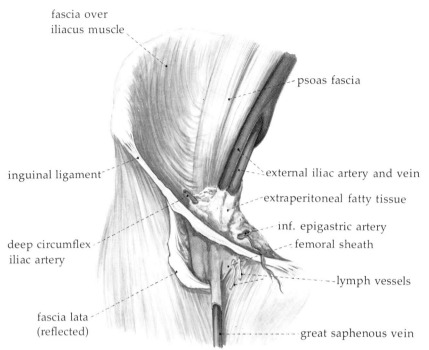

fascia over
iliacus muscle

psoas fascia

inguinal ligament

external iliac artery and vein

extraperitoneal fatty tissue

inf. epigastric artery

deep circumflex
iliac artery

femoral sheath

lymph vessels

fascia lata
(reflected)

great saphenous vein

Right femoral sheath.

Note the following point:

¶ The *femoral sheath* is an extension of the transversalis fascia and the extraperitoneal
fibrous tissue that surrounds the vessels in the abdomen. It is funnel-shaped and contains the femoral artery, the femoral vein and (medially) a lymph node and lymph
vessels. When the lymph node is removed, the femoral ring becomes visible.

lat. femoral cutaneous nerve
inguinal ligament
femoral nerve
iliacus
femoral artery and vein
femoral ring
lacunar ligament
psoas
pectineus

A. Contents and relationship of the right femoral sheath.

psoas major and minor
iliac crest
iliacus
ant. superior iliac spine
origin of psoas
fascia lata over sartorius
inguinal ligament
intestinal loop (cut)
falciform margin
femoral vein
fascia lata over pectineus
femoral hernia
great saphenous vein

B. Location of the right femoral hernia.

¶ The *femoral ring* is bound by the inguinal ligament anteriorly, the pubic bone and pectineus muscle posteriorly, the lacunar ligament medially and the femoral vein laterally. It is covered by a thin membrane consisting of extraperitoneal tissue and is a weak spot. The ring in the female is larger than that in the male and is a preferred site for the *femoral hernia.*

¶ When a portion of the intestine or greater omentum is forced through the ring, it is always surrounded by peritoneum, which forms the sac of the hernia. Usually the hernia descends inside the femoral sheath toward the saphenous opening; the space from the ring to the saphenous opening is called the *femoral canal.* The hernia frequently breaks through the thin cribriform fascia into the superficial fascia. A femoral hernia is often dangerous because the blood supply to its contents is easily closed off by the bony ligamentous walls of the femoral ring. When this occurs, necrosis of the intestinal loop or omentum may result.

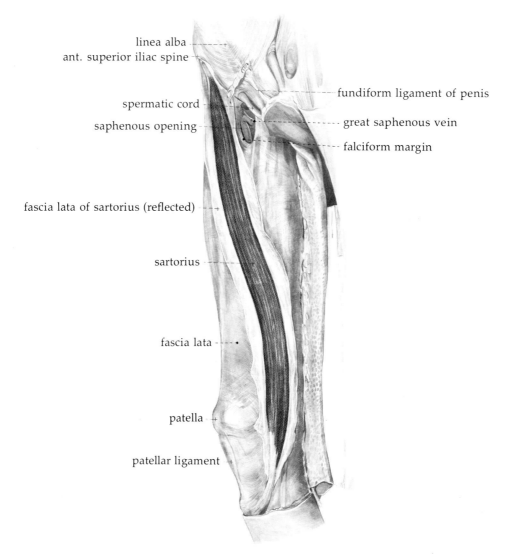

linea alba
ant. superior iliac spine

fundiform ligament of penis

spermatic cord

saphenous opening

great saphenous vein

falciform margin

fascia lata of sartorius (reflected)

sartorius

fascia lata

patella

patellar ligament

Fascia lata and right sartorius muscle.

The fascia lata is the deep fascia of the thigh and surrounds all muscles. By means of intermuscular septa the fascia divides the musculature into three compartments: (a) an anterior compartment (extensor group); (b) a medial compartment (adductor group); and (c) a posterior compartment (flexor group).

Two particular points should be noted:

¶ On the lateral side of the thigh the fascia forms the iliotibial tract, which is so strong that it serves as a site of insertion for the tensor fasciae latae and part of the gluteus maximus (see LL22).

¶ Deep to the sartorius the fascia lata forms a heavy membrane, the subsartorial membrane, which covers the vessels in the adductor canal (see LL15 and LL18).

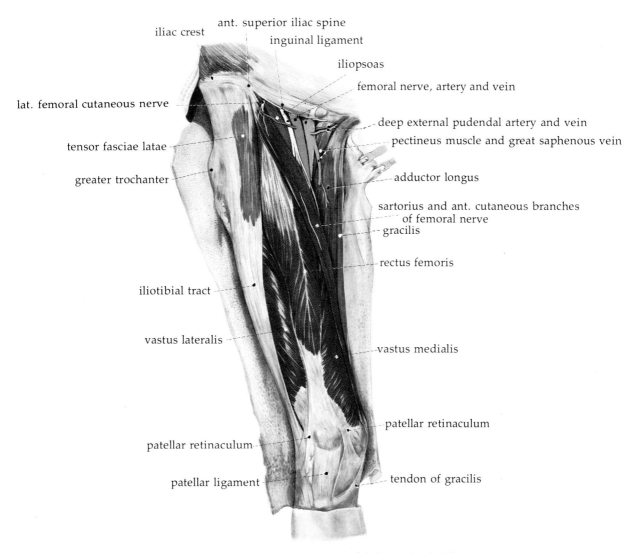

iliac crest

ant. superior iliac spine

inguinal ligament

iliopsoas

femoral nerve, artery and vein

lat. femoral cutaneous nerve

deep external pudendal artery and vein

pectineus muscle and great saphenous vein

tensor fasciae latae

greater trochanter

adductor longus

sartorius and ant. cutaneous branches
of femoral nerve

gracilis

rectus femoris

iliotibial tract

vastus lateralis

vastus medialis

patellar retinaculum

patellar retinaculum

patellar ligament

tendon of gracilis

Muscles on the anterior side of the right thigh.
Note the structures in the femoral triangle.

Note the femoral triangle (see LL15 for a more detailed view). The superficial boundaries
of this triangle are formed by (a) the inguinal ligament; (b) the medial border of the sartorius; and (c) the lateral border of the adductor longus. The floor is formed by the iliopsoas
and pectineus muscles.

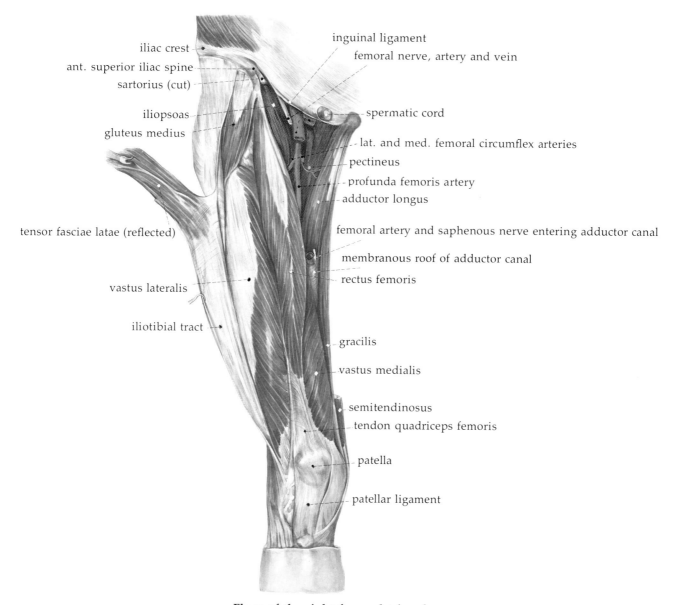

iliac crest
ant. superior iliac spine
sartorius (cut)
iliopsoas
gluteus medius

tensor fasciae latae (reflected)

vastus lateralis

iliotibial tract

inguinal ligament
femoral nerve, artery and vein

spermatic cord

lat. and med. femoral circumflex arteries
pectineus
profunda femoris artery
adductor longus

femoral artery and saphenous nerve entering adductor canal
membranous roof of adductor canal
rectus femoris

gracilis

vastus medialis

semitendinosus
tendon quadriceps femoris

patella

patellar ligament

Floor of the right femoral triangle.
The femoral artery and vein have been removed to expose the profunda femoris artery.

Note:

¶ The profunda femoris artery arises from the femoral artery about 4 cm below the inguinal ligament. It passes behind the adductor longus.

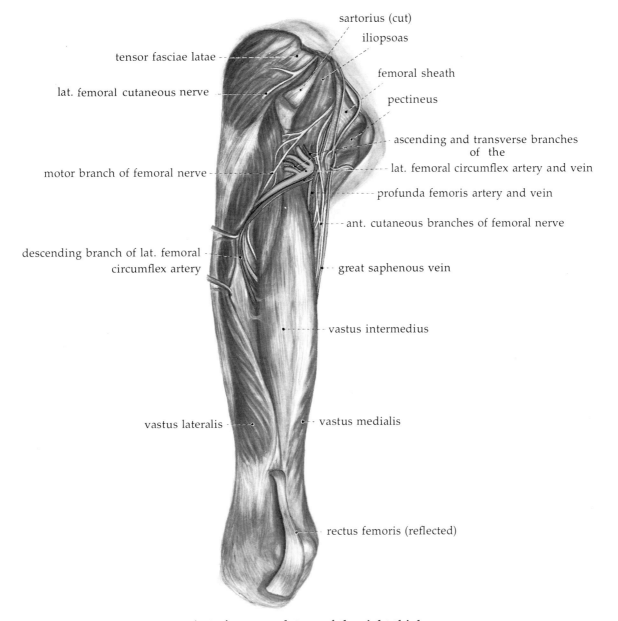

sartorius (cut)

iliopsoas

tensor fasciae latae

femoral sheath

lat. femoral cutaneous nerve

pectineus

ascending and transverse branches
of the

lat. femoral circumflex artery and vein

motor branch of femoral nerve

profunda femoris artery and vein

ant. cutaneous branches of femoral nerve

descending branch of lat. femoral
circumflex artery

great saphenous vein

vastus intermedius

vastus lateralis

vastus medialis

rectus femoris (reflected)

Anterior musculature of the right thigh.
The sartorius and rectus femoris have been removed
and the lateral femoral circumflex
artery is exposed.

¶ The lateral femoral circumflex artery is probably the most important branch of the
profunda femoris artery. Its ascending and transverse branches send several twigs to
the neck and head of the femur (see LL36 C). The descending branch reaches the area of
the knee, where it forms anastomoses with branches of the popliteal artery.

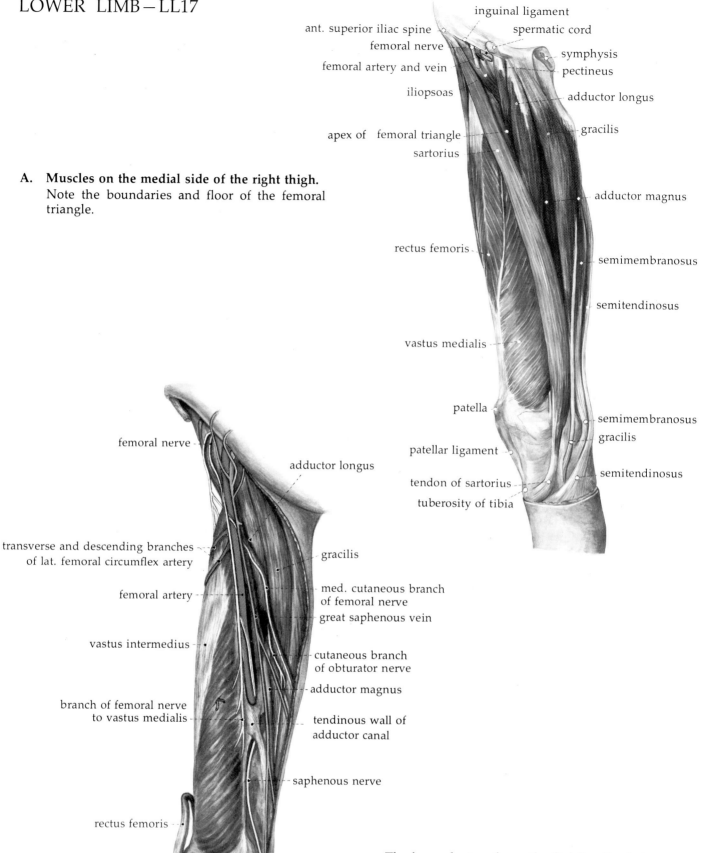

ant. superior iliac spine
femoral nerve
femoral artery and vein
iliopsoas
apex of femoral triangle
sartorius

inguinal ligament
spermatic cord
symphysis
pectineus
adductor longus
gracilis

adductor magnus
semimembranosus
semitendinosus

rectus femoris

vastus medialis

patella

patellar ligament
tendon of sartorius
tuberosity of tibia

semimembranosus
gracilis
semitendinosus

A. Muscles on the medial side of the right thigh.
Note the boundaries and floor of the femoral triangle.

femoral nerve

adductor longus

transverse and descending branches
of lat. femoral circumflex artery

gracilis

femoral artery

med. cutaneous branch
of femoral nerve
great saphenous vein

vastus intermedius

cutaneous branch
of obturator nerve
adductor magnus

branch of femoral nerve
to vastus medialis

tendinous wall of
adductor canal

saphenous nerve

rectus femoris

B. The right femoral artery in its course toward the adductor hiatus.
The sartorius and rectus femoris have been removed, but the subcutaneous nerves and veins have been preserved.

The femoral artery forms the dividing line between two motor nerve territories: (a) the medial territory formed by the adductor group and innervated by the obturator nerve and (b) the muscles on the lateral side (quadriceps and sartorius), innervated by the femoral nerve. The artery is not crossed by motor branches, but several sensory branches of the femoral nerve pass over it to innervate the skin on the medial side of the thigh. The cutaneous branch of the obturator nerve emerges between the adductor longus and the adductor magnus.

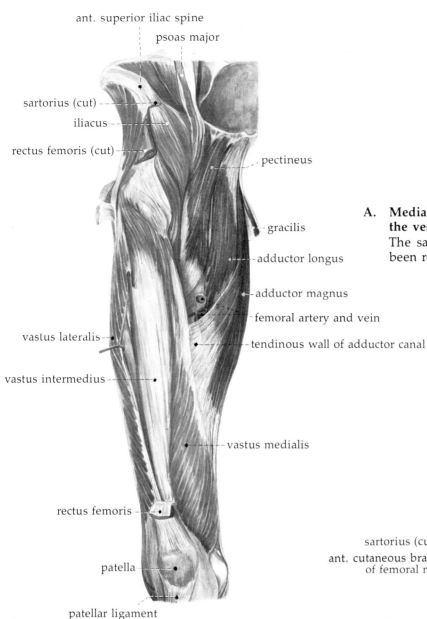

ant. superior iliac spine

psoas major

sartorius (cut)

iliacus

rectus femoris (cut)

pectineus

gracilis

adductor longus

adductor magnus

femoral artery and vein

tendinous wall of adductor canal

vastus lateralis

vastus intermedius

vastus medialis

rectus femoris

patella

patellar ligament

A. Medial aspect of the right thigh after removal of the vessels.
The sartorius and rectus femoris muscles have been removed.

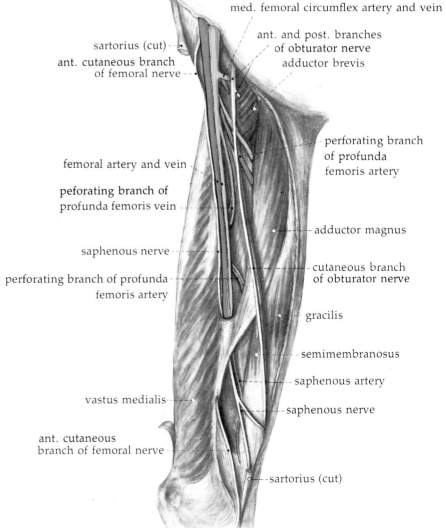

med. femoral circumflex artery and vein

ant. and post. branches of obturator nerve

adductor brevis

sartorius (cut)

ant. cutaneous branch of femoral nerve

perforating branch of profunda femoris artery

femoral artery and vein

peforating branch of profunda femoris vein

adductor magnus

saphenous nerve

cutaneous branch of obturator nerve

perforating branch of profunda femoris artery

gracilis

semimembranosus

saphenous artery

vastus medialis

saphenous nerve

ant. cutaneous branch of femoral nerve

sartorius (cut)

B. Deep dissection of the medial aspect of the right thigh showing the obturator nerve.
The pectineus and adductor longus have been removed.

From the femoral triangle to the adductor hiatus the femoral artery passes through an intermuscular canal. This canal, the subsartorial or adductor canal, is bounded laterally by the vastus medialis and posteriorly by the adductor longus and part of the adductor magnus. The roof of the canal is formed by the sartorius and a strong fascial layer—the subsartorial fascia. This fascia stretches from the fascial coverings of the adductor longus and adductor magnus to the fascia of the vastus medialis, and is not to be confused with the adductor hiatus (see LL19 A), which forms the opening in the insertion of the adductor magnus through which the femoral artery leaves the adductor compartment to enter the popliteal region.

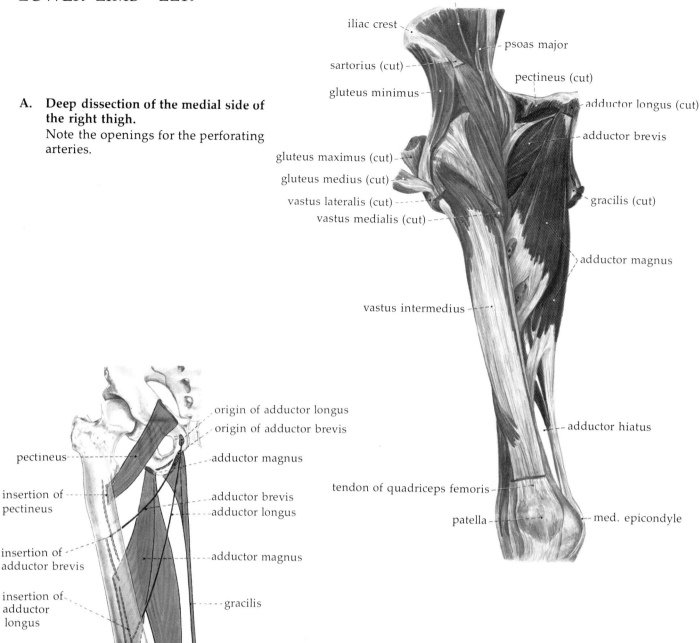

A. Deep dissection of the medial side of the right thigh.
Note the openings for the perforating arteries.

iliacus
iliac crest
sartorius (cut)
gluteus minimus
psoas major
pectineus (cut)
adductor longus (cut)
adductor brevis
gluteus maximus (cut)
gluteus medius (cut)
vastus lateralis (cut)
vastus medialis (cut)
gracilis (cut)
adductor magnus
vastus intermedius
adductor hiatus
tendon of quadriceps femoris
patella
med. epicondyle

origin of adductor longus
origin of adductor brevis
pectineus
adductor magnus
insertion of pectineus
adductor brevis
adductor longus
insertion of adductor brevis
adductor magnus
insertion of adductor longus
gracilis
adductor magnus
insertion of adductor magnus
med. femoral epicondyle
gracilis

B. Schematic drawing of origin and insertion of the right adductors.

¶ One of the main characteristics of spastic paraplegia is spasms of the adductor muscles. The thighs are tightly pulled toward the midline, making walking impossible. To relieve the spasms the obturator nerve is usually cut.

¶ The obturator nerve reaches the adductor compartment after passing through the obturator foramen in the obturator membrane. Sometimes a small loop of the intestinal tract forms a hernia through the obturator foramen, leading to compression of the obturator nerve. As a result, the patient may complain about pain in the area supplied by the sensory branches of the obturator nerve (see LL9 C). Pain over the medial side of the thigh, combined with symptoms of intestinal obstruction, is probably caused by a strangulated obturator hernia.

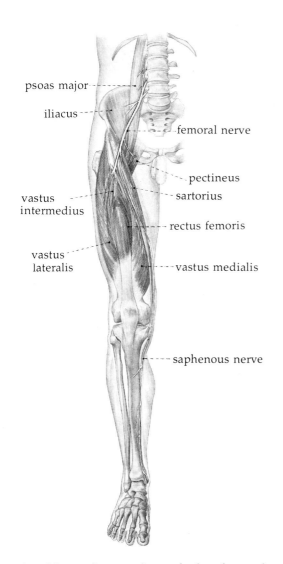

psoas major

iliacus

femoral nerve

pectineus

sartorius

vastus intermedius

rectus femoris

vastus lateralis

vastus medialis

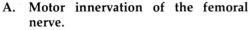

saphenous nerve

femoral nerve

ant. and med. cutaneous branches of femoral nerve

B. Sensory innervation of the femoral nerve.

infrapatellar branch of saphenous nerve

saphenous nerve

A. Motor innervation of the femoral nerve.

obturator canal

ant. branch obturator nerve

post. branch obturator nerve

adductor brevis

adductor magnus

adductor longus

gracilis

cutaneous branch obturator nerve

C. Motor innervation of the obturator nerve.

Because peripheral injuries to the femoral and obturator nerves are not uncommon, it is important to know the motor and sensory functions of these nerves.

¶ The femoral nerve enters the thigh about midway between the anterior superior iliac spine and the pubic tubercle and may be injured by stabs, cuts and gunshot wounds in the inguinal region. Complete severance is not common, but when it does occur the quadriceps and sartorius muscles are paralyzed (the pectineus receives a branch from the obturator nerve as well as from the femoral nerve). As a result, the knee cannot be extended. Walking, however, is not impossible, since the leg can be brought forward by gravity and by some compensatory action of the adductor muscles. Sensory loss is extensive because the anterior and medial sides of the thigh as well as the medial side of the leg and foot are innervated by femoral branches (B).

¶ Injuries of the obturator nerve are less common. Occasionally, however, when the nerve is injured by deep wounds or by an anterior dislocation of the hip joint, adduction of the lower limb becomes difficult. In such patients all adductors, with the exception of the pectineus and the hamstring part of the adductor magnus, are paralyzed. Loss of sensation is restricted to a small area on the medial aspect of the thigh (see also LL9 C).

293

sup. cluneal nerves

cutaneous branch of iliohypogastric nerve

middle cluneal nerves

inf. cluneal nerves

cutaneous branch of genitofemoral nerve

lat. femoral cutaneous nerve

med. cutaneous branch of femoral nerve

post. femoral cutaneous nerve

cutaneous branch of obturator nerve

saphenous nerve

A. Sensory supply of the posterior aspect of the right thigh.

post. femoral cutaneous nerve

perineal branches

cluneal branches

B. Sensory area of the right posterior femoral cutaneous nerve.

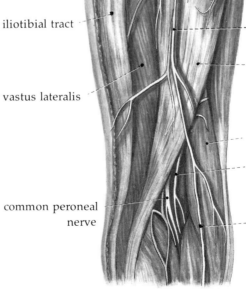

gluteus maximus

inf. cluneal nerves

semitendinosus

iliotibial tract

post. femoral cutaneous nerve

biceps femoris (long head)

vastus lateralis

semimembranosus

tibial nerve

C. Superficial nerves and veins on the posterior aspect of the left thigh.
The fascia lata has been removed.

common peroneal nerve

terminal branch of post. femoral cutaneous nerve

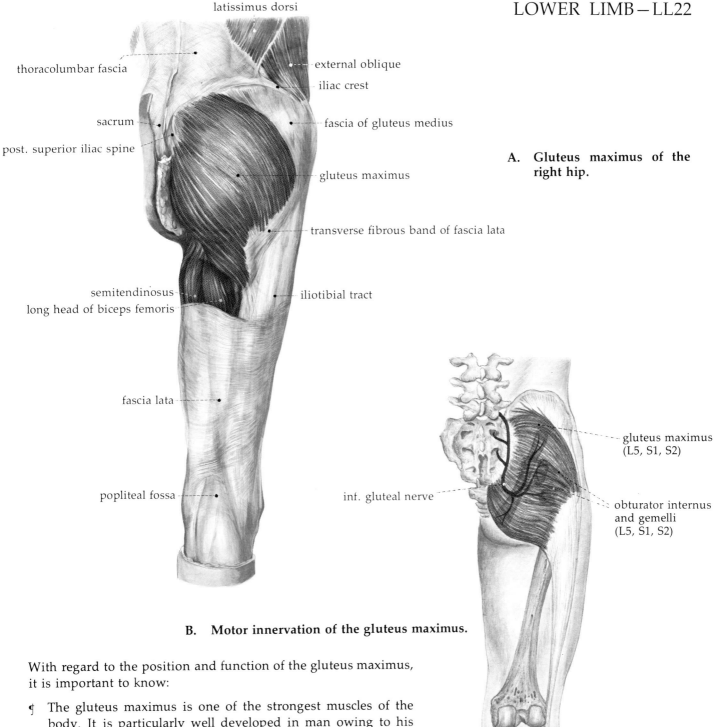

latissimus dorsi

thoracolumbar fascia

external oblique

iliac crest

sacrum

fascia of gluteus medius

post. superior iliac spine

gluteus maximus

transverse fibrous band of fascia lata

semitendinosus
long head of biceps femoris

iliotibial tract

fascia lata

popliteal fossa

inf. gluteal nerve

gluteus maximus
(L5, S1, S2)

obturator internus
and gemelli
(L5, S1, S2)

A. Gluteus maximus of the right hip.

B. Motor innervation of the gluteus maximus.

With regard to the position and function of the gluteus maximus, it is important to know:

- The gluteus maximus is one of the strongest muscles of the body. It is particularly well developed in man owing to his upright position. Its main function is to bring the thigh from a flexed position into line with the body. Since a large part of the muscle inserts in the iliotibial tract, it also helps to keep the knee in extension, thus securing stability in the knee joint.

- In an upright position the lower border of the muscle courses across the ischial tuberosity to the femur. In a sitting position the muscle does not cover the ischial tuberosity but slides to the side.

- Since the gluteal region is frequently a site of intramuscular injections, the position of the sciatic nerve (LL23) in relation to the muscle is important. The nerve first courses midway between the posterior superior iliac spine and the ischial tuberosity, and then it lies midway between the tip of the greater trochanter and the ischial tuberosity. Hence, when giving intramuscular injections the medial half of the muscle should be avoided, and preferences should be given to the outer and upper quadrant.

- The gluteus maximus is innervated by the inferior gluteal nerve. When the nerve is severed and the muscle paralyzed, the patient experiences great difficulty in walking up an incline or standing upright from a sitting position. In addition, stability in the knee joint and lower limb is greatly impaired.

295

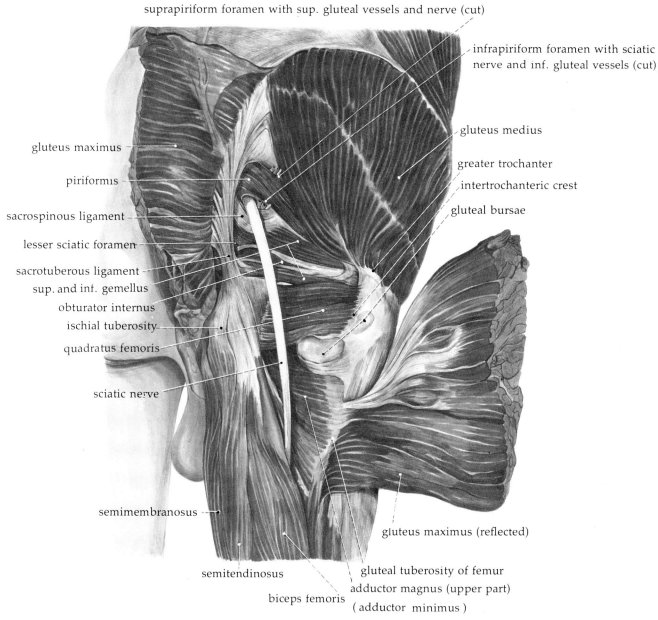

suprapiriform foramen with sup. gluteal vessels and nerve (cut)

infrapiriform foramen with sciatic nerve and inf. gluteal vessels (cut)

gluteus medius

greater trochanter

intertrochanteric crest

gluteal bursae

gluteus maximus

piriformis

sacrospinous ligament

lesser sciatic foramen

sacrotuberous ligament

sup. and inf. gemellus

obturator internus

ischial tuberosity

quadratus femoris

sciatic nerve

semimembranosus

gluteus maximus (reflected)

semitendinosus

gluteal tuberosity of femur

biceps femoris

adductor magnus (upper part)

(adductor minimus)

I.   Dissection of the right gluteal region.
The gluteus maximus has been cut and is reflected.

When the gluteus maximus is cut and pulled to the side, note:

¶ The sciatic nerve leaves the pelvis through the infrapiriform foramen (see LL28 *B*) and courses over the superior gemellus, the obturator internus, the inferior gemellus, the quadratus femoris and the upper part of the adductor magnus to reach the muscles of the thigh.

¶ Three bursae are usually found beneath the gluteus maximus; they are located (a) between the muscle and the greater trochanter; (b) between the muscle and the femur in the area of the lesser trochanter; and (c) between the muscle and the ischial tuberosity. In sedentary people the bursa over the ischial tuberosity may be inflamed (weaver's bottom). Sometimes the bursa is absent and is replaced by a thick mass of fatty fibrous tissue.

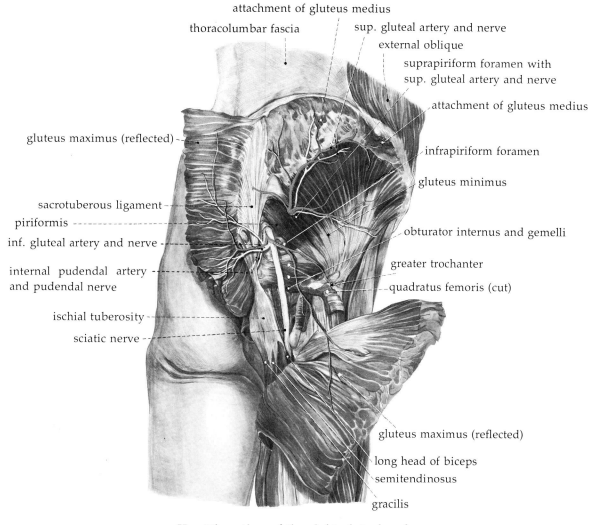

attachment of gluteus medius

thoracolumbar fascia

sup. gluteal artery and nerve

external oblique

suprapiriform foramen with
sup. gluteal artery and nerve

attachment of gluteus medius

gluteus maximus (reflected)

infrapiriform foramen

gluteus minimus

sacrotuberous ligament

piriformis

inf. gluteal artery and nerve

obturator internus and gemelli

internal pudendal artery
and pudendal nerve

greater trochanter

quadratus femoris (cut)

ischial tuberosity

sciatic nerve

gluteus maximus (reflected)

long head of biceps

semitendinosus

gracilis

II. Dissection of the right gluteal region.
The gluteus maximus has been cut and is reflected;
the gluteus medius has been removed.

Note the following structures emerging from the inside of the pelvis:

¶ The *superior gluteal vessels and nerve* leave the pelvis through the suprapiriform foramen. The nerve and the major arterial branches course between the gluteus medius and
gluteus minimus in an anterior direction and terminate in the tensor fasciae latae. Some
branches of the artery supply the gluteus maximus.

¶ The *inferior gluteal vessels and nerve* leave the pelvis through the infrapiriform foramen.
The nerve innervates the gluteus maximus.

¶ The *internal pudendal vessels and pudendal nerve* also leave the pelvis through the infrapiriform foramen. They pass over the sciatic spine and the origin of the sacrospinous
ligament and subsequently course through the lesser sciatic foramen to enter the ischiorectal fossa. The nerve and the vessels do not supply any structures in the gluteal region
but innervate the perineal musculature and external genitalia exclusively (see also P39).

¶ The *posterior femoral cutaneous nerve* emerges as a separate nerve from the infrapiriform
foramen and lies medial and posterior to the sciatic nerve. It has some cluneal branches
and a perineal branch to the medial side of the thigh and the scrotum. Its main area of
innervation, however, is the back and medial side of the thigh, the popliteal fossa and
part of the back of the leg (see LL21).

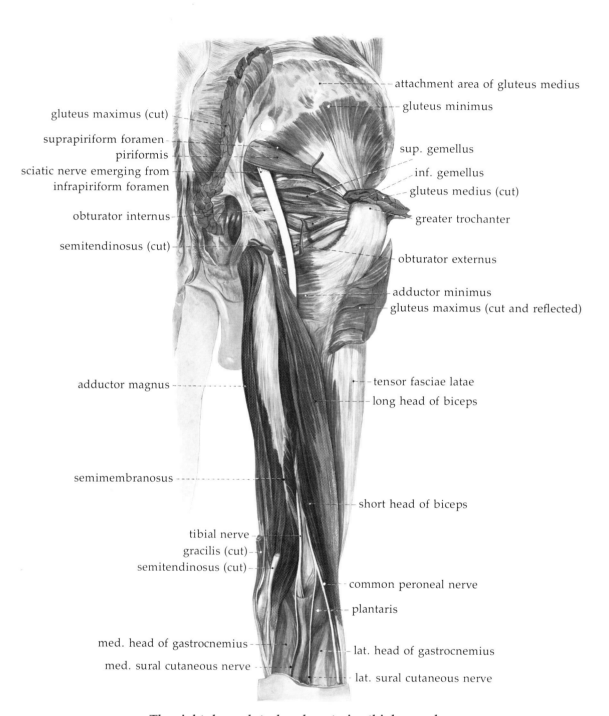

gluteus maximus (cut)

suprapiriform foramen
piriformis
sciatic nerve emerging from
infrapiriform foramen

obturator internus

semitendinosus (cut)

adductor magnus

semimembranosus

tibial nerve
gracilis (cut)
semitendinosus (cut)

med. head of gastrocnemius
med. sural cutaneous nerve

attachment area of gluteus medius
gluteus minimus

sup. gemellus
inf. gemellus
gluteus medius (cut)
greater trochanter

obturator externus

adductor minimus
gluteus maximus (cut and reflected)

tensor fasciae latae
long head of biceps

short head of biceps

common peroneal nerve
plantaris

lat. head of gastrocnemius
lat. sural cutaneous nerve

The right deep gluteal and posterior thigh muscles.
The quadratus femoris has been removed to show the obturator externus.

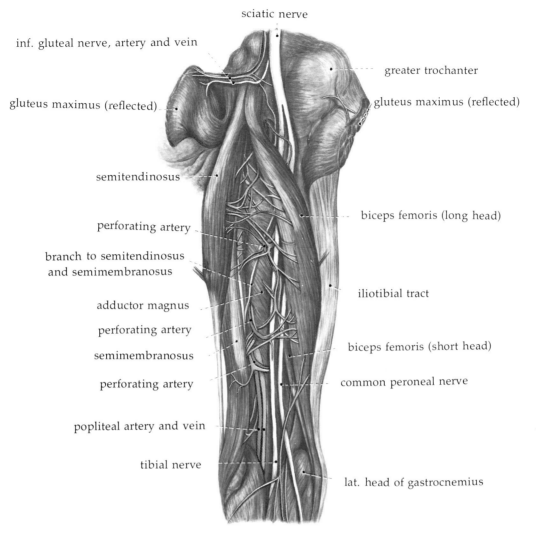

sciatic nerve

inf. gluteal nerve, artery and vein

greater trochanter

gluteus maximus (reflected)

gluteus maximus (reflected)

semitendinosus

biceps femoris (long head)

perforating artery

branch to semitendinosus
and semimembranosus

adductor magnus

iliotibial tract

perforating artery

semimembranosus

biceps femoris (short head)

perforating artery

common peroneal nerve

popliteal artery and vein

tibial nerve

lat. head of gastrocnemius

Superficial dissection of the right posterior thigh muscles.
The long head of the biceps femoris has been pulled laterally, and the semitendinosus and
semimembranosus have been pulled medially to expose the sciatic nerve and perforating
vessels.

Note:

¶ The sciatic nerve is formed by the ventral rami of L4 and L5 and those of S1, S2 and S3.
When the nerve leaves the pelvis through the greater sciatic foramen, below the piriform muscle, its diameter is about 2 cm. During its course along the posterior aspect of
the hip joint, it provides small articular branches for the joint. The muscular branches
of the sciatic nerve are distributed to the biceps femoris, semitendinosus, semimembranosus and the ischial head of the adductor magnus. Usually the sciatic nerve divides
into its ventral branches (tibial nerve) and dorsal branches (common peroneal nerve) in
the lower half of the thigh. Sometimes, however, the nerve divides in the upper half of
the thigh or even before it leaves the pelvis. The common peroneal nerve then perforates the piriform muscle and innervates the short head of the biceps, and the tibial
nerve passes through the infrapiriform foramen and supplies the other muscles.

¶ The posterior side of the thigh does not have a large artery. All the muscles are supplied
by the perforating branches of the profunda femoris artery.

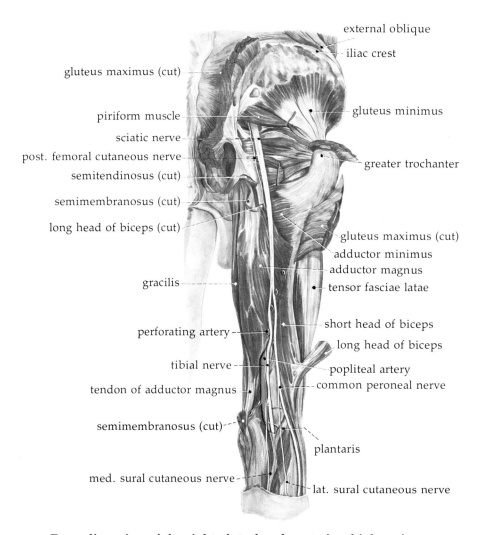

external oblique

iliac crest

gluteus maximus (cut)

gluteus minimus

piriform muscle

sciatic nerve

post. femoral cutaneous nerve

greater trochanter

semitendinosus (cut)

semimembranosus (cut)

long head of biceps (cut)

gluteus maximus (cut)

adductor minimus

adductor magnus

gracilis

tensor fasciae latae

short head of biceps

perforating artery

long head of biceps

tibial nerve

popliteal artery

common peroneal nerve

tendon of adductor magnus

semimembranosus (cut)

plantaris

med. sural cutaneous nerve

lat. sural cutaneous nerve

Deep dissection of the right gluteal and posterior thigh regions.
The biceps femoris, semitendinosus and semimembranosus have been removed.

Note:

¶ The sciatic nerve is separated from the posterior aspect of the hip joint by the small muscles of the hip. Whenever a nerve passes a joint, small nerve branches are provided for the joint. Since the sciatic nerve as well as the femoral and obturator nerves cross the hip joint, all three nerves provide branches for its innervation. The knee joint similarly is innervated by branches of the obturator, femoral, tibial and common peroneal nerves. It is not uncommon for patients with diseases of the hip joint to complain of pain in the knee.

¶ The femoral artery leaves the adductor compartment through the hiatus in the adductor magnus to enter the popliteal fossa. On occasion the hiatus is narrow, and the artery may be compressed. It has been suggested that arteriosclerotic changes and occlusion in the lower part of the femoral artery may result from compression in the hiatus. Usually a good collateral circulation is established via the branches of the profunda femoris artery and the popliteal artery.

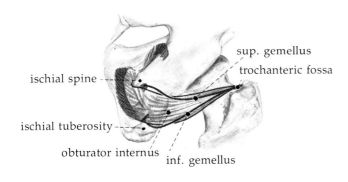

A. Origin and insertion of the gemelli and obturator internus.

Obturator internus
  Origin: Pelvic surface of the obturator membrane and adjoining part of hip bone.
  Insertion: Greater trochanter.
Superior gemellus
  Origin: Ischial spine.
  Insertion: Greater trochanter.
Inferior gemellus
  Origin: Upper margin of ischial tuberosity.
  Insertion: Greater trochanter.

B. Origin and insertion of the piriformis.

Piriformis
  Origin: Front of the sacrum.
  Insertion: Posterior side of the greater trochanter.

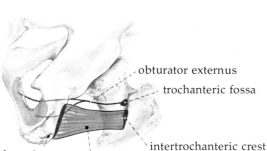

C. Origin and insertion of the obturator externus and quadratus femoris.

Obturator externus
  Origin: Outer surface of obturator membrane; adjacent margin of pubic and ischial rami.
  Insertion: Medial aspect of greater trochanter.
Quadratus femoris
  Origin: Lateral border of ischial tuberosity.
  Insertion: Intertrochanteric crest.

¶ The piriformis and obturator internus originate inside the true pelvis and leave the pelvis through the greater and lesser sciatic foramina, respectively. The piriformis is said to divide the greater sciatic foramen into a suprapiriform foramen and an infrapiriform foramen. Both muscles are lateral rotators of the femur at the hip joint.

¶ The two gemelli join the tendon of the obturator internus to insert with a common tendon at the greater trochanter.

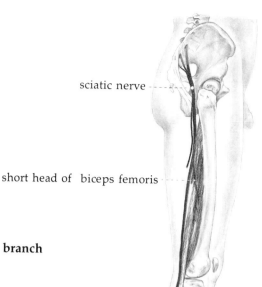

sciatic nerve

short head of biceps femoris

A. Motor function of the common peroneal branch of the sciatic nerve.

deep peroneal nerve

superficial peroneal nerve

peroneus brevis (L4–S1)

peroneus longus

peroneus tertius

extensor digitorum brevis (L4–S1)

tibialis anterior (L4–S1)

extensor digitorum longus (L4–S1)

extensor hallucis longus (L4–S1)

extensor hallucis brevis (L4–S1)

gluteus medius (L4, L5, S1, S2?)

gluteus minimus (L4, L5, S1, S2?)

sup. gluteal nerve

tensor fasciae latae (L4, L5, S1, S2?)

B. Motor function of the superior gluteal nerve.

It is clinically important to know:

¶ The *sciatic nerve* may be injured by dislocations of the hip joint, fractures of the pelvis or badly placed intramuscular injections. If the lesion is complete, which is unusual, the posterior muscles of the thigh and all the muscles below the knee will be paralyzed. Sensibility below the knee will also be lost, except in the area supplied by the saphenous nerve. If the lesion involves the thigh area supplied by the tibial branch of the sciatic nerve, the semimembranosus, semitendinosus, long head of the biceps femoris and ischial head of the adductor magnus will all be paralyzed. Flexion in the knee as well as extension of the hip will be seriously weakened. If the lesion involves the peroneal part of the sciatic nerve, the short head of the biceps and all the muscles on the anterior and lateral sides of the leg and the dorsum of the foot will be paralyzed (see LL39).

¶ The superior gluteal nerve innervates the gluteus medius, gluteus minimus and tensor fasciae latae. The most important function of these muscles is keeping the pelvis in balance when the foot on the opposite side is taken off the ground. When the muscles are paralyzed, the pelvis will tilt downward to the nonaffected, opposite side when that limb is taken off the ground. The patient will walk with a "dipping gait." This symptom, known as a positive Trendelenburg test, is seen not only in patients with lesions of the superior gluteal nerve but also in patients with congenital dislocation of the hip.

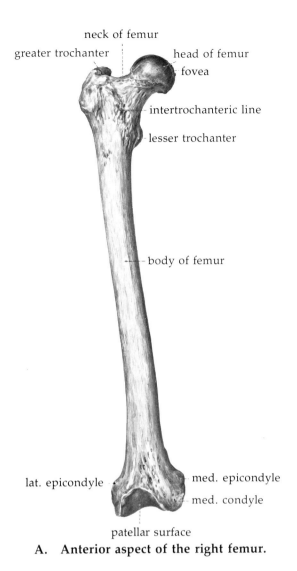

neck of femur
greater trochanter
head of femur
fovea
intertrochanteric line
lesser trochanter

body of femur

lat. epicondyle
med. epicondyle
med. condyle

patellar surface

A. Anterior aspect of the right femur.

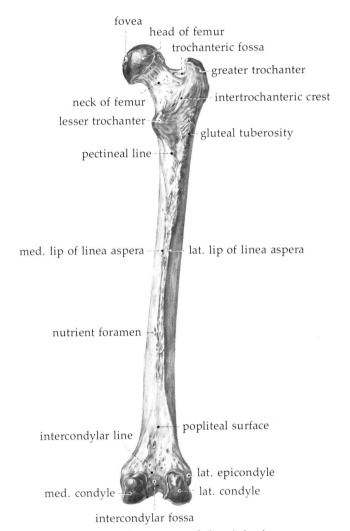

fovea
head of femur
trochanteric fossa
greater trochanter
intertrochanteric crest
neck of femur
lesser trochanter
gluteal tuberosity
pectineal line

med. lip of linea aspera
lat. lip of linea aspera

nutrient foramen

popliteal surface
intercondylar line
lat. epicondyle
med. condyle
lat. condyle
intercondylar fossa

B. Posterior aspect of the right femur.

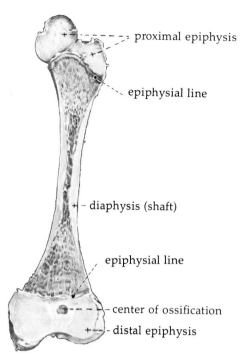

A. Longitudinal section through the femur of a newborn child.

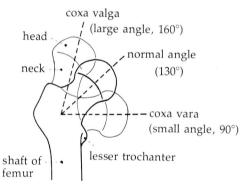

B. Angle between the neck and shaft of the femur.

It is important to know:

¶ In the child the pelvis is narrow, and the neck and shaft of the femur are nearly in line with each other (160 degrees). As the pelvis widens and the weight of the body increases, the angle between the neck and shaft becomes smaller. In the normal male the angle is about 120 to 130 degrees (angle of inclination).

¶ The angle between the neck and shaft of the femur is frequently affected by disease. When the angle is greater than normal it is referred to as *coxa valga*. This condition may occur when the femur is not subjected to normal weight-bearing, as in congenital dislocation of the hip.

¶ When the bone is too soft or when fractures of the neck have occurred, the angle may be much smaller than normal. A small angle between the neck and shaft is referred to as *coxa vara*. This condition occurs when the epiphysis is diseased and the head slips off the neck. This disease—epiphysiolysis—is found not infrequently in children. As can be easily understood, the limb on the affected side is shorter than that on the opposite side.

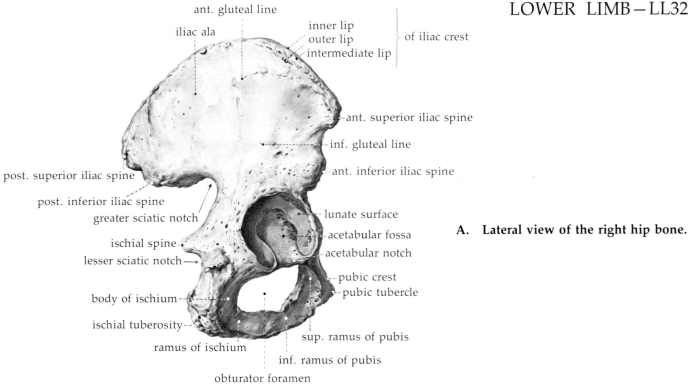

ant. gluteal line

iliac ala

inner lip
outer lip
intermediate lip
} of iliac crest

ant. superior iliac spine

inf. gluteal line

post. superior iliac spine

post. inferior iliac spine

greater sciatic notch

ant. inferior iliac spine

lunate surface

acetabular fossa

ischial spine

acetabular notch

lesser sciatic notch →

pubic crest
pubic tubercle

body of ischium

ischial tuberosity

ramus of ischium

sup. ramus of pubis

inf. ramus of pubis

obturator foramen

A. Lateral view of the right hip bone.

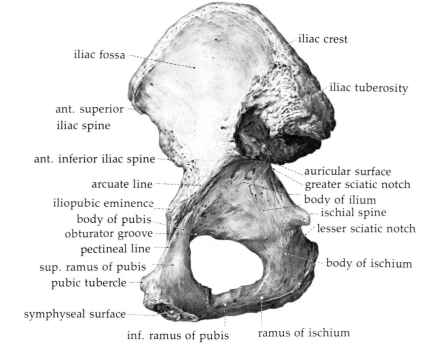

iliac fossa

iliac crest

iliac tuberosity

ant. superior
iliac spine

ant. inferior iliac spine

arcuate line

auricular surface
greater sciatic notch
body of ilium
ischial spine
lesser sciatic notch

iliopubic eminence
body of pubis
obturator groove
pectineal line
sup. ramus of pubis
pubic tubercle

body of ischium

symphyseal surface

inf. ramus of pubis

ramus of ischium

B. Medial view of the right hip bone.

The weight of the body is transmitted to the femora through the sacroiliac joints, the iliac bones and the acetabula. The bony spicules in the head, neck and shaft of the femur are aligned in such a manner that they form a continuation with the weight-bearing arch formed by the pelvis. When one of the lower limbs is shorter than the other, the weight-bearing arch is out of balance. The abnormal strain thus imposed will lead to degeneration of the hip joint in later life.

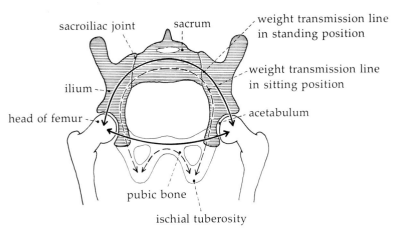

sacroiliac joint

sacrum

weight transmission line
in standing position

ilium

weight transmission line
in sitting position

head of femur

acetabulum

pubic bone

ischial tuberosity

C. Schematic drawing of weight transmission.

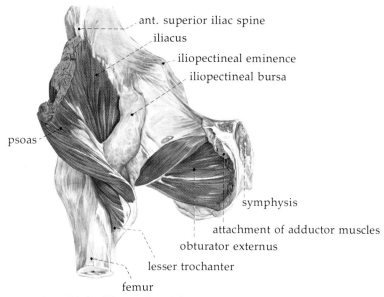

ant. superior iliac spine
iliacus
iliopectineal eminence
iliopectineal bursa
psoas
symphysis
attachment of adductor muscles
obturator externus
lesser trochanter
femur

A. Right iliopectineal bursa.
The psoas and iliacus have been reflected.

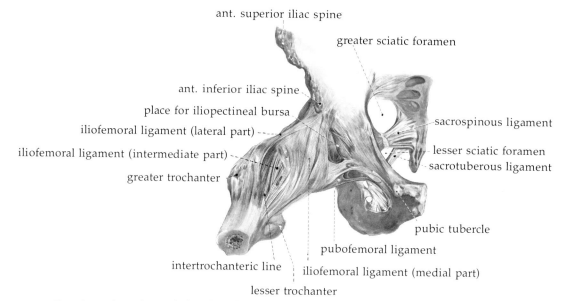

ant. superior iliac spine
greater sciatic foramen
ant. inferior iliac spine
place for iliopectineal bursa
iliofemoral ligament (lateral part)
iliofemoral ligament (intermediate part)
greater trochanter
sacrospinous ligament
lesser sciatic foramen
sacrotuberous ligament
pubic tubercle
pubofemoral ligament
intertrochanteric line
iliofemoral ligament (medial part)
lesser trochanter

B. Anterior view of the right hip joint.
Note the strong ligaments enforcing the anterior aspect of the capsule.

Note:

¶ The fibers of the psoas leave the abdomen by passing under the inguinal ligament. Subsequently they course over the capsule of the hip joint to insert in the lesser trochanter of the femur. A large bursa—the *iliopectineal bursa*— is located between the muscle and the fibrous capsule. This bursa is often in open communication with the synovial cavity of the joint.

¶ Abscesses of the thoracolumbar region of the vertebral column may extend to the fascial sheath of the psoas and subsequently descend in the sheath to the inguinal region (see A73 *A*). Occasionally the abscess may cause a swelling just below the inguinal ligament, and such a swelling is sometimes confused with a femoral hernia. More frequently, the abscess will involve the iliopectineal bursa, expanding into the hip joint from the bursa. Hence, abscesses of the thoracolumbar vertebral column may cause inflammation of the hip joint.

sup. med. genicular artery

sup. lat. genicular artery

genicular arterial network

A. Superficial nerves and vessels on the anterolateral aspect of the left leg.

lat. sural cutaneous nerve

med. crural branches of saphenous nerve

great saphenous vein

superficial peroneal nerve

lat. malleolar network

med. dorsal cutaneous branch of superficial peroneal nerve

lat. dorsal cutaneous branch of superficial peroneal nerve

med. cutaneous branch of femoral nerve

deep peroneal nerve

sup. medial genicular artery

inf. medial genicular artery

great saphenous vein

accessory saphenous vein

saphenous nerve

med. crural cutaneous branches of saphenous nerve

B. Superficial nerves and vessels on the anteromedial aspect of the left leg.

great saphenous vein

terminal branch of saphenous nerve

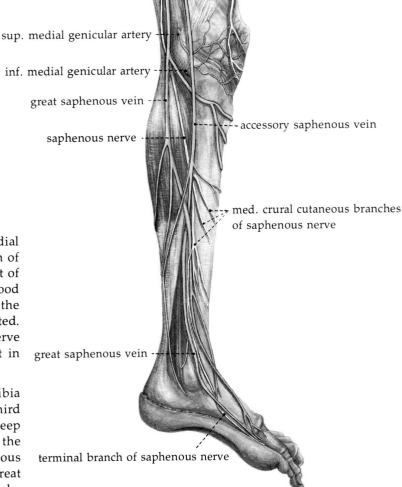

Note:

¶ The great saphenous vein drains the medial part of the venous plexus of the dorsum of the foot. It is found immediately in front of the medial malleolus. When an urgent blood transfusion is necessary, this is one of the sites where a vein can be easily dissected. Sometimes a branch of the saphenous nerve will cross over or behind the vein just in front of the malleolus.

¶ The anterior and medial aspects of the tibia as well as the lateral side of the lower third of the fibula lie immediately under the deep fascia of the leg. They are separated from the skin only by a thin layer of subcutaneous tissue. Wounds over the tibia heal with great difficulty because of the poor blood supply.

A. **Muscles of the anterior aspect of the right leg.**

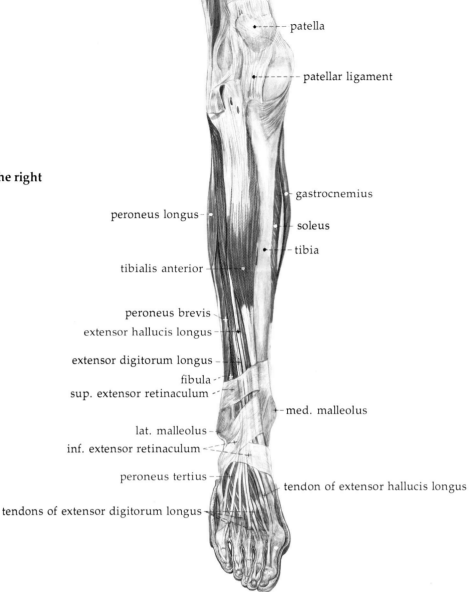

patella
patellar ligament
peroneus longus
gastrocnemius
soleus
tibia
tibialis anterior
peroneus brevis
extensor hallucis longus
extensor digitorum longus
fibula
sup. extensor retinaculum
med. malleolus
lat. malleolus
inf. extensor retinaculum
peroneus tertius
tendon of extensor hallucis longus
tendons of extensor digitorum longus

tuberosity of tibia
deep peroneal nerve
ant. tibial artery and veins
peroneus longus
tibialis anterior
extensor hallucis longus
extensor digitorum longus
superficial peroneal nerve
extensor hallucis longus
fibula
med. dorsal cutaneous nerve
extensor digitorum brevis
deep peroneal nerve
dorsal venous arch

B. **Nerves and arteries in the anterior and lateral compartments of the left leg.**

All the muscles in the anterior and lateral compartments of the leg are supplied by the common peroneal nerve. This nerve reaches the leg by winding around the lateral surface of the neck of the fibula deep to the peroneus longus. At this site it can be rolled under the fingers against the back of the head of the fibula and is most vulnerable to nerve injuries. The deep peroneal nerve passes forward and joins the anterior tibial artery. During its downward course it innervates the tibialis anterior, extensor digitorum longus, extensor hallucis longus and peroneus tertius. On the dorsum of the foot it supplies the short extensor muscles. The superficial peroneal nerve innervates the peroneus longus and brevis. Hence, when the common peroneal nerve is injured at the neck of the fibula all anterior and lateral muscles are paralyzed. As a result, the foot is plantar flexed and slightly inverted (foot drop).

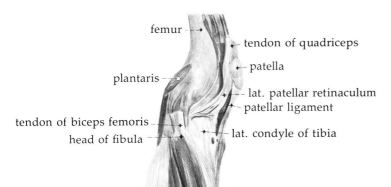

femur
plantaris
tendon of biceps femoris
head of fibula

tendon of quadriceps
patella
lat. patellar retinaculum
patellar ligament
lat. condyle of tibia

A. Muscles of the lateral compartment of the right leg.

gastrocnemius

soleus

tibialis anterior

peroneus longus

peroneus brevis

calcaneal (Achilles) tendon

sup. extensor retinaculum

sup. peroneal retinaculum

lat. malleolus
inf. extensor retinaculum

inf. peroneal retinaculum
calcaneus
tendon of peroneus longus
tendon of peroneus brevis
tendon of peroneus tertius

extensor digitorum brevis

tuberosity of fifth metatarsal

Note:

¶ The peroneus longus arises from the head and the upper two-thirds of the lateral surface of the fibula, from the surrounding fascia and sometimes from the lateral condyle of the tibia. Between its attachments to the head and shaft of the fibula is a gap for the passage of the common peroneal nerve. Here the nerve divides into the superficial and deep peroneal nerves (see *B* and LL39 *B*).

¶ The tendon of the peroneus longus runs behind the lateral malleolus, then passes on the lateral side of the calcaneus, where it is held in place by the inferior peroneal retinaculum. Subsequently it crosses the cuboid and winds around its lateral margin to attach to the base of the first metatarsal and the medial cuneiform bone. It plays an important role in supporting the transverse arch of the foot and the lateral longitudinal arch (see also LL63 *A*). Its active function is eversion and plantar flexion of the foot.

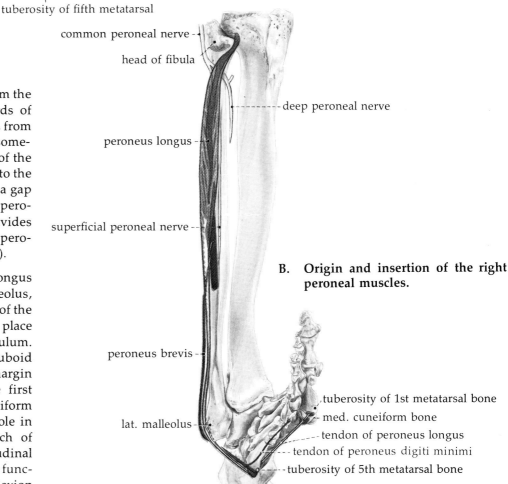

common peroneal nerve
head of fibula

deep peroneal nerve

peroneus longus

superficial peroneal nerve

B. Origin and insertion of the right peroneal muscles.

peroneus brevis

lat. malleolus

tuberosity of 1st metatarsal bone
med. cuneiform bone
tendon of peroneus longus
tendon of peroneus digiti minimi
tuberosity of 5th metatarsal bone

calcaneus

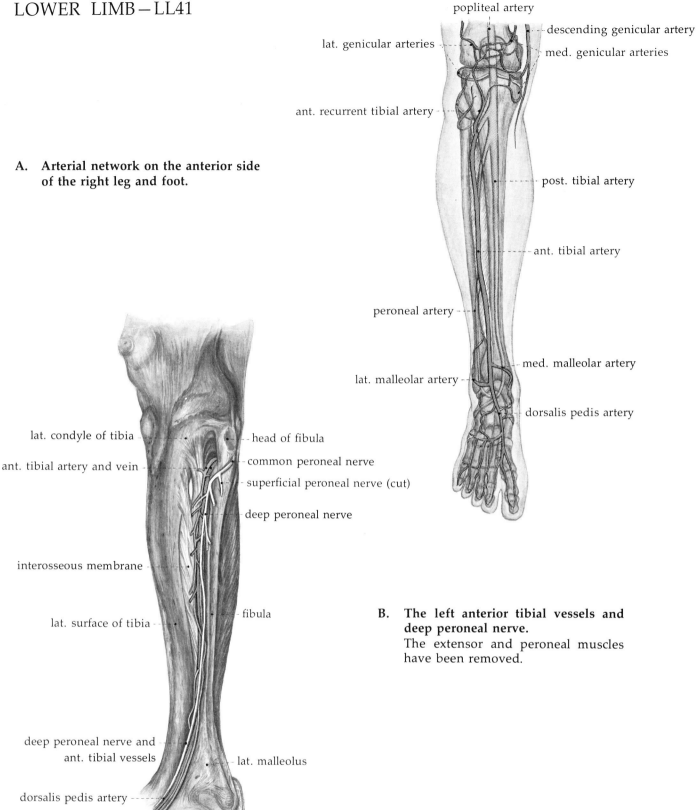

A. Arterial network on the anterior side of the right leg and foot.

popliteal artery

descending genicular artery

lat. genicular arteries

med. genicular arteries

ant. recurrent tibial artery

post. tibial artery

ant. tibial artery

peroneal artery

med. malleolar artery

lat. malleolar artery

dorsalis pedis artery

lat. condyle of tibia

head of fibula

common peroneal nerve

ant. tibial artery and vein

superficial peroneal nerve (cut)

deep peroneal nerve

interosseous membrane

lat. surface of tibia

fibula

B. The left anterior tibial vessels and deep peroneal nerve.
The extensor and peroneal muscles have been removed.

deep peroneal nerve and ant. tibial vessels

lat. malleolus

dorsalis pedis artery

Note:

⁋ The anterior tibial artery enters the anterior compartment of the leg by piercing the interosseous membrane. Its terminal extension is formed by the dorsal artery of the foot (dorsalis pedis artery). This vessel is superficial and can easily be palpated in the region extending from a point halfway between the malleoli to the proximal end of the first intermetatarsal space.

⁋ The deep peroneal nerve joins the anterior tibial artery. The nerve does not pierce the interosseous membrane but winds around the neck of the fibula.

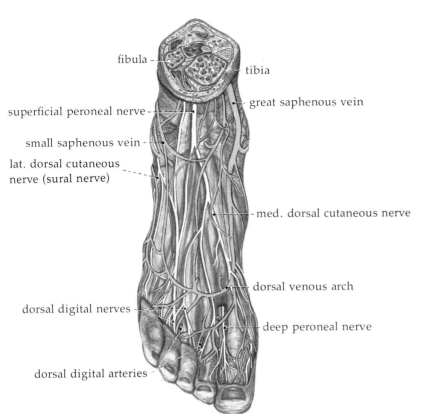

fibula
tibia
great saphenous vein
superficial peroneal nerve
small saphenous vein
lat. dorsal cutaneous nerve (sural nerve)
med. dorsal cutaneous nerve
dorsal venous arch
dorsal digital nerves
deep peroneal nerve
dorsal digital arteries

A. Superficial nerves and veins of the dorsal aspect of the right foot.

ant. tibial artery
peroneal artery
post. tibial artery
perforating branch of peroneal artery
lat. plantar artery
dorsalis pedis artery
med. tarsal arteries
lat. tarsal artery
arcuate artery
plantar arch
dorsal metatarsal arteries
plantar digital arteries
dorsal digital arteries

B. Arteries on the dorsal aspect of the right foot.

Note:

¶ The superficial peroneal nerve is the principal sensory nerve of the dorsum of the foot.

¶ The deep peroneal nerve innervates the adjacent sides of the first and second toes.

¶ The lateral dorsal cutaneous nerve (sural nerve) supplies the skin on the dorsal and lateral aspects of the fifth toe.

¶ A branch of the peroneal artery perforates the interosseous membrane to participate in the blood supply of the ankle joint (see *B*).

315

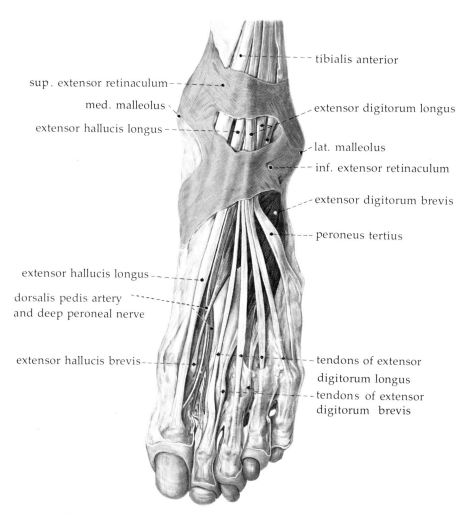

sup. extensor retinaculum

med. malleolus

extensor hallucis longus

tibialis anterior

extensor digitorum longus

lat. malleolus

inf. extensor retinaculum

extensor digitorum brevis

peroneus tertius

extensor hallucis longus

dorsalis pedis artery
and deep peroneal nerve

extensor hallucis brevis

tendons of extensor
digitorum longus

tendons of extensor
digitorum brevis

Muscles and tendons on the dorsal side of the left foot.
The dorsalis pedis artery is accompanied by the deep peroneal nerve.

Note:

¶ As the tendons of the muscles pass downward from the leg to the dorsum of the foot, they are bound by localized thickenings of the deep fascia — the retinacula. Since the tendons are deflected from a straight course, they are enclosed in synovial sheaths. At the sites where the tendons pass over bony points, small bursae are present to diminish the friction (see LL44 *B*).

¶ The pulse of the dorsalis pedis artery is a source of information about vascularization in the leg. The best place to feel it is between the tendons of the extensor hallucis longus and the extensor digitorum longus on the dorsum of the foot. Absence of the pulse usually indicates severe arteriosclerotic changes in the arteries of the leg. Keep in mind, however, that in at least 10 per cent of normal subjects the dorsalis pedis artery is absent.

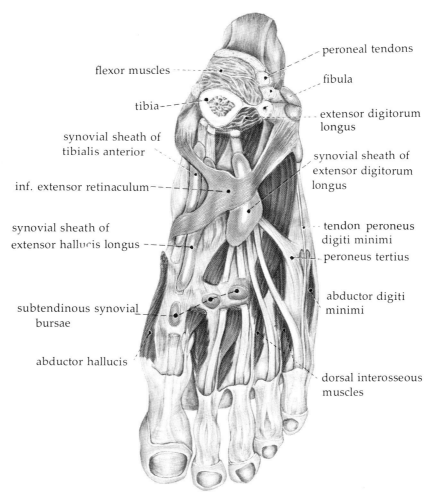

peroneal tendons

flexor muscles

fibula

tibia

extensor digitorum longus

synovial sheath of tibialis anterior

synovial sheath of extensor digitorum longus

inf. extensor retinaculum

synovial sheath of extensor hallucis longus

tendon peroneus digiti minimi

peroneus tertius

subtendinous synovial bursae

abductor digiti minimi

abductor hallucis

dorsal interosseous muscles

A. Tendon sheaths and bursae on the dorsal side of the left foot.

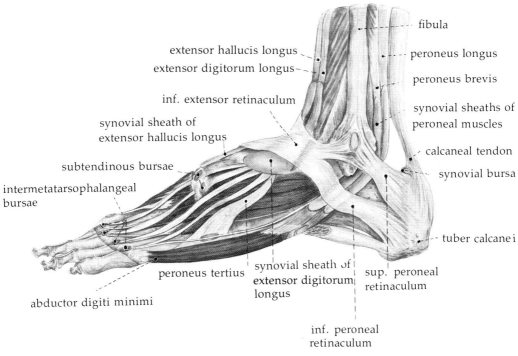

fibula

extensor hallucis longus

peroneus longus

extensor digitorum longus

peroneus brevis

inf. extensor retinaculum

synovial sheaths of peroneal muscles

synovial sheath of extensor hallucis longus

calcaneal tendon

subtendinous bursae

synovial bursa

intermetatarsophalangeal bursae

tuber calcanei

peroneus tertius

synovial sheath of extensor digitorum longus

sup. peroneal retinaculum

abductor digiti minimi

inf. peroneal retinaculum

B. Lateral view of tendon sheaths and bursae on the left foot.

317

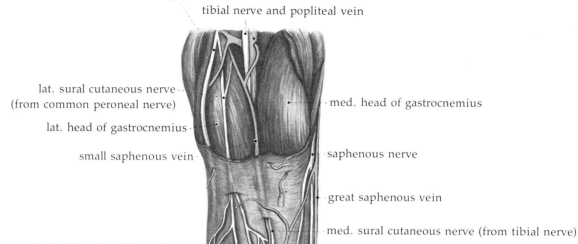

common peroneal nerve

tibial nerve and popliteal vein

lat. sural cutaneous nerve
(from common peroneal nerve)

lat. head of gastrocnemius

small saphenous vein

med. head of gastrocnemius

saphenous nerve

great saphenous vein

med. sural cutaneous nerve (from tibial nerve)

communicating branch with sural nerve

branches of lat. sural cutaneous nerve

small saphenous vein

sural nerve

branches of saphenous nerve

lat. malleolus

Superficial veins and nerves of the posterior side of the left leg.

Note:

¶ Both the great saphenous vein and the small saphenous vein arise from the venous network over the dorsum of the foot. The great saphenous vein then passes just in front of the medial malleolus and ascends on the leg about 3 cm medial to the medial aspect of the tibia. The small saphenous vein passes behind the lateral malleolus and ascends in the superficial fascia on the posterior aspect of the leg, piercing the deep fascia to empty into the popliteal vein. Numerous veins enter the saphenous veins, particularly on the back of the calf.

¶ As a result of increased back pressure, the saphenous network on the calf has a predilection to form varicose veins. Because of the varicosities, the blood flow in the skin of the leg becomes stagnant, causing poor nutrition of the overlying skin. Ulcers may easily develop even after minor injuries. Such ulcers occur particularly over the anteromedial surface of the tibia near the ankle.

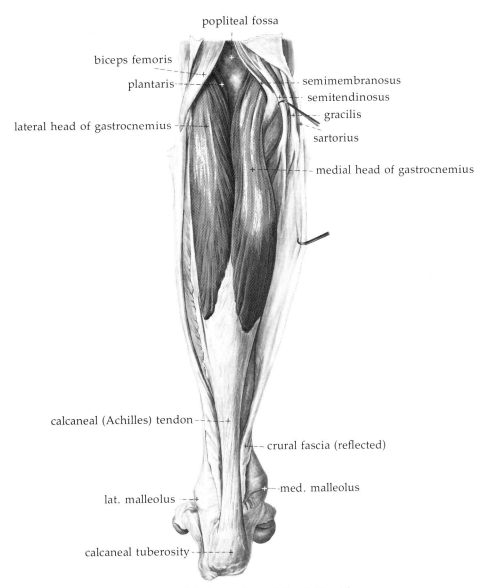

popliteal fossa

biceps femoris

plantaris

lateral head of gastrocnemius

semimembranosus

semitendinosus

gracilis

sartorius

medial head of gastrocnemius

calcaneal (Achilles) tendon

crural fascia (reflected)

med. malleolus

lat. malleolus

calcaneal tuberosity

Superficial muscles of the left calf.

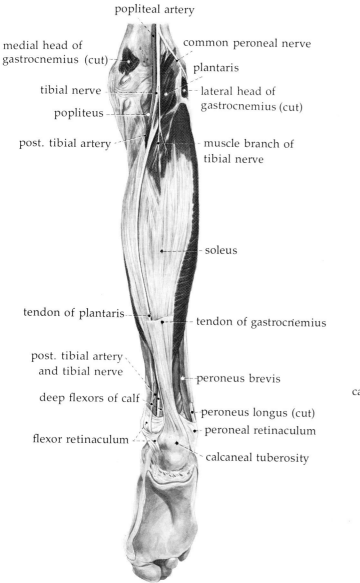

popliteal artery

medial head of
gastrocnemius (cut)

common peroneal nerve

plantaris

tibial nerve

lateral head of
gastrocnemius (cut)

popliteus

post. tibial artery

muscle branch of
tibial nerve

soleus

tendon of plantaris

tendon of gastrocnemius

post. tibial artery
and tibial nerve

deep flexors of calf

peroneus brevis

peroneus longus (cut)

peroneal retinaculum

flexor retinaculum

calcaneal tuberosity

A.   The plantaris and soleus of the right leg.
The gastrocnemius has been removed.

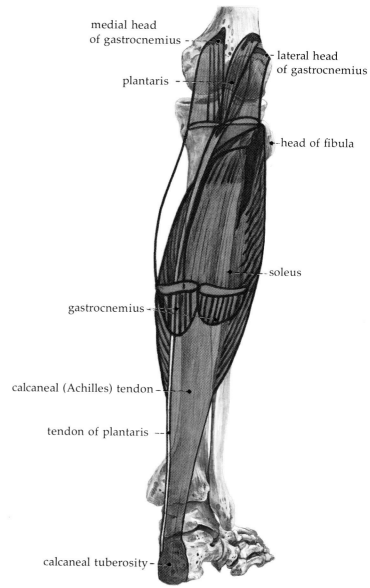

medial head
of gastrocnemius

lateral head
of gastrocnemius

plantaris

head of fibula

soleus

gastrocnemius

calcaneal (Achilles) tendon

tendon of plantaris

calcaneal tuberosity

**B.   Origin and insertion of the right superficial
muscles.**

¶ The medial and lateral heads of the gastrocnemius arise from the medial and lateral femoral condyles, respectively. They insert onto the calcaneal tuberosity by means of the very strong calcaneal tendon (Achilles tendon).

¶ The soleus arises from the posterior surface of the fibula, the intermuscular septum between the superficial and deep flexors and the posterior surface of the tibia. The fibers join the calcaneal tendon.

¶ The plantaris arises from the lateral supracondylar line and the popliteal surface of the femur and also joins the calcaneal tendon.

¶ Both the gastrocnemius and the soleus are strong plantar flexors and invertors of the foot. The gastrocnemius is also able to flex the leg at the knee joint.

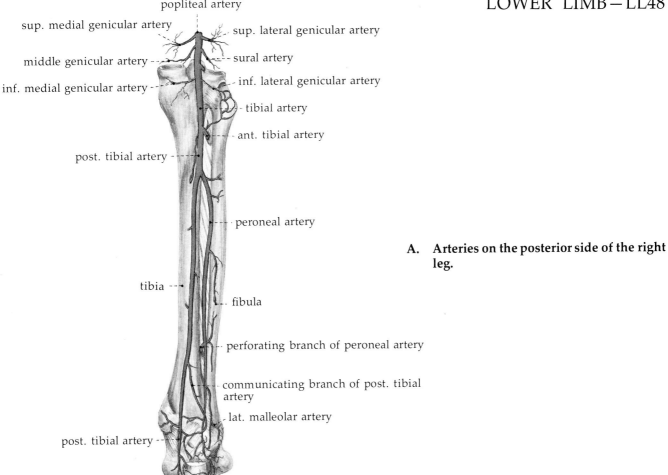

popliteal artery

sup. medial genicular artery — sup. lateral genicular artery

middle genicular artery — sural artery

inf. medial genicular artery — inf. lateral genicular artery

tibial artery

ant. tibial artery

post. tibial artery

peroneal artery

tibia — fibula

perforating branch of peroneal artery

communicating branch of post. tibial artery

lat. malleolar artery

post. tibial artery

A. Arteries on the posterior side of the right leg.

B. Superficial dissection of the posterior aspect of the right leg (medial view).
Note the tibial nerve and the posterior tibial vessels.

Note:

¶ Two arteries pierce the interosseous membrane: (a) the anterior tibial artery, which supplies the front of the leg and the dorsal aspect of the foot, and (b) a small branch of the peroneal artery, which supplies the dorsal aspect of the ankle (talocrural) joint.

¶ The posterior tibial artery is the continuation of the popliteal artery. It descends between the superficial and deep compartments and becomes superficial in the lower third of the leg. The artery, accompanied by the tibial nerve, passes behind the medial malleolus between the tendons of the flexor digitorum longus and the flexor hallucis longus to supply the muscles on the sole of the foot.

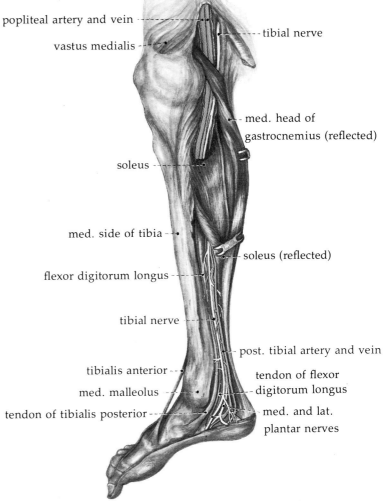

popliteal artery and vein — tibial nerve

vastus medialis

med. head of gastrocnemius (reflected)

soleus

med. side of tibia — soleus (reflected)

flexor digitorum longus

tibial nerve

post. tibial artery and vein

tibialis anterior — tendon of flexor digitorum longus

med. malleolus — med. and lat. plantar nerves

tendon of tibialis posterior

321

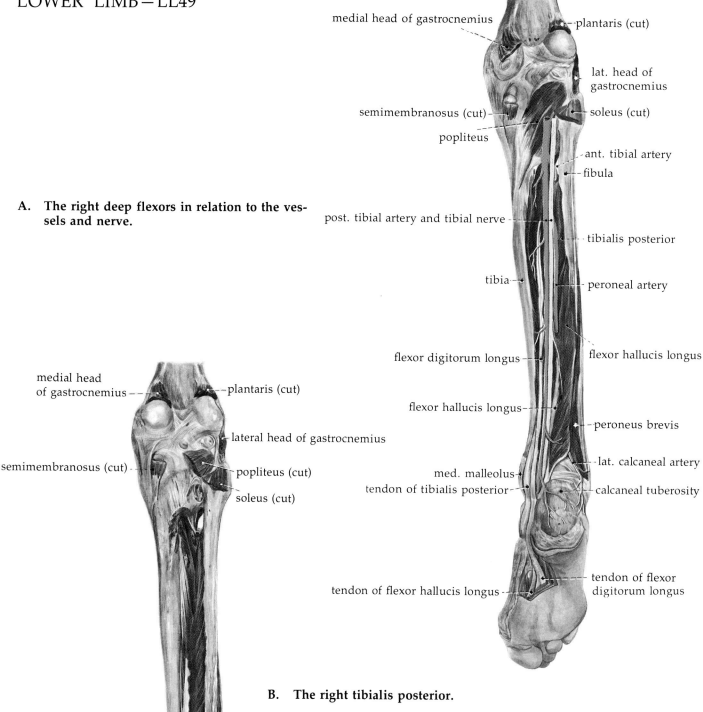

A. The right deep flexors in relation to the vessels and nerve.

medial head of gastrocnemius

plantaris (cut)

lat. head of gastrocnemius

semimembranosus (cut)

soleus (cut)

popliteus

ant. tibial artery

fibula

post. tibial artery and tibial nerve

tibialis posterior

tibia

peroneal artery

flexor digitorum longus

flexor hallucis longus

flexor hallucis longus

peroneus brevis

lat. calcaneal artery

med. malleolus

tendon of tibialis posterior

calcaneal tuberosity

tendon of flexor hallucis longus

tendon of flexor digitorum longus

medial head of gastrocnemius

plantaris (cut)

lateral head of gastrocnemius

semimembranosus (cut)

popliteus (cut)

soleus (cut)

B. The right tibialis posterior.

tibialis posterior

peroneus brevis

tendon of flexor digitorum longus

tendon of peroneus longus

flexor retinaculum

peroneal retinaculum

tendon of flexor hallucis longus

calcaneal tuberosity

Note:

¶ The deep flexor group consists of four muscles: (a) the flexor digitorum longus; (b) the flexor hallucis longus; (c) the tibialis posterior; and (d) the popliteus. Contraction of the muscles produces flexion of the toes, plantar flexion of the foot in the ankle joint and inversion of the foot in the subtalar joint. The popliteus, however, does not participate in this function, but rotates the leg medially and supports flexion of the knee joint (see also LL51).

¶ The posterior tibial artery and the tibial nerve course between the superficial and deep flexors. Note the origin of the anterior tibial artery and the peroneal artery.

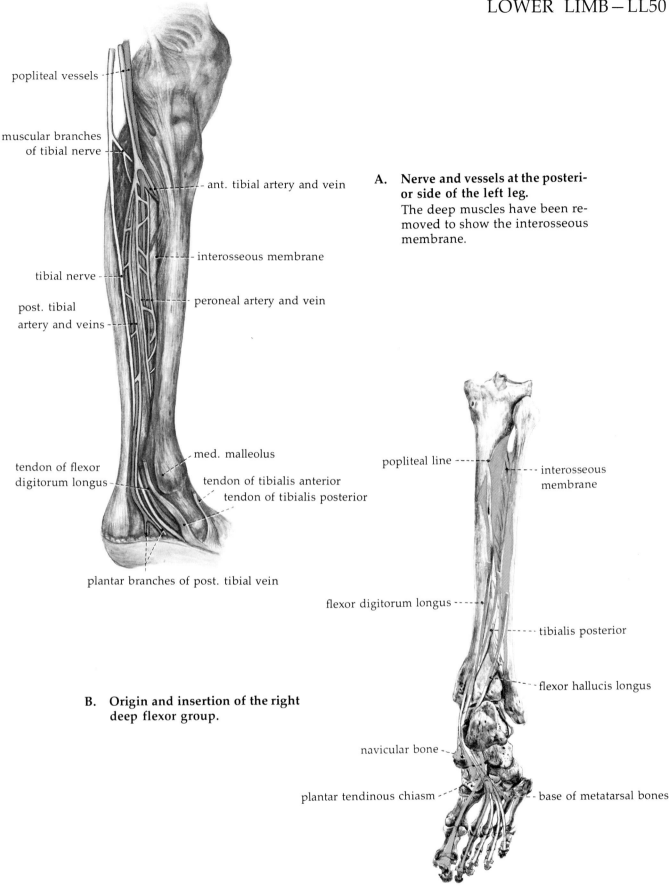

popliteal vessels

muscular branches
of tibial nerve

ant. tibial artery and vein

tibial nerve

post. tibial
artery and veins

interosseous membrane

peroneal artery and vein

A. **Nerve and vessels at the posterior side of the left leg.**
The deep muscles have been removed to show the interosseous membrane.

tendon of flexor
digitorum longus

med. malleolus

tendon of tibialis anterior

tendon of tibialis posterior

plantar branches of post. tibial vein

popliteal line

interosseous
membrane

flexor digitorum longus

tibialis posterior

flexor hallucis longus

B. **Origin and insertion of the right deep flexor group.**

navicular bone

plantar tendinous chiasm

base of metatarsal bones

Note:

The flexor hallucis longus and the flexor digitorum longus cause flexion of the phalanges and plantar flexion of the foot when the foot is off the ground. When the foot is on the ground they act together with the interossei and lumbricals to keep the pads of the toes on the ground, thus enlarging the weight-bearing area. Both muscles contribute little to maintenance of the longitudinal arch of the foot. The tibialis posterior may assist in plantar flexion, but its main function is inversion of the foot.

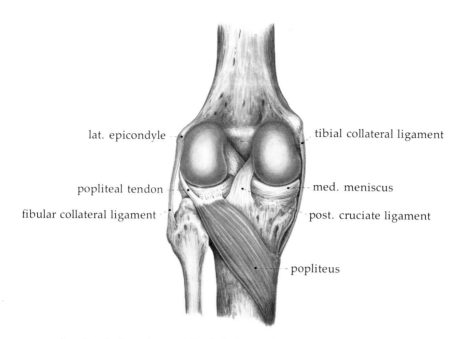

lat. epicondyle

tibial collateral ligament

popliteal tendon

med. meniscus

fibular collateral ligament

post. cruciate ligament

popliteus

A. Posterior view of the left knee showing the popliteus.

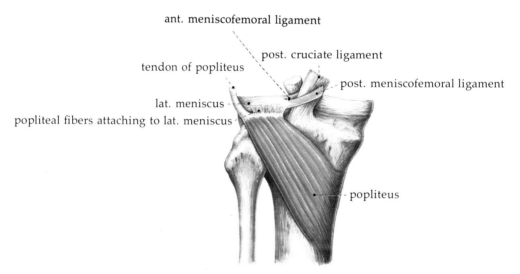

ant. meniscofemoral ligament

post. cruciate ligament

tendon of popliteus

post. meniscofemoral ligament

lat. meniscus

popliteal fibers attaching to lat. meniscus

popliteus

B. Attachment of the popliteus to the lateral meniscus.
Note the meniscofemoral ligaments.

Note:

¶ The lateral part of the popliteus muscle originates with a strong tendon from the lateral condyle of the femur. The medial fibers arise from the arcuate ligament of the capsule (LL54 *B*) and also from the outer margin of the lateral meniscus. When the tibia is fixed, the popliteus muscle rotates the femur laterally. It "unlocks" the joint at the beginning of flexion and pulls the posterior part of the lateral meniscus backward during lateral rotation and flexion of the knee joint. Hence, it protects the meniscus from being crushed between the femur and the tibia.

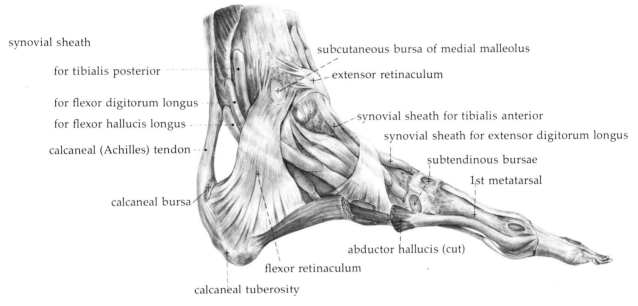

synovial sheath

for tibialis posterior

for flexor digitorum longus

for flexor hallucis longus

calcaneal (Achilles) tendon

calcaneal bursa

subcutaneous bursa of medial malleolus

extensor retinaculum

synovial sheath for tibialis anterior

synovial sheath for extensor digitorum longus

subtendinous bursae

1st metatarsal

abductor hallucis (cut)

flexor retinaculum

calcaneal tuberosity

Tendon sheaths and bursae on the left foot (medial view).

Note:

¶ If shoes or boots fit poorly, some of the bursae of the foot may be prone to inflammation. A subcutaneous bursa may develop over the insertion of the calcaneal tendon, and inflammations of this bursa may spread to the bursa located under the tendon. Another frequently inflamed bursa is that over the head of the first metatarsal bone. This occurs in patients with a hallux valgus, and the bursa is referred to as a bunion.

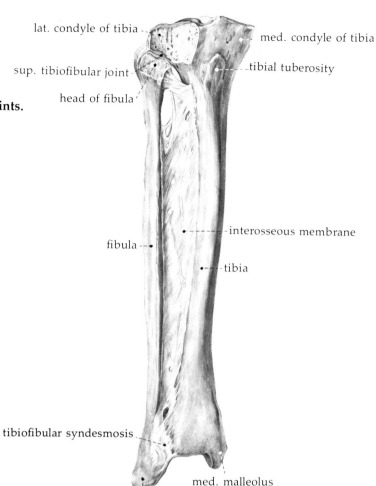

lat. condyle of tibia
med. condyle of tibia
sup. tibiofibular joint
tibial tuberosity
head of fibula
interosseous membrane
fibula
tibia
tibiofibular syndesmosis
med. malleolus
lat. malleolus

A. Right tibia and fibula; tibiofibular joints.

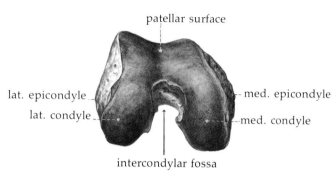

patellar surface
lat. epicondyle
med. epicondyle
lat. condyle
med. condyle
intercondylar fossa

B. Distal end of the right femur.

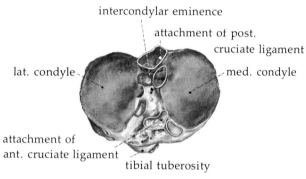

intercondylar eminence
attachment of post. cruciate ligament
lat. condyle
med. condyle
attachment of ant. cruciate ligament
tibial tuberosity

C. Proximal articular surface of the right tibia.
Attachments of the medial meniscus are
indicated in blue, those of the lateral meniscus in red.

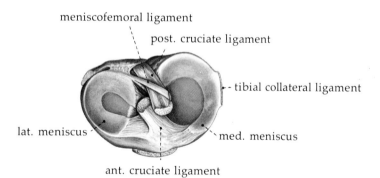

meniscofemoral ligament
post. cruciate ligament
tibial collateral ligament
lat. meniscus
med. meniscus
ant. cruciate ligament

**D. Proximal surface of the right tibia with
menisci and cruciate ligaments.**

Keep in mind:

¶ The entire anteromedial aspect of the tibia
and the lower third of the fibula have a subcutaneous position and are covered only by
skin and the superficial fascia. It is, therefore, not surprising that fractures of the tibia
and fibula occur frequently. If one of the
bones is fractured, the other acts as a splint
and little displacement occurs. Unfortunate-
ly, however, many tibial fractures are compound — that is, fragments of the bone pierce
the skin. In elderly people fractures of the tibia heal with great difficulty owing to the
poor blood supply to the bone and to the overlying skin.

¶ The knee joint is formed by the round condylar surfaces of the femur and the flat condyles of the tibia. The menisci, wedge-shaped in cross section, help to make the flat
surface of the tibia more suitable as a socket for the round condyles of the femur. The
inherent danger, however, is that the menisci may be crushed between the femur and
the tibia.

326

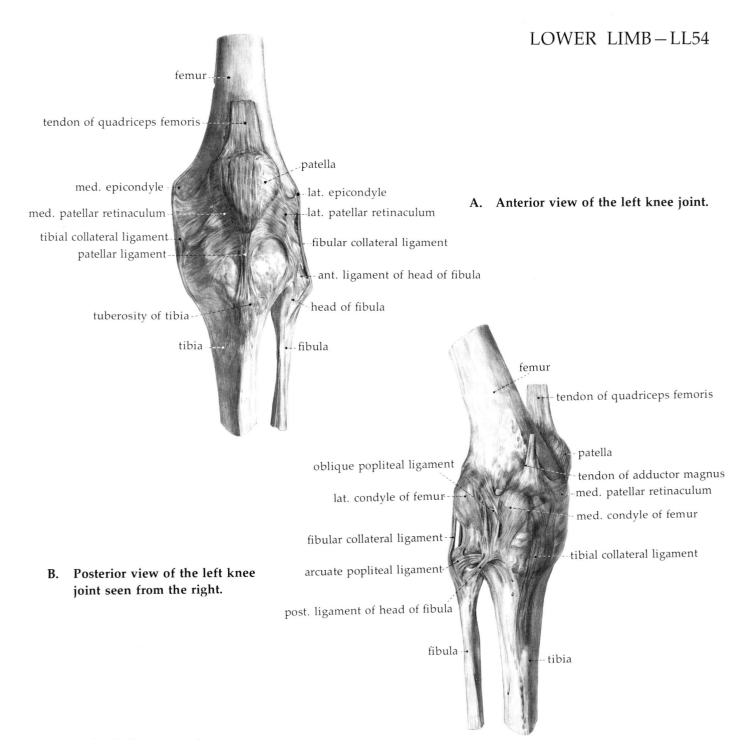

A. **Anterior view of the left knee joint.**

B. **Posterior view of the left knee joint seen from the right.**

Note the following points:

¶ The tibial collateral ligament forms a part of the fibrous capsule; the fibular collateral ligament is not incorporated in the capsule, and the tendon of the popliteus muscle passes between the ligament and the lateral meniscus. The central portion of the tendon of the quadriceps femoris continues from the patella to the tuberosity of the tibia as the patellar ligament. The medial and lateral portions of the tendon—the medial and lateral patellar retinacula—blend with the fibrous capsule.

¶ The rounded condyles of the femur and the flat condyles of the tibia form a hinge joint. Some rotating movement is possible, however, owing to the presence of the menisci. Since the main movements are flexion and extension, the joint is characterized by strong collateral ligaments; the back and particularly the front of the joint capsule, however, are weak. The front is strengthened only by the patellar retinacula.

¶ After trauma to the knee joint or when inflammation occurs, large amounts of fluid usually collect in the joint, and the capsule begins to bulge. Since the collateral ligaments prevent expansion in the lateral and medial directions, the capsule has a particular tendency to bulge anteriorly. When a large amount of fluid is present in the joint, the patella is raised above the patellar surface of the femur. On physical examination the patella can be moved on the underlying fluid cushion of the capsule.

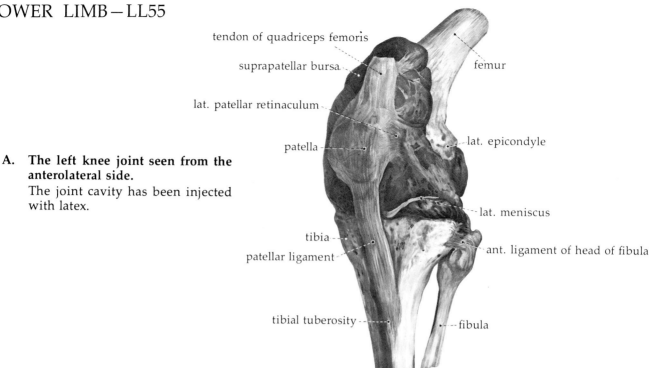

tendon of quadriceps femoris

suprapatellar bursa

femur

lat. patellar retinaculum

lat. epicondyle

patella

lat. meniscus

tibia

patellar ligament

ant. ligament of head of fibula

tibial tuberosity

fibula

A. The left knee joint seen from the anterolateral side.
The joint cavity has been injected with latex.

suprapatellar bursa

femur

intercondylar notch

med. epicondyle

capsule

med. meniscus

med. condyle of tibia

head of fibula

B. The left knee joint seen from the right and behind.
As a result of the latex injection the capsule is distended.

Note:

¶ The synovial capsule is attached to the margins of the articular surfaces and also to the outer margins of the menisci. Hence, when the capsule bulges outward, it does so between the femur and the menisci, and to a small degree between the menisci and the tibia.

¶ The patellar ligament is attached both to the lower border of the patella and to the tibial tuberosity and is a continuation of the quadriceps tendon. The patella is a sesamoid bone embedded in the quadriceps tendon and the patellar ligament. Its posterior surface articulates with the patellar surface of the femur.

¶ When the patella is fractured by a direct blow, it usually breaks into a number of fragments. Since the bone lies within the quadriceps tendon and the patellar ligament, little separation of the fragments occurs. When the fracture is combined with a transverse tear of the quadriceps tendon, the upper and lower parts of the patella are separated from each other owing to traction exerted by the quadriceps muscle. In such cases recombination of the patellar components may be difficult.

¶ When a knock knee (genu valgum) deformity is present, or when the lateral condyle of the femur is underdeveloped, dislocation in a lateral direction may easily occur.

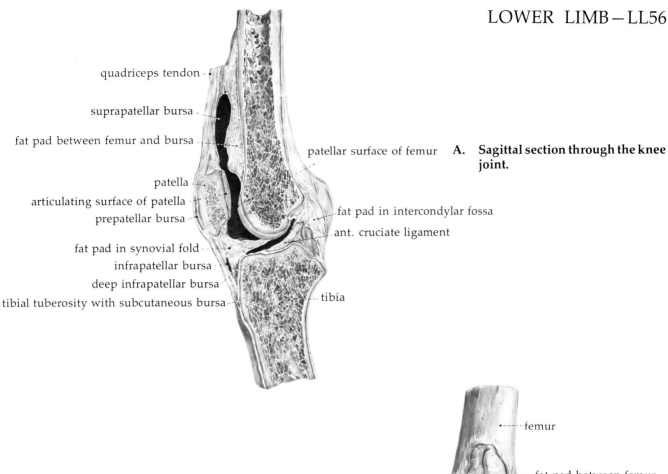

quadriceps tendon

suprapatellar bursa

fat pad between femur and bursa

patellar surface of femur

patella

articulating surface of patella

prepatellar bursa

fat pad in intercondylar fossa

ant. cruciate ligament

fat pad in synovial fold

infrapatellar bursa

deep infrapatellar bursa

tibial tuberosity with subcutaneous bursa

tibia

A. Sagittal section through the knee joint.

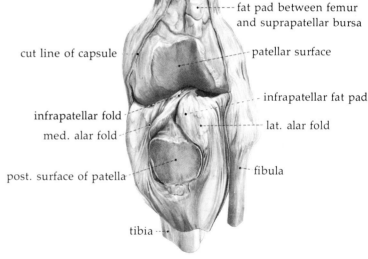

femur

fat pad between femur and suprapatellar bursa

cut line of capsule

patellar surface

infrapatellar fat pad

infrapatellar fold

lat. alar fold

med. alar fold

post. surface of patella

fibula

tibia

B. The left knee joint opened from the front.

The bursae around the knee joint are prone to inflammation. The important bursae are:

¶ The *suprapatellar bursa* extends about three fingerbreadths above the patella under the quadriceps muscle. The bursa is in open communication with the joint cavity, and inflammations of the knee joint usually extend to the suprapatellar bursa. It can be readily understood why the patella will be lifted from its area of contact with the femur when fluid collects in the joint cavity and suprapatellar bursa.

¶ The *prepatellar bursa* is frequently affected by continuous kneeling as in polishing floors. Inflammation of this bursa is known as housemaid's knee.

¶ The *infrapatellar bursae* and the bursa over the tibial tuberosity may be affected by kneeling in a more erect position, as in praying. The inflammation of these bursae is referred to as clergyman's knee.

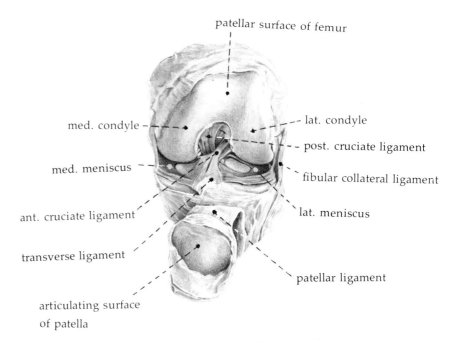

A. Left knee joint opened from the front.
The patella has been pulled distally.

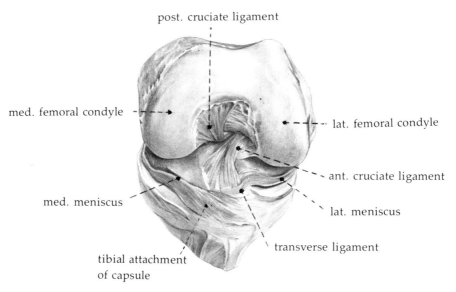

B. Left knee joint seen from the front.
The patella and capsule have been removed.

The cruciate ligaments are frequently injured in sports accidents. Usually the collateral ligaments and the capsule are also damaged, and the joint cavity is filled with blood. To determine whether the cruciate ligaments are intact, remember:

¶ The *anterior cruciate ligament* is attached to the anterior intercondylar area of the tibia. It inserts at the posterior part of the medial surface of the lateral femoral condyle. When the knee is flexed, origin and insertion approach each other, and the ligament is slack. When the ligament is torn, the tibia can be pulled excessively far forward.

¶ The *posterior cruciate ligament* is attached to the posterior intercondylar area of the tibia. It passes upward and forward to insert on the anterior part of the lateral surface of the medial femoral condyle. When the ligament is ruptured, the tibia can be moved excessively backward on the femur.

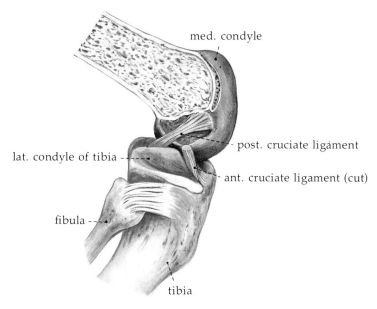

med. condyle

post. cruciate ligament

lat. condyle of tibia

ant. cruciate ligament (cut)

fibula

tibia

A.   Schematic drawing of right posterior cruciate ligament.

lat. condyle of femur

ant. cruciate ligament

med. condyle of tibia

post. cruciate ligament (cut)

tibia

B.   Schematic drawing of right anterior cruciate ligament.

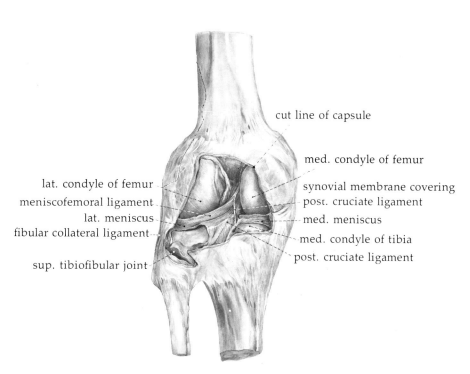

cut line of capsule

med. condyle of femur

lat. condyle of femur

synovial membrane covering

meniscofemoral ligament

post. cruciate ligament

lat. meniscus

med. meniscus

fibular collateral ligament

med. condyle of tibia

sup. tibiofibular joint

post. cruciate ligament

C.   The left knee joint and the tibiofibular joint seen from behind.

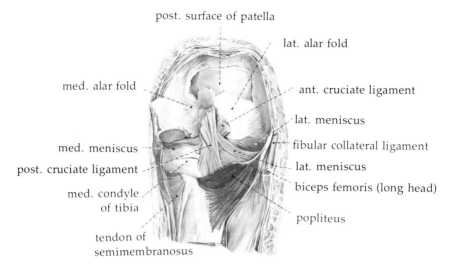

post. surface of patella

lat. alar fold

med. alar fold

ant. cruciate ligament

lat. meniscus

fibular collateral ligament

med. meniscus

post. cruciate ligament

lat. meniscus

med. condyle
of tibia

biceps femoris (long head)

popliteus

tendon of
semimembranosus

A. The right knee joint opened from behind (the femur is removed).

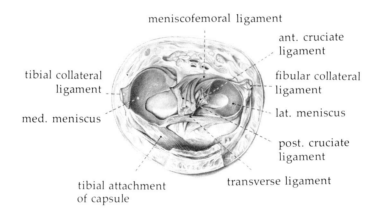

meniscofemoral ligament

ant. cruciate
ligament

tibial collateral
ligament

fibular collateral
ligament

med. meniscus

lat. meniscus

post. cruciate
ligament

tibial attachment
of capsule

transverse ligament

B. Proximal end of the left tibia with semilunar cartilages and cruciate ligaments.

The semilunar cartilages are frequently injured, the medial more often than the lateral.

¶ The *medial semilunar cartilage* (medial meniscus) is semicircular. Its anterior horn is attached to the anterior intercondylar area, the posterior horn to the posterior intercondylar area. The peripheral border is broadly connected with the tibial collateral ligament. When the femur is rotated on the tibia with the knee partially flexed, as in skiing, the meniscus may be pulled between the femoral and tibial condyles owing to forceful rotation of the body. The cartilage may be crushed between the condyles and will then tear or split along its length. Sometimes the cartilage becomes wedged between the articular surfaces—movement then becomes impossible, and the knee is "locked."

¶ The *lateral semilunar cartilage* (lateral meniscus) is almost circular. The posterior horn is attached to the posterior intercondylar area, but usually a fibrous band follows the posterior cruciate ligament to the medial condyle of the femur—the meniscofemoral ligament. The lateral semilunar cartilage is less frequently injured than the medial cartilage because (a) it is not attached to the collateral ligament; (b) the meniscofemoral ligament will pull it away from the condyle in flexion of the knee; and (c) fibers of the popliteal muscle are able to pull the cartilage in a posterior direction (see LL51 *A*).

sup. border of patella

lat. epicondyle

intercondylar fossa

lat. condyle of tibia

head of fibula

neck of fibula

med. epicondyle

intercondylar eminence

med. condyle of tibia

tibial tuberosity

A. Knee, anteroposterior view.
To examine the menisci, absorbable gas or water soluble positive contrast media must be injected in the knee joint.

femur

med. epicondyle

med. condyle

lat. epicondyle

intercondylar fossa

intercondylar eminence

lat. condyle

B. Special view of the intercondylar fossa and eminence.

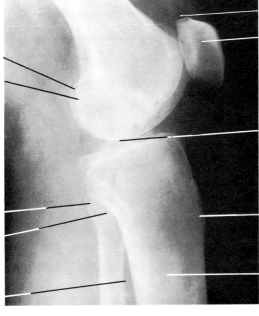

med. condyle

lat. condyle

styloid process

head of fibula

interosseous membrane

quadriceps tendon

areolar tissue

patella

intercondylar eminence

tibial tuberosity

tibia

C. Lateral view of the knee and surrounding soft tissues. (*A* to *C* from Meschan, I.: An Atlas of Anatomy Basic to Radiology. Philadelphia, W. B. Saunders Company, 1975.)

333

A. Superficial vessels and nerves of the sole of the left foot.

proper plantar digital nerves

proper digital arteries

plantar metatarsal arteries

common plantar digital nerves

med. plantar artery

superficial branch of lat. plantar nerve

med. plantar nerve

plantar aponeurosis

med. plantar eminence

lat. plantar eminence

med. calcaneal branches

superficial transverse metatarsal ligament

digital slips of plantar aponeurosis

plantar aponeurosis

plantar fascia

calcaneal tuberosity

B. Plantar aponeurosis on the sole of the left foot.

Note:

¶ There is a close resemblance between the sensory innervation of the sole of the foot and that of the palm of the hand. The lateral side of the sole and the lateral one and a half digits are supplied by the lateral plantar nerve; the medial half of the sole and the medial three and a half digits are supplied by the medial plantar nerve. In the palm of the hand the lateral one and a half fingers are supplied by the ulnar nerve, and the medial three and a half fingers by the median nerve.

¶ The central part of the plantar aponeurosis consists mainly of strong, longitudinally arranged fibers that originate from the medial process of the calcaneal tuberosity and extend with five separate slips toward the toes. The medial and lateral parts are thin and sometimes contain muscle fibers. At the junction lines between the central and the medial and lateral parts of the aponeurosis, intermuscular septa divide the musculature into three compartments. The intermuscular septa are usually incomplete. Although in the hand the three compartments are of clinical significance, in the sole of the foot they are not recognized as such.

synovial sheath for tendon
of flexor hallucis longus

synovial sheaths for
tendons of digital flexors

bursae for tendons
of lumbricals

tendons of flexor
digitorum longus

tendon of flexor
hallucis longus

flexor digitorum brevis

abductor digiti minimi

synovial sheath of tendon
of flexor hallucis longus

plantar aponeurosis (cut)

abductor hallucis

synovial sheath of tendon
of flexor digitorum longus

subcutaneous
calcaneal bursa

A. **First layer of muscles of the sole of the left foot.**
Abductor digiti minimi, flexor digitorum brevis, abductor hallucis.

cruciform part of fibrous sheath
fibrous sheath of flexor tendons
annular part of fibrous sheath
tendons of flexor digitorum brevis

lumbricals

flexor hallucis brevis

flexor hallucis longus

abductor hallucis

tendon of flexor digitorum longus

tendon of flexor hallucis longus

flexor digiti minimi brevis
abductor digiti minimi
tendon of flexor digitorum longus
quadratus plantae (flexor digitorum accessorius)

B. **Second layer of muscles of the sole of the left foot.**
Quadratus plantae and lumbricals.

calcaneal tuberosity

¶ The three muscles comprising the first layer extend from the calcaneal tuberosity to the toes. They form a functional group capable of supporting the long arches of the foot.

¶ The two muscles comprising the second muscular layer both attach to the tendons of the flexor digitorum longus. Since the quadratus plantae acts on the toes by means of the flexor digitorum longus, it is also referred to as the flexor digitorum accessorius. The four lumbricals insert on the medial aspect of the proximal digit of the four lateral toes and into the dorsal aspect of the fibrous sheaths.

335

lumbricals

tendon of flexor hallucis longus

oblique head of adductor hallucis

med. plantar nerve

flexor digiti minimi brevis

part of flexor digiti minimi brevis

deep branch of lat. plantar artery and nerve

tendon of peroneus longus

tendon of flexor digitorum longus

lat. plantar artery and nerve

post. tibial artery and med. plantar nerve

quadratus plantae

tendon of flexor hallucis longus

calcaneal tuberosity

A.   Nerves and vessels in relation to second layer of muscles in the left foot.
The abductor hallucis and the abductor digiti minimi have been removed.

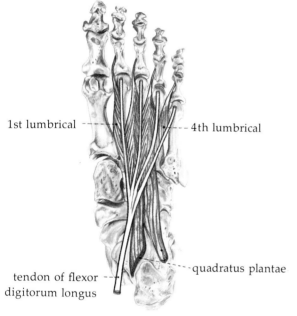

1st lumbrical

4th lumbrical

tendon of flexor
digitorum longus

quadratus plantae

**B.   Schematic drawing of the muscles of the
second layer.**

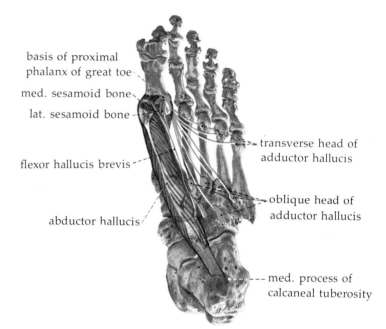

basis of proximal
phalanx of great toe

med. sesamoid bone

lat. sesamoid bone

transverse head of
adductor hallucis

flexor hallucis brevis

abductor hallucis

oblique head of
adductor hallucis

med. process of
calcaneal tuberosity

**C.   Schematic drawing of the short muscles of
the left great toe.**

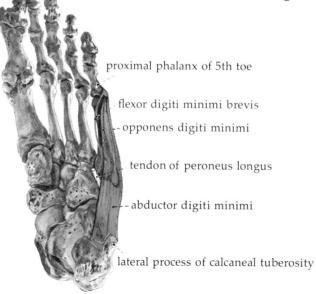

proximal phalanx of 5th toe

flexor digiti minimi brevis

opponens digiti minimi

tendon of peroneus longus

abductor digiti minimi

lateral process of calcaneal tuberosity

D.   Schematic drawing of the short muscles of the left fifth toe.

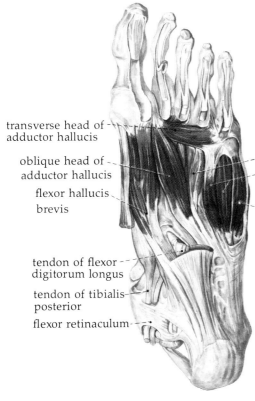

transverse head of adductor hallucis

oblique head of adductor hallucis

flexor hallucis brevis

plantar interosseus

flexor digiti minimi brevis

opponens digiti minimi

tendon of flexor digitorum longus

tendon of tibialis posterior

flexor retinaculum

A. Third layer of muscles of the sole of the left foot.
Flexor hallucis brevis, oblique and transverse heads of the adductor hallucis, flexor and opponens digiti minimi.

fibrous sheath of flexors of digits

tendons of flexors of digits

1st metatarsal

dorsal interossei (four)

plantar interossei (three)

B. Fourth layer of muscles of the sole of the left foot.
Three plantar and four dorsal interossei, tendons of the peroneus longus and tibialis posterior.

C. Schematic drawing of the left plantar and dorsal interossei.

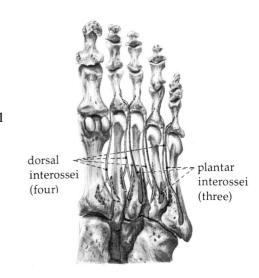

dorsal interossei (four)

plantar interossei (three)

¶ In the hand the axial line on which the interossei act passes through the third finger; in the foot it passes through the second metatarsal bone and second toe. The dorsal interossei abduct the toes from this line; the three plantar interossei adduct the lateral three toes toward the axial line.

¶ The plantar interossei are attached to the medial sides of the bases of the proximal phalanges and to the dorsal digital expansions. The dorsal interossei are attached to the bases of the proximal phalanges and the dorsal digital expansions. All seven interossei are innervated by the lateral plantar nerve (S2 and S3). (Compare with the ulnar nerve in the hand.) The first dorsal interosseus frequently receives a branch from the deep peroneal nerve.

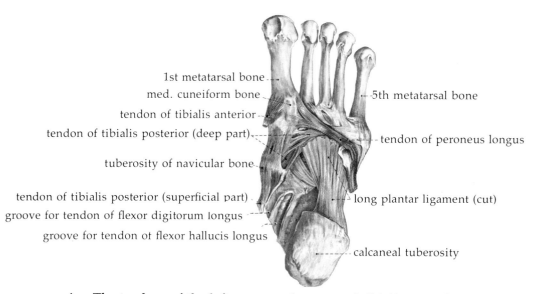

1st metatarsal bone

med. cuneiform bone

5th metatarsal bone

tendon of tibialis anterior

tendon of tibialis posterior (deep part)

tendon of peroneus longus

tuberosity of navicular bone

tendon of tibialis posterior (superficial part)

long plantar ligament (cut)

groove for tendon of flexor digitorum longus

groove for tendon ot flexor hallucis longus

calcaneal tuberosity

A.   The tendons of the left peroneus longus and tibialis posterior.
The long plantar ligament has been cut to expose the tendons.

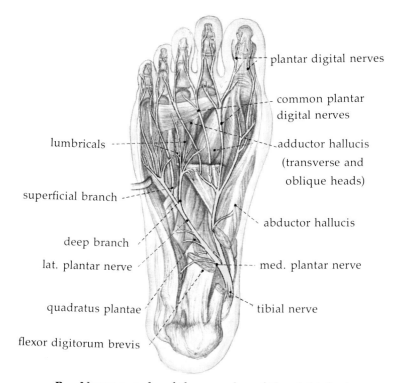

plantar digital nerves

common plantar digital nerves

lumbricals

adductor hallucis (transverse and oblique heads)

superficial branch

abductor hallucis

deep branch

lat. plantar nerve

med. plantar nerve

quadratus plantae

tibial nerve

flexor digitorum brevis

B.   Nerve supply of the muscles of the right foot.

¶   The tibialis anterior and the peroneus longus both insert on the medial aspect of the plantar surface of the foot. Together they form a tendinous sling under the foot that helps to support the transverse arch of the foot. The tendon of the tibialis posterior also helps to support the transverse arch.

¶   The distribution of the lateral plantar nerve is very similar to that of the ulnar nerve: it innervates the skin of the most lateral one and a half toes, and it supplies the abductor digiti minimi, the flexor digiti minimi brevis, the opponens digiti minimi, the quadratus plantae and, with its deep branch, the adductor hallucis, the second, third and fourth lumbricals and all the interossei.

¶   The medial plantar nerve innervates the skin of the medial three and a half toes and provides motor innervation to the flexor digitorum brevis, the abductor hallucis, the flexor hallucis brevis and the first lumbrical. Its sensory and motor supply area is very similar to that of the median nerve in the hand. The only difference is in the innervation of the second lumbrical, which in the hand is innervated by the median nerve and in the foot by the lateral plantar nerve.

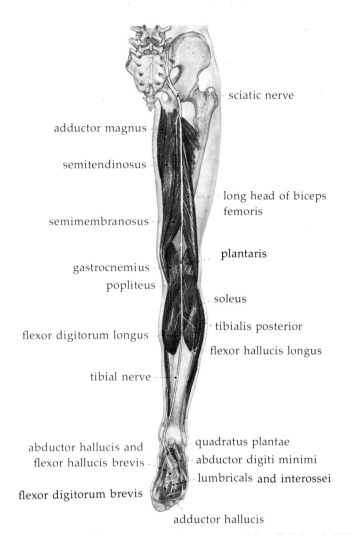

adductor magnus

semitendinosus

semimembranosus

gastrocnemius

popliteus

flexor digitorum longus

tibial nerve

abductor hallucis and
flexor hallucis brevis

flexor digitorum brevis

sciatic nerve

long head of biceps
femoris

plantaris

soleus

tibialis posterior

flexor hallucis longus

quadratus plantae

abductor digiti minimi

lumbricals and interossei

adductor hallucis

Motor innervation of the right sciatic nerve and its tibial subdivision.

The sciatic nerve and its branches may be injured at several places along its course.

¶ Intramuscular injections in the gluteal region, dislocations of the hip and fractures of the pelvis may affect the *sciatic nerve* directly after it emerges from the pelvis. Fortunately, the injuries are usually partial. When the sciatic nerve is totally severed, the loss of the hamstrings causes problems with flexion of the knee (part of that function, however, is maintained by the sartorius and the gracilis). Below the knee, however, all muscles are paralyzed, and the weight of the foot causes it to assume a plantar-flexed position (foot drop).

¶ The *common peroneal nerve* (see LL39) is most frequently injured at the place where it winds around the neck of the fibula. Injury may occur after fractures of the neck of the fibula or by pressure from casts. All the muscles of the anterior and peroneal compartments of the leg are paralyzed, as well as the muscles on the dorsal aspect of the foot. Because of the paralysis the flexors and invertors pull the foot into a plantar-flexed and inverted position (pes equinovarus).

¶ The *tibial nerve* lies in a deep and protected position and is rarely injured. When it is severed, all the muscles in the posterior compartment of the leg as well as those in the sole of the foot are paralyzed. Owing to the action of the antagonists, the foot is kept in a dorsiflexed, everted position.

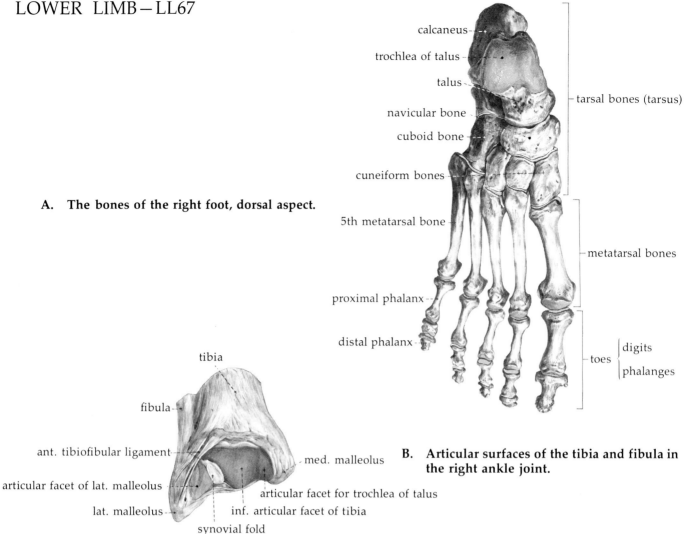

A. The bones of the right foot, dorsal aspect.

calcaneus
trochlea of talus
talus
navicular bone
cuboid bone
cuneiform bones
5th metatarsal bone
proximal phalanx
distal phalanx
tarsal bones (tarsus)
metatarsal bones
toes — digits / phalanges

tibia
fibula
ant. tibiofibular ligament
articular facet of lat. malleolus
lat. malleolus
med. malleolus
articular facet for trochlea of talus
inf. articular facet of tibia
synovial fold

B. Articular surfaces of the tibia and fibula in the right ankle joint.

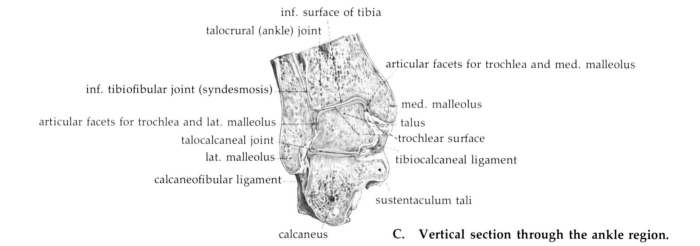

inf. surface of tibia
talocrural (ankle) joint
inf. tibiofibular joint (syndesmosis)
articular facets for trochlea and lat. malleolus
talocalcaneal joint
lat. malleolus
calcaneofibular ligament
calcaneus
articular facets for trochlea and med. malleolus
med. malleolus
talus
trochlear surface
tibiocalcaneal ligament
sustentaculum tali

C. Vertical section through the ankle region.

Note:

¶ The superior surface of the trochlea of the talus is much broader in front than behind. Hence, in dorsiflexion of the foot the front part of the trochlea will tend to force the tibial and fibular malleoli apart. In this position the trochlea becomes tightly placed between the malleoli. In plantar flexion the smaller posterior part of the trochlea moves between the malleoli, and some side to side tilting is possible.

¶ The talocrural (ankle) joint is a typical hinge joint, which is responsible for dorsiflexion and plantar flexion of the foot. To prevent abduction and adduction it is enforced by strong collateral ligaments (see LL70). The anterior and posterior aspects of the capsule must be slack, since otherwise dorsiflexion and plantar flexion would be inhibited.

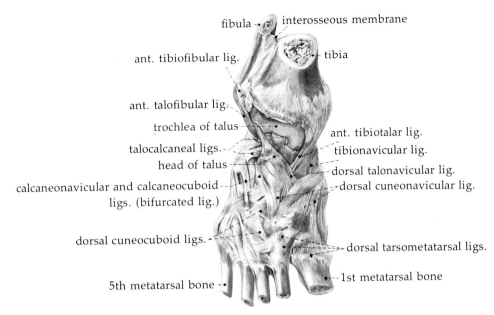

fibula · interosseous membrane
ant. tibiofibular lig.
tibia
ant. talofibular lig.
trochlea of talus
ant. tibiotalar lig.
talocalcaneal ligs.
tibionavicular lig.
head of talus
dorsal talonavicular lig.
calcaneonavicular and calcaneocuboid
ligs. (bifurcated lig.)
dorsal cuneonavicular lig.
dorsal cuneocuboid ligs.
dorsal tarsometatarsal ligs.
5th metatarsal bone
1st metatarsal bone

A. Dorsal view of the right ankle joint and joints of the foot.
The anterior part of the capsule has been removed.

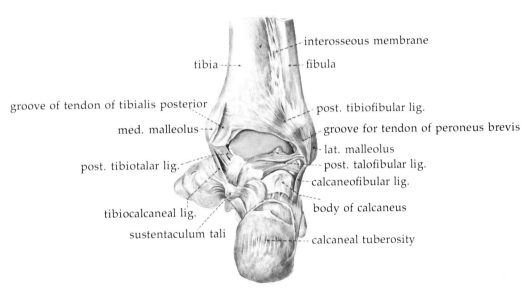

interosseous membrane
tibia
fibula
groove of tendon of tibialis posterior
post. tibiofibular lig.
med. malleolus
groove for tendon of peroneus brevis
lat. malleolus
post. tibiotalar lig.
post. talofibular lig.
calcaneofibular lig.
tibiocalcaneal lig.
body of calcaneus
sustentaculum tali
calcaneal tuberosity

B. The right ankle joint seen from the back.
The thin posterior part of the capsule has been removed.

¶ The anterior part of the capsule of the ankle joint is slack and permits considerable movement for plantar flexion. It is not strengthened by ligamentous structures. When fluid collects in the joint, as in sprains or fracture–dislocations, the anterior part bulges more than any other part of the capsule.

¶ Similarly, the posterior part of the capsule is weak and permits dorsiflexion (toes pointing upward) to a considerable degree. Dorsiflexion, however, is far more restricted than plantar flexion owing to the fact that in dorsiflexion the anterior, broader part of the talus is tightly wedged between the tibia and the fibula.

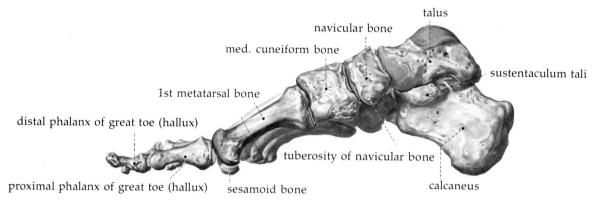

A. Medial view of the bones of the right foot.

talus

navicular bone

med. cuneiform bone

sustentaculum tali

1st metatarsal bone

distal phalanx of great toe (hallux)

tuberosity of navicular bone

proximal phalanx of great toe (hallux) sesamoid bone

calcaneus

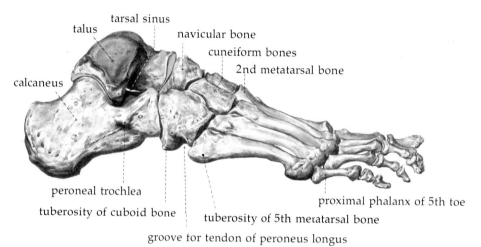

tarsal sinus

talus

navicular bone

cuneiform bones

2nd metatarsal bone

calcaneus

peroneal trochlea

proximal phalanx of 5th toe

tuberosity of cuboid bone

tuberosity of 5th metatarsal bone

groove for tendon of peroneus longus

B. Lateral view of the bones of the right foot.

In studying the skeleton of the foot, keep in mind:

❡ The various bones of the foot act together as a weight-bearing structure and are there-fore arranged in the form of arches. In the adult foot three arches can be recognized: (a) the medial longitudinal arch; (b) the lateral longitudinal arch; and (c) the transverse arch. In a normal standing person the heel, the lateral margin of the foot, the metatarsal heads and the distal phalanges are in contact with the ground. The medial arch from the calcaneus to the head of the first metatarsal is high above the ground.

❡ The medial longitudinal arch, formed by the calcaneus, talus, navicular, three cunei-forms and the three medial metatarsal bones, is partially maintained by the shape of the bones. The rounded head of the talus forms the keystone in the center of the arch. The lateral longitudinal arch, formed by the calcaneus and cuboid and the lateral two metatarsal bones, is considerably lower than the medial arch. The cuboid forms the keystone of the arch.

❡ The wedge shape of some of the bones (talus, navicular and cuboid) plays an important role in maintaining the longitudinal arches. In addition, however, several strong liga-ments support the arches (see LL74).

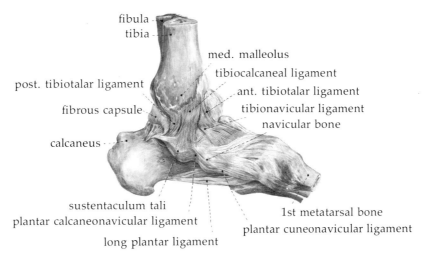

A. Medial view of the ligaments of the ankle joint of the left foot.

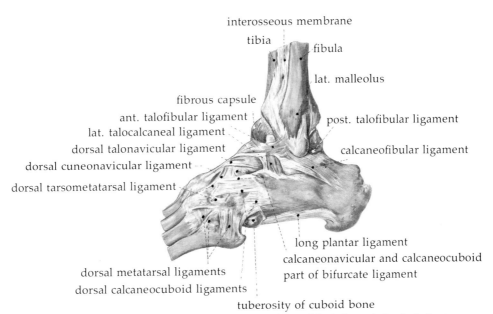

B. Lateral view of the ligaments of the ankle joint of the left foot.

The collateral ligaments of the ankle joint prevent abduction and adduction of the foot, but more importantly they serve to stabilize the body when the feet are fixed. The deltoid (medial collateral) ligament has four parts: (a) the *anterior tibiotalar ligament*, which passes from the tibia to the talus; (b) the *tibionavicular ligament*, which passes from the tibia to the navicular bone; (c) the very strong *tibiocalcaneal ligament*, which is attached to the sustentaculum tali of the calcaneus; and (d) the *posterior tibiotalar ligament*.

The lateral collateral ligament is not as strong as the deltoid ligament and consists of the anterior and posterior talofibular ligaments and the calcaneofibular ligament.

The ligaments of the ankle are of great importance:

¶ The ankle may easily be sprained by excessive inversion of the foot. The anterior talofibular ligament and the calcaneofibular ligament are then injured or torn, resulting in swelling and pain of the joint. Ruptures of the deltoid components following excessive eversion are less frequent. Sometimes the ligament will tear off the tip of the medial malleolus before rupturing itself.

¶ When excessive eversion of the ankle occurs, with or without rotation, dislocations and fractures result. When the talus is externally rotated in an everted position, it is pushed against the lateral malleolus, and the malleolus may fracture. At the same time, the deltoid ligament may become so taut that the tip of the medial malleolus is pulled off.

343

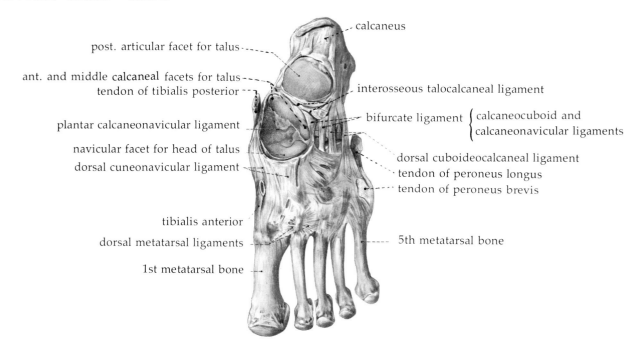

post. articular facet for talus

ant. and middle calcaneal facets for talus
tendon of tibialis posterior

plantar calcaneonavicular ligament

navicular facet for head of talus
dorsal cuneonavicular ligament

tibialis anterior
dorsal metatarsal ligaments

1st metatarsal bone

calcaneus

interosseous talocalcaneal ligament

bifurcate ligament { calcaneocuboid and
calcaneonavicular ligaments

dorsal cuboideocalcaneal ligament
tendon of peroneus longus
tendon of peroneus brevis

5th metatarsal bone

A. The left posterior talocalcaneal and talocalcaneonavicular joints. The talus has been removed.

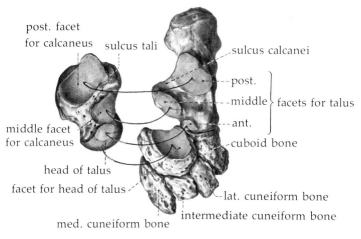

post. facet
for calcaneus   sulcus tali

middle facet
for calcaneus

head of talus
facet for head of talus

med. cuneiform bone

sulcus calcanei

post.
middle } facets for talus
ant.

cuboid bone

lat. cuneiform bone
intermediate cuneiform bone

B. Surfaces of bony contact between the left talus and the calcaneus and navicular.

Inversion and eversion of the foot are produced by movement of the talus in both the posterior talocalcaneal and the talocalcaneonavicular joints. Either movement always involves both joints, and the two are, therefore, sometimes referred to as the *infratalar joint*.

Note:

¶ The posterior talocalcaneal joint is separated from the talocalcaneonavicular joint by the interosseous talocalcaneal ligament. This ligament is very strong and is the main band between the talus and calcaneus. It is attached in the sulcus calcanei.

¶ The space between the navicular bone and the midtalar facet of the sustentaculum is bridged by the *plantar calcaneonavicular ligament* (spring ligament). This ligament forms part of the socket for the head of the talus and is covered with fibrous cartilage.

¶ The head of the talus forms the important keystone of the medial longitudinal arch. The body weight transmitted through the head of the talus presses the talus deep into its socket, pushing the calcaneus and navicular bones apart. Hence, the important function of the plantar calcaneonavicular ligament is to tie the two bones together. If the ligament weakens, the medial arch of the foot will collapse, resulting in a flat foot.

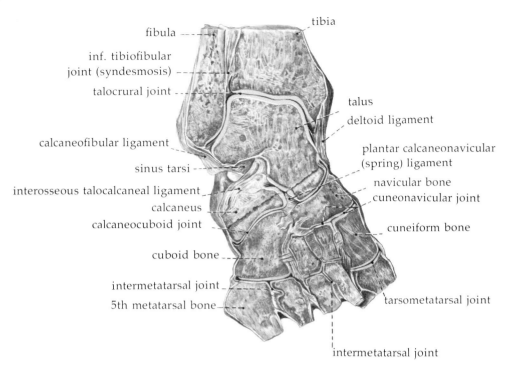

A. Section through the intertarsal and tarsometatarsal joints.

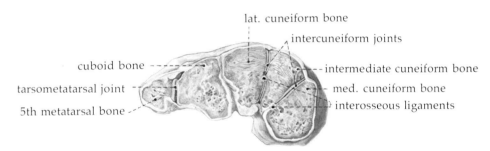

B. Transverse section through the distal row of tarsal bones.

Note:

¶ The intertarsal joint is formed by two separate joints: the calcaneocuboid joint and the talonavicular joint. The two joints combined permit some dorsal and plantar flexion of the anterior part of the foot with respect to the posterior part.

¶ The tarsometatarsal joints also form a transverse joint line across the foot. The cuboid articulates with the head of the two lateral metatarsal bones; the cuneiform bones each articulate with a metatarsal bone.

¶ The two transverse joint lines are used in amputations of the foot. Depending on the level of the amputation, the cut is made through the tarsometatarsal joints or through the intertarsal joints.

¶ The transverse arch of the foot consists of the cuboid, the three cuneiform bones and the bases of the metatarsal bones. This arch is maintained not only by the marked wedge shape of the cuneiform bones but also by deep transverse ligaments. In addition, the tendon of the peroneus longus ties the ends of the arch together (LL65 *A*).

345

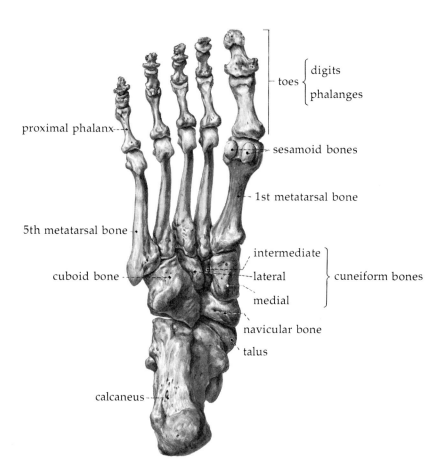

proximal phalanx

toes { digits
phalanges }

sesamoid bones

1st metatarsal bone

5th metatarsal bone

intermediate
lateral
medial } cuneiform bones

cuboid bone

navicular bone

talus

calcaneus

The bones of the right foot seen from the plantar side.

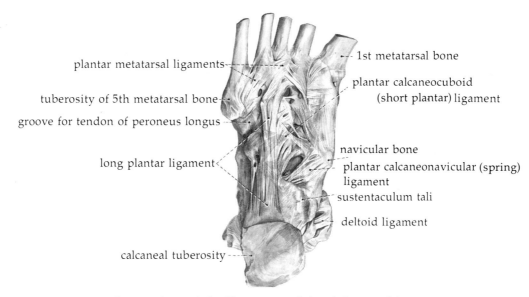

plantar metatarsal ligaments

1st metatarsal bone

plantar calcaneocuboid
(short plantar) ligament

tuberosity of 5th metatarsal bone

groove for tendon of peroneus longus

navicular bone

plantar calcaneonavicular (spring)
ligament

long plantar ligament

sustentaculum tali

deltoid ligament

calcaneal tuberosity

Plantar view of the ligaments of the right tarsal bones.

Although the longitudinal arches are maintained by the shape of the bones of the foot, the ligaments also play an important role.

¶ The *plantar aponeurosis* extends from the medial and lateral tubercles of the calcaneus to the fibrous flexor sheaths of the toes and the deep transverse ligaments (see LL61 *B*).

¶ The *long plantar ligament* is attached to the undersurface of the calcaneus and extends to the cuboid and the bases of the three lateral metatarsal bones. It bridges the tendon of the peroneus longus (see LL65 *A*).

¶ The *short plantar ligament* is attached to the anterior tubercle of the calcaneus and extends to the adjoining part of the cuboid bone (*plantar calcaneocuboid ligament*).

¶ The *plantar calcaneonavicular ligament*, which is probably the most important and strongest of the group, extends from the anterior margin of the sustentaculum tali to the inferior surface and tuberosity of the navicular bone (see LL71 *A*). If this ligament becomes slack, the head of the talus moves down between the calcaneus and navicular bone, resulting in a flat foot.

347

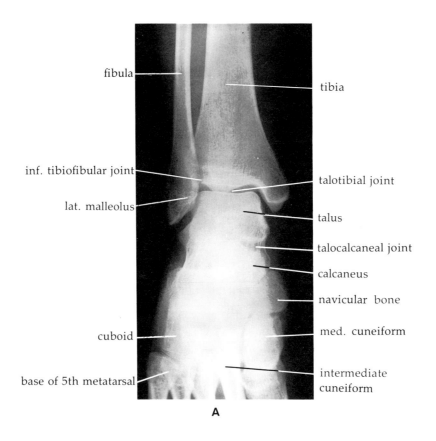

fibula

tibia

inf. tibiofibular joint

talotibial joint

lat. malleolus

talus

talocalcaneal joint

calcaneus

navicular bone

cuboid

med. cuneiform

base of 5th metatarsal

intermediate cuneiform

A

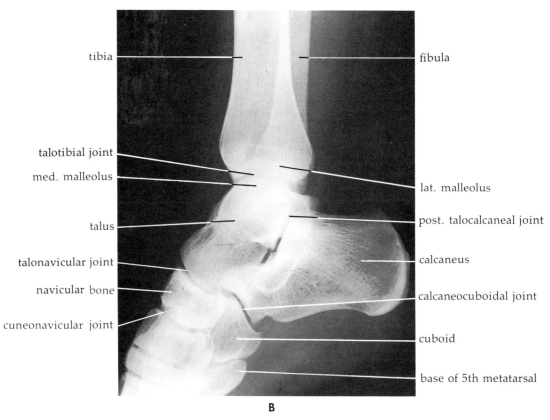

tibia

fibula

talotibial joint

med. malleolus

lat. malleolus

talus

post. talocalcaneal joint

talonavicular joint

calcaneus

navicular bone

calcaneocuboidal joint

cuneonavicular joint

cuboid

base of 5th metatarsal

B

A. **Anteroposterior view of the right ankle.**

B. **Lateral view of the right ankle.**
   (*A* and *B* from Meschan, I.: An Atlas of Anatomy Basic to Radiology. Philadelphia, W. B. Saunders Company, 1975.)

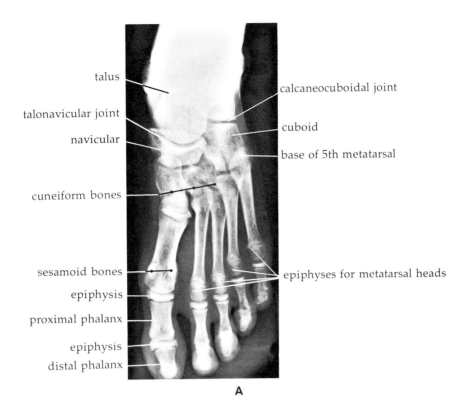

talus
talonavicular joint
navicular
cuneiform bones
sesamoid bones
epiphysis
proximal phalanx
epiphysis
distal phalanx

calcaneocuboidal joint
cuboid
base of 5th metatarsal
epiphyses for metatarsal heads

A

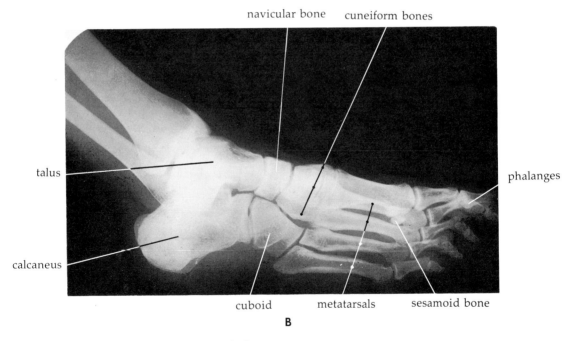

navicular bone   cuneiform bones

talus

phalanges

calcaneus

cuboid   metatarsals   sesamoid bone

B

A. **Anteroposterior view of the left foot.**
   In younger people the epiphyses have not yet united with the shafts of the metatarsals and phalanges. Differentiation from fracture lines may therebefore be difficult.

B. **Lateral view of the left foot.** (*A* and *B* from Meschan, I.: An Atlas of Anatomy Basic to Radiology. Philadelphia, W. B. Saunders Company, 1975.)

HEAD
AND NECK

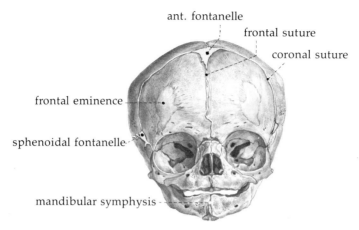

A. Skull of newborn; anterior aspect (norma frontalis).

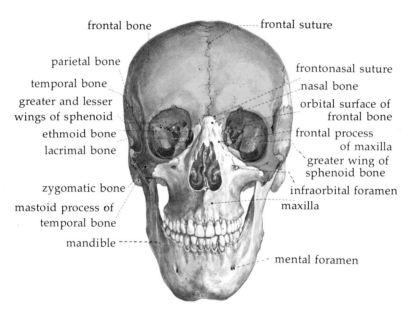

B. Skull of adult; anterior aspect (norma frontalis).

When studying and comparing the bony skull of an adult with that of a newborn or young child, keep in mind:

¶ In young children the flat bones of the skull are separated from each other by narrow seams of connective tissue, the *sutures*. When more than two bones meet, the sutures are wide and triangular and are known as *fontanelles*. In adults some of the sutures disappear completely, while others remain as immobile joints with interlocking, serrated edges.

¶ The viscerocranium (skeleton of the face) is mainly derived from the bony and cartilaginous components of the first two pharyngeal arches. It is small at birth due to the absence of teeth, the small size of the jaws (maxilla and mandible) and the absence of the paranasal air sinuses. Hence, most of the growth of the skull in the postnatal period and in puberty occurs in the bones of the face.

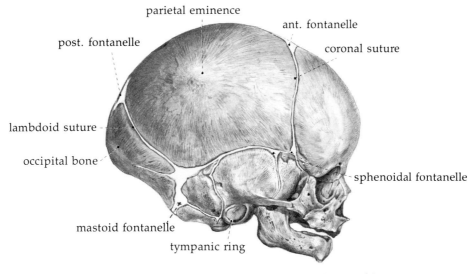

A. Lateral aspect of the fetal skull (8th month).

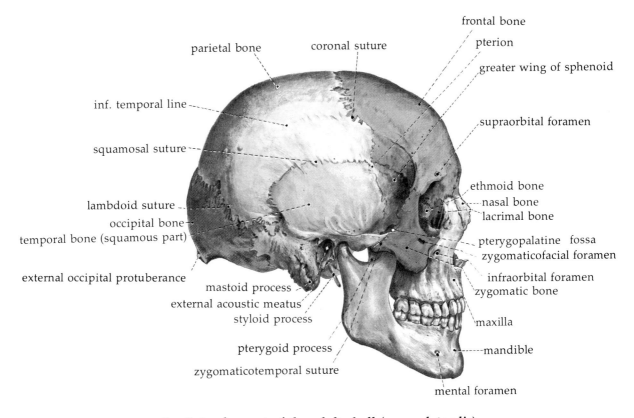

B. Lateral aspect of the adult skull (norma lateralis).

¶ The skull of the infant is characterized by the anterior fontanelle between the frontal and parietal bones and the posterior fontanelle between the occipital and parietal bones. In addition, it has a sphenoidal and a mastoid fontanelle on each lateral side.

¶ The thinnest part of the adult skull is found where the anteroinferior corner of the parietal bone comes in contact with the greater wing of the sphenoid. In the newborn this region is known as the sphenoidal fontanelle; in the adult it is referred to as the pterion (HN21). Clinically, the pterion is an important reference point because it overlies the anterior branch of the middle meningeal artery (see HN21 and HN22 *A*). A blow on the head in the region of the pterion frequently results in a fracture of the skull and a rupture of the artery.

¶ The mastoid process, so characteristic in the adult skull, is virtually absent in the newborn infant. For this reason, the facial nerve runs close to the surface as it emerges from the stylomastoid foramen and may easily be damaged in a difficult forceps delivery.

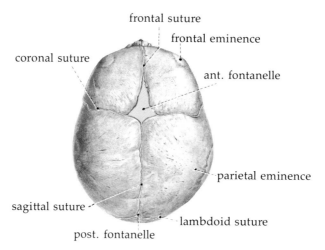

frontal suture

frontal eminence

coronal suture

ant. fontanelle

parietal eminence

sagittal suture

lambdoid suture

post. fontanelle

A. Skull of the newborn (superior aspect).

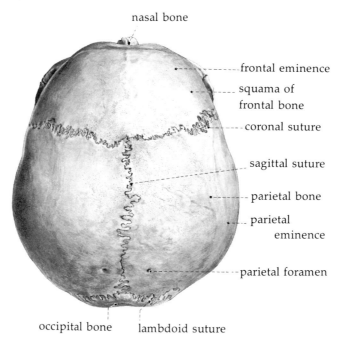

nasal bone

frontal eminence

squama of
frontal bone

coronal suture

sagittal suture

parietal bone

parietal
eminence

parietal foramen

occipital bone   lambdoid suture

B. Skull of the adult, superior aspect (norma verticalis).
Note the serrated sutures.

When comparing the superior aspect of the skull of the newborn with that of an adult, remember:

¶ The sutures and fontanelles of the newborn skull allow the bones to overlap during the birth process. Most of the fontanelles close during the first postnatal year, but the anterior fontanelle remains open at least until the eighteenth month after birth.

¶ Palpation of the fontanelles in babies is important to determine whether growth of the bones is proceeding at a normal rate. In some cases the sutures and fontanelles close prematurely (craniosynostosis), which results in an abnormal skull. Palpation of the fontanelles may also provide information about intracranial pressure and dehydration. Increased intracranial pressure causes the fontanelles to bulge; when the fontanelles are depressed below the surface, the child is usually dehydrated.

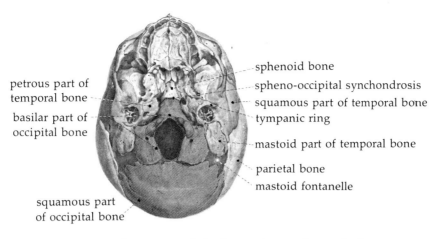

petrous part of
temporal bone

basilar part of
occipital bone

sphenoid bone

spheno-occipital synchondrosis

squamous part of temporal bone

tympanic ring

mastoid part of temporal bone

parietal bone

mastoid fontanelle

squamous part
of occipital bone

A. Exterior aspect of the base of a newborn skull.

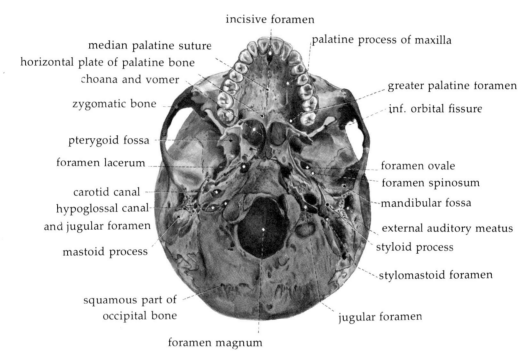

incisive foramen

median palatine suture

horizontal plate of palatine bone

choana and vomer

zygomatic bone

pterygoid fossa

foramen lacerum

carotid canal

hypoglossal canal
and jugular foramen

mastoid process

squamous part of
occipital bone

palatine process of maxilla

greater palatine foramen

inf. orbital fissure

foramen ovale

foramen spinosum

mandibular fossa

external auditory meatus

styloid process

stylomastoid foramen

jugular foramen

foramen magnum

B. Exterior aspect of the base of an adult skull (norma basalis).
See also HN104.

When comparing the exterior aspect of the base of the skull in a newborn with that in an adult, some striking differences are apparent:

¶ In the adult skull the basilar and squamous portions of the occipital bone are completely fused. In the newborn, however, the basilar part surrounding the foramen magnum is separated from the squamous part by a suture line. Similarly, the petrous and squamous portions of the temporal bone are fused in the adult but separated from each other in the newborn. This explains why parts of some bones are characterized by membranous ossification, while other parts exhibit endochondral ossification.

¶ The mastoid process in the newborn skull is absent. It develops during childhood in response to the pull of the muscles (mainly the sternocleidomastoid) attached to this part of the temporal bone.

¶ In the newborn the tympanic membrane (eardrum) lies close to the surface, and the tympanic part of the temporal bone forms a flat C-shaped ring. During childhood the tympanic ring grows laterally, forming the bony part of the external auditory meatus.

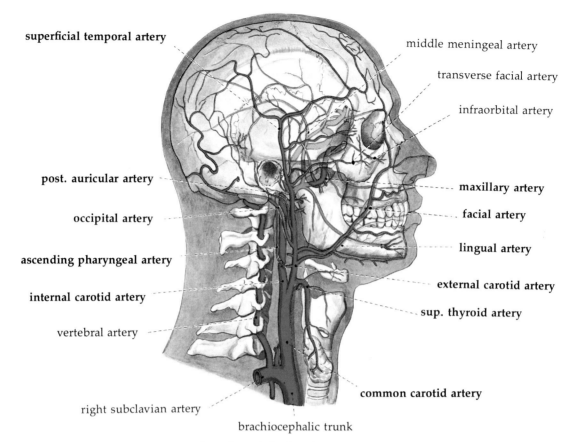

Arteries of the head and neck.

The common carotid arteries are the main arteries supplying the head and neck. They ascend in the neck and split at the level of C4 into the external and internal carotid arteries. The common carotid and internal carotid arteries do not have any branches in the neck and face. The external carotid provides the main arterial supply for the neck and face; the internal carotid artery supplies the brain. Details of the arterial supply will be shown in the following figures of each specific area, but the general pattern of the branches of the external carotid artery should be remembered:

◖ *Anterior branches* (three in number)

1. The superior thyroid artery supplies the structures in the neck (hyoid bone, larynx and thyroid gland)

2. The lingual artery supplies the tongue

3. The facial artery supplies the superficial tissues of the face. It loops over the mandible where its pulsations can be felt. Subsequently, it ascends obliquely over the face to the angle between the nose and eye.

◖ *Posterior branches* (three in number)

1. The ascending pharyngeal artery

2. The occipital artery

3. The posterior auricular artery.

◖ *Terminal branches* (two in number)

1. The maxillary artery supplies the upper and lower jaws, the muscles of mastication, the nasal cavity and the paranasal sinuses.

2. The superficial temporal artery supplies the scalp. Its pulsations can be felt over the zygomatic process.

356

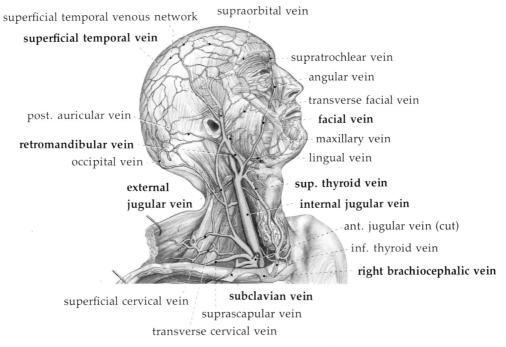

superficial temporal venous network
supraorbital vein
superficial temporal vein
supratrochlear vein
angular vein
transverse facial vein
post. auricular vein
facial vein
maxillary vein
retromandibular vein
lingual vein
occipital vein
sup. thyroid vein
external jugular vein
internal jugular vein
ant. jugular vein (cut)
inf. thyroid vein
right brachiocephalic vein
superficial cervical vein
subclavian vein
suprascapular vein
transverse cervical vein

A. The veins of the right side of the head and neck.
The platysma and part of the sternocleidomastoid have been removed.

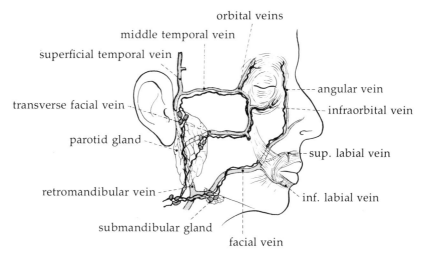

orbital veins
middle temporal vein
superficial temporal vein
angular vein
transverse facial vein
infraorbital vein
parotid gland
sup. labial vein
retromandibular vein
inf. labial vein
submandibular gland
facial vein

B. Superficial veins and lymph vessels of the face.
For lymph vessels, see also HN72.

The internal jugular vein forms the main venous drainage channel for the head and neck. It leaves the skull through the jugular foramen and drains the brain. Unlike the internal carotid artery which supplies blood to the brain, the internal jugular vein also receives blood from the face and neck (the supply area of the external carotid artery) through the following venous channels:

◦ The superficial veins of the scalp (superficial temporal veins) and those of the face (the facial and transverse facial veins) unite to enter the internal jugular vein through the retromandibular vein.

◦ The deep vein of the face (maxillary vein), which drains the mandible, maxilla and nasal region, joins the temporal vein in the substance of the parotid gland and also enters the internal jugular vein through the retromandibular vein (see also HN24).

◦ The external jugular vein runs superficially and can be clearly seen in the neck. It receives blood from the posterior parts of the scalp and neck. The vein originates from the retromandibular vein and empties into the right subclavian vein, thus forming a bypass to the internal jugular vein.

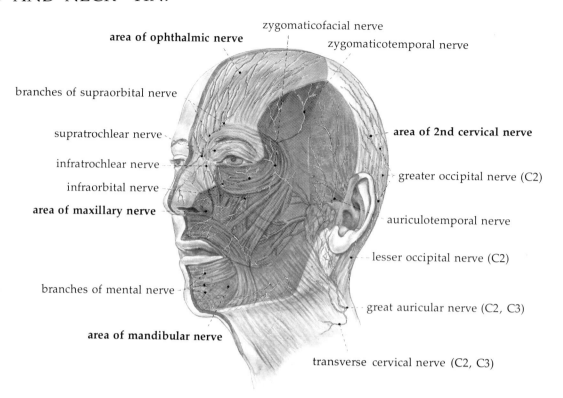

zygomaticofacial nerve

area of ophthalmic nerve

zygomaticotemporal nerve

branches of supraorbital nerve

supratrochlear nerve

infratrochlear nerve

infraorbital nerve

area of maxillary nerve

branches of mental nerve

area of mandibular nerve

area of 2nd cervical nerve

greater occipital nerve (C2)

auriculotemporal nerve

lesser occipital nerve (C2)

great auricular nerve (C2, C3)

transverse cervical nerve (C2, C3)

Trigeminal nerve—sensory innervation of the head.
Note the specific branches of the trigeminal divisions.

The three divisions of the trigeminal nerve supply the anterior and lateral aspects of the face and head; the nerves of C2 and C3 supply mainly the posterior side of the head. When examining the face to determine whether the trigeminal nerve is intact, it is important to know:

¶ The ophthalmic nerve innervates the skin of the tip and bridge of the nose, the forehead to the top of the vault, the upper eyelid and the medial angle of the eye. Most important, it also innervates the cornea. When the cornea has lost its sensory innervation, dust and other particles will not be noticed and inflammations and ulcerations of the cornea may occur. Ulceration of the cornea frequently results in blindness.

¶ The maxillary nerve innervates the skin of the upper lip, the lateral aspect of the nose, the lower eyelid and its conjunctival sac, the cheek and part of the temporal region. However, it also sends branches to the inside of the mouth, the teeth of the upper jaw and the paranasal air sinuses.

¶ The mandibular nerve innervates the lower lip, the skin over the lower jaw (except its angle) and part of the temporal region. It also supplies part of the external auditory meatus and the outside surface of the tympanic membrane. Similarly, the nerve carries sensory branches to the inside of the mouth, the tongue and the teeth of the lower jaw. (Keep in mind that the mandibular nerve is the only division of the trigeminal nerve with a motor component (see HN85).

¶ When a lesion affects one of the branches of the trigeminal nerve, the sensory loss is well defined. Unlike the sensory components of the spinal nerves, which overlap each other considerably, overlapping of the trigeminal divisions is minimal. (For details of the spinal nerves of C2 and C3, see HN20 *A* and HN69).

¶ A most common disease of the trigeminal nerve is trigeminal neuralgia. The patient experiences spontaneous, excruciating pain in the area innervated by the mandibular or maxillary nerve. The ophthalmic nerve is usually not involved. The pain may involve the skin of the face as well as the teeth, paranasal and nasal cavities or eardrum. Pain is frequently referred from one area to another, and pain originating in the tongue (lingual nerve) may be referred to the ear (auriculotemporal nerve) (see HN90).

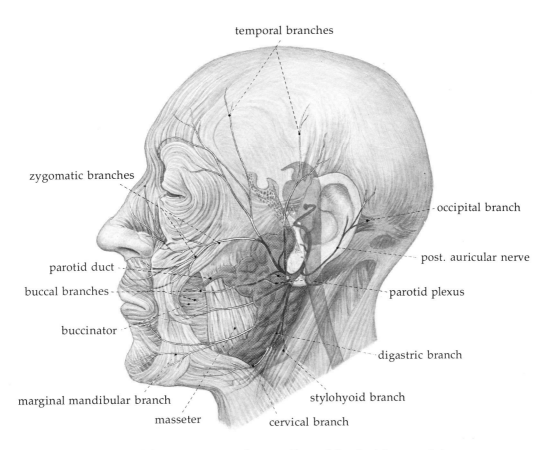

temporal branches

zygomatic branches

occipital branch

post. auricular nerve

parotid duct

buccal branches

parotid plexus

buccinator

digastric branch

marginal mandibular branch

stylohyoid branch

masseter

cervical branch

Facial nerve—motor innervation of the facial musculature.
The shaded area outlines the brain stem.

The facial or seventh cranial nerve emerges from the skull through the stylomastoid foramen. The main branches course forward through the parotid gland. Originally the gland covers only the lateral surface of the nerve, but with further development the glandular tissue extends between the branches of the nerve in a medial direction, surrounding them completely. This fact is important in surgical procedures on the parotid gland (see HN13). Keep in mind:

¶ The facial nerve is the nerve of the second pharyngeal arch, and therefore it innervates all the muscles derived from this arch. Since the muscles have migrated a considerable distance, the nerve branches are distributed over a large area that reaches from the auricularis posterior behind the ear to the platysma in the neck. According to the distribution area, five main branches are recognized: (a) temporal branches; (b) zygomatic branches; (c) buccal branches; (d) mandibular branches; and (e) cervical branch.

¶ The motor branches to the stylohyoid and posterior belly of the digastric as well as those to the auricularis posterior and occipital part of the occipitofrontalis arise from the main nerve stem *before* it enters the parotid gland.

The effects of lesions of the facial nerve are discussed with the facial musculature (see HN10).

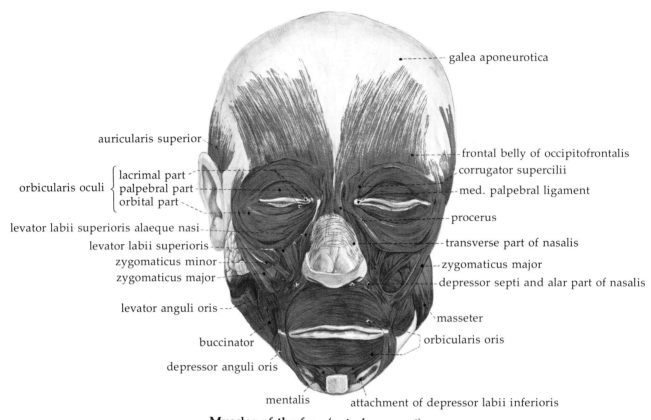

galea aponeurotica

auricularis superior

frontal belly of occipitofrontalis

corrugator supercilii

lacrimal part

orbicularis oculi { palpebral part

orbital part

med. palpebral ligament

procerus

levator labii superioris alaeque nasi

transverse part of nasalis

levator labii superioris

zygomaticus minor

zygomaticus major

zygomaticus major

depressor septi and alar part of nasalis

levator anguli oris

masseter

buccinator

orbicularis oris

depressor anguli oris

mentalis

attachment of depressor labii inferioris

Muscles of the face (anterior aspect).

¶ The muscles of the face are embedded in the superficial fascia and insert into the skin. Their main function is to guard the orifices of the mouth and orbit, where they form sphincters and dilators. An equally important function is to translate thoughts and emotions into facial expressions.

¶ The facial muscles are grouped into: (a) those of the scalp (occipitofrontalis); (b) those of the ear (auricularis anterior, posterior, and superior); (c) those of the eye (orbicularis oculi with its lacrimal, palpebral and orbital parts and the corrugator supercilii); (d) those of the nose (procerus and nasalis with its alar and transverse parts); (e) those of the mouth and lips (the orbicularis oris acts as a sphincter; several muscles act as dilators: the levator labii superioris and levator of the nasal ala, zygomaticus major and minor, levator anguli oris and risorius; pulling down the lower lip are the depressor anguli oris, depressor labii inferioris and mentalis); (f) the muscle of the cheek (buccinator); and (g) the muscle of the neck (platysma).

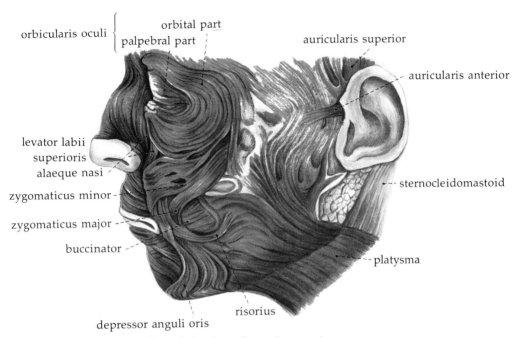

orbicularis oculi {
orbital part
palpebral part

auricularis superior

auricularis anterior

levator labii
superioris
alaeque nasi

zygomaticus minor

zygomaticus major

buccinator

sternocleidomastoid

platysma

risorius

depressor anguli oris

Muscles of the face (lateral aspect).

The muscles of the face, particularly those around the eye and mouth, are of considerable clinical importance, since they are frequently paralyzed.

¶ Paralysis of the facial musculature, involving all or part of the musculature, may occur after operations on or infections of the middle ear (see HN63); in patients with cancers of the parotid gland (see HN13); after cuts on the face; and in the newborn after a difficult forceps delivery.

¶ When the facial nerve is injured after it has emerged from the skull through the stylomastoid foramen, the following symptoms may be expected:

1. On the affected side the eye cannot be tightly closed (owing to loss of function of orbicularis oculi), and the lower eyelid will droop (not the upper eyelid, which receives its motor innervation from the oculomotor nerve). As the eye cannot be closed, there is a risk that the cornea will dry out, resulting in corneal ulceration.

2. On the affected side the angle of the mouth will droop, and saliva will flow from the drooping corner. The patient is unable to show the teeth on the affected side. In addition, he is unable to whistle and will have difficulty in pronouncing labial sounds.

3. Normally, the buccinator presses the cheeks and lips against the teeth, thereby preventing food from accumulating in the oral vestibule. When this muscle is paralyzed, the affected cheek will sag and food will accumulate in the vestibule.

361

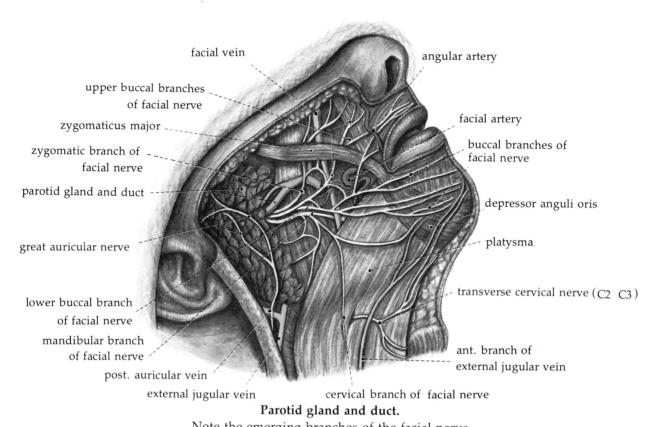

facial vein

angular artery

upper buccal branches
of facial nerve

zygomaticus major

facial artery

zygomatic branch of
facial nerve

buccal branches of
facial nerve

parotid gland and duct

depressor anguli oris

great auricular nerve

platysma

transverse cervical nerve (C2 C3)

lower buccal branch
of facial nerve

mandibular branch
of facial nerve

ant. branch of
external jugular vein

post. auricular vein

external jugular vein

cervical branch of facial nerve

Parotid gland and duct.
Note the emerging branches of the facial nerve.

Note:

⁋ The parotid gland is situated in front and below the external auditory meatus and fills the deep hollow between the ramus of the mandible anteriorly and the sternocleido-mastoid posteriorly (see also HN13). The anterior part of the gland may extend super-ficially onto the masseter.

⁋ The parotid duct passes over the masseter, pierces the buccinator and opens into the vestibule of the mouth opposite the upper first molar tooth (see HN12 *B*). The bucci-nator acts as a valve for the duct, preventing air from entering the duct system during heavy blowing (as in playing a trumpet).

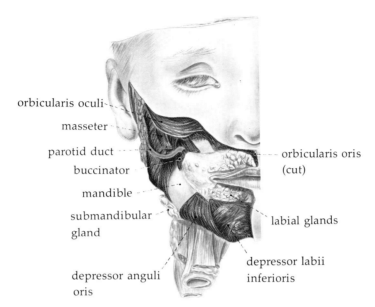

orbicularis oculi

masseter

parotid duct

buccinator

mandible

submandibular
gland

depressor anguli
oris

orbicularis oris
(cut)

labial glands

depressor labii
inferioris

A. Relation of parotid duct to masseter and buccinator (right half of face).

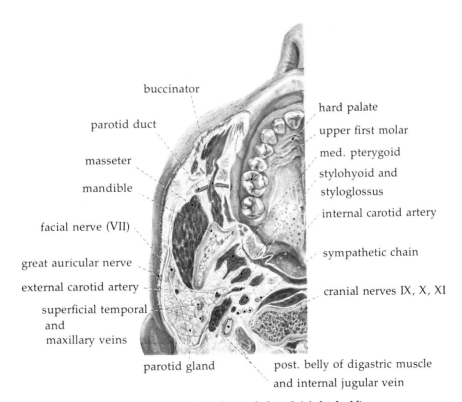

buccinator

parotid duct

masseter

mandible

facial nerve (VII)

great auricular nerve

external carotid artery

superficial temporal
and
maxillary veins

hard palate

upper first molar

med. pterygoid

stylohyoid and
styloglossus

internal carotid artery

sympathetic chain

cranial nerves IX, X, XI

parotid gland

post. belly of digastric muscle
and internal jugular vein

B. Transverse section through head (right half).
Note the relationship of the parotid gland to the surrounding structures.

A. Facial nerve and vessels after removal of the right parotid gland.

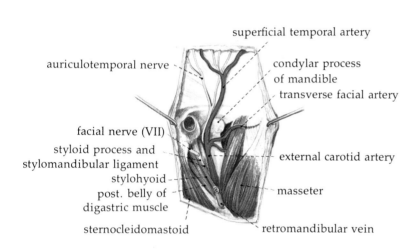

superficial temporal artery and vein

temporal nerves

zygomatic nerves

transverse facial artery and vein

maxillary artery and vein

retromandibular vein

post. belly of digastric muscle

buccal nerves

facial vein

stylomandibular ligament

internal jugular vein

marginal mandibular nerve

external carotid artery

facial artery

superficial temporal artery

auriculotemporal nerve

condylar process of mandible

transverse facial artery

facial nerve (VII)

styloid process and stylomandibular ligament

stylohyoid

post. belly of digastric muscle

external carotid artery

masseter

sternocleidomastoid

retromandibular vein

B. Right external carotid artery and its branches (see also HN76 B). Note the emergence of the facial nerve through the stylomastoid foramen.

Benign and malignant tumors of the parotid gland are relatively common. These malignant tumors are invasive and frequently involve one or more branches of the facial nerve. When the tumor is removed, the surgeon must keep in mind:

¶ (a) The sensory branches of the great auricular nerve pass superficial to the gland (see HN11); (b) the five main branches of the facial nerve (see HN8) pass through the gland; (c) the retromandibular vein is formed in the deeper portion of the gland by the superficial temporal and maxillary veins; (d) the external carotid artery in the deeper part of the gland divides into the superficial temporal and maxillary arteries (see also HN76 B and HN85 B).

¶ The posterior belly of the digastric, the stylohyoid, the auricularis posterior and the occipital belly of the occipitofrontalis receive their branches from the facial nerve before it enters the parotid gland (see also HN8).

¶ Inflammations of the parotid gland are common and are most frequently caused by mumps. Infections of the mouth, however, may also enter the glandular tissue through the parotid duct. Swelling of the gland is usually painful, since the surrounding deep cervical fascia is rather tight (see HN81).

¶ The auriculotemporal nerve, a branch of the mandibular division of the trigeminal nerve, carries postganglionic parasympathetic secretomotor fibers to the parotid gland (see HN91).

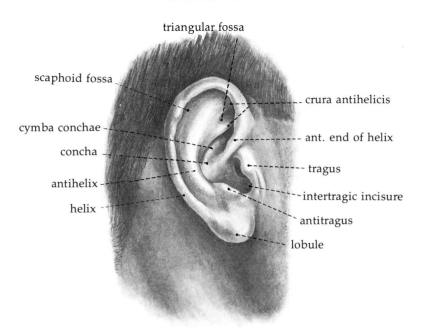

A. Lateral view of the right external ear.

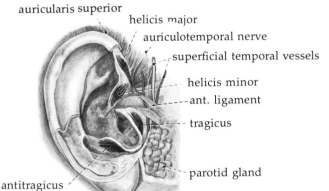

B. Intrinsic muscles of the external ear.

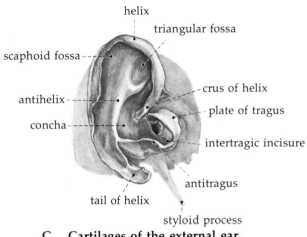

C. Cartilages of the external ear.

Note the following points:

¶ The external ear (auricle) consists of elastic fibrocartilage covered by skin. The lobule contains mainly connective and fatty tissue and can therefore be easily pierced. It is sometimes used to obtain blood for a blood count.

¶ The muscles of the ear are divided into the extrinsic muscles (auricularis anterior, superior and posterior) and four small intrinsic muscles. Although in most mammals the ears can be moved, in humans this musculature is insignificant, and only a few people are able to move the ears to a small extent.

¶ The auricular cartilages that give shape to the external ear are attached to the temporal bone. These attachments are strengthened by the anterior and posterior auricular ligaments.

¶ Note the relation of the parotid gland to the ear. In swellings of the gland the lobule of the ear is frequently pushed laterally. The superficial temporal artery and vein and the auriculotemporal nerve pass just in front of the external auditory meatus.

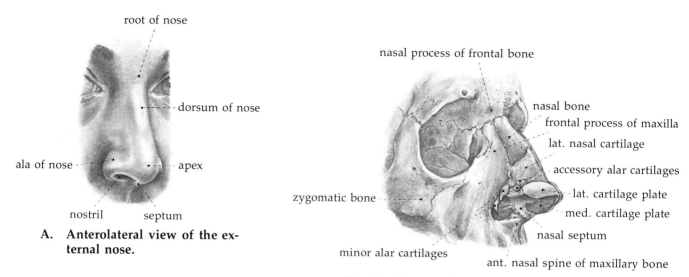

root of nose

dorsum of nose

ala of nose

apex

nostril   septum

A. Anterolateral view of the external nose.

nasal process of frontal bone

nasal bone
frontal process of maxilla
lat. nasal cartilage
accessory alar cartilages
lat. cartilage plate
med. cartilage plate

zygomatic bone

nasal septum

minor alar cartilages

ant. nasal spine of maxillary bone

B. Cartilages and bones of the external nose.

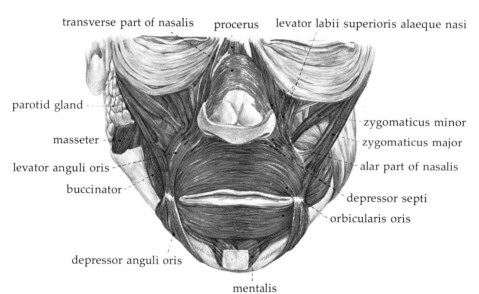

transverse part of nasalis   procerus   levator labii superioris alaeque nasi

parotid gland

masseter

levator anguli oris

buccinator

zygomaticus minor
zygomaticus major
alar part of nasalis
depressor septi
orbicularis oris

depressor anguli oris

mentalis

C. Superficial muscles of the nasal and oral regions.

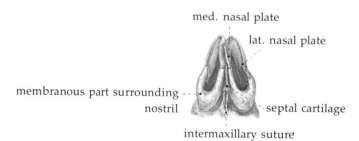

med. nasal plate

lat. nasal plate

membranous part surrounding
nostril

septal cartilage

intermaxillary suture

D. Cartilages of the external nares (nostrils).

The bony components of the root and dorsum of the nose are formed by the nasal bones and the nasal processes of the frontal and maxillary bones. The distal and lateral portions of the nose consist of nasal cartilages bound together by tough connective tissue. The cartilages of the nose consist of hyaline cartilage, unlike those of the ear, which are composed of elastic cartilage.

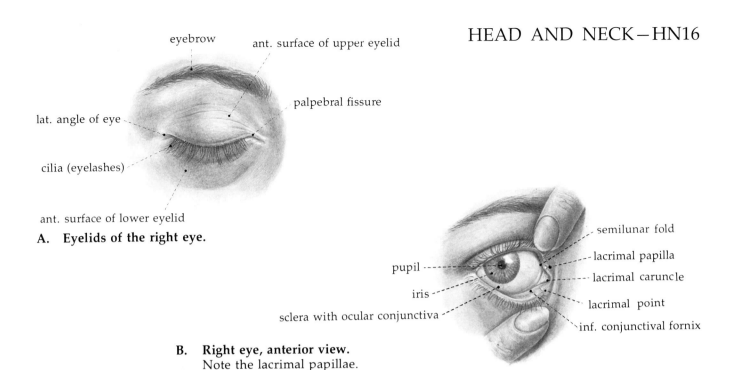

eyebrow
ant. surface of upper eyelid
palpebral fissure
lat. angle of eye
cilia (eyelashes)
ant. surface of lower eyelid

A. Eyelids of the right eye.

semilunar fold
lacrimal papilla
pupil
lacrimal caruncle
iris
lacrimal point
sclera with ocular conjunctiva
inf. conjunctival fornix

B. Right eye, anterior view.
Note the lacrimal papillae.

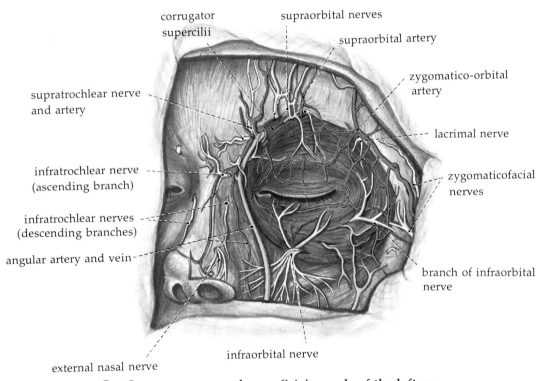

corrugator supercilii
supraorbital nerves
supraorbital artery
zygomatico-orbital artery
supratrochlear nerve and artery
lacrimal nerve
infratrochlear nerve (ascending branch)
zygomaticofacial nerves
infratrochlear nerves (descending branches)
angular artery and vein
branch of infraorbital nerve
external nasal nerve
infraorbital nerve

C. Sensory nerves and superficial vessels of the left eye.

The skin of the eyelids has an extremely rich supply of vessels and sensory nerves. Remember the following points (see also HN7):

¶ The upper eyelid and the root, dorsum and tip of the nose are supplied by the ophthalmic division of the trigeminal nerve, consisting of: (a) external nasal nerve; (b) infratrochlear nerve; (c) supratrochlear nerve; (d) supraorbital nerve; and (e) lacrimal nerve.

¶ The lower eyelid and side of the nose are supplied by the maxillary division of the trigeminal nerve, consisting of: (a) infraorbital nerve and (b) zygomaticofacial nerve.

¶ The palpebral and orbital parts of the orbicularis oculi as well as the corrugator supercilii are supplied by the facial nerve. Under normal conditions the upper eyelid closes the eye by gravity; parts of the orbicularis oculi are used to close the eye tightly.

¶ Note the angular vein, the terminal part of the facial vein (see HN6). From a clinical standpoint this vein is important because it communicates with the ophthalmic vein, which drains into the intracranial venous network. (For details, see HN24.)

367

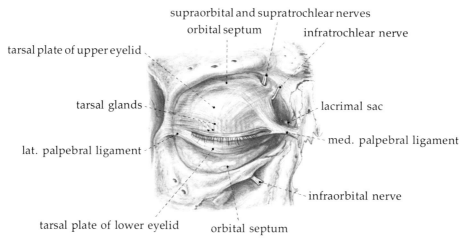

supraorbital and supratrochlear nerves

orbital septum

infratrochlear nerve

tarsal plate of upper eyelid

tarsal glands

lacrimal sac

lat. palpebral ligament

med. palpebral ligament

infraorbital nerve

tarsal plate of lower eyelid   orbital septum

A.   The orbital septa and tarsal plates.

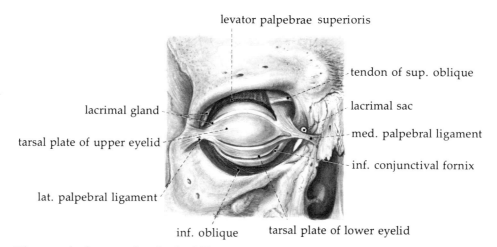

levator palpebrae superioris

tendon of sup. oblique

lacrimal gland

lacrimal sac

tarsal plate of upper eyelid

med. palpebral ligament

inf. conjunctival fornix

lat. palpebral ligament

inf. oblique   tarsal plate of lower eyelid

B.   The tarsal plates and palpebral ligaments.
The orbital septum, the underlying fat pads and the tendon of the levator palpebrae superioris have been removed.

Note:

¶ The orbital septum becomes visible after removal of the skin, superficial fascia and muscle fibers of the orbicularis oculi. It is attached to the periosteum of the bones surrounding the orbit and centrally to the tarsal plates of the eyelids. The septum covers some fatty tissue. In patients with severe malnutrition, the eyes lie deep in their sockets owing to the disappearance of the fatty tissue in the orbit and under the septa (see HN41).

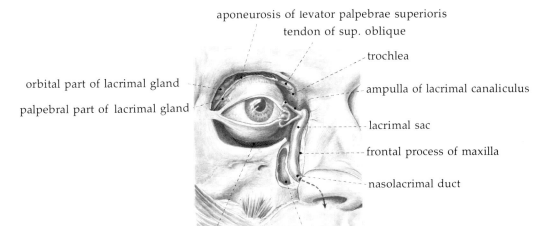

aponeurosis of levator palpebrae superioris

tendon of sup. oblique

trochlea

orbital part of lacrimal gland

palpebral part of lacrimal gland

ampulla of lacrimal canaliculus

lacrimal sac

frontal process of maxilla

nasolacrimal duct

inf. oblique   maxillary sinus

A.   The lacrimal apparatus of the right eye.

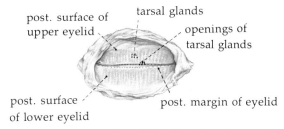

post. surface of
upper eyelid

tarsal glands

openings of
tarsal glands

post. surface
of lower eyelid

post. margin of eyelid

B.   The inner surface of eyelids showing the tarsal glands.

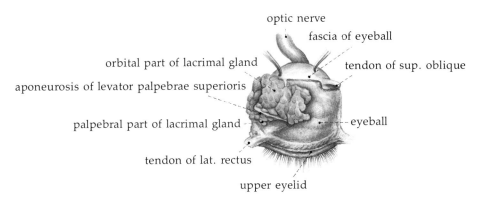

optic nerve

fascia of eyeball

orbital part of lacrimal gland

tendon of sup. oblique

aponeurosis of levator palpebrae superioris

palpebral part of lacrimal gland

eyeball

tendon of lat. rectus

upper eyelid

C.   The lacrimal gland.

¶ The lacrimal gland consists of palpebral and orbital portions, separated by the aponeurosis of the levator palpebrae superioris. It enters the lateral part of the superior conjunctival fornix with about ten little ducts. The tears flow over the cornea and then enter the lacrimal canaliculi through the puncta lacrimalia. The canaliculi open into the lacrimal sac, and from there the tears pass through the nasolacrimal duct to the inferior meatus of the nose. The entrance into the nose is guarded by a mucous fold, the lacrimal fold, which prevents air from entering the lacrimal system. When the nasolacrimal duct or the lacrimal canaliculi are obstructed, tears flow out of the eye. The duct system can usually be opened by carefully blowing air through the puncta into the canaliculi. (For innervation of the lacrimal gland, see HN36.)

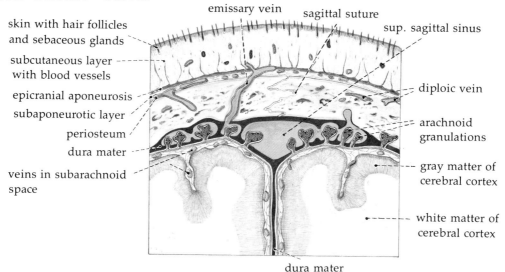

skin with hair follicles and sebaceous glands

subcutaneous layer with blood vessels

epicranial aponeurosis

subaponeurotic layer

periosteum

dura mater

veins in subarachnoid space

emissary vein

sagittal suture

sup. sagittal sinus

diploic vein

arachnoid granulations

gray matter of cerebral cortex

white matter of cerebral cortex

dura mater

A. Coronal section through the scalp.
Note the venous connections.

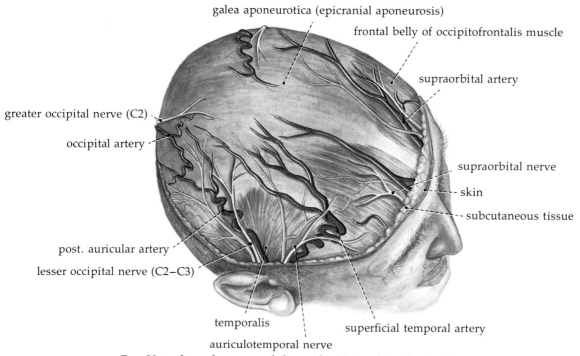

galea aponeurotica (epicranial aponeurosis)

frontal belly of occipitofrontalis muscle

supraorbital artery

greater occipital nerve (C2)

occipital artery

supraorbital nerve

skin

subcutaneous tissue

post. auricular artery

lesser occipital nerve (C2–C3)

temporalis

auriculotemporal nerve

superficial temporal artery

B. Vessels and nerves of the scalp (anterolateral view).

The following layers of the scalp should be identified:

¶ The *skin* is richly supplied with sebaceous glands and is the most common site for sebaceous cysts.

¶ The *subcutaneous layer* is characterized by tough fibrous septa that connect the skin with the underlying aponeurosis. The vessels and nerves are found in this subcutaneous layer. Lacerations of the scalp cause profuse bleeding that is difficult to stop, since the vessels withdraw between the fibrous septa. Therefore, wounds of the scalp must be carefully sutured, and when arteries have been cut they must be ligated. Some of the veins connect with the diploic veins between the two tables of the bone and even with the intracranial venous sinuses. Hence, infection of the scalp may spread to the bone (causing osteomyelitis), to the meninges and even to the venous sinuses, causing thrombus formation.

¶ The *epicranial aponeurosis* or *galea aponeurotica* is the third layer of the scalp. The occipital and frontal bellies of the occipitofrontalis muscle lie between two layers of the aponeurosis (see HN20). The skin, subcutaneous layer and epicranial aponeurosis together form a unit, which can be moved over the bones of the skull by the bellies of the occipitofrontalis.

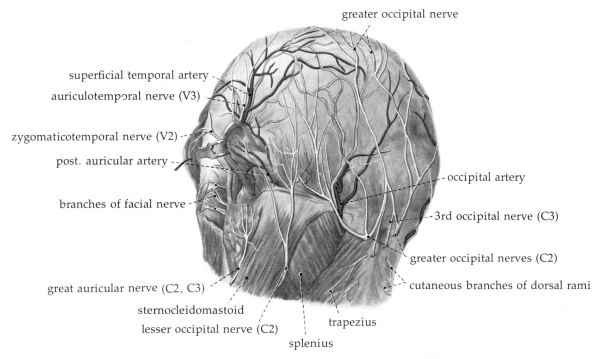

greater occipital nerve

superficial temporal artery

auriculotemporal nerve (V3)

zygomaticotemporal nerve (V2)

post. auricular artery

branches of facial nerve

occipital artery

3rd occipital nerve (C3)

greater occipital nerves (C2)

cutaneous branches of dorsal rami

great auricular nerve (C2, C3)

sternocleidomastoid

lesser occipital nerve (C2)

trapezius

splenius

A. Posterolateral view of the vessels and nerves of the scalp.

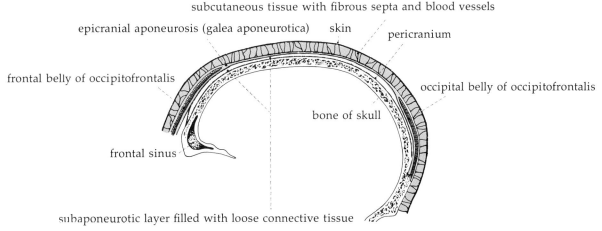

subcutaneous tissue with fibrous septa and blood vessels

epicranial aponeurosis (galea aponeurotica)   skin

pericranium

frontal belly of occipitofrontalis

occipital belly of occipitofrontalis

bone of skull

frontal sinus

subaponeurotic layer filled with loose connective tissue

B. Paramedian section through the scalp.

¶ The *subaponeurotic layer,* the fourth layer of the scalp, is located between the epicranial aponeurosis and the pericranium (periosteum of the bones). It is filled with very loose connective
tissue that permits the scalp to move over the underlying bones. Blood and pus collecting in this
space will spread rapidly, and the subaponeurotic layer is, therefore, called the "dangerous
layer." The blood does not penetrate the temporal and occipital regions, since in these regions
the epicranial aponeurosis is directly attached to the periosteum and the bone. In the region of
the orbits, however, the epicranial aponeurosis is not attached to bone; this explains the orbital
hematomas seen after severe head injuries and head operations.

¶ The *periosteum* or *pericranium* covers the outer surface of the bones. It adheres tightly to the suture
lines between the various bones. When blood collects under the periosteum, it will not spread
beyond the surface area of that particular bone. Subperiosteal bleeding sometimes occurs as a
result of birth injuries.

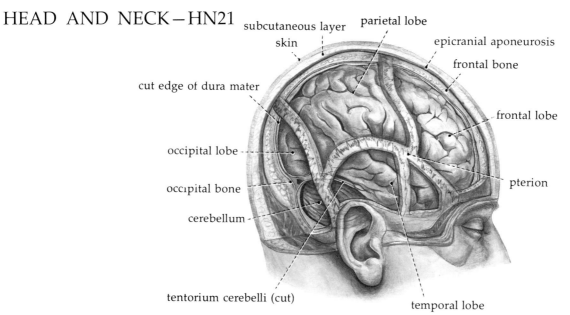

subcutaneous layer
skin
parietal lobe
epicranial aponeurosis
frontal bone
cut edge of dura mater
frontal lobe
occipital lobe
occipital bone
pterion
cerebellum
tentorium cerebelli (cut)
temporal lobe

A. Position of the brain in the skull.
The areas of the suture lines have been left intact.

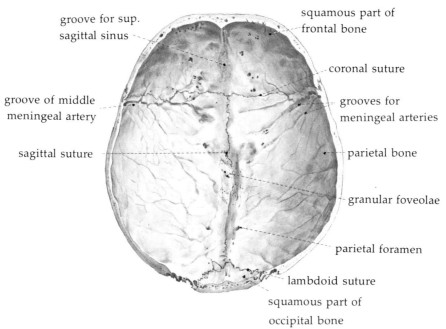

groove for sup.
sagittal sinus
squamous part of
frontal bone
coronal suture
groove of middle
meningeal artery
grooves for
meningeal arteries
sagittal suture
parietal bone
granular foveolae
parietal foramen
lambdoid suture
squamous part of
occipital bone

B. Inside view of the skull cap.

Note:

¶ The deep grooves in the inner table of the flat bones of the skull are caused by the pulsations of the meningeal arteries. Occasionally the arteries are fixed in the bony grooves, and fractures of the bones will therefore also cause ruptures of the arteries.

¶ The most dangerous area for fractures of the bones of the skull is at the pterion, where the temporal, parietal, frontal and sphenoid bones meet. When the meningeal artery is severed, blood accumulates between the dura mater and the endosteal layer of the bone. Since the artery runs parallel to the underlying precentral gyrus, the accumulating blood presses on the motor area. Gradual drowsiness and twitching of the facial musculature are followed by weakness and paralysis of the muscles of the face and upper extremity. As the intracranial pressure increases, the patient frequently becomes comatose. The diagnosis may be difficult, since often no external bleeding or wound of the skull is visible. The patient's life may be saved by releasing the pressure through a hole in the skull and ligating the artery.

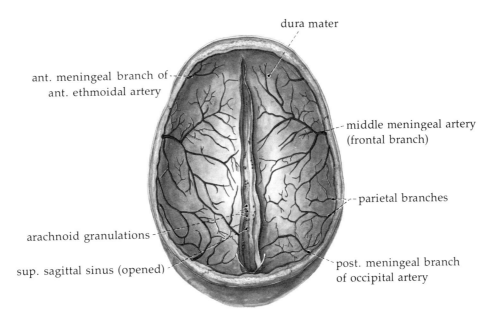

ant. meningeal branch of ant. ethmoidal artery

dura mater

middle meningeal artery (frontal branch)

parietal branches

arachnoid granulations

post. meningeal branch of occipital artery

sup. sagittal sinus (opened)

A. External surface of the dura mater.
The skull cap has been removed and the superior sagittal sinus has been opened.

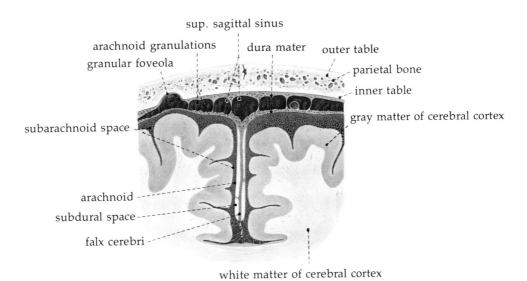

sup. sagittal sinus

arachnoid granulations
granular foveola

dura mater

outer table

parietal bone

inner table

gray matter of cerebral cortex

subarachnoid space

arachnoid

subdural space

falx cerebri

white matter of cerebral cortex

B. Frontal section of the skull, showing the arachnoid granulations.

¶ The dura is supplied by numerous arteries, of which the middle meningeal is the most important. It enters the cranial cavity through the foramen spinosum and subsequently runs forward and laterally in a groove on the squamous part of the temporal bone. The frontal branch may be enclosed in a bony canal for part of its course. The artery lies between the meningeal and the endosteal layer of the dura mater and runs nearly parallel to the underlying precentral (motor) gyrus of the brain (see HN21 A).

¶ The arachnoid granulations project into the superior sagittal sinus, which is located between the two layers of the dura mater. The granulations are extensions of the arachnoid membrane and pierce the inner layer of the dura. The tufts of arachnoid are separated from the venous blood in the sinus by endothelium. Since the subarachnoid space is filled with cerebrospinal fluid, the arachnoid granulations allow the cerebrospinal fluid to pass into the venous blood stream. Sometimes the arachnoid granulations press against the inner table of the parietal bone, causing small indentations known as granular foveolae (see also HN21 B).

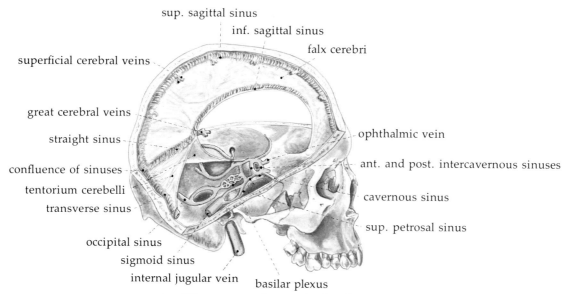

sup. sagittal sinus
inf. sagittal sinus
falx cerebri
superficial cerebral veins
great cerebral veins
straight sinus
confluence of sinuses
tentorium cerebelli
transverse sinus
occipital sinus
sigmoid sinus
internal jugular vein
basilar plexus
ophthalmic vein
ant. and post. intercavernous sinuses
cavernous sinus
sup. petrosal sinus

A. The venous sinuses in the dura mater.

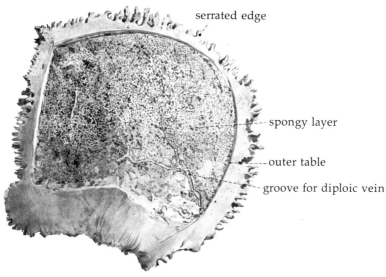

serrated edge
spongy layer
outer table
groove for diploic vein

B. Parietal bone, outer table removed to show diploic veins.
Note the serrated edges at the suture lines.

Note:

¶ The venous sinuses lie between the two layers of the dura and receive blood from: (a) the superficial cerebral veins, which drain the cortex of the cerebrum and cerebellum; (b) the great cerebral vein, which drains the deep structures on each side of the brain and joins the inferior sagittal sinus to form the straight sinus; and (c) the diploic veins, which drain the bones of the skull (see HN19 *A*).

¶ The cavernous sinus differs from all other venous sinuses (see HN31 and HN32). It is traversed by numerous trabeculae, which give it a spongelike appearance. The flow of the blood is relatively slow, and thrombus formation under pathologic conditions is not uncommon. Under normal conditions the cavernous sinus drains through the superior and inferior petrosal sinuses. The former enters the transverse sinus and the latter the root of the internal jugular vein (see HN24).

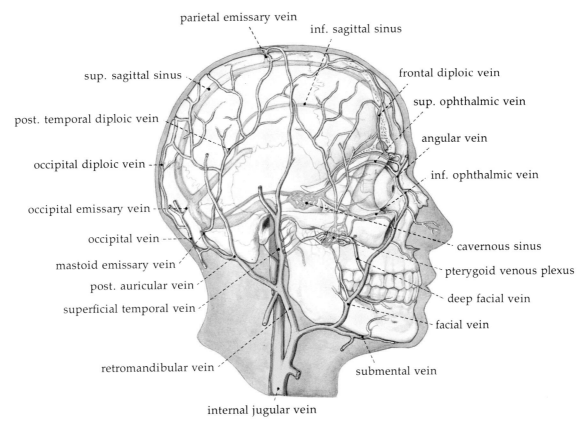

parietal emissary vein

inf. sagittal sinus

sup. sagittal sinus

frontal diploic vein

sup. ophthalmic vein

post. temporal diploic vein

angular vein

occipital diploic vein

inf. ophthalmic vein

occipital emissary vein

occipital vein

cavernous sinus

mastoid emissary vein

pterygoid venous plexus

post. auricular vein

superficial temporal vein

deep facial vein

facial vein

retromandibular vein

submental vein

internal jugular vein

The intracranial and extracranial veins.
Note the diploic and emissary veins.

¶ The facial vein is the major venous channel of the face. It drains the eyelids, eyebrows, forehead, nose and nasal cavities, lips and cheeks. The absence of valves in the veins of the face allows the venous blood to flow either by the normal route toward the internal jugular vein or, in abnormal conditions, toward the beginning of the facial vein at the medial angle of the eye. In this region the angular vein not only receives tributaries from the forehead, the eyelids, the lips and the side of the nose but is also connected to the superior ophthalmic vein. This vein in turn drains into the cavernous sinus.

¶ In patients with infections of the eye, nose and lips, the surrounding tissues will be swollen, and the blood in the facial vein may flow toward the ophthalmic vein. Infections may thus spread to the cavernous sinus. However, the facial vein does not necessarily drain via the ophthalmic vein. Through the deep facial vein it also drains into the pterygoid plexus, which in turn is connected with the cavernous sinus by means of emissary veins. Infections and thrombus formation in the cavernous sinus are frequently fatal (see HN32).

¶ The emissary veins are clinically important, since infections in the superficial regions of the head may spread into the intracranial cavity to the venous sinuses. Note the mastoid, occipital and parietal emissary veins. There are similar veins traversing the foramen ovale and uniting the cavernous sinus with the pterygoid plexus, and coursing through the foramen lacerum to connect the pharyngeal plexus with the cavernous sinus.

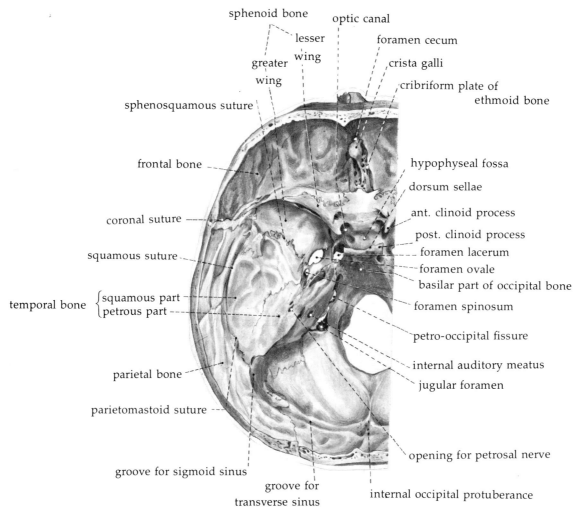

sphenoid bone
optic canal
lesser
foramen cecum
greater   wing
crista galli
wing
cribriform plate of
ethmoid bone
sphenosquamous suture
frontal bone
hypophyseal fossa
dorsum sellae
ant. clinoid process
coronal suture
post. clinoid process
squamous suture
foramen lacerum
foramen ovale
basilar part of occipital bone
temporal bone { squamous part
petrous part
foramen spinosum
petro-occipital fissure
parietal bone
internal auditory meatus
jugular foramen
parietomastoid suture
groove for sigmoid sinus
opening for petrosal nerve
groove for
transverse sinus
internal occipital protuberance

The inside of the base of the cranial cavity in the adult.
Note the foramina and the sutures.

Before the brain itself is dissected, the inside of the base of the cranial cavity should be examined. Three separate cavities are recognized (see also HN26).

¶ The *anterior cranial fossa* is bounded anteriorly by the inner surface of the frontal bone and posteriorly by the lesser wings of the sphenoid. The floor of the fossa is formed by the orbital plates of the frontal bones and the ethmoid bone. The fossa contains the frontal lobes of the cerebral hemispheres.

¶ The *middle cranial fossa* consists of a median part formed by the body of the sphenoid and two lateral parts containing the temporal lobes of the cerebral hemispheres. The anterior border is formed by the lesser wings of the sphenoid, and the posterior border is formed by the superior rims of the petrous parts of the temporal bones. The lateral borders as well as the floor are formed by the squamous parts of the temporal and parietal bones and the greater wings of the sphenoid bones.

¶ The *posterior cranial fossa* is bounded anteriorly by the superior borders of the petrous parts of the temporal bones, posteriorly by the squamous part of the occipital bone. The floor is formed by the basilar and squamous parts of the occipital bone and the mastoid part of the temporal bone. The roof is formed by the tentorium cerebelli. The fossa contains the occipital lobes, the cerebellum, the pons and the medulla oblongata.

¶ The nerves and vessels passing through the foramina are shown in HN28 and HN30.

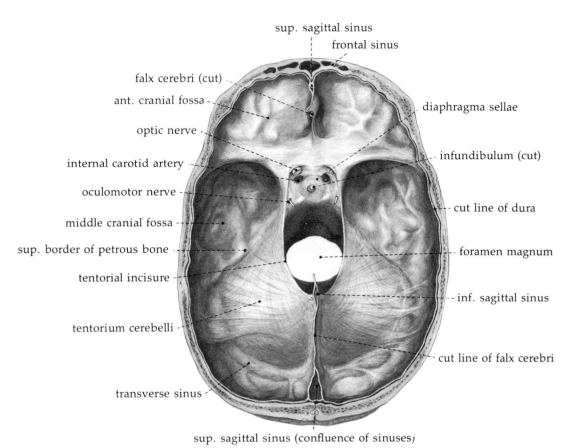

sup. sagittal sinus

frontal sinus

falx cerebri (cut)

ant. cranial fossa

diaphragma sellae

optic nerve

internal carotid artery

infundibulum (cut)

oculomotor nerve

cut line of dura

middle cranial fossa

sup. border of petrous bone

foramen magnum

tentorial incisure

inf. sagittal sinus

tentorium cerebelli

cut line of falx cerebri

transverse sinus

sup. sagittal sinus (confluence of sinuses)

The dura mater after removal of the falx cerebri.

The dura mater consists of the endosteal layer (periosteum covering the inner surface of the bones) and the meningeal layer, the dura mater proper. In many places the two layers are closely united; in other places they are separated from each other. The cranial cavity is incompletely divided into various compartments by four meningeal septa:

¶ The *tentorium cerebelli* forms the roof of the posterior cranial fossa. Its anterior border is attached along the superior borders of the petrous parts of the temporal bones toward the posterior clinoid process of the sphenoid bone. Its lateral border is attached along the margin of the grooves for the transverse sinuses (see HN27). In front it has a free border for the passage of the brainstem. The free rim, called the tentorial notch or tentorial incisure, extends forward on each side and is attached to the anterior clinoid processes.

¶ The *diaphragma sellae* is a layer of the dura mater that forms a roof over the hypophyseal fossa. In its center is a small opening for passage of the stalk (infundibulum) of the hypophysis.

¶ The *falx cerebri* forms a septum between the cerebral hemispheres (note the cut lines of its attachment) (see also HN27).

¶ The *falx cerebelli* forms a septum between the hemispheres of the cerebellum (see HN27).

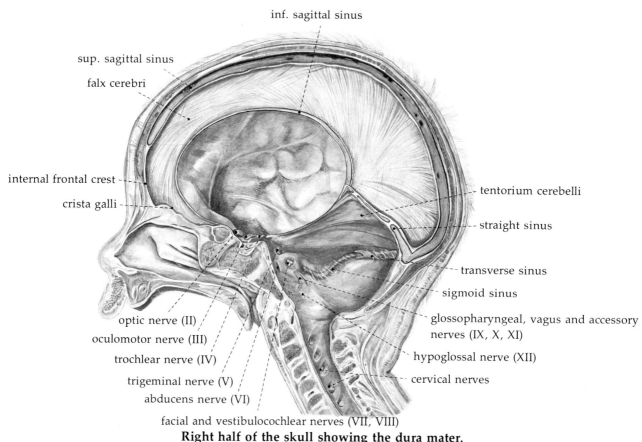

inf. sagittal sinus

sup. sagittal sinus

falx cerebri

internal frontal crest

crista galli

tentorium cerebelli

straight sinus

transverse sinus

sigmoid sinus

optic nerve (II)

oculomotor nerve (III)

trochlear nerve (IV)

trigeminal nerve (V)

abducens nerve (VI)

glossopharyngeal, vagus and accessory nerves (IX, X, XI)

hypoglossal nerve (XII)

cervical nerves

facial and vestibulocochlear nerves (VII, VIII)

Right half of the skull showing the dura mater.
Note the cranial and cervical nerves.

In addition to the tentorium cerebelli and the diaphragma sellae, the dura mater forms two vertical septa:

¶ The *falx cerebri* is a sickle-shaped fold in the midline, located between the two cerebral hemispheres. In front it is attached to the crista galli of the ethmoid bone and to the internal frontal crest. Its posterior end blends with the upper surface of the tentorium cerebelli. In the lower free margin of the falx cerebri is the inferior sagittal sinus; the straight sinus is in the line of attachment with the tentorium.

¶ The *falx cerebelli* is a small sickle-shaped fold that projects forward between the two cerebellar hemispheres. It is posteriorly attached to the internal occipital crest.

Another important point to remember is that the dura mater proper surrounds the cranial nerves with tubular sheaths that extend through the foramina of the skull. Outside the foramina these sheaths are continuous with the epineurium of the nerves. The optic nerve, however, is sheathed along its entire length by a dural sleeve that finally blends with the fascia of the eyeball (see HN42).

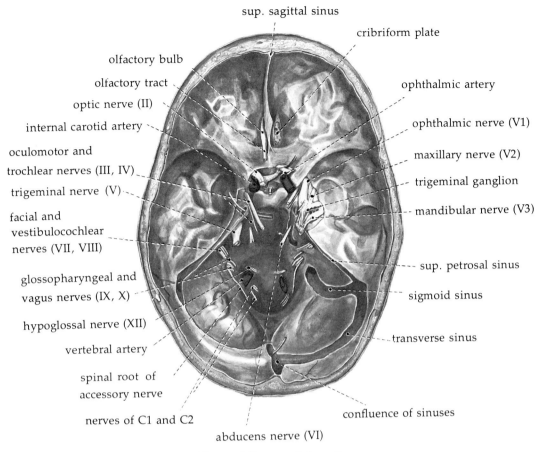

sup. sagittal sinus
cribriform plate
olfactory bulb
olfactory tract
optic nerve (II)
internal carotid artery
oculomotor and
trochlear nerves (III, IV)
trigeminal nerve (V)
facial and
vestibulocochlear
nerves (VII, VIII)
glossopharyngeal and
vagus nerves (IX, X)
hypoglossal nerve (XII)
vertebral artery
spinal root of
accessory nerve
nerves of C1 and C2
abducens nerve (VI)
ophthalmic artery
ophthalmic nerve (V1)
maxillary nerve (V2)
trigeminal ganglion
mandibular nerve (V3)
sup. petrosal sinus
sigmoid sinus
transverse sinus
confluence of sinuses

Base of the cranial cavity.
The tentorium cerebelli has been removed; the cranial arteries and nerves have been cut; the dural sinuses have been opened. See also HN25 and HN30.

Note the structures that pass through the openings at the base of the cranial cavity:

1. The nerve fibers of the olfactory (I) nerve originate in the mucous membrane of the upper part of the nose and pierce the cribriform plate of the ethmoid bone.

2. The optic (II) nerve, accompanied by the ophthalmic artery, passes through the optic canal (see HN43).

3. The oculomotor (III) and trochlear (IV) nerves enter the orbit through the superior orbital fissure (see HN33).

4. The trigeminal (V) ganglion lies in a double fold of the dura on the apex of the temporal bone. The ophthalmic division of the trigeminal nerve enters the orbit through the superior orbital fissure; the maxillary nerve pierces the foramen rotundum; and the mandibular nerve passes through the foramen ovale.

5. The abducens (VI) nerve leaves the cranial cavity through the superior orbital fissure.

6. The facial (VII) and vestibulocochlear (VIII) nerves leave the posterior cranial fossa through the internal acoustic meatus.

7. The glossopharyngeal (IX) and vagus (X) nerves leave the posterior cranial fossa through the jugular foramen.

8. The accessory (XI) nerve also leaves the cranial cavity through the jugular foramen. Its spinal root, which arises from the upper segments of the spinal cord (see HN29), enters the skull through the foramen magnum and then joins the cranial root to leave through the jugular foramen.

9. The hypoglossal (XII) nerve leaves the skull through the hypoglossal canal in the occipital bone.

10. The vertebral arteries enter the cranial cavity through the foramen magnum; the internal carotid arteries emerge from the cavernous sinus on the medial side of the anterior clinoid process by perforating the dura mater.

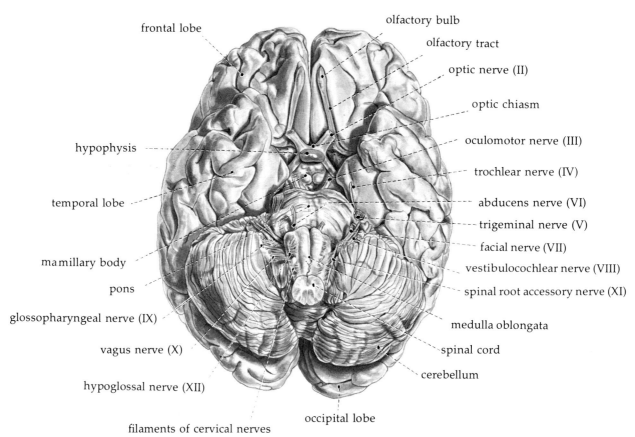

frontal lobe

olfactory bulb

olfactory tract

optic nerve (II)

optic chiasm

hypophysis

oculomotor nerve (III)

trochlear nerve (IV)

temporal lobe

abducens nerve (VI)

trigeminal nerve (V)

facial nerve (VII)

mamillary body

vestibulocochlear nerve (VIII)

pons

spinal root accessory nerve (XI)

glossopharyngeal nerve (IX)

medulla oblongata

vagus nerve (X)

spinal cord

cerebellum

hypoglossal nerve (XII)

occipital lobe

filaments of cervical nerves

Inferior surface of the brain with cranial nerves.

Some of the cranial nerves are affected by pathological processes when leaving the skull through the foramina.

¶ The vestibulocochlear nerve may be affected by the so-called acoustic neurinoma, a tumor originating from the Schwann cells close to or in the internal acoustic meatus. The tumor will gradually exert pressure on the cochlear, the vestibular, the facial and the intermediate nerves. The deeper in the meatus the tumor starts its growth, the earlier it will produce symptoms, owing to compression of the nerves and circulatory disturbances. Deafness, loss of taste in the anterior two-thirds of the tongue and facial paralysis are the most common complaints.

¶ Aneurysms close to or in the cranial foramina may also cause compression of the nerves. When the optic nerve is compressed, unilateral impairment of vision may result. Similarly, paralysis of the third, fourth or sixth cranial nerves may occur as a result of slowly expanding aneurysms.

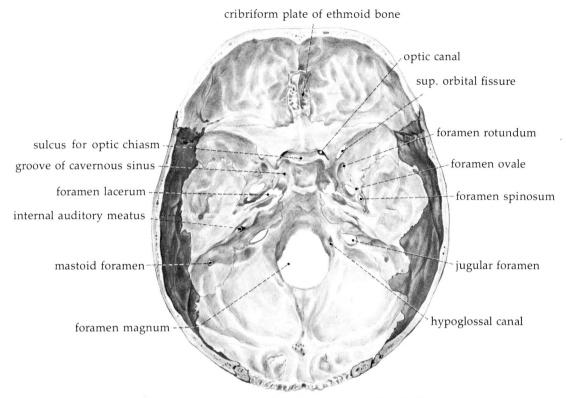

cribriform plate of ethmoid bone

optic canal

sup. orbital fissure

foramen rotundum

sulcus for optic chiasm

groove of cavernous sinus

foramen ovale

foramen lacerum

foramen spinosum

internal auditory meatus

mastoid foramen

jugular foramen

hypoglossal canal

foramen magnum

Foramina on the inside of the base of the skull.

Note:

¶ In the *anterior cranial fossa:*

1. Foramina in the cribriform plate. Filaments of the olfactory nerves enter through these foramina.

¶ In the *middle cranial fossa:*

1. Optic canal. Through this canal pass the optic nerve and the ophthalmic artery.

2. Superior orbital fissure. Through this large fissure pass the oculomotor (III) nerve, the trochlear (IV) nerve, the ophthalmic (V_1) nerve, the abducens (VI) nerve, sympathetic fibers, ophthalmic veins and branches of the middle meningeal artery (see HN40 C).

3. Foramen rotundum. Through this foramen passes the maxillary nerve (V_2).

4. Foramen ovale. Through this foramen pass the mandibular nerve (V_3) and an accessory meningeal artery.

5. Foramen spinosum. Through this foramen enters the middle meningeal artery.

6. Foramen lacerum. The internal carotid artery passes across the superior part of the foramen and subsequently enters the cavernous sinus; the meningeal branch of the ascending pharyngeal artery also enters this opening.

¶ In the *posterior cranial fossa:*

1. Internal auditory meatus. Through this opening pass the facial (VII) nerve, the vestibulocochlear (VIII) nerve and the labyrinthine artery.

2. Jugular foramen. The internal jugular vein, the glossopharyngeal (IX) nerve, the vagus (X) nerve and the accessory (XI) nerve all pass through this foramen.

3. Hypoglossal canal. The hypoglossal (XII) nerve leaves the cranial cavity through this opening.

4. Foramen magnum. The medulla oblongata, vertebral arteries, the spinal part of the accessory nerve, and the anterior and posterior spinal arteries pass through this opening.

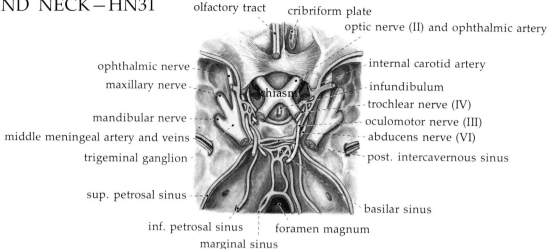

olfactory tract

cribriform plate

optic nerve (II) and ophthalmic artery

ophthalmic nerve

maxillary nerve

chiasm

internal carotid artery

infundibulum

trochlear nerve (IV)

mandibular nerve

oculomotor nerve (III)

middle meningeal artery and veins

abducens nerve (VI)

trigeminal ganglion

post. intercavernous sinus

sup. petrosal sinus

basilar sinus

inf. petrosal sinus

foramen magnum

marginal sinus

A. The nerves in the middle cranial fossa.

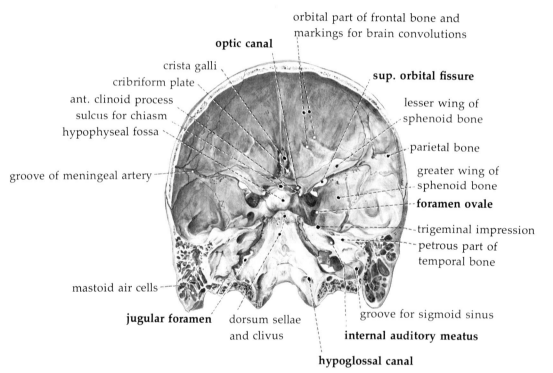

orbital part of frontal bone and markings for brain convolutions

optic canal

crista galli

cribriform plate

ant. clinoid process

sulcus for chiasm

hypophyseal fossa

sup. orbital fissure

lesser wing of sphenoid bone

parietal bone

greater wing of sphenoid bone

foramen ovale

groove of meningeal artery

trigeminal impression

petrous part of temporal bone

mastoid air cells

jugular foramen

dorsum sellae and clivus

groove for sigmoid sinus

internal auditory meatus

hypoglossal canal

B. Frontal section through the base of the cranial cavity showing the anterior part.

Note the following clinically important points:

¶ The optic nerves enter the middle cranial fossa through the optic canals. As soon as they have entered the fossa the fibers carrying impulses from the medial half of the retina (temporal visual field) cross the midline, thus forming the optic chiasm. The chiasm is located on the dorsum of the body of the sphenoid. The optic nerve fibers carrying impulses from the lateral halves of the retina do not cross the midline.

¶ Just behind the optic chiasm is the hypophysis. It lies in the hypophyseal fossa and is covered by the diaphragma sellae. The infundibulum of the hypophysis pierces the diaphragma. When a tumor of the anterior lobe of the hypophysis is present, the glandular tissue expands out of the fossa and may exert pressure on the optic chiasm. The optic fibers crossing the midline in the chiasm are compressed, and a loss of vision in both temporal visual fields then becomes gradually apparent.

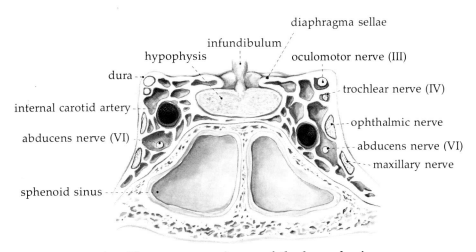

A. The cavernous sinus and the hypophysis.

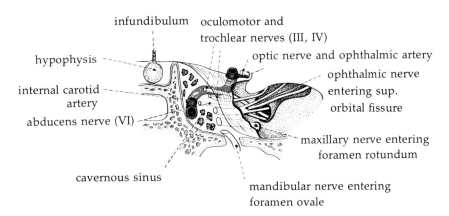

B. Diagram of the cavernous sinus with vessels and nerves.

¶ The cavernous sinus, one on each side of the body of the sphenoid, lies against the lateral wall of the hypophyseal fossa and rests inferiorly on the greater wing of the sphenoid. It consists of a large plexus of communicating veins forming a cavernous, almost trabeculated structure. The blood flow is often sluggish. The anterior and posterior intercavernous sinuses connect the right and left cavernous sinus (see HN31 A).

¶ Traversing the cavernous sinus are: (a) the internal carotid artery, and (b) the abducens nerve. In the lateral wall of the sinus are: (a) the oculomotor nerve; (b) the trochlear nerve; and (c) the ophthalmic and maxillary divisions of the trigeminal nerve. The mandibular nerve usually courses just below the sinus.

¶ The cavernous sinus is sometimes affected by infections from the lip, nose and eye through connections of the ophthalmic veins with the facial vein or via the deep facial vein and pterygoid plexus (see HN23 A). Owing to the cavernous structure of the sinus and the sluggishness of the blood stream, thrombosis may occur, thus blocking the venous drainage of the orbit. This causes edema of the eyelids and conjunctiva, exophthalmos, and engorgement and hemorrhages in the retina. The fundus of the retina shows papilledema, and the pulsations of the retinal arteries are striking (see HN45). When the pressure increases, the nerves traversing the sinus become compressed, and paralysis of the musculature may result. Sometimes thrombus formation in the cavernous sinus occurs after infections of the middle ear and mastoid bone. In these cases the infection is transmitted via the sigmoid and petrosal sinuses.

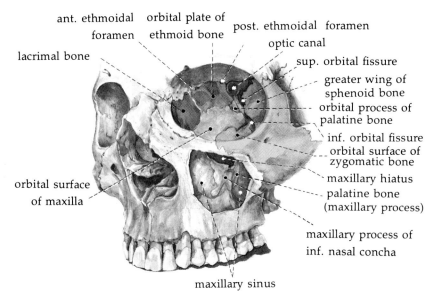

ant. ethmoidal foramen
orbital plate of ethmoid bone
post. ethmoidal foramen
optic canal
sup. orbital fissure
greater wing of sphenoid bone
orbital process of palatine bone
inf. orbital fissure
orbital surface of zygomatic bone
maxillary hiatus
palatine bone (maxillary process)
maxillary process of inf. nasal concha
lacrimal bone
orbital surface of maxilla
maxillary sinus

A. The bony components of the left orbit.
Part of the maxilla has been removed to expose the maxillary sinus.

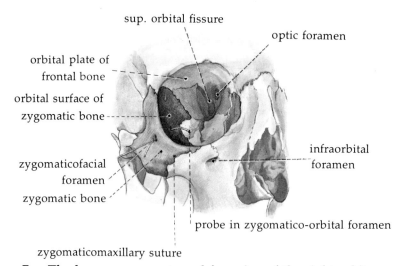

sup. orbital fissure
optic foramen
orbital plate of frontal bone
orbital surface of zygomatic bone
infraorbital foramen
zygomaticofacial foramen
zygomatic bone
probe in zygomatico-orbital foramen
zygomaticomaxillary suture

B. The bony components and foramina of the right orbit.

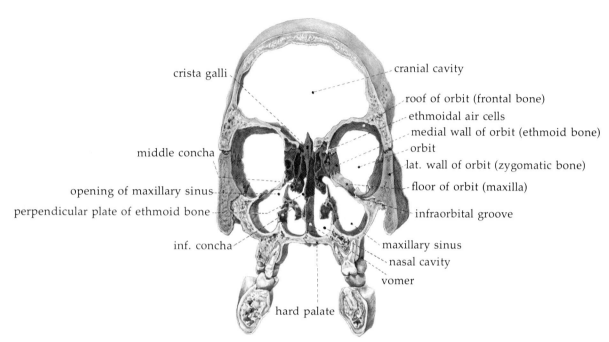

crista galli

cranial cavity

roof of orbit (frontal bone)

ethmoidal air cells

medial wall of orbit (ethmoid bone)

orbit

lat. wall of orbit (zygomatic bone)

floor of orbit (maxilla)

middle concha

opening of maxillary sinus

perpendicular plate of ethmoid bone

infraorbital groove

inf. concha

maxillary sinus

nasal cavity

vomer

hard palate

Frontal section through the skull.
Note the relationship of the orbit to the cranial cavity and the maxillary and ethmoid sinuses.

Note:

¶ The roof of the orbit is formed by the orbital plate of the frontal bone, a thin bony plate which fractures easily. In some places the bone is so thin that infections of the eye penetrate the bone, causing meningitis and brain abscesses in the frontal lobe.

¶ The lateral wall is formed by the zygomatic bone and the greater wing of the sphenoid. This is the strongest wall of the orbit (see HN33 *A*).

¶ The floor is formed by the paper-thin orbital plate of the maxilla and bony plates of the zygomatic and palatine bones. The thin orbital plate separates the maxillary sinus from the orbit, and inflammations of the sinus sometimes expand through this plate into the orbital cavity.

¶ The medial wall is formed by the frontal process of the maxilla, the lacrimal bone, the orbital plate of the ethmoid, and the body of the sphenoid. The thin bony plate separating the orbital cavity from the ethmoidal air cells permits infections from the air cells to penetrate the orbital cavity.

385

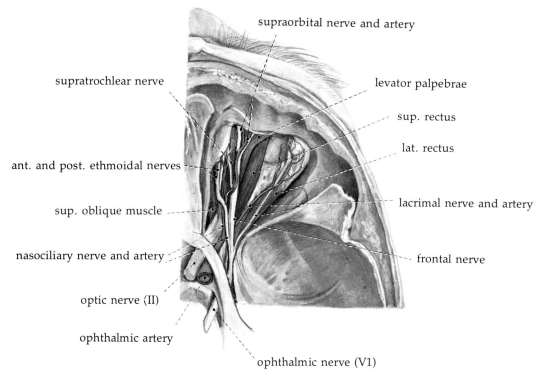

supraorbital nerve and artery

supratrochlear nerve

levator palpebrae

sup. rectus

lat. rectus

ant. and post. ethmoidal nerves

sup. oblique muscle

lacrimal nerve and artery

nasociliary nerve and artery

frontal nerve

optic nerve (II)

ophthalmic artery

ophthalmic nerve (V1)

A. The muscles of the right eye.
The roof of the orbit has been removed.

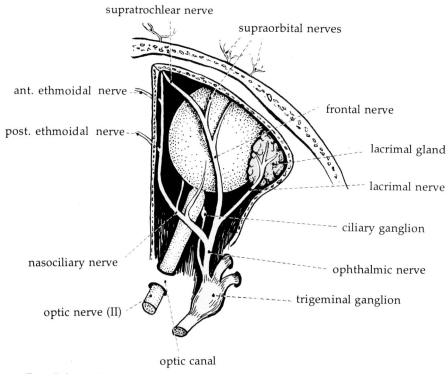

supratrochlear nerve

supraorbital nerves

ant. ethmoidal nerve

post. ethmoidal nerve

frontal nerve

lacrimal gland

lacrimal nerve

ciliary ganglion

nasociliary nerve

ophthalmic nerve

trigeminal ganglion

optic nerve (II)

optic canal

B. Schematic drawing of the ophthalmic nerve (seen from above).

The ophthalmic nerve and its branches (nasociliary, frontal and lacrimal) enter the orbit through the superior orbital fissure. The nerve supplies the sensory innervation to the skin of the forehead and most of the nose but carries no motor fibers. In addition, it has a number of other functions (see also HN36):

¶ It innervates the cornea and the upper eyelid. Loss of sensation of the cornea, which prevents the patient from awareness of dust and other foreign particles, may result in ulceration of the cornea and subsequent blindness (see HN7).

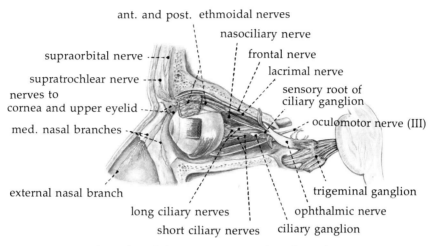

ant. and post. ethmoidal nerves

nasociliary nerve

supraorbital nerve

frontal nerve

supratrochlear nerve

lacrimal nerve

nerves to
cornea and upper eyelid

sensory root of
ciliary ganglion

med. nasal branches

oculomotor nerve (III)

external nasal branch

trigeminal ganglion

long ciliary nerves

ophthalmic nerve

short ciliary nerves   ciliary ganglion

A.   The left ophthalmic nerve and its branches.
The orbit has been opened from the lateral side.

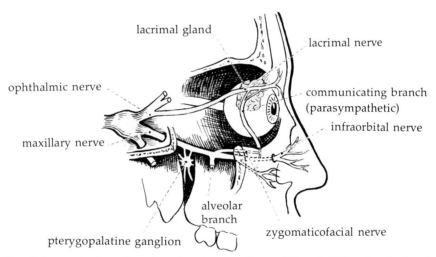

lacrimal gland

lacrimal nerve

ophthalmic nerve

communicating branch
(parasympathetic)

infraorbital nerve

maxillary nerve

alveolar
branch

pterygopalatine ganglion

zygomaticofacial nerve

B.   Schematic drawing showing innervation of the right lacrimal gland.

¶ Postganglionic parasympathetic fibers reach the lacrimal gland through the lacrimal nerve. These fibers originate in the pterygopalatine ganglion, travel for a short distance with the zygomatic nerve and finally reach the lacrimal nerve through a communicating branch. The fibers are secretomotor to the gland. The preganglionic parasympathetic fibers reach the ganglion through the greater petrosal nerve and the nerve of the pterygoid canal (see HN51).

¶ The postganglionic sympathetic fibers of the lacrimal gland originate in the superior cervical ganglion and travel to the gland by way of a plexus around the internal carotid artery, the deep petrosal nerve and the nerve of the pterygoid canal. From there the fibers reach the gland through the lacrimal artery and nerve (see HN51).

¶ The nasociliary nerve receives sensory fibers from the eyeball through the long ciliary nerves that pass uninterrupted through the ciliary ganglion.

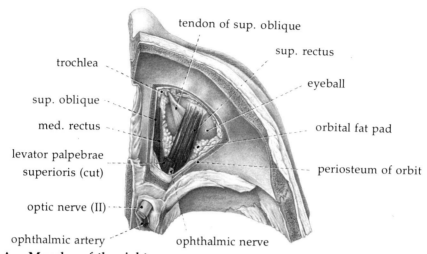

trochlea

sup. oblique

med. rectus

levator palpebrae
superioris (cut)

optic nerve (II)

ophthalmic artery

tendon of sup. oblique

sup. rectus

eyeball

orbital fat pad

periosteum of orbit

ophthalmic nerve

A. Muscles of the right eye.
The levator palpebrae and part of the fat body have been removed.

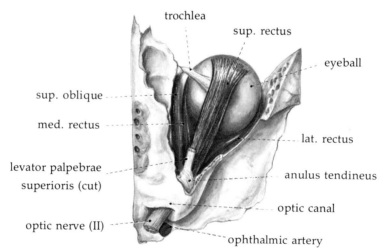

trochlea

sup. rectus

eyeball

sup. oblique

med. rectus

levator palpebrae
superioris (cut)

optic nerve (II)

lat. rectus

anulus tendineus

optic canal

ophthalmic artery

B. Muscles of the right eye.
The lacrimal gland and the fat body have been removed.

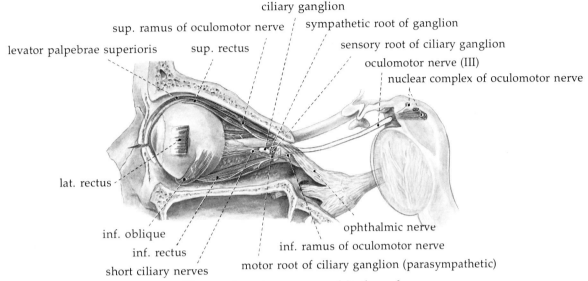

The oculomotor nerve and its branches.
The orbit is opened from the lateral aspect.

¶ The oculomotor nerve supplies all the extrinsic muscles of the eye except the lateral rectus and the superior oblique. In addition, it carries preganglionic parasympathetic fibers from the nuclear complex in the midbrain to the ciliary ganglion, where they synapse. The postganglionic parasympathetic fibers pass through the short ciliary nerves to the sphincter pupillae and the ciliary muscles (see HN91).

¶ The ciliary ganglion also receives postganglionic sympathetic fibers from the sympathetic plexus around the ophthalmic artery. These fibers innervate the dilator pupillae, the orbitalis and the palpebral or tarsal muscles (HN41 and HN44) through the short ciliary nerves and the plexus around the arteries.

¶ When the oculomotor nerve is injured, the following symptoms may be expected: (a) drooping of the eyelid (ptosis) due to paralysis of the levator palpebrae superioris; (b) a divergent squint caused by the unopposed action of the superior oblique and lateral rectus; (c) double vision; (d) dilation of the pupil due to paralysis of the sphincter pupillae; (e) loss of accommodation due to paralysis of the ciliary muscle.

¶ The dilation of the pupil is under the control of the postganglionic sympathetic fibers of the superior cervical ganglion (see HN78). The preganglionic fibers originate in the spinal cord at the level of T1. When disease is present at this level of the spinal cord or in the superior cervical ganglion, an interesting eye syndrome results (Horner's syndrome), characterized by (a) a narrow pupil (miosis) due to paralysis of the dilator pupillae; (b) ptosis of the upper eyelid due to paralysis of the tarsalis (see HN41); and (c) dryness (absence of sweating) and flushing of the affected side of the face as a result of vasoconstrictor denervation.

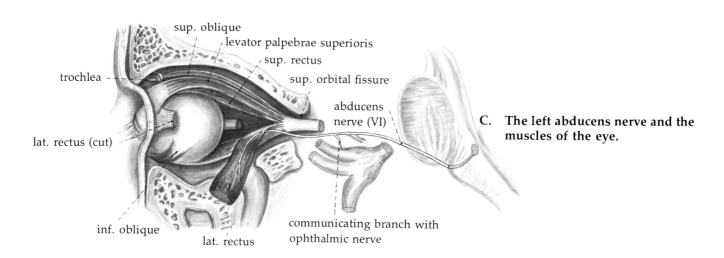

A. The left trochlear nerve and the muscles of the eye.

trochlea

tendon of sup. oblique

sup. oblique

sup. orbital fissure

trochlear nerve (IV)

lat. rectus

communicating branch with ophthalmic nerve

inf. oblique

inf. rectus

aponeurosis levator palpebrae superioris

palpebral part of lacrimal gland

orbital part of lacrimal gland

ocular conjunctiva (cut)

lat. rectus

inf. conjunctival fornix

B. Muscles of the right eye.
The lateral wall of the orbit has been removed.

fat pad of orbit

tendon of inf. oblique

sup. oblique

levator palpebrae superioris

sup. rectus

trochlea

sup. orbital fissure

abducens nerve (VI)

lat. rectus (cut)

C. The left abducens nerve and the muscles of the eye.

inf. oblique

lat. rectus

communicating branch with ophthalmic nerve

¶ The trochlear nerve supplies only the superior oblique. Under normal conditions the superior oblique pulls the eyeball laterally and downward. Hence, patients who have a lesion of the nerve experience double vision when they attempt to turn the eye downward and laterally.

¶ The abducens nerve is frequently injured in fractures of the base of the skull. Loss of nerve action causes double vision, and a convergent squint results. When the eyes are directed straight ahead, the unopposed medial rectus pulls the eyeball medially. Due to its long intracranial course, the nerve is often damaged by long-lasting intracranial pressure.

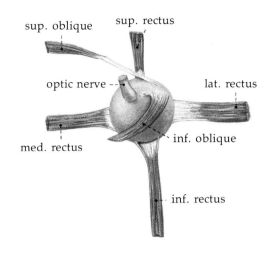

sup. oblique   sup. rectus

optic nerve

lat. rectus

med. rectus

inf. oblique

inf. rectus

A. The right eyeball and its muscles (posterior view).

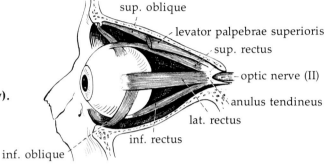

sup. oblique

levator palpebrae superioris

sup. rectus

optic nerve (II)

anulus tendineus

lat. rectus

inf. rectus

inf. oblique

B. The muscles of the left eye (lateral view).

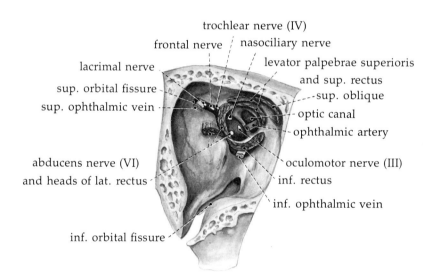

trochlear nerve (IV)

frontal nerve   nasociliary nerve

lacrimal nerve

levator palpebrae superioris
and sup. rectus

sup. orbital fissure

sup. oblique

sup. ophthalmic vein

optic canal

ophthalmic artery

abducens nerve (VI)
and heads of lat. rectus

oculomotor nerve (III)

inf. rectus

inf. ophthalmic vein

inf. orbital fissure

C. The anulus tendineus.
Apex of the right orbit with the origin of
the extrinsic eye muscles.

Note:

¶ The four rectus muscles originate from the anulus tendineus, which surrounds the optic canal and bridges the medial part of the superior orbital fissure. The other three muscles originate from the wall of the orbit: the levator palpebrae superioris from the lesser wing of the sphenoid, the superior oblique from the body of the sphenoid and the inferior oblique from the anterior part of the floor of the orbit.

¶ The movements of the eye are complicated, and all muscles participate to a greater or lesser degree in each movement of the eyeball. Three axes are recognized: (a) a vertical axis through the center of the eye that permits adduction and abduction of the center of the cornea; (b) a lateromedial axis around which upward (elevation) and downward (depression) movements occur; and (c) an anteroposterior axis for lateral rotation (extorsion) and medial rotation (intorsion). In summary:

Medial rectus: adduction.
Lateral rectus: abduction.
Inferior rectus: depression, adduction, lateral rotation.
Superior rectus: elevation, adduction, medial rotation.
Superior oblique: depression, abduction, medial rotation.
Inferior oblique: elevation, abduction, lateral rotation.

Since most muscles carry out movements on all three axes, it is often difficult to determine which of the eye muscles is paralyzed.

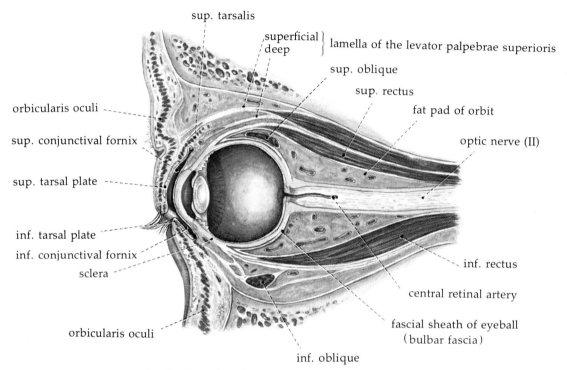

sup. tarsalis

superficial ⎫
deep ⎭ lamella of the levator palpebrae superioris

sup. oblique

sup. rectus

orbicularis oculi

fat pad of orbit

sup. conjunctival fornix

optic nerve (II)

sup. tarsal plate

inf. tarsal plate

inf. conjunctival fornix

sclera

inf. rectus

central retinal artery

orbicularis oculi

fascial sheath of eyeball
(bulbar fascia)

inf. oblique

Sagittal section through the orbit and eyeball.
Note the large amount of fat in the orbital cavity.

Note:

¶ The bulbar fascia is a thin membrane separating the eyeball from the orbital fat. It is pierced by and sheathes the tendons of the ocular muscles which insert in the sclera. After removal of an eye, the fascia is used as a socket for the prosthesis.

¶ The fibrous coat of the eyeball consists of an anterior transparent part, the cornea, and a tough posterior part, the sclera. The sclera maintains the shape of the eyeball and is continuous with the dura around the optic nerve. Posteriorly, the fibers of the optic nerve pierce the sclera, thus causing a weak spot known as the cribriform area of the sclera.

¶ In patients with severe malnutrition the eyes lie deep in the socket. In patients with hyperthyroidism (Graves' disease) the eyeball protrudes (exophthalmos). The protrusion is caused by an enlargement of the retro-orbital fat body.

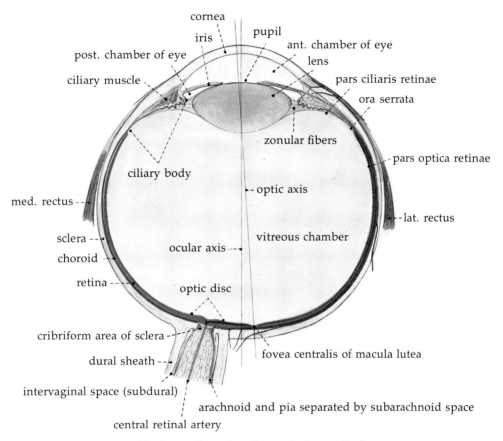

Horizontal section through the eyeball.

¶ The optic nerve is surrounded by the dura mater as well as by the arachnoid, the pia mater and an extension of the subarachnoid space. Whenever the intracranial pressure is increased by growing tumors, bleeding or infections, the pressure of the cerebrospinal fluid in the subarachnoid space will extend in the sheath of the optic nerve. In such cases the papilla of the optic nerve, also known as the optic disc, becomes edematous. If the intraocular pressure is increased, the perforated area of the sclera in the region of the optic disc will bulge outward.

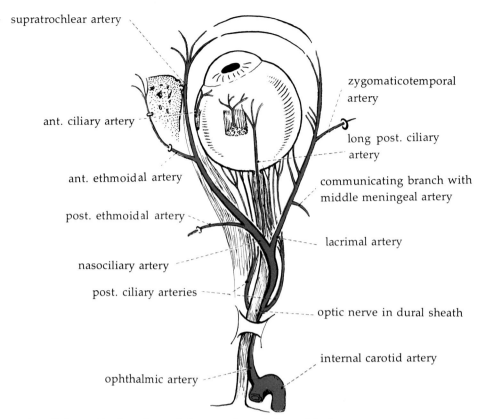

supratrochlear artery

zygomaticotemporal artery

ant. ciliary artery

long post. ciliary artery

ant. ethmoidal artery

communicating branch with middle meningeal artery

post. ethmoidal artery

nasociliary artery

lacrimal artery

post. ciliary arteries

optic nerve in dural sheath

internal carotid artery

ophthalmic artery

A. Schematic drawing of the arteries of the orbital cavity and eyeball.

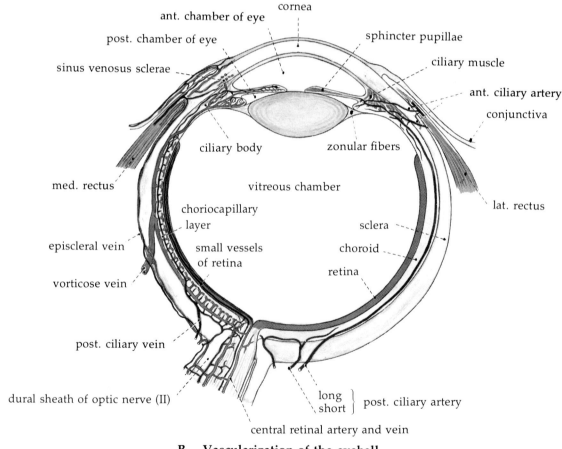

cornea

ant. chamber of eye

post. chamber of eye

sphincter pupillae

sinus venosus sclerae

ciliary muscle

ant. ciliary artery

conjunctiva

ciliary body

zonular fibers

med. rectus

vitreous chamber

lat. rectus

choriocapillary layer

sclera

episcleral vein

choroid

small vessels of retina

retina

vorticose vein

post. ciliary vein

dural sheath of optic nerve (II)

long
short } post. ciliary artery

central retinal artery and vein

B. Vascularization of the eyeball.

¶ The aqueous humor is a plasma filtrate secreted by the vessels of the iris and ciliary body into the posterior chamber of the eye. Through the pupillary aperture it passes into the anterior chamber and is reabsorbed into the ciliary veins by way of the sinus venosus sclerae. When the drainage of the aqueous humor is impeded, the intraocular pressure rises (glaucoma). The intraocular pressure is determined in every routine examination of the eye, since glaucoma produces rapid degenerative changes in the retina.

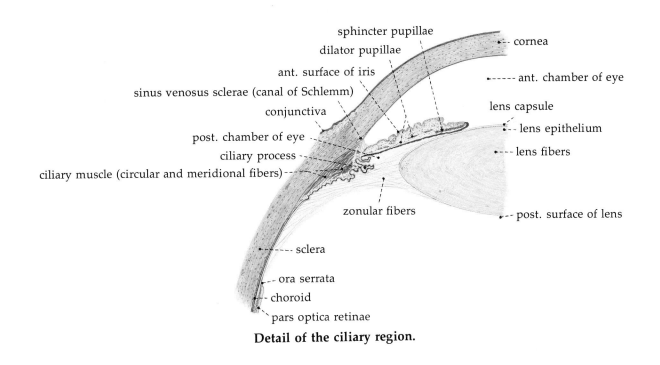

sphincter pupillae

dilator pupillae

ant. surface of iris

sinus venosus sclerae (canal of Schlemm)

conjunctiva

post. chamber of eye

ciliary process

ciliary muscle (circular and meridional fibers)

cornea

ant. chamber of eye

lens capsule

lens epithelium

lens fibers

post. surface of lens

zonular fibers

sclera

ora serrata

choroid

pars optica retinae

Detail of the ciliary region.

¶ The circular and meridional fibers of the ciliary muscle act on the lens through the zonular fibers. Contraction of both fiber groups pulls the ciliary body forward, relaxes the tension of the zonular fibers and allows the lens to become more convex. This increases the refractive power of the lens. The muscle receives postganglionic parasympathetic fibers from the ciliary ganglion through the oculomotor nerve. The sphincter pupillae constricts the pupil, and the radiating fibers—the dilator pupillae—open the pupil. (For paralysis of the parasympathetic and sympathetic innervation, see HN38.)

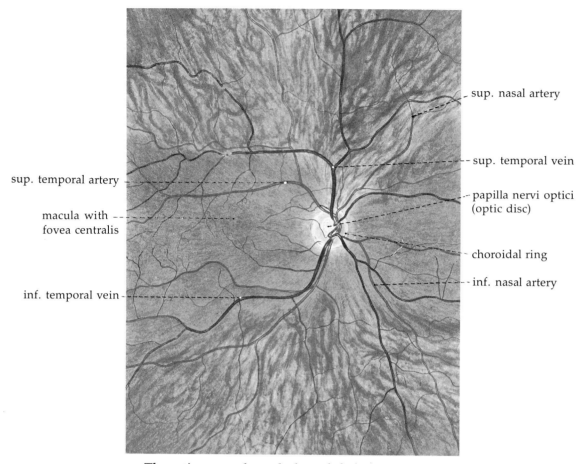

sup. nasal artery

sup. temporal vein

papilla nervi optici
(optic disc)

choroidal ring

inf. nasal artery

sup. temporal artery

macula with
fovea centralis

inf. temporal vein

The retina seen through the ophthalmoscope.
Note that the pigment of the choroid is visible through the retina.

A number of important observations should be made:

¶ The central artery of the retina passes through the optic nerve and can be seen to emerge from the papilla of the optic nerve. It then divides into upper and lower branches, which subsequently divide into nasal and temporal rami. The arteries and veins can be clearly seen through the ophthalmoscope, and their appearance may reflect a systemic disease such as arteriosclerosis.

¶ Near the center of the posterior part of the retina is a yellowish area, the macula. It is somewhat depressed and is, therefore, referred to as the fovea centralis. This area, lying exactly in the center of the optic axis of the eye, is the site of highest visual resolution. The pigment of the choroid can be seen through the fovea.

¶ Since the papilla of the nerve forms a weak spot in the posterior wall of the retina, it will protrude slightly forward in patients with increased intraorbital pressure, as caused by retrobulbar tumors.

¶ Increased intracranial pressure is also reflected at the papilla through the subarachnoid space around the optic nerve. The papilla may become edematous.

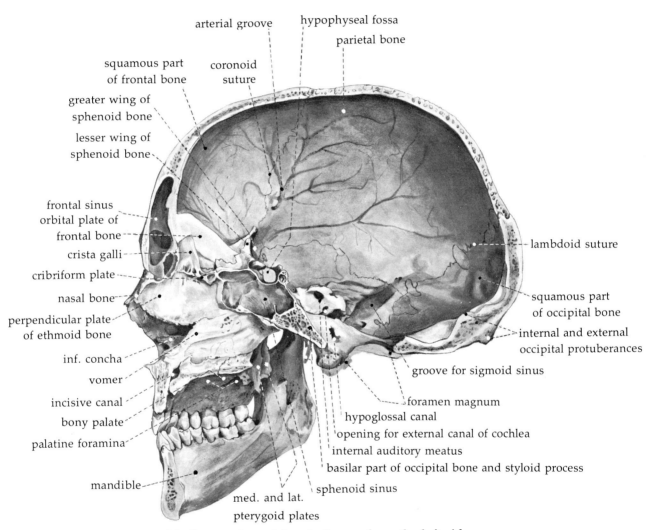

arterial groove

hypophyseal fossa

parietal bone

squamous part
of frontal bone

coronoid
suture

greater wing of
sphenoid bone

lesser wing of
sphenoid bone

frontal sinus

orbital plate of
frontal bone

crista galli

cribriform plate

nasal bone

perpendicular plate
of ethmoid bone

inf. concha

vomer

incisive canal

bony palate

palatine foramina

mandible

lambdoid suture

squamous part
of occipital bone

internal and external
occipital protuberances

groove for sigmoid sinus

foramen magnum

hypoglossal canal

opening for external canal of cochlea

internal auditory meatus

basilar part of occipital bone and styloid process

sphenoid sinus

med. and lat.
pterygoid plates

Median section of the skull seen from the left side.

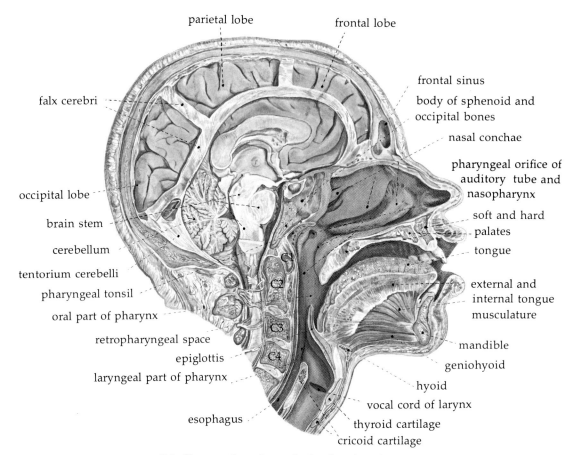

Median section through the head and neck.

Make the following observations:

¶ The oral cavity is mainly occupied by the tongue. When the uvula is lifted, the cavity of the mouth is in open communication with the oropharynx. From here food will descend into the laryngeal portion of the pharynx and the esophagus. Note the opening of the larynx into the laryngopharynx. The mechanism of swallowing is discussed at HN113.

¶ Superiorly, the oropharynx opens into the nasopharynx, in which are located the openings of the auditory tubes from the middle ear and the posterior nasal apertures, also known as the choanae. Hence, infections of the nasopharynx may easily spread to the middle ear and the nasal cavities.

¶ When the posterior wall of the pharynx is examined through the oral cavity, it is important to realize that the body of the axis and the anterior arch of the atlas are located immediately behind the pharyngeal wall. Between the two structures, however, is the retropharyngeal space, through which infections from the cervical region may descend into the thorax (see HN81).

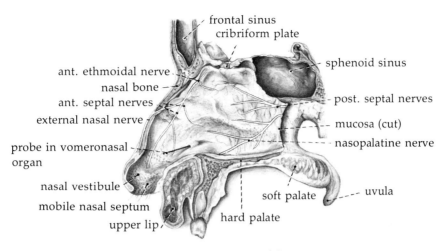

A. The nasal septum and its nerves.

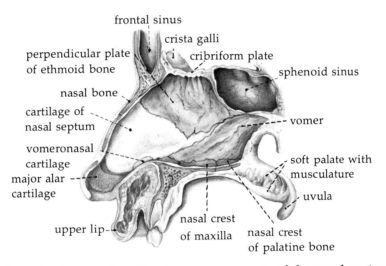

B. The bony and cartilaginous components of the nasal septum.

Note:

¶ The nasal septum is innervated by branches of the anterior ethmoidal nerve, a branch of the nasociliary nerve (V_1) (anterior septal and external nasal nerves) and the nasopalatine nerve, a branch of the maxillary nerve (V_2). The nasopalatine nerve runs obliquely over the septum toward the incisive canal (see HN49), through which it passes to innervate the oral surface of the palate.

¶ The mucous membrane lining the septum and conchae is firmly attached to the underlying periosteum, forming a so-called mucoperiosteum. As is well known, the mucosa contains numerous mucous glands and a rich vascular network. The mucosa of the nose is continuous with that of the paranasal sinuses, and inflammation of the nasal mucosa frequently expands into the paranasal cavities.

¶ The vomeronasal organ is present in reptiles and receives twigs of the olfactory nerve. In man it is rudimentary and usually consists of a little pouch (2 to 6 mm long) supported by a small piece of cartilage, the vomeronasal cartilage. The vomeronasal organ probably represents a chemoreceptive area with a narrow range of chemical reception.

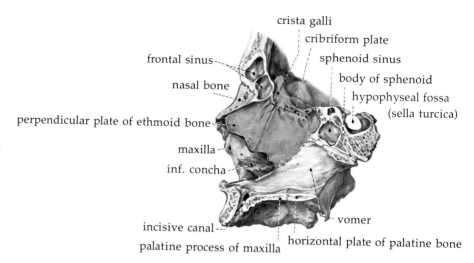

crista galli
cribriform plate
sphenoid sinus
frontal sinus
body of sphenoid
nasal bone
hypophyseal fossa
(sella turcica)
perpendicular plate of ethmoid bone
maxilla
inf. concha

incisive canal
vomer
palatine process of maxilla
horizontal plate of palatine bone

A. The bony components of the nasal septum.

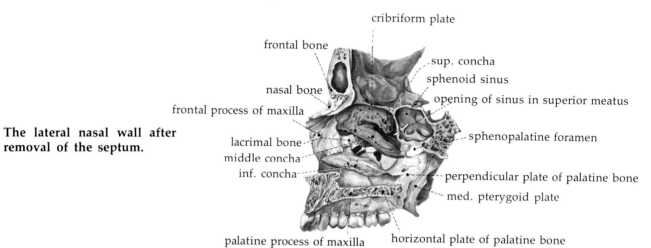

cribriform plate
frontal bone
sup. concha
sphenoid sinus
nasal bone
opening of sinus in superior meatus
frontal process of maxilla
lacrimal bone
sphenopalatine foramen
middle concha
inf. concha
perpendicular plate of palatine bone
med. pterygoid plate
palatine process of maxilla
horizontal plate of palatine bone

B. The lateral nasal wall after removal of the septum.

frontal bone
nasal bone
sphenoid bone
lacrimal bone
orbital cavity

inf. concha
ethmoid process
maxilla
lat. pterygoid plate

C. The lateral nasal wall after removal of the ethmoid bone.

probe in nasolacrimal
duct
nasal bone
lacrimal bone

D. The lateral nasal wall after removal of the inferior concha.
Note the entrance of the nasolacrimal duct.

Note:

¶ The superior and middle conchae are parts of the ethmoid bone; the inferior concha is an independent bone closely related to the maxilla (see HN34).

¶ The hard palate is formed by the palatine processes of the maxilla and by the horizontal plates of the palatine bones.

¶ The nasolacrimal duct passes through the lacrimal bone and enters the inferior meatus under the inferior concha (see HN18 *A*).

¶ The cribriform plates are part of the ethmoid bone. Special olfactory cells in the mucous membrane form axons, which ascend through the foramina in the cribriform plate to reach the olfactory bulb.

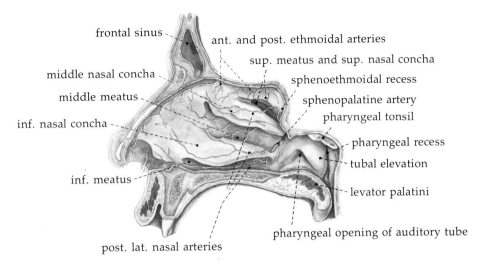

frontal sinus

ant. and post. ethmoidal arteries

sup. meatus and sup. nasal concha

middle nasal concha

sphenoethmoidal recess

middle meatus

sphenopalatine artery

pharyngeal tonsil

inf. nasal concha

pharyngeal recess

tubal elevation

inf. meatus

levator palatini

pharyngeal opening of auditory tube

post. lat. nasal arteries

A. Arteries of the lateral wall of the nasal cavity.

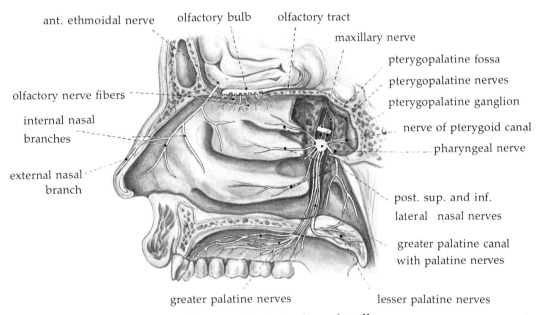

ant. ethmoidal nerve   olfactory bulb   olfactory tract

maxillary nerve

pterygopalatine fossa

pterygopalatine nerves

olfactory nerve fibers

pterygopalatine ganglion

internal nasal branches

nerve of pterygoid canal

pharyngeal nerve

external nasal branch

post. sup. and inf. lateral nasal nerves

greater palatine canal with palatine nerves

greater palatine nerves   lesser palatine nerves

B. Nerves of the lateral nasal wall.

Note:

⁋ The most important arteries of the nasal cavity are the sphenopalatine and the anterior and posterior ethmoidal arteries. Bleeding of the nose usually occurs at the septum, where the septal branches of the sphenopalatine meet the superior labial artery (branch of the facial artery). If the bleeding arteries are cauterized, an area of septal necrosis may result.

⁋ Although the pterygopalatine ganglion (see also HN51) is the largest parasympathetic ganglion, many sensory branches pass through it without interruption before joining the maxillary nerve: (a) the posterior superior and inferior lateral nasal nerves, which supply the nasal cavity; (b) the nasopalatine nerve, which descends obliquely over the nasal septum to the median incisive foramen and innervates the anterior part of the palate (see HN48 *A*); (c) the greater palatine nerves, which emerge through the greater palatine foramen to innervate the hard palate; (d) the lesser palatine nerve, which emerges through the lesser palatine foramen to innervate the soft palate and uvula; (e) the pharyngeal nerve, which supplies the roof of the pharynx and the sphenoid sinus.

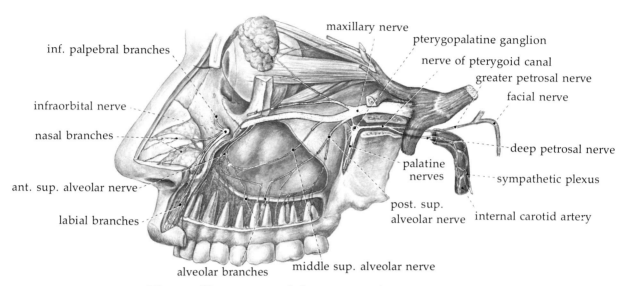

The maxillary nerve and the pterygopalatine ganglion.

The pterygopalatine ganglion is situated in the pterygopalatine fossa, just below the maxillary nerve. If necessary, the ganglion can be injected through the mandibular notch of the pterygopalatine fossa.

It has several roots:

¶ The *preganglionic parasympathetic (motor) fibers* originate from the facial nerve and reach the ganglion through the greater petrosal nerve, which passes through the pterygoid canal. These preganglionic fibers synapse in the ganglion, and the postganglionic fibers pass in various directions to their target organs. Some go to the lacrimal gland by way of the maxillary, zygomatic and lacrimal nerves (see also HN36 *B*); others pass to the mucous glands of the nasal cavity and palate as components of the branches of the maxillary nerve.

¶ The *sympathetic root* is derived from the plexus surrounding the internal carotid artery. These fibers travel by way of the deep petrosal nerve, then join the greater petrosal nerve to reach the ganglion. The two are known as the nerve of the pterygoid canal. The sympathetic fibers, which arise in the superior cervical ganglion, are postganglionic fibers. They pass through the ganglion without synapsing to join the parasympathetic fibers to the various glands.

¶ The *sensory root* has already been described (see HN50). In addition to the maxillary branches which pass through the sphenopalatine foramen, a number of other branches are sensory to the skin of the face (zygomaticotemporal, zygomaticofacial and infraorbital nerves). Another important group of nerves is formed by the posterior, middle and anterior superior alveolar branches. They supply the teeth, gums, cheeks and the wall of the maxillary sinus.

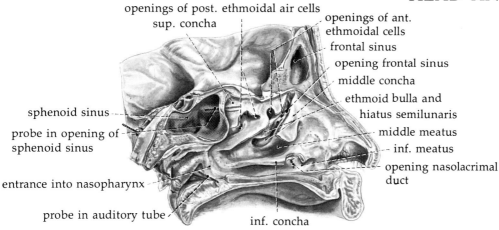

openings of post. ethmoidal air cells
sup. concha
openings of ant. ethmoidal cells
frontal sinus
opening frontal sinus
middle concha
ethmoid bulla and hiatus semilunaris
sphenoid sinus
probe in opening of sphenoid sinus
middle meatus
inf. meatus
opening nasolacrimal duct
entrance into nasopharynx
probe in auditory tube
inf. concha

A. Lateral wall of the left nasal cavity.

The conchae have been partially removed to show the openings of the paranasal sinuses. Note the ethmoid bulla caused by the medial expansion of the ethmoidal air cells and the hiatus semilunaris, through which the maxillary sinus drains into the middle meatus.

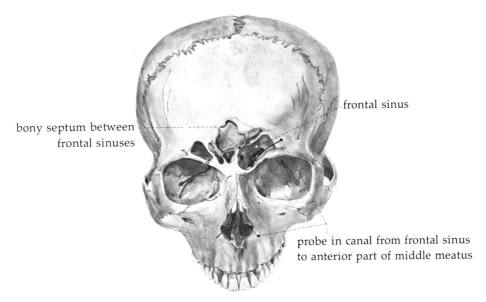

frontal sinus
bony septum between frontal sinuses
probe in canal from frontal sinus to anterior part of middle meatus

B. Frontal sinuses with subdivisions.

The paranasal sinuses (ethmoidal, frontal, maxillary, sphenoid) come to full development at the time of puberty (see also HN53 and HN54). They are large air-containing spaces lined with ciliated epithelium that communicate with the nasal cavity through narrow canals. When the mucous membranes of the nose are swollen because of infections or allergic reactions, the canals to the paranasal sinuses may easily become occluded.

The paranasal sinuses are clinically of great importance:

¶ The frontal sinuses, one located on each side of the midline, are frequently broken up into a number of subdivisions, which make drainage especially difficult. The sinuses are separated from the frontal lobes, the orbits and the ethmoidal cells by thin bony plates. Each frontal sinus drains directly into the anterior part of the middle meatus or through a narrow canal, the frontonasal duct (see *A*).

¶ When the frontal sinus is inflamed, the infection sometimes penetrates through the thin spots in the frontal bone and causes meningitis or a frontal lobe abscess. Another important point to remember is that when the bones of the frontal sinus fracture after severe trauma, the dura mater may be torn, and cerebrospinal fluid may then enter the frontal sinus and subsequently the nasal cavity. Cerebrospinal fluid leaking out of the nose usually indicates a severe fracture in the wall of the anterior cranial fossa.

¶ The sphenoid sinuses lie one on either side of the midline in the body of the sphenoid bone. Each sinus drains into the nasal cavity in the sphenoethmoidal recess. They are less frequently inflamed than the frontal sinuses (see also HN49 *B*).

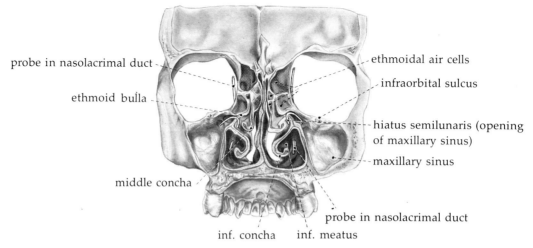

probe in nasolacrimal duct

ethmoid bulla

middle concha

ethmoidal air cells

infraorbital sulcus

hiatus semilunaris (opening of maxillary sinus)

maxillary sinus

probe in nasolacrimal duct

inf. concha   inf. meatus

A. Frontal section through the anterior part of the nasal cavity.

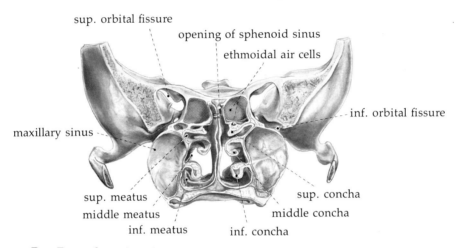

sup. orbital fissure

opening of sphenoid sinus

ethmoidal air cells

inf. orbital fissure

maxillary sinus

sup. meatus
middle meatus
inf. meatus

sup. concha
middle concha
inf. concha

B. Frontal section through the posterior part of the nasal cavity.

The maxillary sinus is the most potentially dangerous of the paranasal sinuses. It is pyramid-shaped and occupies the cavity of the maxilla. It is separated by thin bony plates from the orbit, from the roots of the upper premolar and molar teeth (see HN51) and from the ethmoidal air cells. The medial expansion of the ethmoid bulla may compress the drainage canal, which extends from the roof of the sinus into the middle meatus by means of the hiatus semilunaris. This makes the drainage of the sinus especially difficult.

¶ The maxillary sinus may easily become inflamed by infections originating in the nasal cavity or the roots of the upper molar and premolar teeth. Since the orifice of the maxillary sinus is close to that of the frontal sinus (HN52 *A*), infections of the frontal sinus are also frequently accompanied by inflammations of the maxillary sinus.

¶ The sinus is innervated by branches of the infraorbital nerve. In addition, several branches of the maxillary nerve to the teeth pass under the mucoperiosteum of the walls of the sinus. Hence, inflammations of the maxillary sinus may affect the nerves and cause severe toothache. The sinus can be drained relatively easily by opening the medial wall of the sinus below the inferior concha.

¶ Cancer of the maxillary sinus may cause various symptoms, depending on its location in the sinus: (a) it may invade the orbit, displace the eyeball and cause diplopia; (b) it may involve the infraorbital nerve and cause facial pain over the skin of the maxilla; (c) it may involve the nasal cavity, producing obstruction and blockage of the nasolacrimal duct; or (d) it may affect the palatine and superior alveolar nerves and cause severe pain in the palate and upper teeth (see HN51).

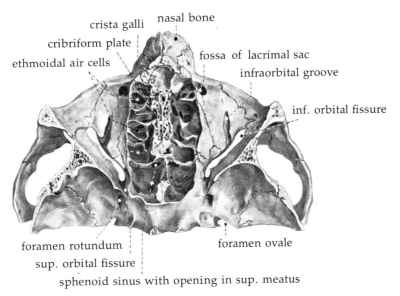

crista galli   nasal bone
cribriform plate
ethmoidal air cells
fossa of lacrimal sac
infraorbital groove
inf. orbital fissure
foramen rotundum   foramen ovale
sup. orbital fissure
sphenoid sinus with opening in sup. meatus

A. Ethmoidal air cells seen from above.

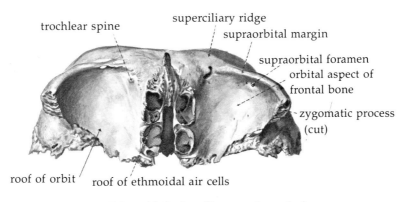

trochlear spine   superciliary ridge
supraorbital margin
supraorbital foramen
orbital aspect of
frontal bone
zygomatic process
(cut)
roof of orbit   roof of ethmoidal air cells

B. Ethmoidal air cells seen from below.

¶ The ethmoidal sinuses form a group of eight to ten air cells in the lateral part of the ethmoid bone. They are located between the orbit and the upper part of the nasal cavity. Superiorly they lie on each side of the cribriform plate, and their thin bony roofs are related to the frontal lobes.

¶ Infections of the ethmoidal air cells may result in meningitis and abscesses of the frontal lobes of the cerebral hemispheres. Similarly, since the air cells are separated from the orbit only by paper-thin bony septa, inflammations may spread to the orbit.

¶ Fractures of the base of the skull in the ethmoid region may cause leakage of cerebro-spinal fluid into the nasal cavity.

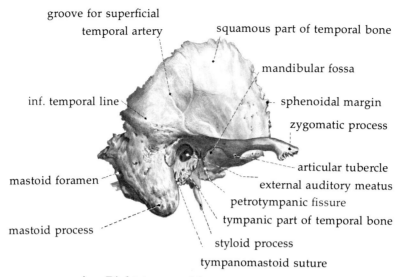

groove for superficial
temporal artery

squamous part of temporal bone

mandibular fossa

inf. temporal line

sphenoidal margin

zygomatic process

mastoid foramen

articular tubercle

external auditory meatus

petrotympanic fissure

tympanic part of temporal bone

mastoid process

styloid process

tympanomastoid suture

A. Right temporal bone, external aspect.

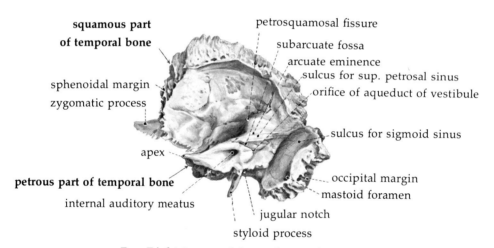

**squamous part
of temporal bone**

petrosquamosal fissure

subarcuate fossa

arcuate eminence

sulcus for sup. petrosal sinus

sphenoidal margin

zygomatic process

orifice of aqueduct of vestibule

sulcus for sigmoid sinus

apex

occipital margin

mastoid foramen

petrous part of temporal bone

internal auditory meatus

jugular notch

styloid process

B. Right temporal bone, internal aspect.

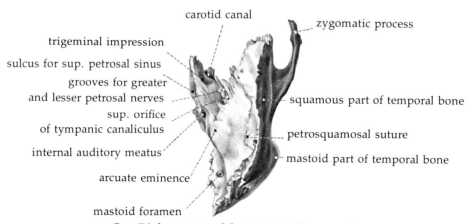

carotid canal

zygomatic process

trigeminal impression

sulcus for sup. petrosal sinus

grooves for greater
and lesser petrosal nerves

sup. orifice
of tympanic canaliculus

squamous part of temporal bone

petrosquamosal suture

internal auditory meatus

mastoid part of temporal bone

arcuate eminence

mastoid foramen

C. Right temporal bone, superior aspect.

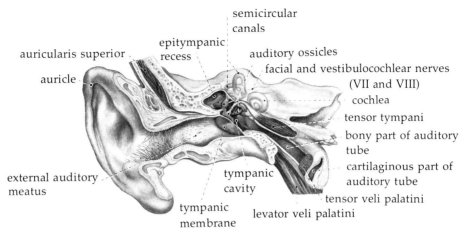

semicircular canals

epitympanic recess

auricularis superior

auricle

auditory ossicles

facial and vestibulocochlear nerves (VII and VIII)

cochlea

tensor tympani

bony part of auditory tube

cartilaginous part of auditory tube

tensor veli palatini

levator veli palatini

tympanic cavity

external auditory meatus

tympanic membrane

A. Frontal section through external, middle and inner ear.

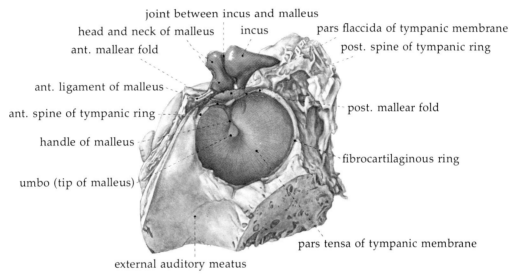

joint between incus and malleus

head and neck of malleus

incus

pars flaccida of tympanic membrane

ant. mallear fold

post. spine of tympanic ring

ant. ligament of malleus

ant. spine of tympanic ring

post. mallear fold

handle of malleus

fibrocartilaginous ring

umbo (tip of malleus)

pars tensa of tympanic membrane

external auditory meatus

B. Left tympanic membrane, external aspect.

In examining the external auditory meatus and eardrum, keep in mind:

¶ It is important to realize that the walls of the external auditory meatus consist of an external cartilaginous part and an inner bony part. By pulling the auricle upward and backward, the two parts can be brought somewhat in line with each other, and the otoscope can be inserted in a medial and slightly forward and downward direction to view the eardrum.

¶ The entire external auditory meatus is lined with skin. In the bony part the skin adheres tightly to the bony wall, but in the outer part it is separated from the cartilage by many sebaceous and ceruminous glands. These modified sweat glands secrete a yellowish brown wax.

¶ The eardrum consists of three layers: an outer membrane of ectodermal origin; an inner membrane of entodermal origin (first entodermal pharyngeal pouch), which is continuous with the mucoperiosteum of the tympanic cavity; and a middle fibrous layer of mesodermal origin which contains some small blood vessels.

¶ Inflammation of the tympanic membrane is extremely painful. The external surface is innervated by the auriculotemporal nerve (V_3) and the auricular branch of the vagus. The inner surface receives its sensory innervation from the tympanic branch of the glossopharyngeal nerve. When inflamed, the membrane becomes reddish and bulges outward. Spontaneous perforations are not uncommon.

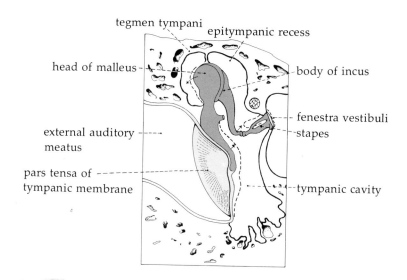

tegmen tympani
epitympanic recess
head of malleus
body of incus
external auditory meatus
fenestra vestibuli
stapes
pars tensa of tympanic membrane
tympanic cavity

A. **Schematic drawing of the auditory ossicles and their movements.**

post. ligament of incus
short limb of incus
epitympanic recess
incus
sup. ligament of incus
sup. ligament of malleus
joint between incus and malleus
malleus
ant. mallear fold
pars tensa of tympanic membrane
fibrocartilaginous ring

mastoid antrum
chorda tympani nerve
stapes
tip of manubrium of malleus (umbo)

floor of tympanic cavity

B. **Lateral wall of the left tympanic cavity.**
Viewed from within the tympanic cavity.

pars flaccida of tympanic membrane
epitympanic recess
tympanic notch
ant. mallear fold
mastoid antrum
post. mallear fold
attachment of tensor tympani
manubrium of malleus
tympanic orifice of auditory tube
pars tensa of tympanic membrane
umbo
fibrocartilaginous ring

C. **Right tympanic membrane.**
Seen from within the tympanic cavity.

¶ The handle of the malleus is displaced medially when sound waves reach the tympanic membrane (eardrum). The head of the malleus then moves laterally, since the neck is fixed by the anterior ligament. As a result, the body of the incus is pulled laterally. At the same time the long process of the incus moves medially, thereby pushing the base of the stapes medially onto the vestibular window. The vibrations of the ossicles thus cause waves in the perilymph which in turn stimulate the auditory receptors in the cochlea.

¶ The lateral wall of the tympanic cavity is formed by the tympanic membrane and the squamous part of the temporal bone forming the wall of the epitympanic recess. Since most of the wall of the tympanic cavity is bony, inflammations of the middle ear result in accumulation of fluid and pus, which causes the eardrum to bulge laterally.

¶ The tympanic membrane is fixed peripherally through a fibrocartilaginous ring in a bony groove, the tympanic sulcus. The groove is deficient superiorly where it forms a notch. Two bands, the anterior and posterior mallear folds, pass from the edges of the notch to the lateral process of the malleus. The triangular area bounded by the folds is slack and is called the "pars flaccida" of the eardrum.

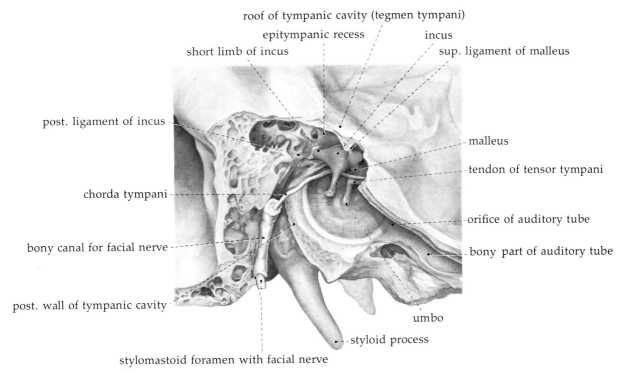

roof of tympanic cavity (tegmen tympani)

epitympanic recess

incus

short limb of incus

sup. ligament of malleus

post. ligament of incus

malleus

tendon of tensor tympani

chorda tympani

orifice of auditory tube

bony canal for facial nerve

bony part of auditory tube

post. wall of tympanic cavity

umbo

styloid process

stylomastoid foramen with facial nerve

A. The tympanic cavity and the chorda tympani.

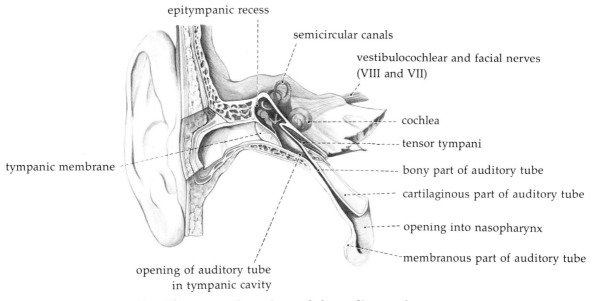

epitympanic recess

semicircular canals

vestibulocochlear and facial nerves (VIII and VII)

cochlea

tensor tympani

tympanic membrane

bony part of auditory tube

cartilaginous part of auditory tube

opening into nasopharynx

membranous part of auditory tube

opening of auditory tube in tympanic cavity

B. The tympanic cavity and the auditory tube.

Note the following important points:

¶ The chorda tympani leaves the facial canal to enter the tympanic cavity and passes between the malleus and the incus. Subsequently, it enters the temporal bone which it leaves again through the petrotympanic fissure to join the lingual nerve (see HN90). The chorda tympani contains gustatory fibers from the anterior two-thirds of the tongue and preganglionic parasympathetic fibers to the submandibular ganglion for secretomotor innervation of the submandibular and sublingual glands (for further details, see HN91).

¶ The relation of the auditory tube to the tympanic cavity is of great clinical importance. The tube courses from the anterior part of the tympanic cavity in a medial, forward and downward direction to enter the nasopharynx (see HN47). It is about 1½ inches long and functions to keep the air pressure on each side of the membrane equal. In patients with inflammations of the nose, tonsils and pharynx, the tissues around the pharyngeal entrance of the tube become edematous, and the duct may be closed off. Infections from the nose and throat also ascend to the tympanic cavity and frequently cause otitis media. Small babies and children are particularly prone to this complication, since the course of the duct in children is more horizontal than it is in adults.

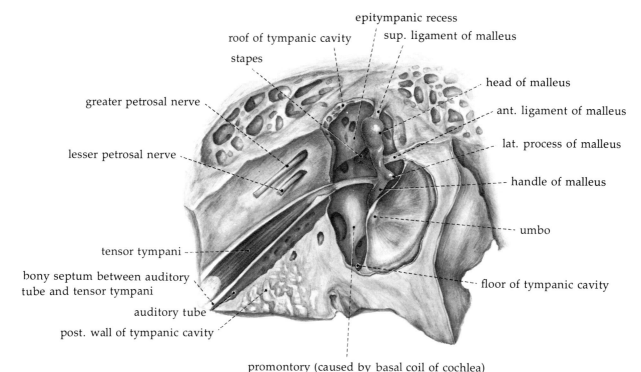

epitympanic recess

roof of tympanic cavity

sup. ligament of malleus

stapes

head of malleus

greater petrosal nerve

ant. ligament of malleus

lesser petrosal nerve

lat. process of malleus

handle of malleus

umbo

tensor tympani

bony septum between auditory
tube and tensor tympani

floor of tympanic cavity

auditory tube

post. wall of tympanic cavity

promontory (caused by basal coil of cochlea)

A. The medial wall of the left tympanic cavity and the tensor tympani.
Part of the eardrum has been removed.

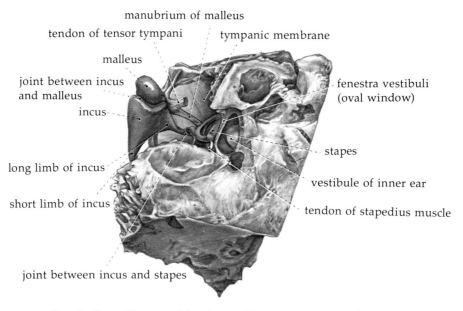

manubrium of malleus

tendon of tensor tympani

tympanic membrane

malleus

joint between incus
and malleus

incus

fenestra vestibuli
(oval window)

long limb of incus

stapes

vestibule of inner ear

short limb of incus

tendon of stapedius muscle

joint between incus and stapes

B. Left auditory ossicles in position; posterosuperior view.
The roof of the tympanic cavity has been removed.

Note:

¶ The tensor tympani muscle runs parallel to the auditory tube. It attaches to the handle of the malleus with a small tendon, and its function is to dampen vibrations of the malleus by making the tympanic membrane more tense. Since the malleus and the incus are derivatives of the first pharyngeal arch, the muscle is innervated by the mandibular branch of the trigeminal nerve.

¶ The stapedius muscle (only the tendon is visible in *B*) attaches to the stapes. Since the stapes is derived from the second pharyngeal arch, the stapedius is innervated by a small branch of the facial nerve.

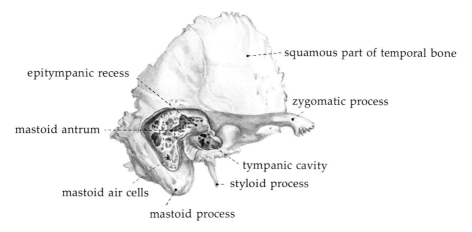

epitympanic recess

squamous part of temporal bone

zygomatic process

mastoid antrum

tympanic cavity

styloid process

mastoid air cells

mastoid process

A. Right temporal bone showing epitympanic recess, mastoid antrum and air cells.

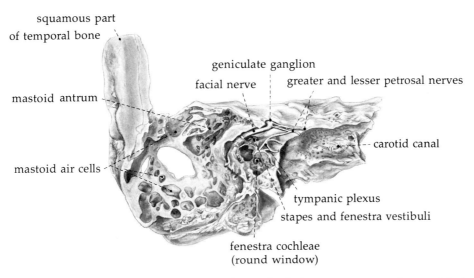

squamous part
of temporal bone

geniculate ganglion

facial nerve

greater and lesser petrosal nerves

mastoid antrum

carotid canal

mastoid air cells

tympanic plexus

stapes and fenestra vestibuli

fenestra cochleae
(round window)

B. Medial wall of the right tympanic cavity and relation to antrum and mastoid air cells.

Note:

¶ The mastoid antrum is the first portion of the mastoid bone to be formed. After formation of the mastoid process, it gradually attains a deeper position. The antrum is continuous with the epitympanic recess, but the connection between the two, the aditus to the antrum, is often narrow.

¶ The relation of the mastoid antrum to its surrounding structures is of utmost importance. When infections of the nose and throat enter the tympanic cavity through the auditory tube, they spread easily to the epitympanic recess and through the aditus into the antrum. From the antrum the infection may spread to the mastoid air cells. More dangerous, however, is the extension of the infection through the bony walls of the antrum. When spreading posteriorly, the infection may cause thrombus formation in the transverse sinus, meningitis or an abscess in the cerebellum. When spreading superiorly, it may cause meningitis or an abscess in the temporal lobe.

¶ The tympanic plexus is formed by the tympanic branch of the glossopharyngeal nerve. It lies in grooves in the promontory and innervates the mucosa of the tympanic cavity. The plexus gives off the lesser petrosal nerve (HN89) which contains secretomotor fibers for the parotid gland. The nerve leaves the skull through the foramen ovale and joins the otic ganglion (see HN91).

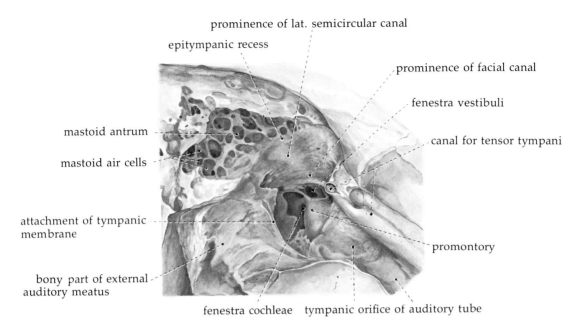

prominence of lat. semicircular canal

epitympanic recess

prominence of facial canal

fenestra vestibuli

mastoid antrum

canal for tensor tympani

mastoid air cells

attachment of tympanic membrane

promontory

bony part of external auditory meatus

fenestra cochleae   tympanic orifice of auditory tube

A. Lateral view of the medial wall of the right tympanic cavity.

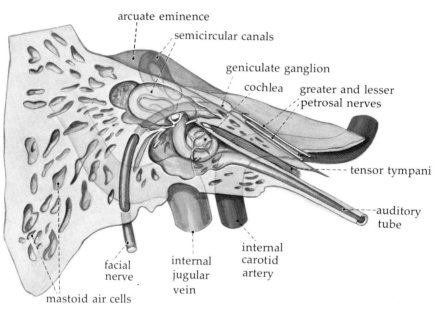

arcuate eminence

semicircular canals

geniculate ganglion

cochlea   greater and lesser petrosal nerves

tensor tympani

auditory tube

facial nerve   internal jugular vein   internal carotid artery

mastoid air cells

B. Relation of the right internal ear to the middle ear cavity.
The medial wall of the tympanic cavity has been partially removed.

When examining the medial wall of the tympanic cavity, a number of points should be noted:

¶ The promontory is the most prominent feature of the medial wall. It is caused by the large basal coil of the cochlea.

¶ Just above the fenestra vestibuli (oval window) is a ridge-shaped prominence caused by the canal of the facial nerve.

¶ The prominence in the wall of the epitympanic recess is caused by the lateral semicircular canal.

¶ The fenestra vestibuli gives access to the vestibule of the inner ear and the scala vestibuli (see HN64).

¶ The fenestra cochleae (round window) gives access to the scala tympani (HN64).

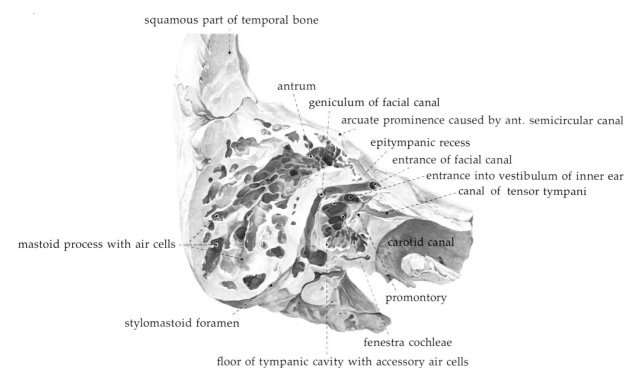

squamous part of temporal bone

antrum

geniculum of facial canal

arcuate prominence caused by ant. semicircular canal

epitympanic recess

entrance of facial canal

entrance into vestibulum of inner ear

canal of tensor tympani

mastoid process with air cells

carotid canal

promontory

stylomastoid foramen

fenestra cochleae

floor of tympanic cavity with accessory air cells

A. Medial wall of the right tympanic cavity with facial canal opened.

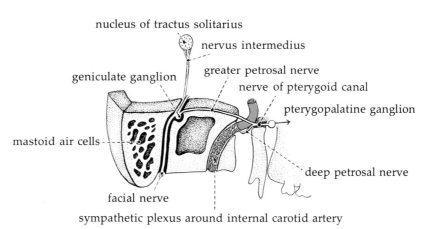

nucleus of tractus solitarius

nervus intermedius

geniculate ganglion

greater petrosal nerve

nerve of pterygoid canal

pterygopalatine ganglion

mastoid air cells

deep petrosal nerve

facial nerve

sympathetic plexus around internal carotid artery

B. The geniculate ganglion and greater petrosal nerve.

The course of the facial nerve through the temporal bone is complicated and should be examined carefully. A precise knowledge of its course and the various branches it gives off in the bone is of great diagnostic value (see HN63).

¶ The facial nerve enters the internal auditory meatus accompanied by the vestibulocochlear nerve. At the bottom of the meatus the two nerves separate, and the facial nerve enters the facial canal (see HN66).

¶ In the facial canal the nerve extends at first laterally above the vestibule of the inner ear. When it reaches the epitympanic recess, it bends sharply posteriorly and then runs inferiorly in the medial wall of the tympanic antrum. Finally, the nerve emerges through the stylomastoid foramen.

¶ In the petrous part of the temporal bone the greater petrosal nerve emerges at the geniculate ganglion. It lies on the superior surface of the petrous part of the temporal bone (HN59 A, HN61 B) and carries preganglionic parasympathetic fibers to the pterygopalatine ganglion (see also HN51).

¶ In its further course through the bone the facial nerve gives off the chorda tympani (HN58 A) and a motor branch to the stapedius muscle.

¶ Keep in mind that the smaller part of the facial nerve is formed by the nervus intermedius. This nerve contains the taste fibers of the chorda tympani and the secretomotor fibers for the lacrimal and salivary glands. The cells of origin of the gustatory fibers are located in the geniculate ganglion.

413

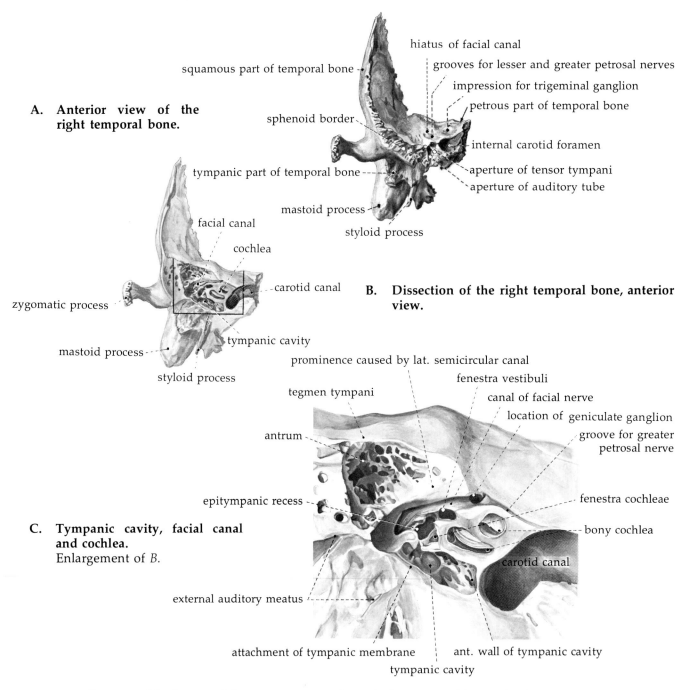

A. Anterior view of the right temporal bone.

hiatus of facial canal

squamous part of temporal bone

grooves for lesser and greater petrosal nerves

impression for trigeminal ganglion

petrous part of temporal bone

sphenoid border

internal carotid foramen

tympanic part of temporal bone

aperture of tensor tympani

aperture of auditory tube

mastoid process

styloid process

facial canal

cochlea

zygomatic process

carotid canal

B. Dissection of the right temporal bone, anterior view.

mastoid process

tympanic cavity

styloid process

prominence caused by lat. semicircular canal

fenestra vestibuli

tegmen tympani

canal of facial nerve

location of geniculate ganglion

antrum

groove for greater petrosal nerve

epitympanic recess

fenestra cochleae

C. Tympanic cavity, facial canal and cochlea.
Enlargement of B.

bony cochlea

carotid canal

external auditory meatus

attachment of tympanic membrane

ant. wall of tympanic cavity

tympanic cavity

Because of its long and dangerous course through the temporal bone, the facial nerve is susceptible to damage by infections and surgical procedures in the middle ear. A thorough knowledge of the course of the nerve and its relation to other cranial nerves makes it relatively easy to diagnose the place of a nerve injury.

¶ If the facial musculature and the lateral rectus of the eye are paralyzed, the lesion is probably in the pons of the brain, where the nuclei of the facial and abducens nerves lie close together.

¶ If the facial musculature is nonfunctional and the patient is deaf, the lesion is probably close to the internal auditory meatus. At this point the seventh and eighth nerves enter the petrous part of the temporal bone together.

¶ If the lesion involves the nerve to the stapedius, the patient will be extremely sensitive to sound, since the stapedius will be unable to prevent extreme vibrations of the vestibular window.

¶ Sometimes the lesion of the facial nerve is below the origin of the branch to the stapedius, and in such cases the chorda tympani is affected. The characteristic complaint of these patients is loss of taste on the anterior two-thirds of the tongue.

¶ If the facial nerve is damaged below the origin of the chorda tympani, the facial musculature will be paralyzed (HN10), but taste sensations from the anterior two-thirds of the tongue will be unaffected.

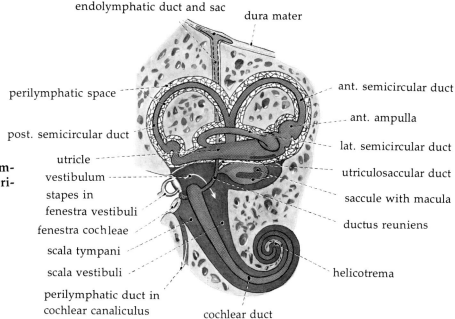

endolymphatic duct and sac

dura mater

perilymphatic space

ant. semicircular duct

ant. ampulla

post. semicircular duct

lat. semicircular duct

utricle

vestibulum

utriculosaccular duct

stapes in
fenestra vestibuli

saccule with macula

fenestra cochleae

ductus reuniens

scala tympani

scala vestibuli

perilymphatic duct in
cochlear canaliculus

helicotrema

cochlear duct

A. Schematic drawing of the membranous labyrinth and perilymphatic space.

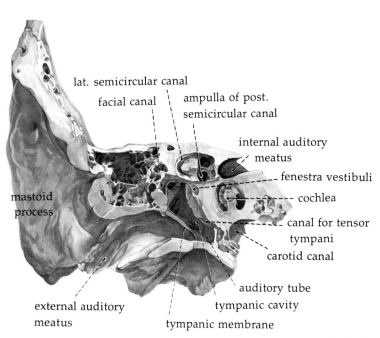

lat. semicircular canal

facial canal

ampulla of post.
semicircular canal

internal auditory
meatus

fenestra vestibuli

mastoid
process

cochlea

canal for tensor
tympani

carotid canal

auditory tube

external auditory
meatus

tympanic cavity

tympanic membrane

B. Right tympanic cavity and its relation to the labyrinth.

¶ When sound vibrations move the tympanic membrane, the base of the stapes is pushed medially in the fenestra vestibuli. The vibrations are thus communicated to the perilymph in the vestibulum and scala vestibuli. Since the perilymph cannot be compressed, the vibrations travel through the scala vestibuli and then return via the scala tympani, thus causing the membrane in the fenestra cochleae to bulge and dissipating the wave of energy.

¶ Occasionally the membrane in the fenestra vestibuli becomes sclerotic and may even ossify. The result is deafness. In such patients the ossified membrane may be replaced with an artificial membrane. In these operations great care must be taken to avoid damaging the facial nerve and the chorda tympani.

A. Right temporal bone, anterior view.
The bone is dissected to show the cochlea and semicircular canals.

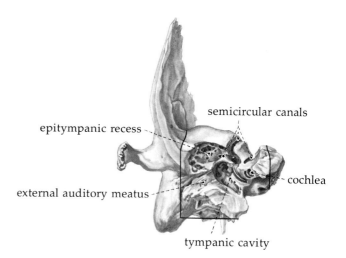

epitympanic recess

semicircular canals

external auditory meatus

cochlea

tympanic cavity

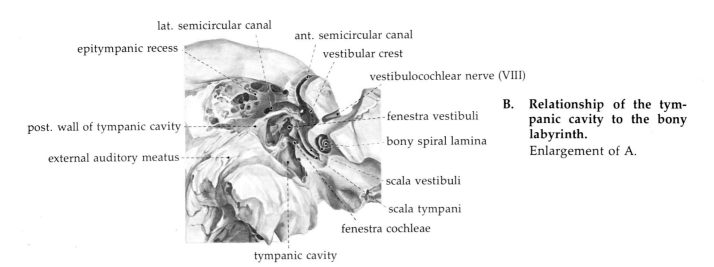

lat. semicircular canal

epitympanic recess

ant. semicircular canal

vestibular crest

vestibulocochlear nerve (VIII)

post. wall of tympanic cavity

fenestra vestibuli

bony spiral lamina

external auditory meatus

scala vestibuli

scala tympani

fenestra cochleae

tympanic cavity

B. Relationship of the tympanic cavity to the bony labyrinth.
Enlargement of A.

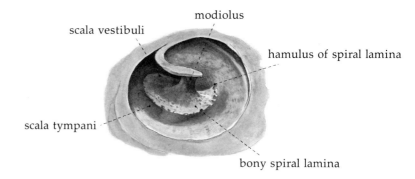

scala vestibuli

modiolus

hamulus of spiral lamina

scala tympani

bony spiral lamina

C. The right bony cochlea (opened).

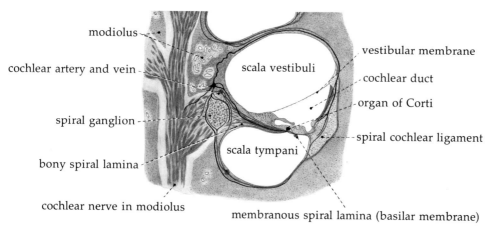

modiolus

cochlear artery and vein

scala vestibuli

vestibular membrane

cochlear duct

organ of Corti

spiral ganglion

spiral cochlear ligament

bony spiral lamina

scala tympani

cochlear nerve in modiolus

membranous spiral lamina (basilar membrane)

D. Section through the cochlea.

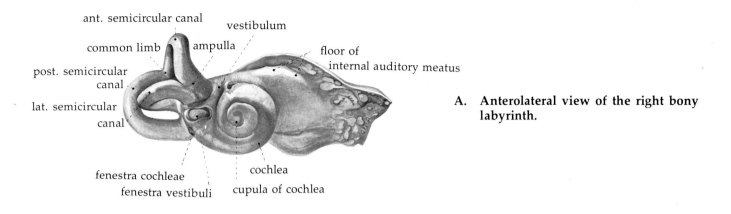

ant. semicircular canal
vestibulum
common limb
ampulla
floor of
internal auditory meatus
post. semicircular
canal
lat. semicircular
canal
fenestra cochleae
cochlea
fenestra vestibuli
cupula of cochlea

A. Anterolateral view of the right bony labyrinth.

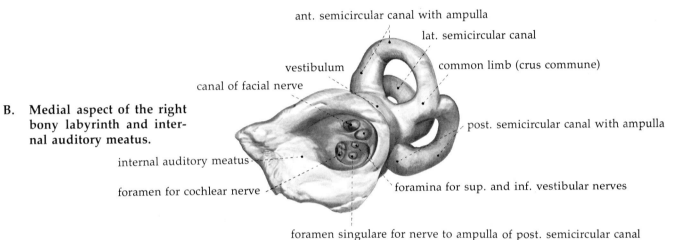

ant. semicircular canal with ampulla
lat. semicircular canal
vestibulum
common limb (crus commune)
canal of facial nerve
post. semicircular canal with ampulla
internal auditory meatus
foramen for cochlear nerve
foramina for sup. and inf. vestibular nerves
foramen singulare for nerve to ampulla of post. semicircular canal

B. Medial aspect of the right bony labyrinth and internal auditory meatus.

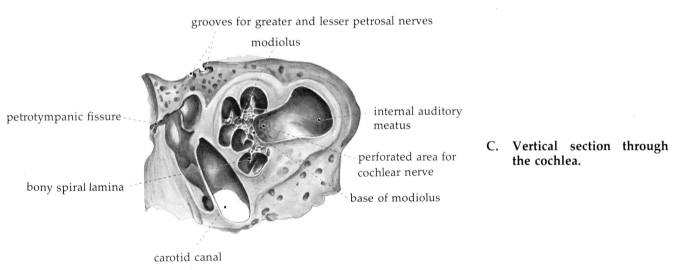

grooves for greater and lesser petrosal nerves
modiolus
petrotympanic fissure
internal auditory meatus
perforated area for cochlear nerve
bony spiral lamina
base of modiolus
carotid canal

C. Vertical section through the cochlea.

Although the vestibulocochlear and facial nerves enter the internal auditory meatus together, they separate almost immediately. Each nerve then enters its own canal (see *B*).

¶ The facial nerve enters the facial canal.

¶ The cochlear portion of the vestibulocochlear nerve splits from the main trunk and enters its canal to the modiolus.

¶ The vestibular portion splits into the superior and inferior vestibular nerves, each entering its own canal to supply part of the vestibular apparatus (see HN67*A*).

¶ A small portion of the vestibular nerve follows its own course and enters the foramen singulare to innervate the ampulla of the posterior semicircular canal.

A. Vestibulocochlear nerve and its branches.

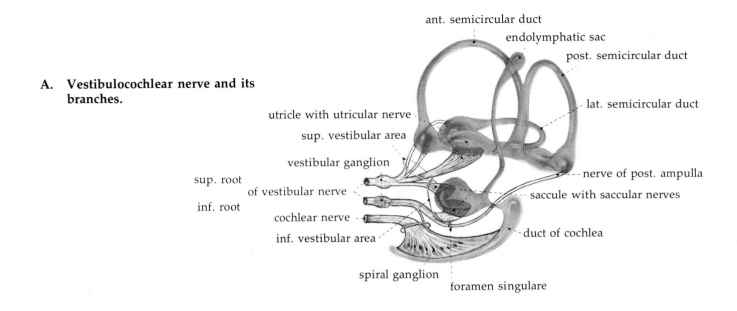

ant. semicircular duct
endolymphatic sac
post. semicircular duct
lat. semicircular duct
utricle with utricular nerve
sup. vestibular area
vestibular ganglion
sup. root
of vestibular nerve
inf. root
nerve of post. ampulla
saccule with saccular nerves
cochlear nerve
inf. vestibular area
duct of cochlea
spiral ganglion
foramen singulare

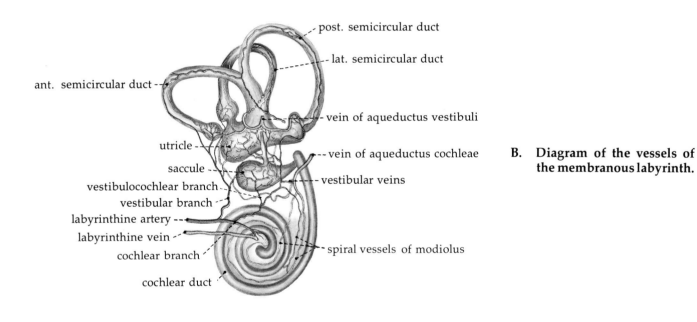

post. semicircular duct
lat. semicircular duct
ant. semicircular duct
vein of aqueductus vestibuli
utricle
saccule
vein of aqueductus cochleae
vestibulocochlear branch
vestibular branch
vestibular veins
labyrinthine artery
labyrinthine vein
cochlear branch
spiral vessels of modiolus
cochlear duct

B. Diagram of the vessels of the membranous labyrinth.

¶ Although the vestibulocochlear nerve enters the petrous bone as a single nerve, it soon divides into four branches, each with its own area of innervation: (a) the cochlear nerve supplies the organ of Corti; (b) the superior vestibular division supplies the utricle, the ampullae of the anterior and lateral semicircular canals and part of the saccule; (c) the inferior vestibular division innervates the saccule and part of the cochlea; and (d) the nerve for the ampulla of the posterior semicircular canal is a separate nerve which enters through the foramen singulare.

¶ Sometimes infection of the tympanic cavity spreads to the internal ear, causing labyrinthitis with vertigo and deafness. Usually, however, the cause of vertigo (giddiness) is found in the vestibulocochlear nerve. Disturbances of the vestibular function cause vertigo, vomiting and nystagmus, an uncontrollable pendular movement of the eyeballs. Lesions of the cochlear nerve become apparent as deafness and tinnitus.

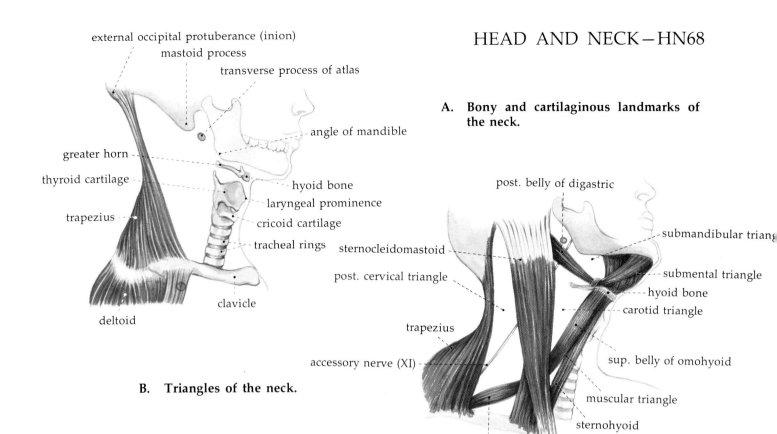

external occipital protuberance (inion)

mastoid process

transverse process of atlas

angle of mandible

greater horn

thyroid cartilage

trapezius

hyoid bone

laryngeal prominence

cricoid cartilage

tracheal rings

deltoid

clavicle

A. Bony and cartilaginous landmarks of the neck.

post. belly of digastric

sternocleidomastoid

post. cervical triangle

submandibular triangle

submental triangle

hyoid bone

carotid triangle

trapezius

accessory nerve (XI)

sup. belly of omohyoid

muscular triangle

sternohyoid

inf. belly of omohyoid

B. Triangles of the neck.

Palpate the following important landmarks:

¶ The *mastoid process.* In the newborn child the mastoid process is underdeveloped but comes to full development under the influence of the pull of the sternocleidomastoid during childhood.

¶ The *mandible.* The posterior border of the mandible is overlapped by the parotid gland, but its angle and the lower part of the posterior border can easily be palpated. Pulsations of the facial artery can be felt over the lower border of the mandible just in front of the masseter (see HN75 and HN82 *B*).

¶ The *transverse process of the atlas.* By pressing the fingertip upward between the mastoid process and the angle of the jaw, the most prominent of the transverse processes of the cervical vertebrae can be felt. Note that the atlas (C1) lies at the same level as the roof of the mouth.

¶ The *hyoid bone.* The hyoid lies at the angle between the floor of the mouth and the front of the neck. The greater horns of the hyoid bone can be felt by moving the thumb and index finger toward the sides of the body of the bone.

¶ The *laryngeal prominence* (Adam's apple). This structure is formed by the thyroid cartilage and is readily visible in men. It can be seen to move upward and downward during swallowing. The prominence lies opposite C4 (see HN47).

¶ The *cricoid cartilage.* The cricoid cartilage lies at the level of C6. The isthmus of the thyroid gland is situated below the cricoid cartilage in front of the second to fourth tracheal rings (see also HN123).

¶ The *rings of the trachea.* The first ring can be felt just below the cricoid cartilage.

Note the following important regions in the neck:

¶ The *posterior triangle* is bounded by the trapezius, sternocleidomastoid and the middle third of the clavicle. Its floor is formed by the scalenus muscles and the levator scapulae. Since the accessory nerve and the nerves of the brachial plexus traverse the lower half of the triangle, wounds in this region may cause serious nerve damage (see HN75).

¶ The *anterior triangle* is bounded by the sternocleidomastoid, the midline of the neck and the lower border of the mandible. It is subdivided into: (a) the carotid triangle, in which the pulse of the carotid arteries can easily be felt; (b) the submandibular triangle, which contains the submandibular gland and many submandibular lymph nodes; (c) the muscular triangle; and (d) the submental triangle with the submental lymph nodes.

419

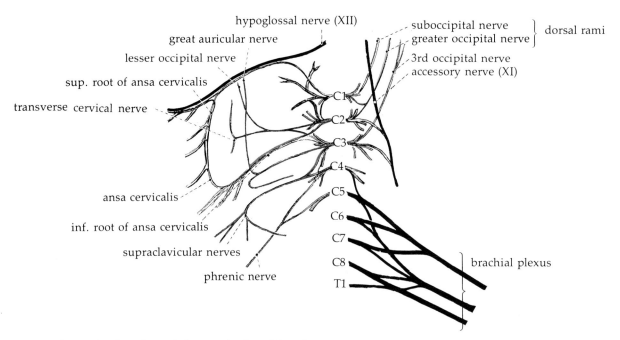

Schematic drawing of the cervical and brachial plexuses.
Cutaneous nerves of the ventral rami are shown in red, the motor nerves in yellow; the dorsal rami are blue.

The cervical plexus is formed by the ventral rami of the first four cervical nerves. Like all other ventral rami, these contain sensory cutaneous as well as motor branches.

¶ *Cutaneous nerves* (keep in mind the ventral ramus of C1 has no cutaneous branch)

1. Lesser occipital nerve: branch of ventral ramus of C2 (C3?).

2. Great auricular nerve: branch of ventral rami of C2 and C3.

3. Transverse cutaneous nerve of the neck (transverse cervical nerve): branch of ventral rami of C2 and C3.

4. Supraclavicular nerves: branches of ventral rami of C3 and C4.

¶ *Motor (muscular) nerves*

1. An important motor branch from C1 joins the hypoglossal nerve, but a portion of it leaves the nerve again to form the *superior root* of the ansa cervicalis (see HN76 *A*).

2. Motor branches of C2 and C3 unite to form the *inferior root* of the ansa cervicalis. The two roots form the *ansa cervicalis,* which in turn provides branches to the sternohyoid, omohyoid and sternothyroid muscles. Other fibers of C1 continue with the hypoglossal nerve to innervate the thyrohyoid and geniohyoid muscles. (The hypoglossal nerve itself supplies the extrinsic and intrinsic muscles of the tongue [see HN92 and HN93].)

3. The phrenic nerve originates from C4 but frequently receives branches from C3 and C5.

4. Cervical branches of C2 and C3 join the accessory nerve to the sternocleidomastoid and the trapezius muscles. These cervical components are probably proprioceptive.

The dorsal rami of the cervical segments carry motor as well as sensory fibers. They supply the dorsal musculature and small areas of the skin close to the midline. Note:

¶ The suboccipital nerve (C1) supplies motor innervation to the suboccipital musculature (see B17), but usually has no cutaneous distribution.

¶ The greater occipital nerve (C2) supplies mainly the skin of the suboccipital and occipital regions extending to the vertex (see HN20 *A*).

¶ The third occipital nerve (C3) supplies sensory innervation to the suboccipital region.

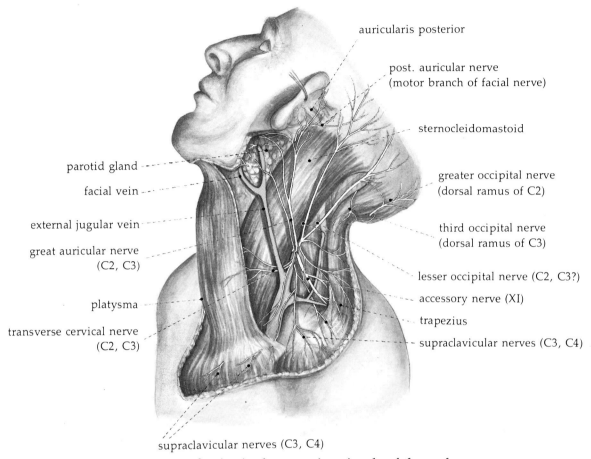

Nerves and veins in the posterior triangle of the neck.

Labels on the figure:

auricularis posterior

post. auricular nerve (motor branch of facial nerve)

sternocleidomastoid

greater occipital nerve (dorsal ramus of C2)

third occipital nerve (dorsal ramus of C3)

lesser occipital nerve (C2, C3?)

accessory nerve (XI)

trapezius

supraclavicular nerves (C3, C4)

parotid gland

facial vein

external jugular vein

great auricular nerve (C2, C3)

platysma

transverse cervical nerve (C2, C3)

supraclavicular nerves (C3, C4)

¶ The external jugular vein, located within the superficial fascia of the neck, courses from the angle of the mandible over the sternocleidomastoid toward the midpoint of the clavicle to drain into the subclavian vein. Clinically it serves as a venous manometer. In the supine position the level of the blood in the vein reaches about one-third of the way into the neck. In patients with right heart failure and high venous pressure the level may reach much higher, and in extreme cases it reaches almost to the angle of the mandible.

¶ The accessory nerve emerges from the posterior border of the sternocleidomastoid muscle, passes in a superficial position through the posterior triangle (HN68 B) and then enters the trapezius. When the nerve in the posterior triangle is cut during surgery or as a result of penetrating wounds, the trapezius will be paralyzed. The muscle will atrophy, and the patient will be unable to raise his arm above the horizontal position on the affected side. The sternocleidomastoid will not be affected.

¶ Note the sensory branches of the cervical plexus. Remember also that the posterior auricular nerve is a motor branch of the facial nerve and innervates the auricularis posterior and the occipital belly of the occipitofrontalis.

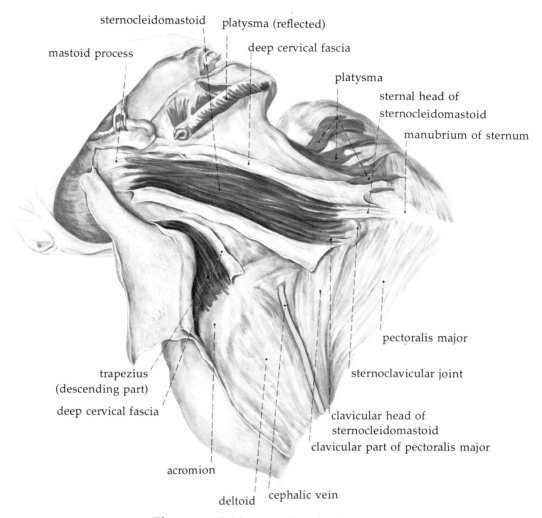

The sternocleidomastoid and platysma.

Note the following interesting points:

⸭ The platysma forms a thin muscular sheet in the superficial fascia. It is of little importance, but in a transverse incision in the neck, the platysma should be sutured as a separate layer. If not, the muscle fibers may pull the wound open again. The platysma belongs to the musculature of the second arch and is, therefore, innervated by the facial nerve (see also HN10).

⸭ The sternocleidomastoid in the fetus is sometimes excessively stretched during a difficult birth, which results in a hemorrhage in the muscle. During the healing process the hemorrhagic area is invaded by fibrous tissue, and the muscle contracts and shortens. The mastoid process and the head are pulled down toward the affected side, the cervical spine becomes somewhat flexed and rotated, and the face is turned upward to the opposite side. The syndrome is known as *congenital torticollis.*

⸭ The sternocleidomastoid is innervated by the accessory nerve. Some branches of C2 and C3 also enter the muscle, but these are probably proprioceptive. When the muscle is paralyzed, the action of the sternocleidomastoid on the opposite side causes the same symptoms as in torticollis.

⸭ Note the investing layer of the deep cervical fascia that sheathes the sternocleidomastoid and trapezius and forms the floor of the posterior triangle of the neck.

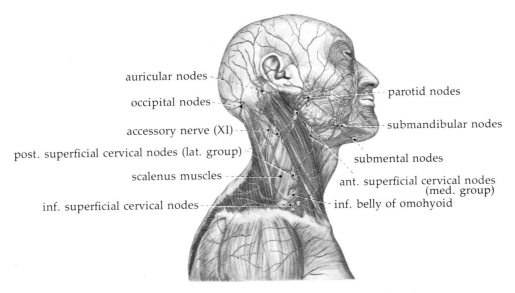

A. Superficial lymph nodes of the head and neck.

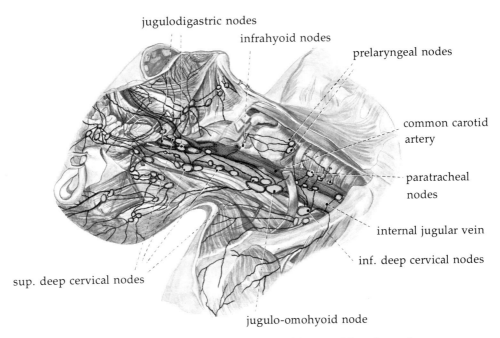

B. Deep cervical lymph nodes and internal jugular vein.
The sternocleidomastoid has been reflected.

¶ Enlargement of the submandibular lymph nodes may be caused by infections of the face, including infections in the region of the eye, the maxillary sinus, the tongue and lips, the submandibular and sublingual glands, and the teeth of the upper and lower jaws. The submental nodes drain mainly the central part of the lower lip and the tip of the tongue.

¶ The occipital, posterior auricular and parotid nodes drain the scalp, mastoid process, external meatus, tympanic cavity, parotid gland, lateral orbital regions and part of the nasal cavity. Inflammations in these regions may cause swellings of the nodes.

¶ Ultimately, most of the lymph of the head and neck drains to the deep cervical nodes along the internal jugular vein. When these nodes are invaded by metastases, the primary cancer is not always easy to find. Keep in mind that metastases of cancers of the larynx, pharynx, esophagus and external auditory meatus may settle in the deep cervical lymph nodes.

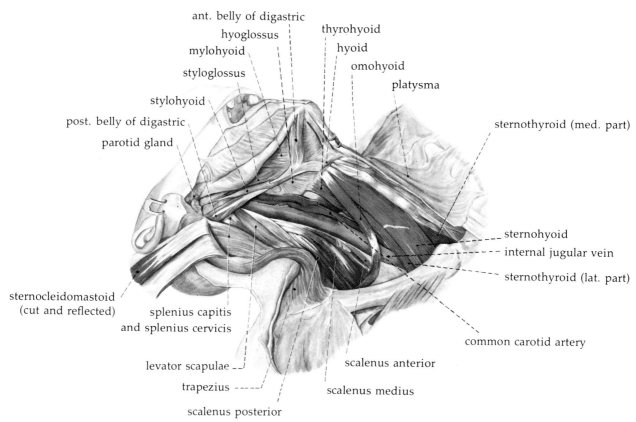

ant. belly of digastric
hyoglossus
mylohyoid
styloglossus
stylohyoid
post. belly of digastric
parotid gland
thyrohyoid
hyoid
omohyoid
platysma
sternothyroid (med. part)
sternohyoid
internal jugular vein
sternothyroid (lat. part)
common carotid artery
sternocleidomastoid
(cut and reflected)
splenius capitis
and splenius cervicis
levator scapulae
trapezius
scalenus posterior
scalenus medius
scalenus anterior

Muscles of the neck.
The sternocleidomastoid has been cut and reflected.

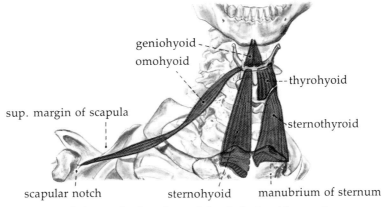

A. Schematic drawing of the infrahyoid muscles.

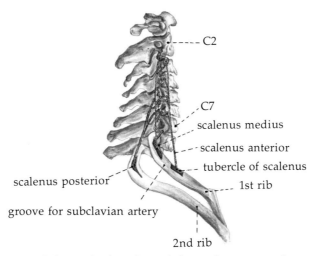

B. Schematic drawing of the scalenus muscles.

Before starting the dissection of the nerves and vessels of the neck, it is useful to study the innervation of the muscles (see also HN93):

¶ The *infrahyoid muscles*

1. The sternohyoid	
2. The omohyoid	Innervated by the ventral rami of C1, C2 and C3.
3. The sternothyroid	
4. The thyrohyoid	

¶ The *scalenus muscles*

1. The scalenus anterior to the first rib	
2. The scalenus medius to the first rib	Innervated by the ventral rami of C4, C5 and C6.
3. The scalenus posterior to the second rib	

4. The levator scapulae to the medial border of the scapula (innervated by the ventral rami of C3 and C4).

5. The splenius capitis and cervicis (innervated by the dorsal rami of C3, C4 and C5).

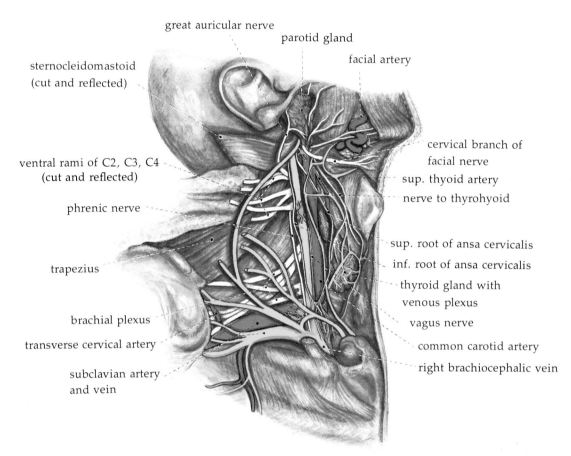

Great vessels in the neck and cervical and brachial plexuses.
The sternocleidomastoid has been cut and reflected. The omohyoid has been removed.

Make the following observations:

¶ Keep in mind that the carotid sheath containing the large vessels of the neck is covered by the sternocleidomastoid muscle and partially by the superior belly of the omohyoid (see HN71 and HN73). Cuts and wounds of the neck in suicide attempts frequently fail to damage the vein and arteries because of the large protective sternocleidomastoid.

¶ The internal jugular vein, the common and internal carotid arteries and the vagus nerve have a common fascia known as the carotid sheath (see HN81). The deep cervical lymph nodes form a chain on both sides of the internal jugular vein and are located in the carotid sheath (see HN72 *B*).

¶ The vagus nerve emerges from the jugular foramen and passes vertically downward between the internal jugular vein and the common carotid artery (usually under cover of the internal jugular vein). During its course it provides branches to the pharynx, larynx, palatal musculature and heart (for details, see HN78). Isolated lesions of the vagus are uncommon.

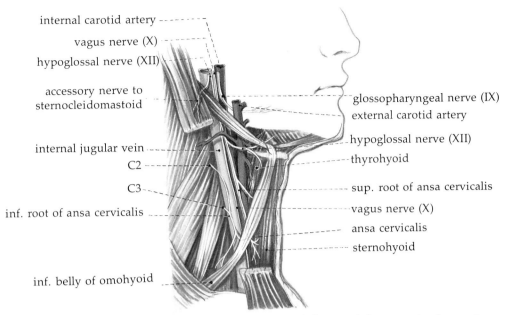

A. Schematic drawing of the great vessels and the cranial nerves in the neck.

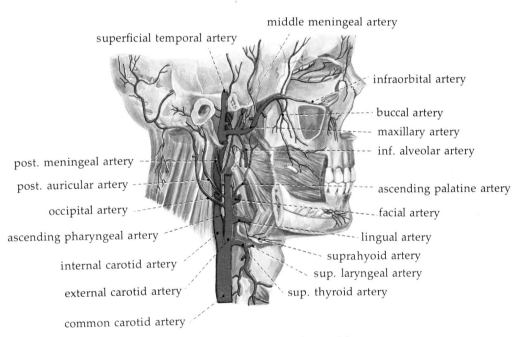

B. Branches of the external carotid artery.

¶ The superior root of the ansa cervicalis leaves the hypoglossal nerve and descends over the internal and common carotid arteries (see HN69). It carries fibers from C1 and is not affected by hypoglossal lesions. The inferior root of the ansa cervicalis contains fibers from C2 and C3. It descends over the internal jugular vein to join the superior root. Together they innervate the infrahyoid musculature and the geniohyoid (see HN74).

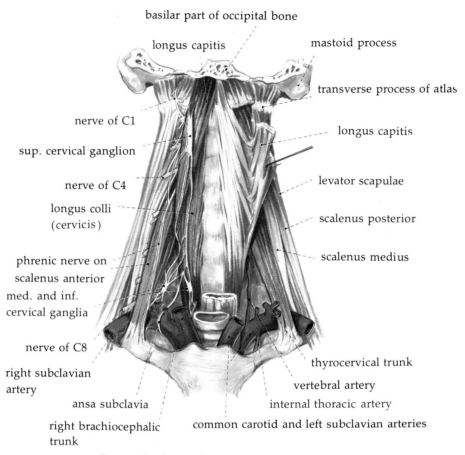

basilar part of occipital bone

longus capitis

mastoid process

transverse process of atlas

nerve of C1

longus capitis

sup. cervical ganglion

nerve of C4

levator scapulae

longus colli
(cervicis)

scalenus posterior

scalenus medius

phrenic nerve on
scalenus anterior
med. and inf.
cervical ganglia

nerve of C8

right subclavian
artery

thyrocervical trunk

vertebral artery

ansa subclavia

internal thoracic artery

right brachiocephalic
trunk

common carotid and left subclavian arteries

Sympathetic trunk and ganglia in the neck.
The large vessels and nerves have been removed.

Note the following points:

¶ The phrenic nerve originates from the ventral ramus of C4 but frequently contains contributions from C3 and C5 also. The nerve contains motor fibers to the diaphragm and also carries sensory fibers from the pleural and peritoneal covering on the upper and lower surfaces of the diaphragm. Other fibers supply the pericardium and mediastinal pleura. (For referred pain in the shoulder region, see T31). In patients with pathologic processes in the lower lobe of the lung, the nerve is sometimes cut in the neck to paralyze the diaphragm. This is not always successful because the contribution of C3 or C5 may form an independent branch (accessory phrenic nerve), which takes over the function of the phrenic nerve.

¶ The sympathetic trunk (see HN78) lies directly behind the internal and common carotid arteries between the carotid sheath and the fascia of the prevertebral muscles (see HN81). The superior cervical ganglion lies immediately below the skull, the middle cervical ganglion at the level of the cricoid cartilage and the inferior cervical ganglion at the level of the transverse process of C7 (see also HN79 A). The inferior ganglion is frequently fused with the first thoracic ganglion to form the cervicothoracic (stellate) ganglion.

¶ Many connections exist between the middle and inferior ganglia. One of these bundles is the ansa subclavia which crosses in front of the subclavian artery.

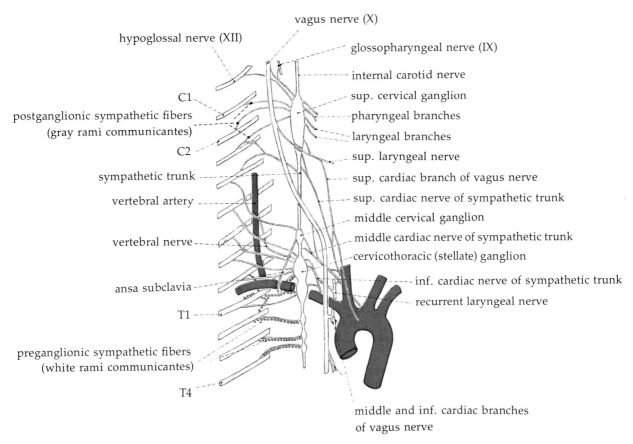

hypoglossal nerve (XII)

vagus nerve (X)

glossopharyngeal nerve (IX)

internal carotid nerve

C1

sup. cervical ganglion

postganglionic sympathetic fibers
(gray rami communicantes)

pharyngeal branches

laryngeal branches

C2

sup. laryngeal nerve

sympathetic trunk

sup. cardiac branch of vagus nerve

vertebral artery

sup. cardiac nerve of sympathetic trunk

middle cervical ganglion

middle cardiac nerve of sympathetic trunk

vertebral nerve

cervicothoracic (stellate) ganglion

ansa subclavia

inf. cardiac nerve of sympathetic trunk

recurrent laryngeal nerve

T1

preganglionic sympathetic fibers
(white rami communicantes)

T4

middle and inf. cardiac branches
of vagus nerve

The sympathetic trunk and ganglia.
Preganglionic sympathetic fibers are indicated by red dotted lines;
postganglionic sympathetic fibers are shown by blue lines.

¶ In the thoracic region each sympathetic ganglion receives preganglionic fibers (white rami communicantes) from its corresponding spinal segment. The preganglionic fibers for the head and neck, however, arise only from T1 and T2 and sometimes from C8. They leave by way of the first thoracic ventral root and sometimes from the roots of T2 and C8. The preganglionic fibers synapse in the cervical ganglia. Loss of the sympathetic nerve supply to the head and neck resulting from a lesion at T1 causes Horner's syndrome (see HN38).

¶ The superior cervical ganglion provides postganglionic fibers (gray rami communicantes) to C1, C2, C3, C4 and to the ninth, tenth, eleventh and twelfth cranial nerves. In addition, it provides branches to the pharynx, larynx and heart. An important branch, the *internal carotid nerve,* joins the internal carotid artery to form the carotid plexus inside the skull (see HN51).

¶ The middle cervical ganglion is highly variable in its position. It provides postganglionic fibers to C4, C5 and C6 and the middle cardiac branch to the heart.

¶ The inferior cervical ganglion or cervicothoracic ganglion provides postganglionic fibers to C7, C8, T1 and the heart, as well as a branch to the vertebral artery to form the vertebral plexus.

¶ Note the vagus nerve with the superior laryngeal nerve and the recurrent laryngeal nerve (see also HN121).

429

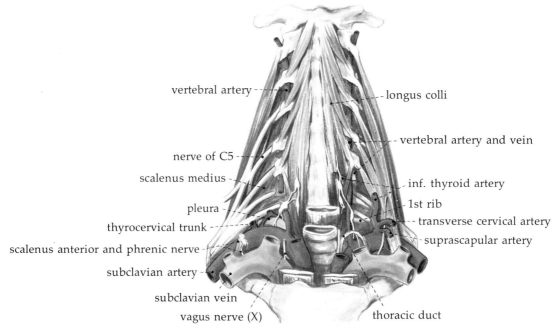

A. Relation of the subclavian vessels to the scalenus anterior.

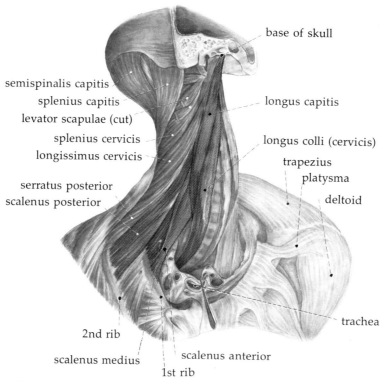

B. The prevertebral muscles in the neck.
The trachea, larynx and esophagus have been removed.

¶ Under normal conditions the subclavian artery and brachial plexus pass behind the scalenus anterior and in front of the scalenus medius. The subclavian vein passes in front of the scalenus anterior. Sometimes the space between the scalenus anterior and scalenus medius is narrow, and this results in compression of the subclavian artery and brachial plexus (usually the medial cord). This compression causes pain, numbness, prickling, weakness and sometimes swelling and ulceration of the upper extremity. The symptoms are known as the *neurovascular compression syndrome*.

¶ The neurovascular syndrome is usually caused by compression between the scaleni but may also result from the presence of a cervical rib. Such a rib is formed by a long transverse process of C7. The cervical rib may end freely but may also be connected to the first rib by a strong ligamentous band.

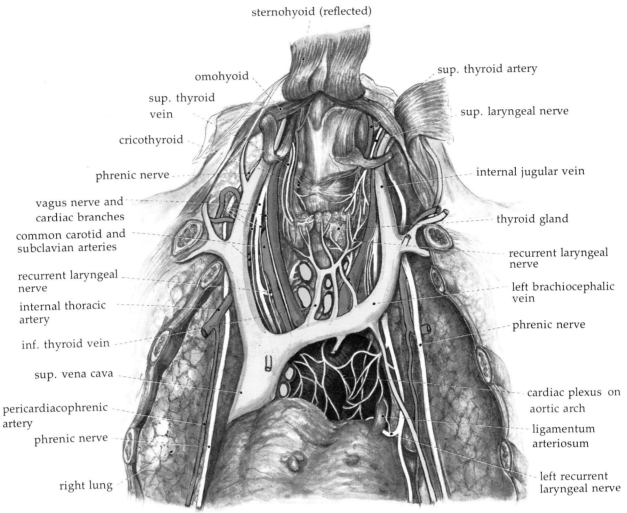

sternohyoid (reflected)

omohyoid

sup. thyroid vein

cricothyroid

phrenic nerve

vagus nerve and cardiac branches

common carotid and subclavian arteries

recurrent laryngeal nerve

internal thoracic artery

inf. thyroid vein

sup. vena cava

pericardiacophrenic artery

phrenic nerve

right lung

sup. thyroid artery

sup. laryngeal nerve

internal jugular vein

thyroid gland

recurrent laryngeal nerve

left brachiocephalic vein

phrenic nerve

cardiac plexus on aortic arch

ligamentum arteriosum

left recurrent laryngeal nerve

Anterior view of the great vessels and nerves of the root of the neck and upper part of the thorax.

Note:

¶ The laryngeal muscles are innervated by branches of the vagus. The superior laryngeal nerve supplies the cricothyroid muscle and the sensory innervation of the larynx above the vocal cords. The inferior laryngeal nerve on the right side passes under the subclavian artery, but on the left side it passes around the ligamentum arteriosum. (For details see HN121.)

¶ The thyroid gland is drained by the superior and inferior thyroid veins. The latter drains into the left brachiocephalic vein.

¶ The cardiac plexus contains sympathetic and parasympathetic fibers. The parasympathetic fibers originate from the vagus nerve, and the sympathetic fibers arise from the cervical and upper thoracic ganglia. The parasympathetic vagal fibers slow the rate of the heartbeat and constrict the coronary arteries. The function of the sympathetic fibers is acceleration of the heart and dilation of the coronary arteries.

431

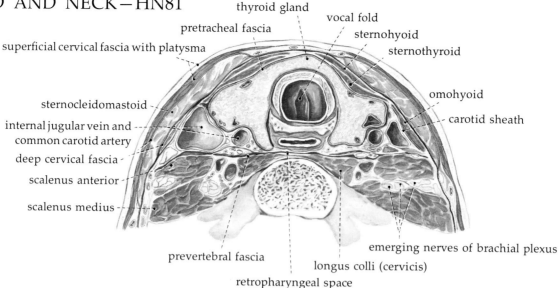

superficial cervical fascia with platysma
pretracheal fascia
thyroid gland
vocal fold
sternohyoid
sternothyroid

sternocleidomastoid
internal jugular vein and
common carotid artery
deep cervical fascia
scalenus anterior
scalenus medius

omohyoid
carotid sheath

prevertebral fascia
longus colli (cervicis)
retropharyngeal space
emerging nerves of brachial plexus

A. Fascial layers as seen in transverse section through the neck.

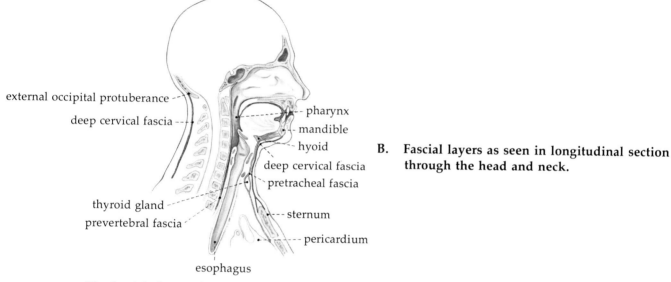

external occipital protuberance
deep cervical fascia

pharynx
mandible
hyoid
deep cervical fascia
pretracheal fascia

thyroid gland
prevertebral fascia

sternum
pericardium

esophagus

B. Fascial layers as seen in longitudinal section through the head and neck.

The fascial planes of the neck are clinically important because they determine the extent of spread of abscesses and infections in the neck. In addition, they provide the planes of cleavage in surgical procedures. Note the following fascial planes:

¶ The *superficial cervical fascia* contains the platysma, superficial veins and cutaneous nerves.

¶ The *deep cervical fascia* invests all the muscles of the neck and is posteriorly attached to the ligamentum nuchae. It splits to enclose the trapezius and sternocleidomastoid muscles. Superiorly the fascia is attached to the lower border of the mandible and the zygomatic arch. It sheathes the parotid and submandibular glands and descends to the manubrium of the sternum. The external jugular vein passes through the deep fascia, and when the vein is cut during surgical procedures or wounds, the fascia keeps it open. Air may be sucked into the lumen of the vein, and these air bubbles are directly transported to the heart and lungs, where they may cause a fatal air embolism. Inflammations of the submandibular gland are hindered from spreading downward because of the attachment of the deep fascia to the lower border of the mandible and the hyoid bone. Pus and edema caused by inflammation of the gland will push the tongue forward and upward.

¶ The *pretracheal fascia* extends from the hyoid bone to the fibrous pericardium and encloses the trachea, larynx, pharynx, esophagus and thyroid gland.

¶ The *prevertebral fascia* passes behind the esophagus, pharynx and great vessels. Laterally the fascia covers the scalenus muscles, the emerging brachial plexus and the subclavian artery. In the axilla it forms the axillary sheath. Pus from tuberculous cervical vertebrae usually remains behind the fascia in the midline but may expand laterally over the scaleni behind the sternocleidomastoid. It usually does not reach the axillary sheath toward the arm. Sometimes edema and pus reach the mediastinum by moving downward behind the fascia.

¶ The *carotid sheath* is a separate fascial compartment containing the common carotid artery, internal jugular vein and vagus nerve. The sympathetic chain is usually found in its posterior wall.

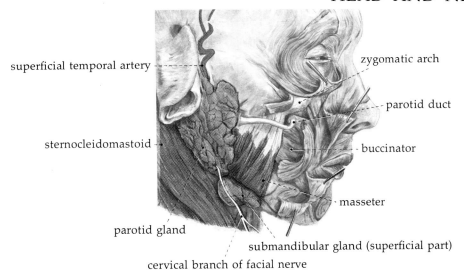

superficial temporal artery

zygomatic arch

parotid duct

sternocleidomastoid

buccinator

masseter

parotid gland

submandibular gland (superficial part)

cervical branch of facial nerve

A. The submandibular gland in relation to the parotid gland.
Note the cervical branch of the facial nerve.

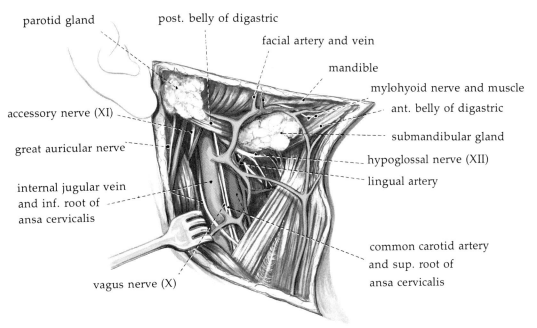

parotid gland

post. belly of digastric

facial artery and vein

mandible

mylohyoid nerve and muscle

accessory nerve (XI)

ant. belly of digastric

submandibular gland

great auricular nerve

hypoglossal nerve (XII)

lingual artery

internal jugular vein
and inf. root of
ansa cervicalis

common carotid artery
and sup. root of
ansa cervicalis

vagus nerve (X)

B. The submandibular gland in relation to the vessels.

¶ The submandibular gland consists of a superficial part and a deep part. The superficial part lies inferior and the deep part superior to the mylohyoid muscle (see HN86); hence the two parts are continuous with each other around the posterior border of the muscle. The submandibular duct passes forward on the side of the tongue and opens on the sublingual papilla at the side of the frenulum (see HN96 C). The opening is visible in the mouth, and saliva can be seen trickling from it.

¶ The submandibular gland is often swollen, in which case it protrudes beyond the angle of the mandible in front of the sternocleidomastoid. A swollen gland can easily be confused with swollen submandibular lymph nodes (see HN72). To distinguish between the two, remember that the deep part of the gland lies on top of the mylohyoid and can be palpated by placing one finger on the side of the tongue and another below the angle of the jaw. The lymph nodes are only felt at the angle of the jaw.

¶ Tumors of the submandibular gland are not uncommon, and in such cases the gland must be removed. As with tumors of the parotid gland, great care must be taken not to damage the surrounding nerves and blood vessels. Note that (a) the cervical branch of the facial nerve crosses over the gland to innervate the platysma; (b) the facial vein passes over the gland; (c) the facial artery arches over its superior aspect; and (d) the lingual and hypoglossal nerves pass over the hyoglossus muscle closely related to the deep part of the gland (see HN92 A).

433

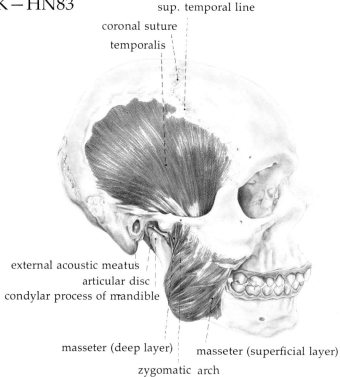

sup. temporal line
coronal suture
temporalis

external acoustic meatus
articular disc
condylar process of mandible

masseter (deep layer)
masseter (superficial layer)
zygomatic arch

A. The masseter and temporalis muscles.

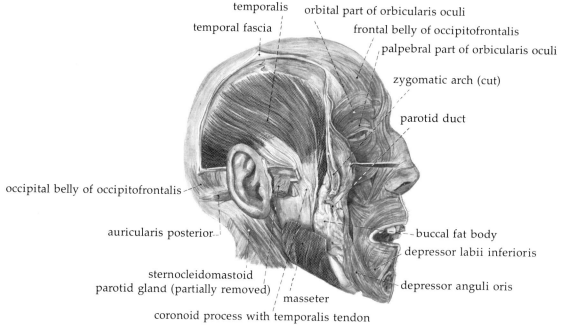

temporalis
temporal fascia
orbital part of orbicularis oculi
frontal belly of occipitofrontalis
palpebral part of orbicularis oculi
zygomatic arch (cut)
parotid duct

occipital belly of occipitofrontalis

auricularis posterior

buccal fat body
depressor labii inferioris

sternocleidomastoid
parotid gland (partially removed)
masseter
depressor anguli oris
coronoid process with temporalis tendon

B. The temporalis after removal of the zygomatic arch.
Part of the masseter and the buccinator have been removed.

Note:

¶ The temporalis muscle originates from the bony floor of the temporal fossa and from the very strong fascia that overlies the muscle. The fibers converge to the coronoid process and the anterior border of the ramus of the mandible. The muscle elevates the mandible with great force, thus closing the mouth. The posterior fibers retract the mandible from a protruded position.

¶ The masseter originates from the zygomatic process of the maxilla and the anterior part of the zygomatic arch. It inserts at the angle and the lower half of the ramus of the mandible. The muscle elevates the mandible to occlude the teeth in mastication. When the teeth are clenched, both the temporalis and the masseter can be palpated. Keep in mind that both muscles are innervated by motor branches of the mandibular nerve (see HN85).

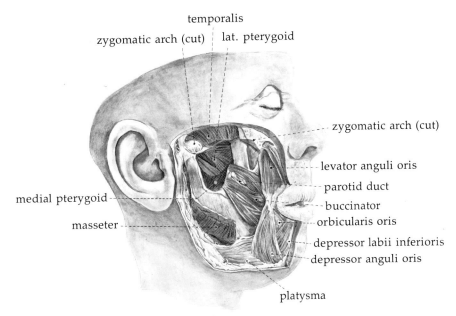

A. The right pterygoid muscles.
Part of the mandible and zygomatic arch have been removed.

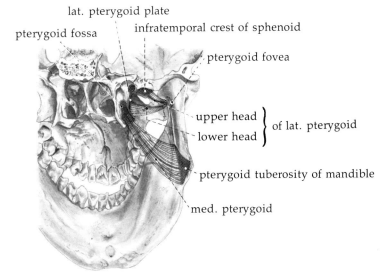

B. Schematic drawing of the origin and insertion of the pterygoid muscles (posterior view).

The course and action of the pterygoid muscles have always been difficult to understand, and careful study of their origin and insertion on the skull is recommended (see also HN85).

¶ The lateral pterygoid originates from: the infratemporal crest of the greater wing of the sphenoid and the lateral surface of the lateral pterygoid plate. The fibers pass laterally and backward to insert into a depression on the front of the neck of the mandible. Some insert into the articular capsule of the temporomandibular joint. When the muscle contracts, it pulls the condylar process of the mandible and the articular disc forward: half of the mandible protrudes, and the mouth is slightly opened.

¶ The medial pterygoid originates from the medial surface of the lateral pterygoid plate and from the tuberosity of the maxilla (see also HN85 A). Its fibers also pass backward and laterally to insert into the medial surface of the ramus and angle of the mandible. Hence, it elevates the mandible but also causes the mandible to protrude on the side of the contraction.

Acting together on both sides, the two pterygoids forcefully protrude the jaw. When the pterygoids act together on one side, that side of the mandible is moved forward and toward the opposite side, while the head of the mandible on the other side rotates slightly. Hence, the pterygoids can protrude the mandible and carry out side to side movements.

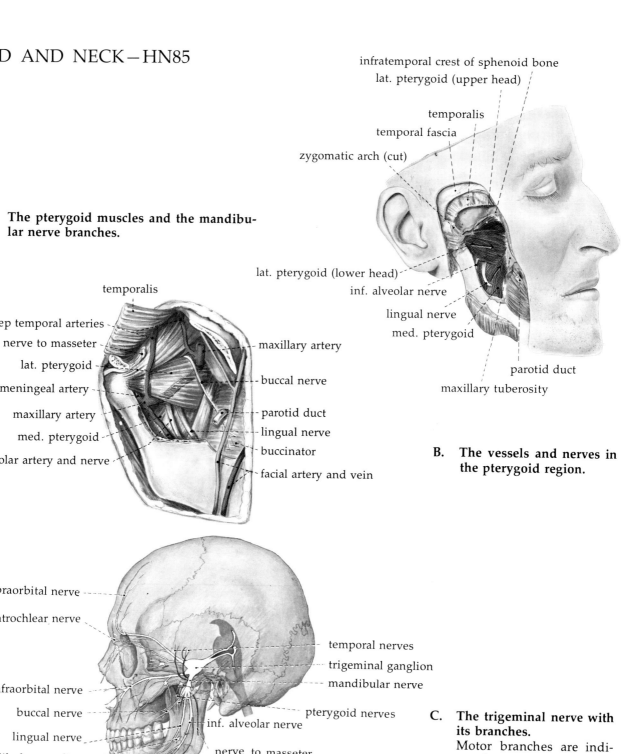

A. The pterygoid muscles and the mandibular nerve branches.

infratemporal crest of sphenoid bone

lat. pterygoid (upper head)

temporalis

temporal fascia

zygomatic arch (cut)

lat. pterygoid (lower head)

inf. alveolar nerve

lingual nerve

med. pterygoid

parotid duct

maxillary tuberosity

temporalis

deep temporal arteries

nerve to masseter

lat. pterygoid

middle meningeal artery

maxillary artery

med. pterygoid

inf. alveolar artery and nerve

maxillary artery

buccal nerve

parotid duct

lingual nerve

buccinator

facial artery and vein

B. The vessels and nerves in the pterygoid region.

supraorbital nerve

supratrochlear nerve

infraorbital nerve

buccal nerve

lingual nerve

submandibular ganglion

temporal nerves

trigeminal ganglion

mandibular nerve

pterygoid nerves

inf. alveolar nerve

nerve to masseter

mylohyoid nerve

mental nerve

C. The trigeminal nerve with its branches.
Motor branches are indicated in red.

Note:

- Both the lingual and the inferior alveolar nerves appear at the inferior border of the lateral pterygoid. The lingual nerve, carrying the chorda tympani, continues over the medial pterygoid and then lies against the mandible just behind the third molar (see HN87 *B*). The inferior alveolar nerve enters the mandibular foramen to innervate the teeth and terminates in the mental nerve. (See HN102.)

- Keep in mind that the buccal nerve supplies the skin over the anterior part of the buccinator and the mucous membrane on the inside of the cheek. Sometimes it provides a small motor branch to the lateral pterygoid. The buccinator muscle is innervated by a buccal nerve, but this nerve is a branch of the facial nerve.

- The motor branches of the mandibular nerve innervate the muscles of mastication: (a) masseter; (b) temporalis; (c) lateral pterygoid; and (d) medial pterygoid. In addition, the anterior belly of the digastric and the mylohyoid are innervated by the mandibular nerve through the mylohyoid nerve.

436

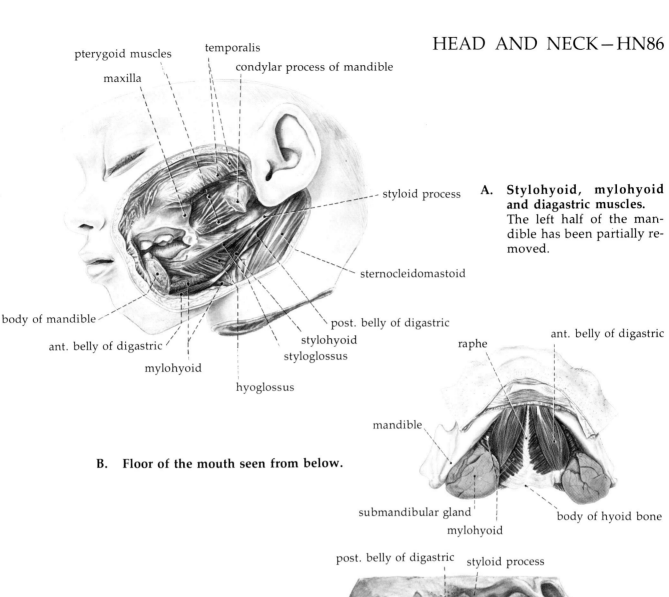

pterygoid muscles
temporalis
condylar process of mandible
maxilla
styloid process
sternocleidomastoid
body of mandible
post. belly of digastric
ant. belly of digastric
stylohyoid
styloglossus
mylohyoid
hyoglossus

A. Stylohyoid, mylohyoid and diagastric muscles.
The left half of the mandible has been partially removed.

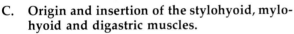

B. Floor of the mouth seen from below.

raphe
ant. belly of digastric
mandible
submandibular gland
mylohyoid
body of hyoid bone

C. Origin and insertion of the stylohyoid, mylohyoid and digastric muscles.

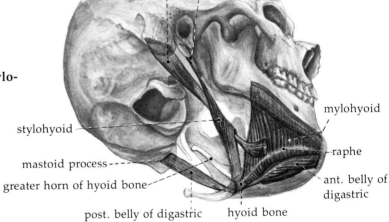

post. belly of digastric
styloid process
stylohyoid
mastoid process
greater horn of hyoid bone
post. belly of digastric
hyoid bone
mylohyoid
raphe
ant. belly of digastric

Note the following points:

¶ The stylohyoid originates from the posterior aspect of the styloid process and inserts into the hyoid bone at the junction of the body and the greater horn. The muscle and tendinous fibers are split close to their insertion to permit passage to the intermediate tendon of the digastric. The muscle is innervated by the facial nerve.

¶ The digastric has two bellies and an intermediate tendon. The posterior belly originates from the medial surface of the mastoid process, passes across and in front of the carotid sheath and then ends in the intermediate tendon. This tendon is kept in position by the stylohyoid and by fibers of the deep fascia which bind it to the junction of the body and the greater horn of the hyoid. The anterior belly runs forward inferior to the mylohyoid and is attached to the mandible near the midline. Keep in mind that the posterior belly is innervated by the facial nerve and the anterior belly by the mylohyoid nerve, a branch of the mandibular nerve.

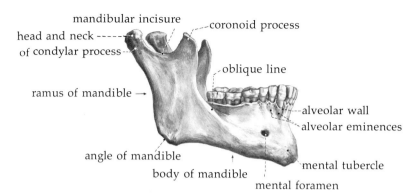

A. The mandible seen from the right side.

mandibular incisure
coronoid process
head and neck ----
of condylar process --
oblique line
ramus of mandible →
alveolar wall
alveolar eminences
angle of mandible
mental tubercle
body of mandible
mental foramen

head of condylar process
pterygoid fovea
coronoid process
lingula of mandible
lingual nerve
inf. alveolar nerve and artery
mandibular foramen
mylohyoid nerve and artery
mylohyoid groove
angle of mandible
submandibular fossa
digastric fossa
mylohyoid
mental spine (genial tubercle)
line
sublingual fossa

B. Medial view of the right half of the mandible.

mandibular canal
interalveolar septum
dental socket

C. Mandible showing right inferior alveolar canal.

mandibular canal opened
mental foramen

Keep in mind:

¶ The mandible develops by membranous ossification in the place of Meckel's cartilage, the mandibular portion of the first branchial arch. Similarly, the sphenomandibular ligament, coursing from the spine of the sphenoid to the lingula of the mandible, represents a part of the first branchial arch (HN88 C).

¶ The inferior alveolar nerve is a branch of the mandibular division of the trigeminal nerve and is accompanied by the inferior alveolar artery (a branch of the maxillary artery) while passing through the mandibular canal. It innervates the teeth of the lower jaw and finally emerges through the mental foramen to become the cutaneous nerve of the chin (mental nerve).

¶ The lingual nerve lies against the mandible just behind the third molar tooth. The nerve is covered only by the mucous membrane, and extraction of the third molar will endanger it.

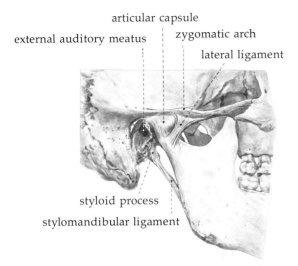

articular capsule
external auditory meatus
zygomatic arch
lateral ligament

styloid process
stylomandibular ligament

A. The right temporomandibular joint (lateral view).

condylar process of mandible
lateral ligament
mandibular fossa
zygomatic arch

articular disc
articular capsule
stylomandibular ligament

B. The temporomandibular joint with part of the capsule removed.

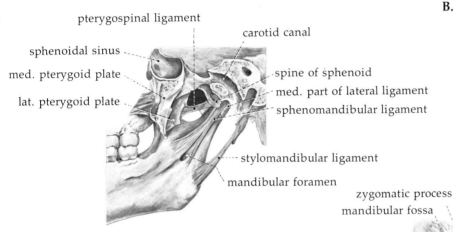

pterygospinal ligament
carotid canal
sphenoidal sinus
med. pterygoid plate
lat. pterygoid plate
spine of sphenoid
med. part of lateral ligament
sphenomandibular ligament
stylomandibular ligament
mandibular foramen

C. The sphenomandibular and stylomandibular ligaments (medial view).

zygomatic process
mandibular fossa
external auditory meatus
external carotid foramen
foramen ovale
pterygoid fossa
lat. pterygoid plate
pterygopalatine fossa
probe in palatine canal
zygomatic bone
probe in inf. orbital fissure
sphenopalatine foramen

D. Lateral view of the infratemporal region after removal of the mandible.

¶ The temporomandibular joint is easily dislocated and is the source of many complaints. The joint is formed by the condylar process of the mandible and the mandibular fossa and tubercle of the temporal bone. A fibrocartilaginous disc separates the two and divides the joint into upper and lower compartments. This permits a considerable range of mandibular movements: (a) protrusion and retraction, (b) elevation and depression and (c) side to side movement.

¶ When the jaw is dislocated, the condylar process slides forward onto the articular tubercle and then over the tubercle into the infratemporal fossa. A yawn or a slight blow on the mandible may cause this rather common type of dislocation. By pressing down on the molar teeth of the mandible with the thumbs placed in the mouth, the mandible can be moved back into position.

¶ When the mandible receives a backward blow, the joint may dislocate posteriorly, thereby fracturing the wall of the bony external auditory meatus. Backward dislocation is rare, but forward dislocation is common and often recurs.

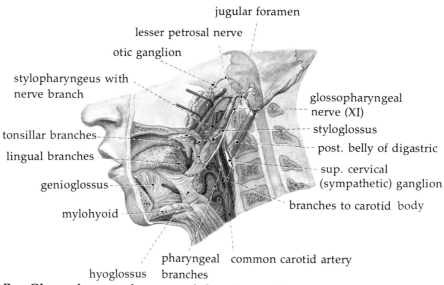

lat. pterygoid (cut)

temporalis

med. pterygoid

lingual nerve

styloglossus

stylopharyngeus

stylohyoid

post. belly of digastric

genioglossus

geniohyoid

mylohyoid

ant. belly of digastric

hyoglossus

A. Muscles of the tongue after removal of the right half of the mandible.

jugular foramen

lesser petrosal nerve

otic ganglion

stylopharyngeus with nerve branch

glossopharyngeal nerve (XI)

tonsillar branches

styloglossus

lingual branches

post. belly of digastric

genioglossus

sup. cervical (sympathetic) ganglion

mylohyoid

branches to carotid body

pharyngeal branches

common carotid artery

hyoglossus

B. Glossopharyngeal nerve and the otic ganglion.
Note that the stylopharyngeus is partially covered by the styloglossus.

Make the following observations:

¶ The glossopharyngeal nerve emerges from the skull through the jugular foramen and gives off the tympanic nerve immediately after its exit. This nerve traverses the middle ear and then continues as the lesser petrosal nerve, which provides preganglionic parasympathetic fibers to the otic ganglion (see HN60 *B* and HN90).

¶ The stylopharyngeus is the only muscle innervated by the glossopharyngeal nerve. From this muscle the nerve descends over the pharynx, its branches intermingling with those of the vagus and the sympathetic trunk to form the pharyngeal plexus. Through this plexus sensory fibers travel to the mucous membranes of the pharynx, tonsil and soft palate (see HN105).

¶ An important branch below the styloglossus supplies the posterior third of the tongue with taste fibers and general sensory fibers (see HN97).

¶ An important branch innervates the carotid body at the bifurcation of the common carotid artery. This body is a chemoreceptor and is particularly sensitive to hypoxia. Decreased oxygen content produces a rise in blood pressure and heart rate and an increase in respiratory movements.

¶ Lesions of the glossopharyngeal nerve cause sensory loss of the pharynx, tonsillar region and posterior palate, combined with a loss of salivation of the parotid gland. Isolated lesions of the nerve, however, are rare.

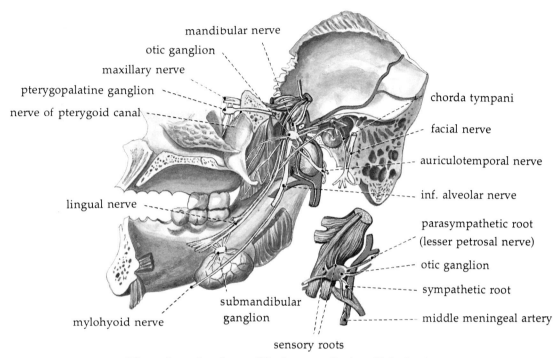

mandibular nerve
otic ganglion
maxillary nerve
pterygopalatine ganglion
nerve of pterygoid canal
chorda tympani
facial nerve
auriculotemporal nerve
inf. alveolar nerve
lingual nerve
parasympathetic root
(lesser petrosal nerve)
otic ganglion
sympathetic root
middle meningeal artery
mylohyoid nerve
submandibular ganglion
sensory roots

The otic and submandibular ganglia (medial view).
Note the location of the otic and pterygopalatine ganglia on the skull.

After the pterygoid muscles have been cut, the important branches of the mandibular nerve can be traced upward. A number of interesting anatomic features are visible:

¶ The lingual nerve is joined by the chorda tympani near the inferior border of the lateral pterygoid. The chorda tympani is a branch of the facial nerve. It traverses the tympanic cavity and emerges from the skull through the petrotympanic fissure (see HN58). The chorda tympani carries taste fibers from the anterior two-thirds of the tongue (see HN91 and HN97).

¶ The chorda tympani also carries preganglionic parasympathetic fibers to the submandibular ganglion. In this ganglion the fibers synapse and the postganglionic (secretomotor) fibers continue to the submandibular and sublingual glands.

¶ The otic ganglion lies on the mandibular nerve immediately below the foramen ovale. Functionally, however, it is related mainly to the glossopharyngeal nerve, although some sensory fibers of the mandibular nerve pass through the ganglion without interruption. The ganglion receives its preganglionic parasympathetic fibers through the lesser petrosal nerve, a branch of the glossopharyngeal nerve (see HN89). These fibers synapse in the ganglion and the postganglionic parasympathetic (secretomotor) fibers join the auriculotemporal nerve to the parotid gland.

Some postganglionic sympathetic fibers surrounding the middle meningeal artery also pass through the ganglion. They do not synapse but join the auriculotemporal nerve to the parotid gland.

441

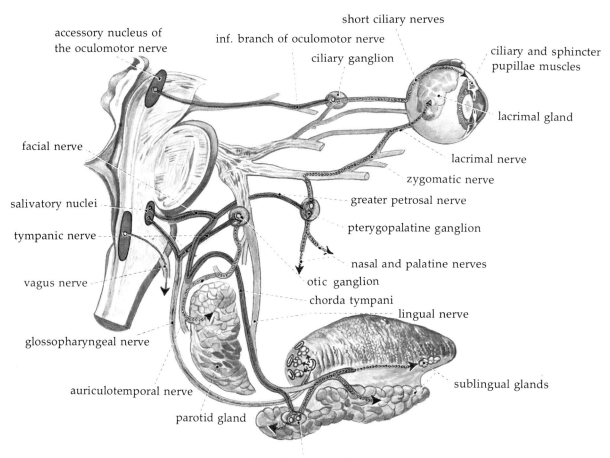

The cranial parasympathetic ganglia.

¶ *Ciliary ganglion.* Preganglionic parasympathetic fibers from the accessory nucleus of the oculomotor nerve reach the ganglion through the inferior branch of the oculomotor nerve. Postganglionic nerves innervate the ciliary and sphincter pupillae muscles through the short ciliary nerves (see HN35 and HN36).

¶ *Pterygopalatine ganglion.* Preganglionic fibers from the facial nerve reach the ganglion through the greater petrosal nerve. Postganglionic fibers pass through the zygomatic and lacrimal nerves to the lacrimal gland and through the nasal and palatine branches of the maxillary nerve to the nasal and palatine glands (see HN50 and HN114).

¶ *Otic ganglion.* Preganglionic parasympathetic fibers from the glossopharyngeal nerve reach the ganglion through the tympanic and lesser petrosal nerves (see HN60 *B*). Postganglionic fibers pass through the auriculotemporal nerve to the parotid gland (see HN90).

¶ *Submandibular ganglion.* Preganglionic parasympathetic fibers from the facial nerve reach the ganglion through the chorda tympani. Postganglionic fibers pass to the submandibular gland and through the lingual nerve to the sublingual and lingual glands (HN92).

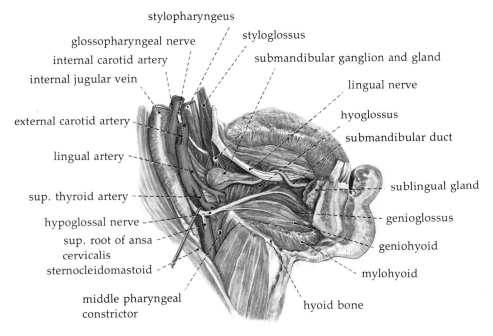

stylopharyngeus
glossopharyngeal nerve
internal carotid artery
internal jugular vein
external carotid artery
lingual artery
sup. thyroid artery
hypoglossal nerve
sup. root of ansa
cervicalis
sternocleidomastoid
middle pharyngeal
constrictor

styloglossus
submandibular ganglion and gland
lingual nerve
hyoglossus
submandibular duct
sublingual gland
genioglossus
geniohyoid
mylohyoid
hyoid bone

A. The hypoglossal and lingual nerves and the submandibular gland.
The three muscles of the extrinsic tongue musculature are shown in color.
The hypoglossal nerve has been pulled down.

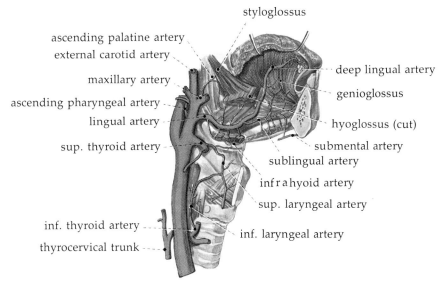

styloglossus
ascending palatine artery
external carotid artery
maxillary artery
ascending pharyngeal artery
lingual artery
sup. thyroid artery
inf. thyroid artery
thyrocervical trunk

deep lingual artery
genioglossus
hyoglossus (cut)
submental artery
sublingual artery
infrahyoid artery
sup. laryngeal artery
inf. laryngeal artery

B. The lingual artery and its branches.
The hyoglossus has been cut to show the artery.

Note:

⁋ The deep part of the submandibular gland lies on the hyoglossus and is in close contact with the hypoglossal and lingual nerves and the submandibular ganglion. The submandibular duct passes over the hyoglossus, subsequently curves over the lingual nerve and then courses over the genioglossus on the side of the tongue, just beneath the mucous membrane on the floor of the mouth. Finally, it lies between the sublingual gland and the genioglossus and opens with a small papilla on the side of the frenulum (see HN96 C).

⁋ The course of the submandibular duct is important. Calculi (stones) in the duct are not uncommon, and surgical removal is sometimes required. In this event, particular attention must be given to the lingual nerve and the deep branch of the lingual artery. The duct can easily be palpated bimanually, with one finger in the mouth and another below the angle of the jaw. (For swellings of the gland, see HN82).

443

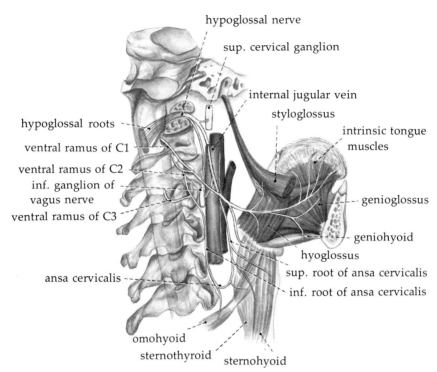

A. The hypoglossal nerve and the extrinsic tongue muscles.

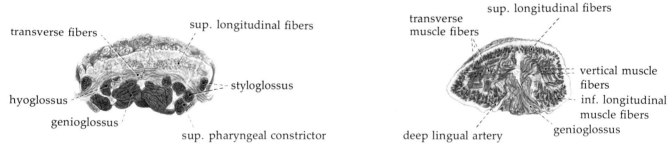

B and C. Frontal sections through the tongue.

¶ The hypoglossal nerve emerges from the hypoglossal canal and subsequently descends between the internal jugular vein and the internal carotid artery. It runs forward over the hyoglossus and then curves upward to supply the extrinsic and intrinsic muscles of the tongue. The extrinsic muscles are: (a) the hyoglossus, (b) the styloglosus and (c) the genioglossus. The intrinsic musculature of the tongue is formed by superior and inferior longitudinal fibers, vertical fibers and transverse fibers.

¶ Contraction of the genioglossus causes protrusion of the tongue. If the hypoglossal nerve is damaged unilaterally, the tongue protrudes toward the side of the lesion when the patient is asked to stick out his tongue. When the paralysis is of long duration, the tongue becomes atrophied and wrinkled on the affected side.

¶ Keep in mind that the sternohyoid, omohyoid, thyrohyoid and sternothyroid are all innervated by the ventral rami of the cervical nerves through the branches of the ansa cervicalis. The geniohyoid is innervated through the branch of C1, which accompanies the hypoglossal nerve until it reaches the muscle (see HN69).

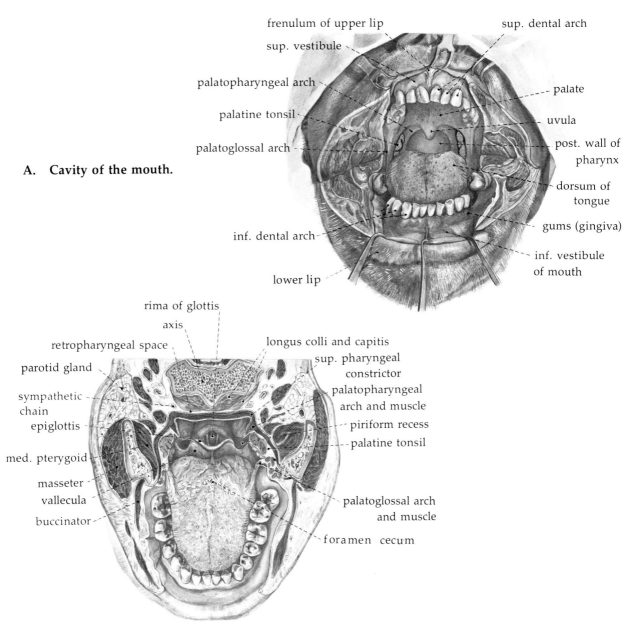

frenulum of upper lip
sup. dental arch
sup. vestibule
palatopharyngeal arch
palatine tonsil
palatoglossal arch
palate
uvula
post. wall of pharynx
dorsum of tongue
gums (gingiva)
inf. vestibule of mouth
inf. dental arch
lower lip

A. Cavity of the mouth.

rima of glottis
axis
retropharyngeal space
parotid gland
sympathetic chain
epiglottis
med. pterygoid
masseter
vallecula
buccinator
longus colli and capitis
sup. pharyngeal constrictor
palatopharyngeal arch and muscle
piriform recess
palatine tonsil
palatoglossal arch and muscle
foramen cecum

B. Horizontal section through the head.
The inferior portion of the oral cavity and the entrance into the larynx are visible.

Inspection of the oral cavity is important, and special attention should be given to:

¶ The superior and inferior vestibule. Note the color of the mucosa, and examine the area for the presence of ulcers or discolorations.

¶ The teeth and gingiva. Determine whether dental cavities, caries or ulcers and inflammations of the gums are present.

¶ The tongue. Note the color and see whether inflammations, ulcers or swellings are present. Also ask the patient to move and protrude the tongue (check for hypoglossal function).

¶ Study the palate, and in newborn infants particularly be careful to determine whether clefts are present.

¶ Under normal conditions the palatine tonsils are barely visible between the palatoglossal and palatopharyngeal arches When they are inflamed, they protrude from between the arches, are swollen and edematous and frequently show yellow-white pus on the surface.

¶ The pharyngeal tonsil is located at the posterior wall of the pharynx. It is frequently swollen and inflamed and may cause difficulty with breathing and swallowing (see HN95 and HN115). The gland regresses during puberty. (Keep in mind that the posterior wall of the oropharynx lies in front of the axis.)

445

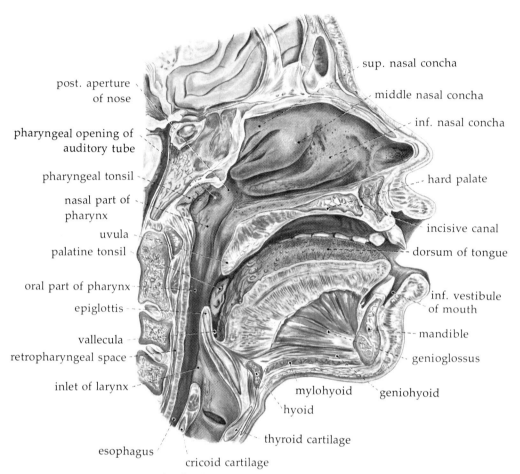

post. aperture of nose

pharyngeal opening of auditory tube

pharyngeal tonsil

nasal part of pharynx

uvula

palatine tonsil

oral part of pharynx

epiglottis

vallecula

retropharyngeal space

inlet of larynx

esophagus

cricoid cartilage

sup. nasal concha

middle nasal concha

inf. nasal concha

hard palate

incisive canal

dorsum of tongue

inf. vestibule of mouth

mandible

genioglossus

mylohyoid

geniohyoid

hyoid

thyroid cartilage

Sagittal section through the head.
The mucosa of the oral and nasal cavities, pharynx and larynx is shown in color.

¶ The posterior part of the oral cavity is in open communication with the oropharynx, which in turn is connected with the nasopharynx and the opening of the auditory tube. Inferiorly the oropharynx is connected to the laryngopharynx. It is evident that infections from the tonsils can spread easily to the oropharynx and then to the auditory tube and nose or to the larynx. Similarly, edema accompanying infections of the lymphoid tissue surrounding the oral part of the pharynx (see HN115) may spread to the epiglottis and into the larynx. Swelling of the epiglottis is dangerous because the passage to the trachea may become blocked, resulting in asphyxia.

¶ Another point of importance is the position of the tongue in the mouth. In unconscious patients or patients under deep anesthesia the tongue musculature is without tonus. When the patient lies in a supine position, the tongue slides back and may block the opening into the larynx. Hence, in all unconscious patients it must be realized that the tongue should be pulled forward. This can be partially accomplished by placing the patient on his side or by pushing the mandible forward. The genioglossus, attached to the mandible in the midline, will then pull the tongue forward. This simple procedure may sometimes save the life of the patient.

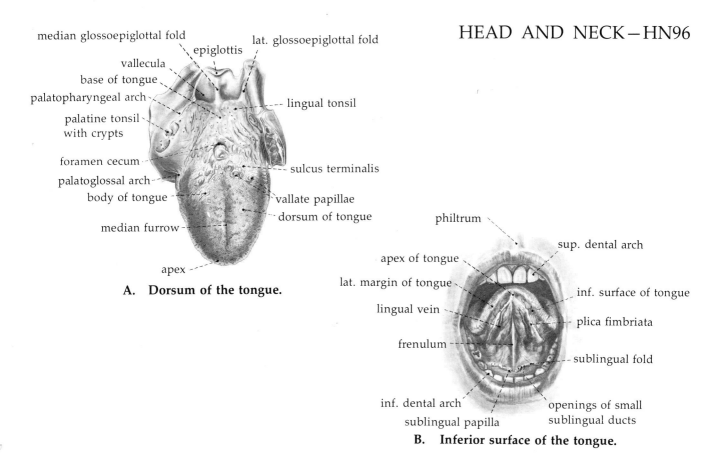

median glossoepiglottal fold
epiglottis
lat. glossoepiglottal fold
vallecula
base of tongue
palatopharyngeal arch
lingual tonsil
palatine tonsil with crypts
foramen cecum
sulcus terminalis
palatoglossal arch
body of tongue
vallate papillae
median furrow
dorsum of tongue
apex

A. Dorsum of the tongue.

philtrum
apex of tongue
sup. dental arch
lat. margin of tongue
inf. surface of tongue
lingual vein
plica fimbriata
frenulum
sublingual fold
inf. dental arch
openings of small sublingual ducts
sublingual papilla

B. Inferior surface of the tongue.

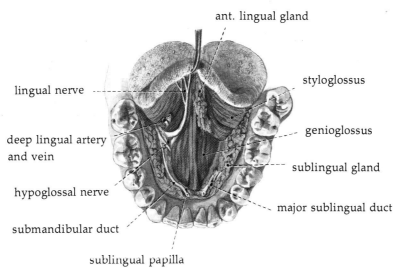

ant. lingual gland
lingual nerve
styloglossus
deep lingual artery and vein
genioglossus
hypoglossal nerve
sublingual gland
submandibular duct
major sublingual duct
sublingual papilla

C. Inferior surface of the tongue after removal of the mucous membrane.

Note:

¶ The V-shaped groove, the sulcus terminalis, with the foramen cecum at its apex, divides the tongue into buccal and pharyngeal portions. The vallate papillae lie immediately in front of the sulcus terminalis. The foramen cecum is clinically important, since the thyroid gland originates from this region, and remnants of the thyroid primordium may be found in the region of the foramen. These remnants may produce swellings and sometimes become malignant (see HN123).

¶ A fimbriated fold can be distinguished at the underside of the tongue. In this fold the lingual vein can be seen through the mucosal surface. Similarly, the submandibular duct and the sublingual gland are located immediately under the mucosa of the floor of the mouth, and the gland and duct can easily be palpated for the presence of tumors or stones.

A. Lymph drainage of the tongue.

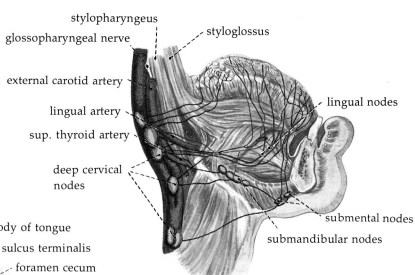

stylopharyngeus
glossopharyngeal nerve
styloglossus
external carotid artery
lingual artery
sup. thyroid artery
lingual nodes
deep cervical nodes
submental nodes
submandibular nodes

B. Sensory innervation of the tongue.

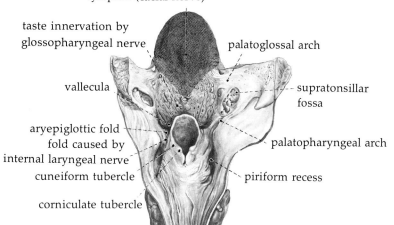

sensory innervation by lingual nerve
body of tongue
sulcus terminalis
foramen cecum
sensory innervation by glossopharyngeal nerve
palatine tonsil with crypts
base of tongue
epiglottis
sensory innervation by internal laryngeal nerve of vagus

C. Taste innervation of the tongue.

taste innervation by chorda tympani (facial nerve)
taste innervation by glossopharyngeal nerve
palatoglossal arch
vallecula
supratonsillar fossa
aryepiglottic fold
fold caused by internal laryngeal nerve
cuneiform tubercle
palatopharyngeal arch
corniculate tubercle
piriform recess

❡ The lymph of the tongue drains into three areas: (a) the lower lip drains to the submental nodes; (b) the tip of the tongue drains mainly to the submental nodes but, like the remaining two-thirds of the tongue, may also drain to the submandibular nodes; (c) the posterior one-third drains to the upper nodes of the deep cervical chain, especially the jugulodigastric and jugulo-omohyoid nodes. Little cross-communication of the lymph vessels occurs in the anterior two-thirds of the tongue, but in the posterior one-third the lymph channels cross the midline. Since inflammations, ulcerations and cancers of the tongue are rather common, it is important to be aware of the patterns of lymph drainage.

❡ Sensory innervation: (a) the anterior two-thirds of the tongue are innervated by the lingual nerve; (b) the posterior one-third receives innervation from the glossopharyngeal nerve; and (c) the most posterior part of the tongue is supplied by the vagus nerve.

❡ Taste innervation: (a) the anterior two-thirds of the tongue are innervated by the chorda tympani of the facial nerve; (b) the posterior one-third is supplied by the glossopharyngeal nerve (see also HN91); and (c) the epiglottis and most posterior part of the tongue is probably innervated by the vagus nerve.

❡ Motor innervation: all intrinsic and extrinsic muscles are supplied by the hypoglossal nerve (see HN93).

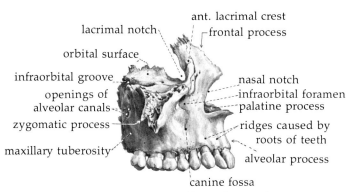

ant. lacrimal crest
lacrimal notch
orbital surface
frontal process
infraorbital groove
nasal notch
openings of
alveolar canals
infraorbital foramen
palatine process
zygomatic process
ridges caused by
roots of teeth
maxillary tuberosity
alveolar process
canine fossa

A.   Right maxilla (lateral aspect).

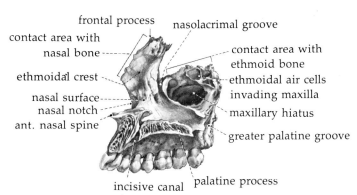

frontal process
nasolacrimal groove
contact area with
nasal bone
contact area with
ethmoid bone
ethmoidal crest
ethmoidal air cells
invading maxilla
nasal surface
maxillary hiatus
nasal notch
ant. nasal spine
greater palatine groove
incisive canal
palatine process

B.   Right maxilla (medial aspect).

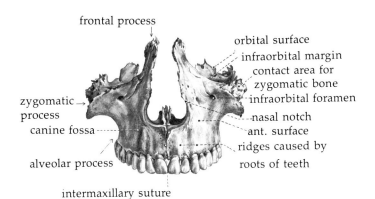

frontal process
orbital surface
infraorbital margin
contact area for
zygomatic bone
zygomatic
process
infraorbital foramen
canine fossa
nasal notch
ant. surface
ridges caused by
roots of teeth
alveolar process
intermaxillary suture

C.   Maxillae (frontal aspect).

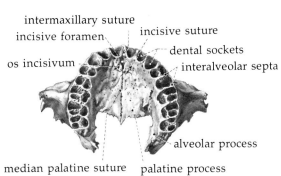

intermaxillary suture
incisive foramen
incisive suture
dental sockets
os incisivum
interalveolar septa
alveolar process
median palatine suture
palatine process

D.   Maxillae (palatine aspect).

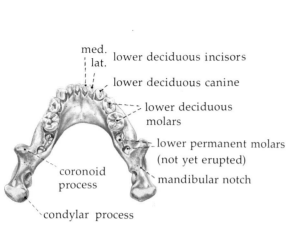

A. Deciduous (milk) dentition in a child of 4 to 5 years (upper jaw).

(upper jaw labels) upper permanent incisors (not yet erupted); med.; lat.; upper deciduous incisors; upper deciduous canine; 1st upper deciduous molar; 2nd upper deciduous molar; palatine process of maxilla; upper 1st permanent molar (not yet erupted); horizontal part of palatine bone; greater and lesser palatine foramina; median palatine suture

(lower jaw labels) med.; lat.; lower deciduous incisors; lower deciduous canine; lower deciduous molars; lower permanent molars (not yet erupted); coronoid process; mandibular notch; condylar process

B. Deciduous (milk) dentition in a child of 4 to 5 years (lower jaw).

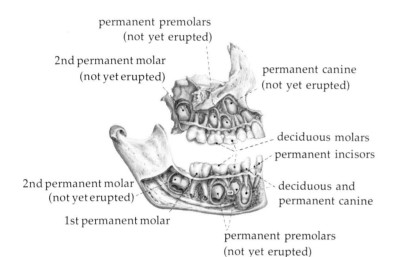

permanent premolars (not yet erupted); 2nd permanent molar (not yet erupted); permanent canine (not yet erupted); deciduous molars; permanent incisors; 2nd permanent molar (not yet erupted); deciduous and permanent canine; 1st permanent molar; permanent premolars (not yet erupted)

C. Replacement of deciduous teeth by permanent teeth in child of 8 to 9 years.

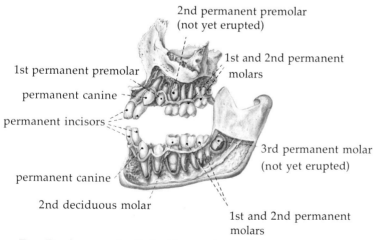

2nd permanent premolar (not yet erupted); 1st and 2nd permanent molars; 1st permanent premolar; permanent canine; permanent incisors; 3rd permanent molar (not yet erupted); permanent canine; 2nd deciduous molar; 1st and 2nd permanent molars

D. Replacement of deciduous teeth by permanent teeth in child of 10 to 11 years.

It is important for a physician to know when the baby's teeth erupt.

¶ The first set of teeth, the deciduous teeth, is temporary. The central or medial incisors erupt at the age of 6 to 8 months; the lateral incisors at 8 to 10 months; the first molars at about 1 year. The canine teeth appear at 1½ years, and finally the second molars erupt at 2 years. The total number of deciduous teeth is 20.

¶ The second, or permanent, set of teeth begins to erupt at the sixth year. The first to appear are the first permanent molars. Subsequently the medial incisors erupt at 7 years, the lateral incisors at 8 years, the first premolars at 9 years, the second premolars at 10 years, the canines at 11 years, the second molars at 12 years and finally, the third permanent molars between 17 and 30 years. It is not uncommon for the third molars to cause great difficulty during eruption because the space in the mandible is restricted. Similarly, the canines erupting between the lateral incisors and the first premolars may find their space restricted by their earlier appearing neighbors.

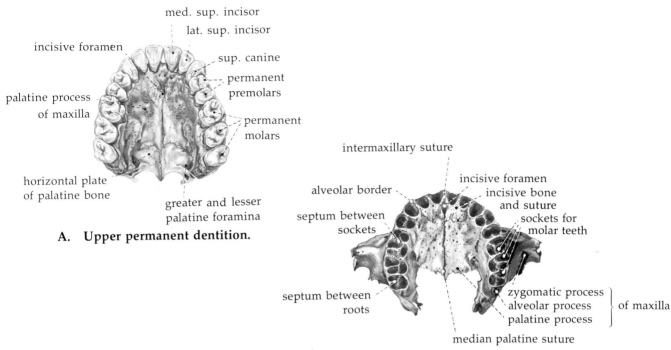

A. Upper permanent dentition.

B. Sockets for upper permanent teeth.

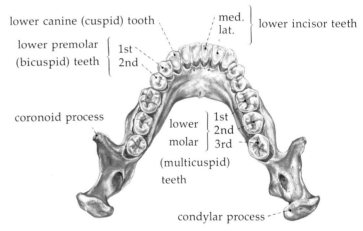

C. Lower permanent dentition.

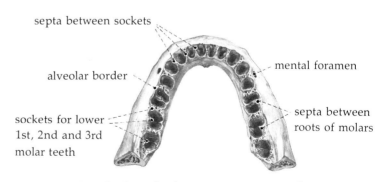

D. Sockets for lower permanent teeth.

¶ Sixteen permanent teeth are present in each dental arch: two incisors, one canine, two premolars and three molars on each side.

¶ The sockets for the lower teeth are closer to the lingual surface, and those of the upper teeth are closer to the labial and buccal surfaces of the mouth. Keep in mind that the roots of the upper molars may extend into the maxillary sinus.

¶ The roots of the molars are frequently curved. Since they are separated from each other in their sockets by bony septa, extraction of the teeth may be difficult. Frequently it cannot be accomplished without fracturing the septa. (Remember the lingual nerve when extracting the lower third molar!) (See HN87 and HN90.)

451

1st upper premolar

1st upper molar

incisive canal

groove for
lingual nerve

mandibular foramen
for inf. alveolar
artery and nerve

1st lower molar

1st lower premolar

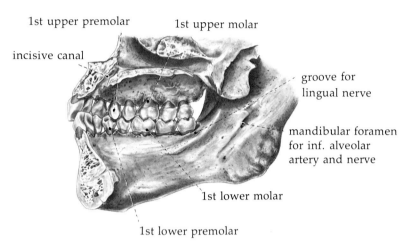

roots of lower
molar teeth

mental foramen

A.   Permanent teeth seen from the right side.
The roots of the teeth have been dissected.

**B.   Normal (centric) occlusion of per-
manent teeth (medial view).**

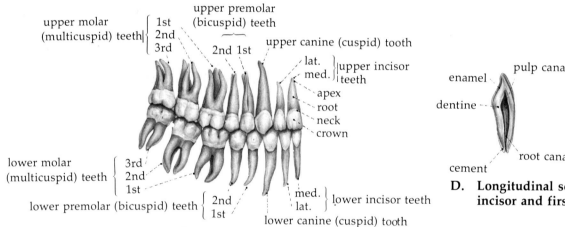

upper molar
(multicuspid) teeth

1st
2nd
3rd

upper premolar
(bicuspid) teeth

2nd 1st

upper canine (cuspid) tooth

lat.
med.

upper incisor
teeth

apex
root
neck
crown

lower molar
(multicuspid) teeth

3rd
2nd
1st

lower premolar (bicuspid) teeth

2nd
1st

med.
lat.

lower incisor teeth

lower canine (cuspid) tooth

**C.   Permanent right teeth (vestibular
view).**

enamel

pulp canal

pulp chamber in crown

cusp

crown
neck
root

dentine

cement

root canal

apical foramen

**D.   Longitudinal section of medial lower
incisor and first lower molar teeth.**

Keep in mind:

ꟼ   Normally the upper dental arch slightly overlaps the lower dental arch. When in occlusion, all
teeth are in contact with two opposing teeth except the lower medial incisor, which is the smallest
of the incisors, and the third upper molar, which is the smallest of the molars.

ꟼ   The incisor teeth have cutting edges and one root. The canine teeth each have one cusp and one
root. The upper premolars each have two (or three) cusps and two roots. The upper molars have
three to four cusps and three roots. The lower molars have three to five cusps and two roots.

ꟼ   The crown of the tooth projecting from the gingiva (gum) is covered with enamel. The root,
covered with a thin layer of cementum, is embedded in the bony socket and secured to the bone
by the periodontal membrane. The pulp cavity contains a branch from the nerve as well as blood
and lymph vessels. Infections of the teeth resulting from caries may penetrate the pulp cavity and
may then cause a periodontal abscess at the root of the teeth. In severe cases osteomyelitis of the
mandible may occur. When the molars of the upper jaw are involved, inflammation of the maxillary sinus may result (see HN51).

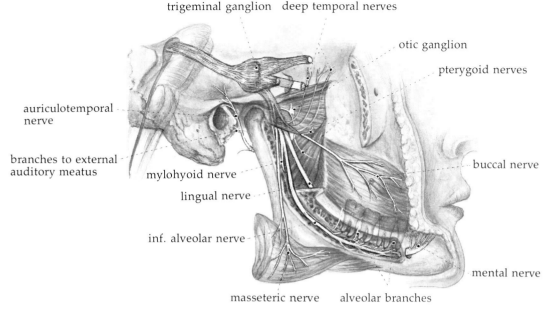

trigeminal ganglion   deep temporal nerves

otic ganglion

pterygoid nerves

auriculotemporal
nerve

branches to external
auditory meatus

buccal nerve

mylohyoid nerve

lingual nerve

inf. alveolar nerve

mental nerve

masseteric nerve   alveolar branches

A.   Innervation of the teeth of the inferior dental arch.

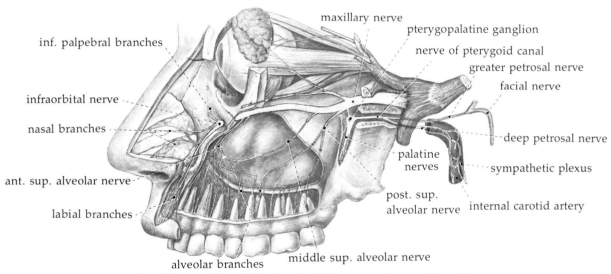

maxillary nerve

pterygopalatine ganglion

inf. palpebral branches

nerve of pterygoid canal

greater petrosal nerve

facial nerve

infraorbital nerve

nasal branches

deep petrosal nerve

palatine
nerves

sympathetic plexus

ant. sup. alveolar nerve

post. sup.
alveolar nerve   internal carotid artery

labial branches

alveolar branches   middle sup. alveolar nerve

B.   Innervation of the teeth of the superior dental arch.

It is important to note:

¶ The inferior alveolar nerve supplies the molar and premolar teeth. At the mental foramen it bi-furcates into a branch to the canine and incisor teeth and the mental nerve to the chin and lower lip. When the entire inferior alveolar nerve must be anesthetized in dental procedures, the best place for injection is just above the mandibular foramen (see HN87 B). Close to the foramen, how-ever, is also found the lingual nerve, which is usually affected by injection in the region of the mandibular foramen, resulting in numbness of the tongue. The mental nerve, of course, is always affected when the inferior alveolar nerve is anesthetized; this results in loss of feeling to the skin over the chin and lower lip.

¶ The teeth of the upper jaw are innervated by the maxillary division of the trigeminal nerve. The posterior superior alveolar nerve arises in the pterygopalatine fossa and supplies the second and third molar teeth and two roots of the first molar. The middle superior alveolar nerve descends in the lateral wall of the maxillary sinus and supplies the mesial root of the first molar and the pre-molar teeth; the anterior superior alveolar nerve descends in the anterior wall of the maxillary sinus and innervates the canine and incisor teeth.

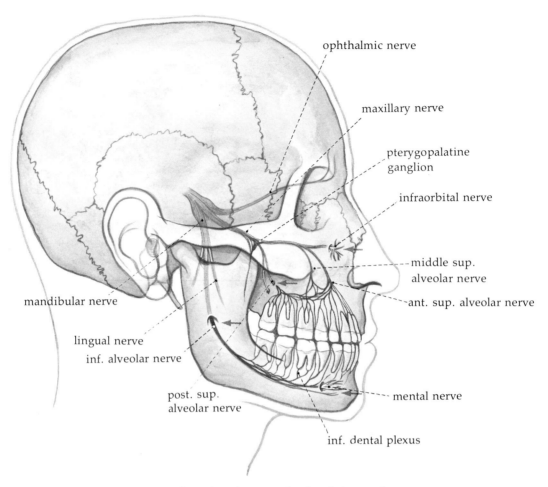

ophthalmic nerve

maxillary nerve

pterygopalatine ganglion

infraorbital nerve

middle sup. alveolar nerve

ant. sup. alveolar nerve

mandibular nerve

lingual nerve

inf. alveolar nerve

post. sup. alveolar nerve

mental nerve

inf. dental plexus

Injection sites for anesthesia of the teeth.

Keep in mind:

¶ To anesthetize the inferior alveolar nerve the injection must be made close to the mandibular foramen, which is bounded by the sphenomandibular ligament medially and the mandible laterally (see HN88). The top of the mandibular foramen lies in a plane level with the occlusal surface of the lower molars. (Before making the injection make sure the needle is not in the inferior alveolar vein or artery!)

¶ To anesthetize the lower canine and incisors, make the injection at the level of the mental foramen, which is located three-fourths of an inch below the crest of the gingiva between the two premolar teeth.

¶ To block the posterior superior alveolar nerve, the needle is introduced above the second maxillary molar and then gently pushed obliquely upward along the maxillary bone.

¶ The anterior and middle superior alveolar nerves branch from the infraorbital nerve in its course through the infraorbital canal. They descend along the wall of the maxillary sinus. To produce a block anesthesia, the nerves are injected through the infraorbital foramen, which is on a vertical plane with the pupil when the eye is fixed straight ahead.

¶ Keep in mind that the buccal nerve innervates the soft tissues on the buccal side of the teeth; the lingual nerve innervates the soft tissues on the lingual side.

¶ The anterior one-third of the palate is innervated by the nasopalatine nerve and the posterior two-thirds by the greater palatine nerve (see HN48 and HN50).

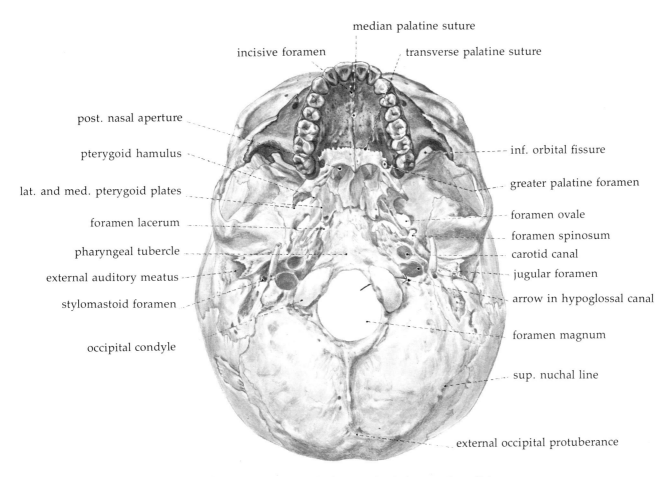

median palatine suture

incisive foramen

transverse palatine suture

post. nasal aperture

pterygoid hamulus

lat. and med. pterygoid plates

foramen lacerum

pharyngeal tubercle

external auditory meatus

stylomastoid foramen

occipital condyle

inf. orbital fissure

greater palatine foramen

foramen ovale

foramen spinosum

carotid canal

jugular foramen

arrow in hypoglossal canal

foramen magnum

sup. nuchal line

external occipital protuberance

The base of the skull (inferior view) (norma basalis).

It is important to examine again the base of the skull before dissecting the pharynx. Note:

¶ The carotid canal through which the internal carotid artery and the sympathetic carotid plexus enter the skull.

¶ The jugular foramen through which the internal jugular vein leaves the cranial cavity. Just before entering the jugular foramen, the vein receives blood from the sigmoid sinus and the inferior petrosal sinus. In addition, the glossopharyngeal, the vagus and the accessory nerves leave the skull through the jugular foramen. Remember that the meningeal branch of the ascending pharyngeal artery as well as the meningeal branch of the occipital artery may also enter the skull through the jugular foramen.

¶ The hypoglossal canal through which the hypoglossal nerve leaves the skull.

¶ The hamulus of the medial pterygoid plate (HN113) from which a portion of the superior pharyngeal constrictor originates.

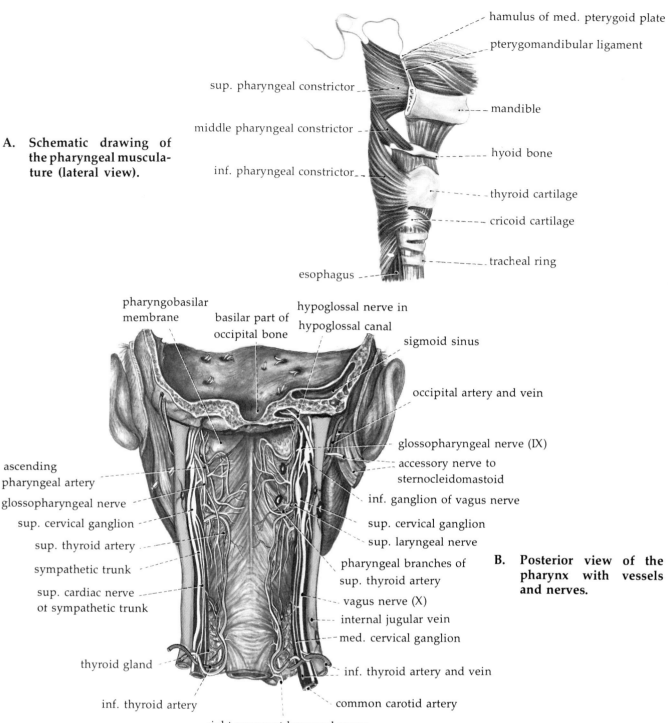

A. Schematic drawing of the pharyngeal musculature (lateral view).

hamulus of med. pterygoid plate

pterygomandibular ligament

sup. pharyngeal constrictor

mandible

middle pharyngeal constrictor

hyoid bone

inf. pharyngeal constrictor

thyroid cartilage

cricoid cartilage

tracheal ring

esophagus

pharyngobasilar membrane

basilar part of occipital bone

hypoglossal nerve in hypoglossal canal

sigmoid sinus

occipital artery and vein

glossopharyngeal nerve (IX)

accessory nerve to sternocleidomastoid

ascending pharyngeal artery

glossopharyngeal nerve

sup. cervical ganglion

inf. ganglion of vagus nerve

sup. cervical ganglion

sup. laryngeal nerve

sup. thyroid artery

sympathetic trunk

pharyngeal branches of sup. thyroid artery

sup. cardiac nerve of sympathetic trunk

vagus nerve (X)

internal jugular vein

med. cervical ganglion

thyroid gland

inf. thyroid artery and vein

inf. thyroid artery

common carotid artery

right recurrent laryngeal nerve

B. Posterior view of the pharynx with vessels and nerves.

¶ The pharynx is a musculomembranous tube. The anterior wall is incomplete, since the posterior nasal apertures, the oral cavity and the larynx enter from the front. The posterior wall, however, is entirely muscular and the fibers sweep from their anterior origin posteriorly to the midline raphe, which is attached above to the pharyngeal tubercle.

¶ According to its place of origin, the superior constrictor is sometimes subdivided into: (a) a pterygopharyngeal part originating from the hamulus of the medial pterygoid plate; (b) a buccopharyngeal part arising from the pterygomandibular ligament; (c) a mylopharyngeal part originating from the mylohyoid line of the mandible; and (d) the glossopharyngeal part arising from the lateral side of the tongue. Similarly, the middle constrictor is divided into a part originating from the lesser horn of the hyoid and the lower part of the stylohyoid ligament (chondropharyngeal part) and a part originating from the greater horn of the hyoid bone (ceratopharyngeal part). The inferior constrictor muscle is divided into the thyropharyngeus and cricopharyngeus, according to their place of origin (see HN109).

¶ The pharynx receives branches from the vagus and glossopharyngeal nerves and from the sympathetic trunk. Together they form a plexus, the pharyngeal plexus.

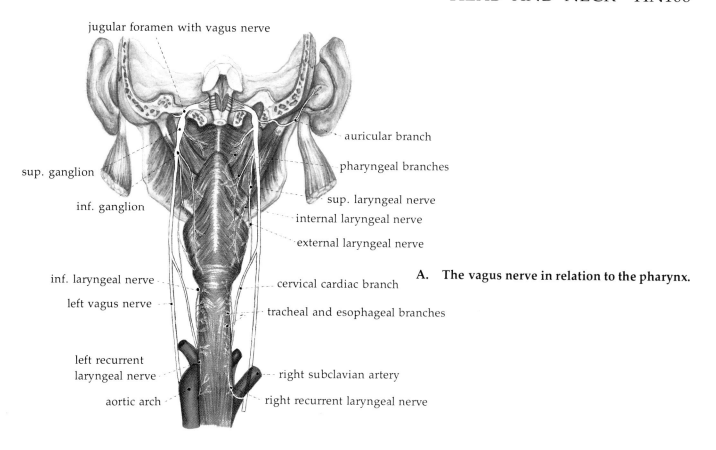

jugular foramen with vagus nerve

auricular branch

pharyngeal branches

sup. ganglion

sup. laryngeal nerve

inf. ganglion

internal laryngeal nerve

external laryngeal nerve

inf. laryngeal nerve

cervical cardiac branch

A. The vagus nerve in relation to the pharynx.

left vagus nerve

tracheal and esophageal branches

left recurrent laryngeal nerve

right subclavian artery

aortic arch

right recurrent laryngeal nerve

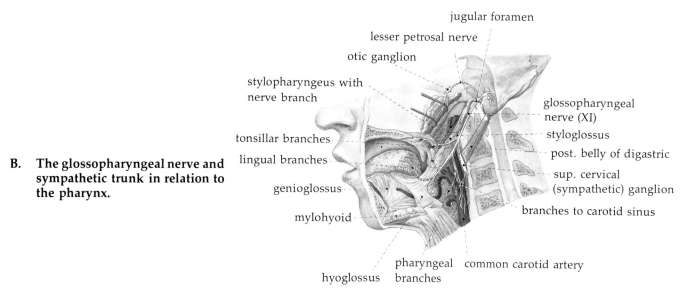

jugular foramen

lesser petrosal nerve

otic ganglion

stylopharyngeus with nerve branch

glossopharyngeal nerve (XI)

styloglossus

tonsillar branches

post. belly of digastric

lingual branches

sup. cervical (sympathetic) ganglion

genioglossus

branches to carotid sinus

mylohyoid

B. The glossopharyngeal nerve and sympathetic trunk in relation to the pharynx.

hyoglossus   pharyngeal branches   common carotid artery

The pharyngeal plexus, supplying the pharyngeal and palate region, contains branches from several sources:

¶ The pharyngeal branches of the vagus carry many fibers of the cranial root of the accessory nerve. They supply all the muscles of the pharynx and palate except the *stylopharyngeus* (glossopharyngeal nerve) and *tensor veli palatini* (motor branch of the mandibular nerve).

¶ The branches of the glossopharyngeal nerve are mainly sensory, with the exception of a motor branch to the stylopharyngeus. They supply sensory fibers to the mucous membranes of the pharynx, the soft palate and the palatine tonsils. The cell bodies of the sensory fibers are found in the ganglia of the glossopharyngeal and vagus nerves.

¶ The branches from the superior cervical ganglion consist of the laryngopharyngeal branches, which pass to the sides of the pharynx, where they join branches from the glossopharyngeal and vagus nerves. Some delicate fibers connect the superior cervical ganglion with the inferior ganglion of the vagus and with that of the glossopharyngeal nerve. (Parasympathetic branches to the pharynx are supplied by the glossopharyngeal nerve.)

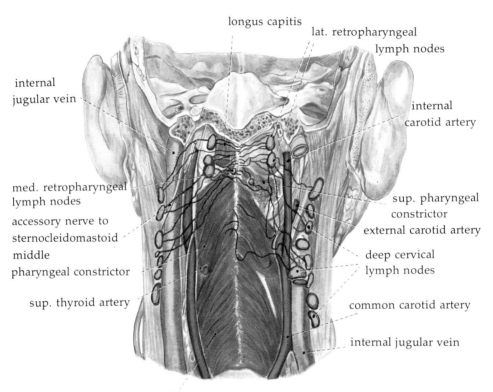

longus capitis

lat. retropharyngeal
lymph nodes

internal
jugular vein

internal
carotid artery

med. retropharyngeal
lymph nodes

accessory nerve to
sternocleidomastoid

middle
pharyngeal constrictor

sup. pharyngeal
constrictor

external carotid artery

deep cervical
lymph nodes

sup. thyroid artery

common carotid artery

internal jugular vein

inf. pharyngeal constrictor

The retropharyngeal and deep cervical lymph nodes.

¶ The retropharyngeal lymph nodes drain the soft palate and to some extent the palatine and pharyngeal tonsils. The lymph channels pierce the superior pharyngeal constrictor to reach the nodes, which lie between the prevertebral and buccopharyngeal fascia. When inflamed and swollen, the nodes cause a swelling in the posterior wall of the pharynx and may eventually rupture into the pharynx. These swellings have to be distinguished from retropharyngeal abscesses, which in front are delineated by the prevertebral fascia. Retropharyngeal abscesses usually originate in the vertebral column, and are generally tuberculous in nature. Their expansion is determined by the plane of the prevertebral fascia (see HN81).

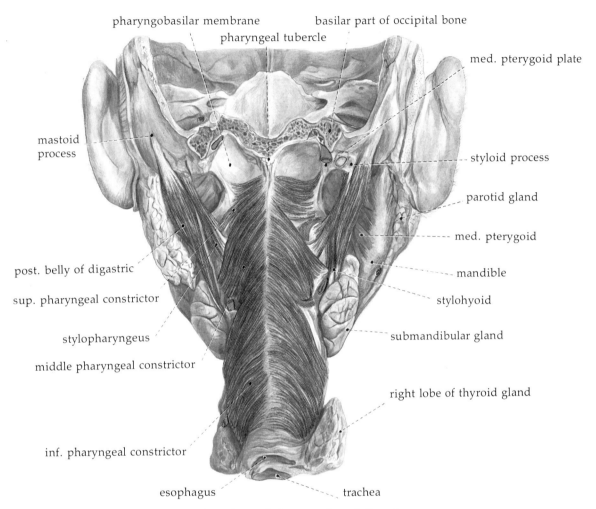

pharyngobasilar membrane

basilar part of occipital bone

pharyngeal tubercle

med. pterygoid plate

mastoid process

styloid process

parotid gland

med. pterygoid

post. belly of digastric

mandible

sup. pharyngeal constrictor

stylohyoid

stylopharyngeus

submandibular gland

middle pharyngeal constrictor

right lobe of thyroid gland

inf. pharyngeal constrictor

esophagus

trachea

Posterior view of the muscles of the pharynx.

¶ The pharyngeal musculature consists of: (a) the superior, middle and inferior constrictors, which have a more or less circular course and (b) the stylopharyngeus and salpingopharyngeus, which have fibers running in a longitudinal direction. The *stylopharyngeus* originates from the medial side of the styloid process and enters the pharyngeal wall between the superior and middle constrictors. It inserts at the posterior border of the thyroid cartilage. The *salpingopharyngeus* originates from the lower margin of the auditory tube and blends with the palatopharyngeus (see HN112). The function of both muscles is to raise the pharynx during swallowing.

¶ The pharyngobasilar membrane helps to keep the nasopharynx patent. It is anchored above to the pharyngeal tubercle on the basilar part of the occipital bone, to the wall of the auditory tube and to the posterior border of the medial pterygoid plate. From here it descends along the pterygomandibular ligament to the posterior end of the mylohyoid line of the mandible.

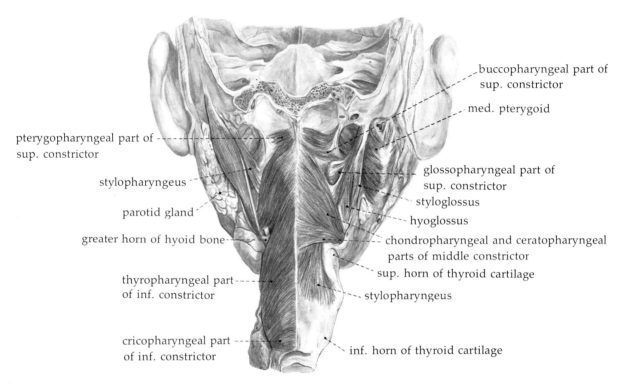

pterygopharyngeal part of
sup. constrictor

stylopharyngeus

parotid gland

greater horn of hyoid bone

thyropharyngeal part
of inf. constrictor

cricopharyngeal part
of inf. constrictor

buccopharyngeal part of
sup. constrictor

med. pterygoid

glossopharyngeal part of
sup. constrictor

styloglossus

hyoglossus

chondropharyngeal and ceratopharyngeal
parts of middle constrictor

sup. horn of thyroid cartilage

stylopharyngeus

inf. horn of thyroid cartilage

Posterior view of the pharynx, showing the various muscle components.
The digastric, stylohyoid and inferior constrictor have been removed on the right side.

The main function of the constrictor muscles is to help in swallowing. They perform three different actions:

¶ The upper fibers of the superior constrictor pull the posterior wall of the pharynx forward. When the soft palate is elevated, it comes in contact with the posterior wall of the pharynx. The nasal part of the pharynx is thus closed, and food is prevented from moving into the nasopharynx.

¶ The contraction of the lower fibers of the superior constrictor followed by that of the middle and inferior constrictors moves the food down toward the esophagus.

¶ The lower fibers of the inferior constrictor are thought to act as a sphincter to prevent air from entering the esophagus between swallowing movements.

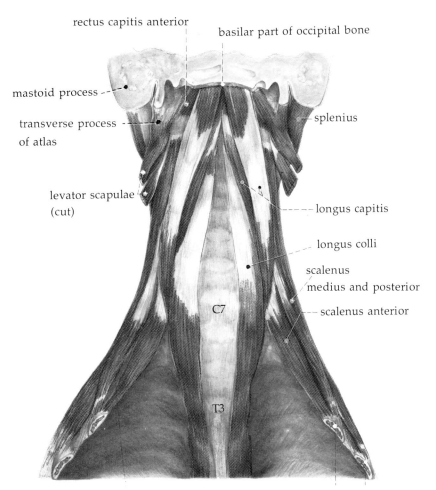

rectus capitis anterior

basilar part of occipital bone

mastoid process

splenius

transverse process
of atlas

levator scapulae
(cut)

longus capitis

longus colli

scalenus
medius and posterior

scalenus anterior

C7

T3

Prevertebral musculature.

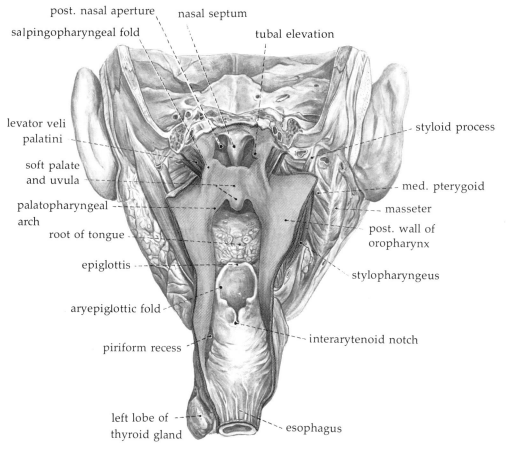

post. nasal aperture nasal septum

salpingopharyngeal fold tubal elevation

levator veli palatini styloid process

soft palate and uvula med. pterygoid

palatopharyngeal arch masseter

root of tongue post. wall of oropharynx

epiglottis stylopharyngeus

aryepiglottic fold interarytenoid notch

piriform recess

left lobe of thyroid gland esophagus

The pharynx opened from behind.

A number of important points should be observed:

¶ When the posterior wall of the pharynx is cut open longitudinally, the mucosa can be seen to be continuous with that of the nasal cavities, mouth, larynx and auditory tube. Hence, inflammations of the pharynx may spread to the nose, palatine tonsils, larynx and even to the middle ear.

¶ The nasopharynx is located above the soft palate and behind the posterior nasal apertures. The roof is attached to the basilar parts of the sphenoid and occipital bones and is rich in lymphatic tissue, the *pharyngeal tonsil* (see HN115). This lymphatic tissue is in contact with the lymphoid tissue around the entrance of the auditory tube (the *tubal tonsil*) and with the lymphoid tissue descending along the salpingopharyngeal folds.

¶ The oropharynx extends from the undersurface of the soft palate to the upper border of the epiglottis. The floor is formed by the posterior third of the tongue, which is irregular in appearance and rich in lymphoid tissue, the *lingual tonsil*. The lateral walls are characterized by the *palatine tonsils* (see HN114 and HN115).

¶ The piriform fossa is a recess on either side of the entrance to the larynx. Medially it is bounded by the aryepiglottic fold and laterally by the thyroid cartilage. Its floor frequently has a little fold caused by the internal ramus of the superior laryngeal nerve (see HN97). The recess is important because fish bones and pieces of peanuts may easily lodge in the recess. It is sometimes difficult to remove the foreign body without technical help.

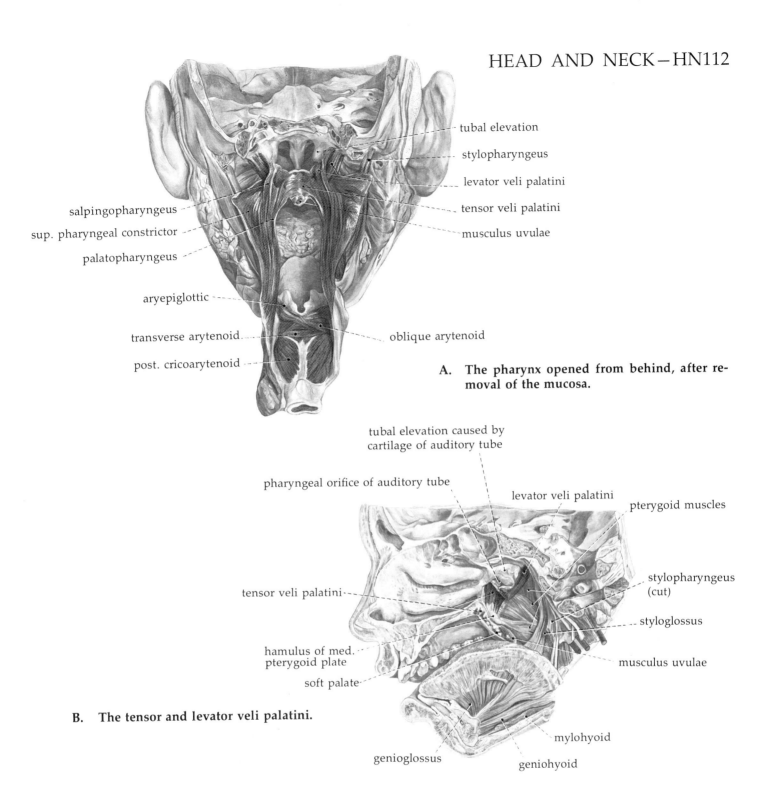

tubal elevation

stylopharyngeus

levator veli palatini

tensor veli palatini

musculus uvulae

salpingopharyngeus

sup. pharyngeal constrictor

palatopharyngeus

aryepiglottic

transverse arytenoid

post. cricoarytenoid

oblique arytenoid

A. The pharynx opened from behind, after removal of the mucosa.

tubal elevation caused by
cartilage of auditory tube

pharyngeal orifice of auditory tube

levator veli palatini

pterygoid muscles

tensor veli palatini

stylopharyngeus
(cut)

styloglossus

hamulus of med.
pterygoid plate

musculus uvulae

soft palate

B. The tensor and levator veli palatini.

mylohyoid

genioglossus

geniohyoid

Note:

¶ The fibers of two pharyngeal muscles, the stylopharyngeus and the salpingopharyngeus, run longitudinally. Both pull the pharynx upward during swallowing.

¶ The levator veli palatini and the tensor veli palatini play an important role in closing off the nasopharynx during swallowing. The *levator veli palatini* originates from the undersurface of the petrous portion of the temporal bone and the medial surface of the auditory tube (see HN113). The muscle inserts into the upper surface of the palatine aponeurosis, and when it contracts, the soft palate is raised toward the posterior wall of the pharynx. The *tensor veli palatini* originates from the lateral side of the auditory tube and from the scaphoid fossa and spine of the sphenoid bone. Its tendon turns medially around the hamulus of the medial pterygoid plate and, with its partner from the opposite side, forms the palatine aponeurosis. Their combined action tightens the soft palate so that the levators can move it upward like a septum. (Keep in mind that the tensor muscle is innervated by the motor branch of the mandibular nerve.)

¶ The *musculus uvulae* originates from the hard palate and palatine aponeurosis and supports the levator and tensor veli palatini in raising the uvula toward the posterior wall of the pharynx.

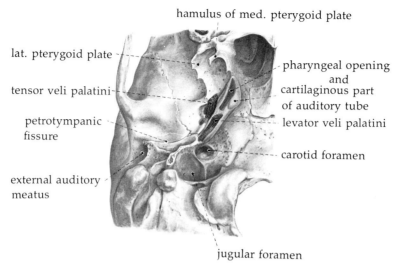

hamulus of med. pterygoid plate

lat. pterygoid plate

tensor veli palatini

petrotympanic fissure

external auditory meatus

pharyngeal opening and cartilaginous part of auditory tube

levator veli palatini

carotid foramen

jugular foramen

A. Origin of the levator and tensor veli palatini.

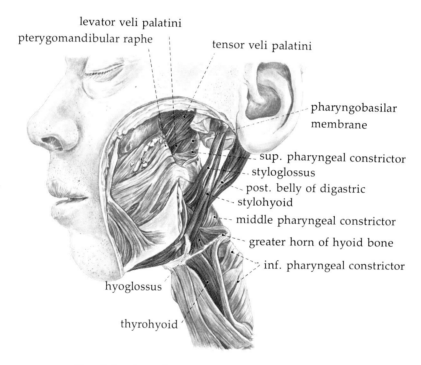

levator veli palatini
pterygomandibular raphe

tensor veli palatini

pharyngobasilar membrane

sup. pharyngeal constrictor

styloglossus

post. belly of digastric

stylohyoid

middle pharyngeal constrictor

greater horn of hyoid bone

inf. pharyngeal constrictor

hyoglossus

thyrohyoid

B. Muscles of the palate, tongue and pharynx.

Swallowing is a complicated function in which many muscles are involved. The main functions of the musculature are: (a) to prevent the food bolus from entering the nasopharynx; (b) to push it down the pharynx to the esophagus; and (c) to prevent it from entering the larynx.

¶ During swallowing the nasopharynx is closed off from the oropharynx by the combined action of the levator veli palatini, tensor veli palatini, musculus uvulae, upper fibers of the superior pharyngeal constrictor and palatopharyngeus (see HN109 and HN112).

¶ To move the food bolus from the mouth into the oropharynx, the hyoid bone is pulled up by the geniohyoid, mylohyoid, digastric and stylohyoid muscles. Simultaneously, the oropharyngeal isthmus is narrowed by the styloglossal and palatoglossal muscles.

¶ Once the food is in the oropharynx, the pharynx is pulled up by the stylopharyngeus, salpingopharyngeus and palatopharyngeus. Simultaneously, the larynx is pulled toward the epiglottis, which serves as its cover. The aryepiglottic folds are then approximated, while the arytenoid cartilages are drawn forward by the aryepiglottic, arytenoid and thyro-arytenoid muscles.

¶ By gravity and by contraction of the pharyngeal constrictors the food bolus slips over the epiglottis and the posterior surfaces of the arytenoid cartilages into the lower part of the pharynx.

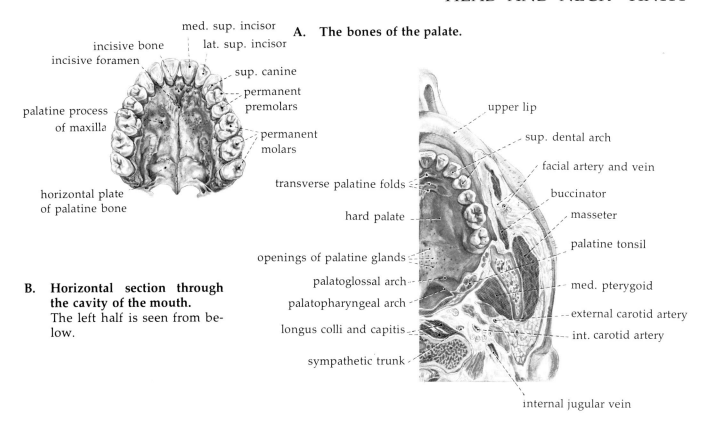

A. The bones of the palate.

med. sup. incisor
incisive bone
lat. sup. incisor
incisive foramen
sup. canine
permanent premolars
palatine process of maxilla
permanent molars
horizontal plate of palatine bone

upper lip
sup. dental arch
facial artery and vein
buccinator
masseter
transverse palatine folds
palatine tonsil
hard palate
med. pterygoid
openings of palatine glands
external carotid artery
palatoglossal arch
int. carotid artery
palatopharyngeal arch
longus colli and capitis
sympathetic trunk
internal jugular vein

B. Horizontal section through the cavity of the mouth.
The left half is seen from below.

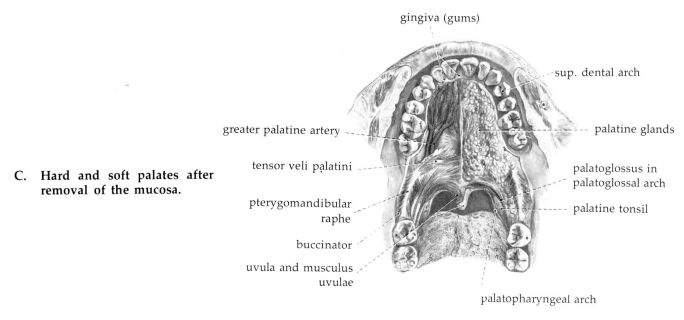

gingiva (gums)
sup. dental arch
greater palatine artery
palatine glands
tensor veli palatini
palatoglossus in palatoglossal arch
pterygomandibular raphe
palatine tonsil
buccinator
uvula and musculus uvulae
palatopharyngeal arch

C. Hard and soft palates after removal of the mucosa.

Inspection of the palate, particularly in the newborn, is very important, since clefts of the palate occur frequently. On the bony palate, note:

¶ The hard palate is formed by the palatine processes of the maxillae and the horizontal plates of the palatine bones. These components fuse in the midline. If the palatine processes (shelves) have failed to fuse, a wide midline cleft will be visible in the newborn.

¶ An additional component of the palate is the incisive bone, a small bone containing the four incisors. Sometimes the palatine processes of the maxillae fail to fuse with the incisive bone. This results in a cleft lip and jaw and a cleft in the palate extending from the lateral border of the second incisor to the incisive foramen.

¶ The soft palate is rich in lymphoid tissue and contains a number of muscles: (a) the tensor veli palatini, spread out as a thin sheet and known as the palatine aponeurosis; it is attached to the posterior border of the bony palate; (b) the levator veli palatini; and (c) the musculus uvulae. A second group of muscles is formed by the palatoglossus and palatopharyngeus, each producing a fold of the same name. The palatine tonsil is found between the folds (see also HN115 A).

465

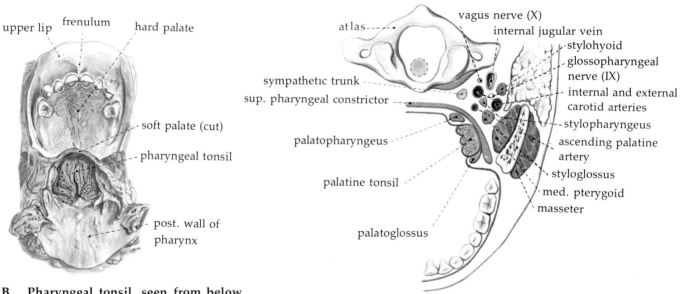

A. Sagittal section through the tongue, larynx and pharynx.

soft palate · palatoglossal arch
supratonsillar fossa · *palatine tonsil* · *pharyngeal tonsil* · palatopharyngeal arch · oral part of pharynx · epiglottis · laryngeal part of pharynx · *lingual tonsil* · hyoid bone · vestibular fold · vocal fold · thyroid cartilage · lamina of cricoid cartilage · arch of cricoid cartilage · esophagus · trachea

upper lip · frenulum · hard palate · soft palate (cut) · pharyngeal tonsil · post. wall of pharynx

B. Pharyngeal tonsil, seen from below, in a child of 2 years.

atlas · vagus nerve (X) · internal jugular vein · stylohyoid · glossopharyngeal nerve (IX) · sympathetic trunk · sup. pharyngeal constrictor · internal and external carotid arteries · stylopharyngeus · palatopharyngeus · ascending palatine artery · styloglossus · palatine tonsil · med. pterygoid · masseter · palatoglossus

C. The palatine tonsil and related structures.

¶ The palatine tonsils consist of lymphoid tissue covered by mucous membrane with a number of small openings leading into tonsillar crypts. Inferiorly, the palatine tonsillar area is continuous with the lingual tonsil; superiorly, it is close to the pharyngeal tonsillar area. Hence, the junction of the nose and the oral cavity is surrounded by a ring of lymphoid tissue.

¶ The collection of lymphoid tissue in the oropharyngeal region is of great clinical importance, particularly in young children. Infections of the palatine tonsils that produce signs of a sore throat spread easily to the pharyngeal tonsil in the roof of the pharynx. The pharyngeal tonsil may become greatly enlarged and is then known as adenoids. The swollen and greatly enlarged tonsil may block the posterior nasal openings, causing the child to breathe through the mouth. Similarly, the pharyngeal entrance of the auditory tubes may be blocked, and this may cause deafness or recurrent middle ear infections.

¶ The lateral surface of the palatine tonsil is covered by a fibrous capsule and separated by a layer of loose areolar tissue from the pharyngeal musculature. Inflammations of the tonsils sometimes expand and break through the capsule to form a peritonsillar abscess. When inflammations occur frequently, tonsillectomy is performed. In removing the tissue of the palatine tonsil, the palatine vessels and other nerves and arteries immediately lateral to the tonsil must be kept in mind.

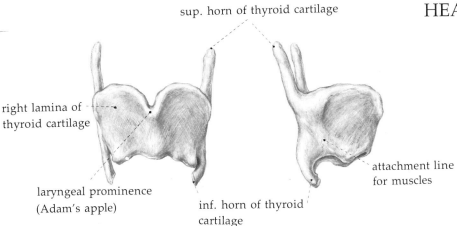

A. Thyroid cartilage seen from the front and from the right.

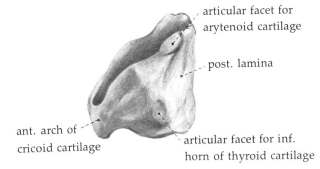

B. Cricoid cartilage seen from the left.

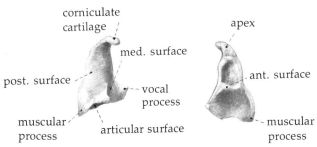

C. Left arytenoid cartilage seen from behind and from the front.

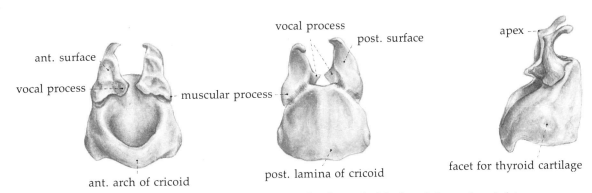

D. Cricoarytenoid joints seen from the front, behind and from the right.

The joints between the arytenoid and cricoid cartilages are important because the width between the vocal cords, as well as their length, is an important factor in the pitch of the voice.

¶ The cricoarytenoid joints allow a horizontal gliding movement of the arytenoids. Since the vocal cords are attached to the vocal processes, the gliding movements permit adduction and abduction of the vocal cords.

¶ The cricoarytenoid joints also allow rotation of the arytenoids around an axis which is nearly vertical. Lateral rotation of the arytenoids results in a lateral anterior displacement of the vocal processes, and medial rotation results in their medial posterior displacement. Hence, medial rotation adducts and lengthens the cords, while lateral rotation abducts and relaxes the cords.

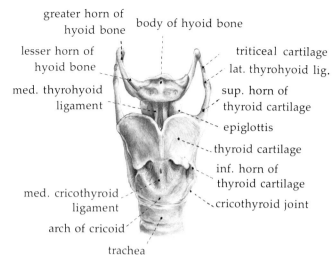

greater horn of
hyoid bone   body of hyoid bone

lesser horn of
hyoid bone

med. thyrohyoid
ligament

triticeal cartilage

lat. thyrohyoid lig.

sup. horn of
thyroid cartilage

epiglottis

thyroid cartilage

inf. horn of
thyroid cartilage

med. cricothyroid
ligament

cricothyroid joint

arch of cricoid

trachea

A. Ligaments of the larynx (front view).
The thyrohyoid membrane has been removed.

greater horn of hyoid bone

hyoepiglottic ligament

lesser horn of
hyoid bone

med. thyrohyoid
ligament

med. cricothyroid
ligament

arch of cricoid
cartilage

triticeal cartilage

lat. thyrohyoid ligament

sup. horn of
thyroid cartilage

cartilage of epiglottis

inf. horn of
thyroid cartilage

fibrous capsule of
cricothyroid joint

B. Ligaments of the larynx (lateral view).
The thyrohyoid membrane has been removed.

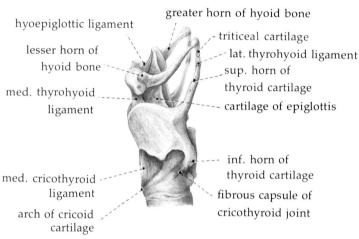

greater horn of hyoid bone   thyrohyoid membrane

lat. thyrohyoid ligament

foramen for sup. laryngeal
vessels and int. laryngeal nerve

sup. thyroid tubercle

inf. thyroid tubercle
cricothyroid joint

body of hyoid bone

med. thyrohyoid ligament

fat body

med. cricothyroid ligament

straight part
oblique part } cricothyroid muscle

C. Thyrohyoid membrane and cricothyroid muscle (lateral view).

Note the connections of the epiglottis to the cartilages of the larynx:

¶ The epiglottis is connected in front to the body of the hyoid bone by the hypoepiglottic ligaments (see *B*); through its stalk it is connected to the back of the thyroid cartilage. The aryepiglottic folds and membranes connect the epiglottis with the top of the arytenoid cartilages (HN118).

¶ The cricothyroid joints permit a rotating movement of the thyroid cartilage around a horizontal axis that passes through the joints on the two sides. This rotating movement permits the thyroid cartilage to move forward and somewhat downward or backward and upward. When the thyroid cartilage is rotated forward by the action of the cricothyroid muscle (see HN119), the origin and insertion of the vocal cords are pulled away from each other, and consequently the cords become tense. The pitch of the voice then becomes higher. The opposite movement in the cricothyroid joints causes relaxation of the vocal cords, and the voice becomes hoarse.

aryepiglottic fold

fat body

cricoarytenoid joint

capsule of cricothyroid joint

lamina of cricoid cartilage

arytenoid cartilage

cricothyroid joint

cricotracheal ligament

fibrous wall of trachea

B. Posterior view of the cavity of the larynx.
The posterior wall of the larynx has been split.

(posterior view).

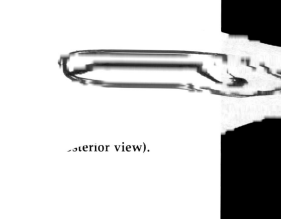

aryepiglottic fold

cuneiform tubercle

corniculate tubercle

vocal fold

transverse arytenoid

lamina of cricoid cartilage

infraglottic cavity

foramen cecum

vallecula

vestibule of larynx

piriform recess

vestibular fold

laryngeal sinus leading into saccule of larynx

trachea

hyoepiglottic ligament

thyrohyoid membrane

epiglottis

hyoid bone

greater horn of hyoid bone

thyrohyoid membrane { superficial layer / deep layer

vestibular ligament

vocal ligament

conus elasticus

cricothyroid ligament

cricotracheal ligament

aryepiglottic fold

quadrangular membrane

arytenoid cartilage

vocal process of arytenoid cartilage

cricoid cartilage

C. Sagittal section through the larynx, viewed from the left.
The left lamina of the thyroid cartilage and the muscles have been removed.

Observe the following important points:

¶ The vocal ligament is attached anteriorly to the deep surface of the thyroid cartilage and posteriorly to the vocal or anterior process of the arytenoid cartilage. The vocal ligaments and the mucosa make up the vocal folds. The rima glottidis is the gap between the vocal folds.

¶ The vestibular ligament is the lower edge of the quadrangular membrane. It is attached to the thyroid cartilage anteriorly and to the side of the arytenoid cartilage posteriorly. The ligaments are covered by mucosa and form the vestibular folds. Between the vestibular and vocal folds is the lateral vestibule (sinus) of the larynx. The rima vestibuli is the gap between the vestibular folds.

469

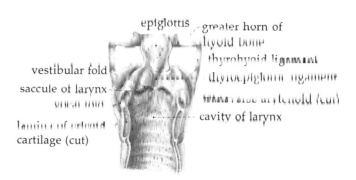

epiglottis — greater horn of hyoid bone

thyrohyoid ligament

thyroepiglottic ligament

vestibular fold

saccule of larynx

vocal fold

muscular process arytenoid (cut)

cavity of larynx

lamina of cricoid cartilage (cut)

A. Cavity of larynx (posterior view).

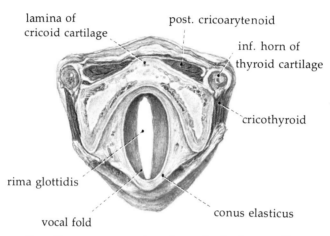

lamina of cricoid cartilage

post. cricoarytenoid

inf. horn of thyroid cartilage

cricothyroid

rima glottidis

vocal fold

conus elasticus

B. Transverse section through the larynx (inferior view).

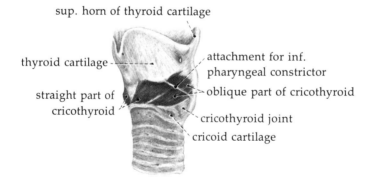

sup. horn of thyroid cartilage

thyroid cartilage

attachment for inf. pharyngeal constrictor

straight part of cricothyroid

oblique part of cricothyroid

cricothyroid joint

cricoid cartilage

C. The cricothyroid seen from the left.

The following points are important to remember:

♪ The cricothyroid is the only muscle innervated by the external branch of the superior laryngeal nerve (see HN121 A). The internal branch of the nerve is sensory and supplies the mucosa of the larynx above the vocal folds. Contraction of the muscle moves the thyroid cartilage forward and slightly downward on the cricoid cartilage. This movement lengthens the distance between the origin and insertion of the vocal cords, and they therefore become tense. Tension of the cords causes a higher pitch of the voice.

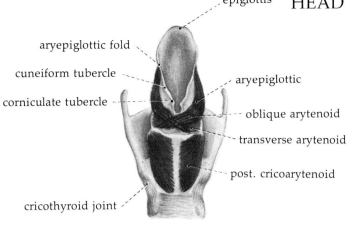

epiglottis

aryepiglottic fold

cuneiform tubercle

corniculate tubercle

aryepiglottic

oblique arytenoid

transverse arytenoid

post. cricoarytenoid

cricothyroid joint

A. The muscles of the larynx seen from behind.

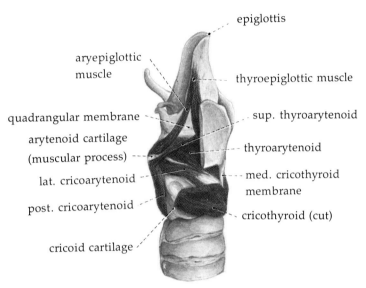

epiglottis

aryepiglottic muscle

thyroepiglottic muscle

quadrangular membrane

sup. thyroarytenoid

arytenoid cartilage (muscular process)

thyroarytenoid

lat. cricoarytenoid

med. cricothyroid membrane

post. cricoarytenoid

cricothyroid (cut)

cricoid cartilage

B. The muscles of the larynx seen from the right.
The right lamina of the thyroid cartilage has been removed.

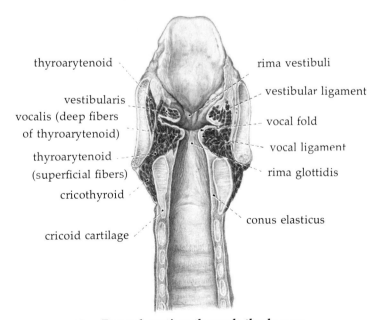

thyroarytenoid

rima vestibuli

vestibularis

vestibular ligament

vocalis (deep fibers of thyroarytenoid)

vocal fold

vocal ligament

thyroarytenoid (superficial fibers)

rima glottidis

cricothyroid

cricoid cartilage

conus elasticus

C. Frontal section through the larynx.

¶ The thyroarytenoid (see *B*) is the antagonist of the cricothyroid. Contraction of the muscle pulls the arytenoid toward the thyroid cartilage, thus shortening the distance between the origin and insertion of the vocal cords. Hence, it relaxes the cords. The most medial part of the muscle is the vocalis. The muscles also provide some adduction of the vocal folds.

¶ Adduction of the vocal folds (narrowing of the rima glottidis) is caused by the lateral cricoarytenoid, the oblique and transverse arytenoid and the cricothyroid muscles. Abduction (widening of the rima glottidis) is caused only by the posterior cricoarytenoids.

471

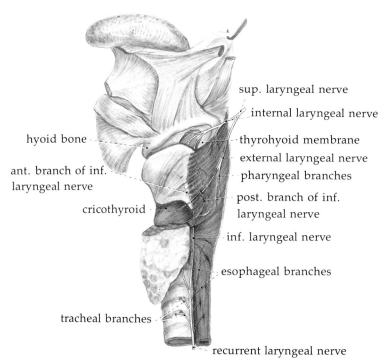

sup. laryngeal nerve

internal laryngeal nerve

hyoid bone

thyrohyoid membrane

external laryngeal nerve

ant. branch of inf. laryngeal nerve

pharyngeal branches

cricothyroid

post. branch of inf. laryngeal nerve

inf. laryngeal nerve

esophageal branches

tracheal branches

recurrent laryngeal nerve

A. Innervation of the laryngeal musculature.

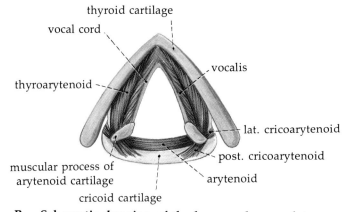

thyroid cartilage

vocal cord

vocalis

thyroarytenoid

lat. cricoarytenoid

post. cricoarytenoid

muscular process of arytenoid cartilage

arytenoid

cricoid cartilage

B. Schematic drawing of the laryngeal musculature.

All the muscles of the larynx are innervated by branches of the vagus. Keep in mind:

¶ The superior laryngeal nerve divides into an external branch, which innervates the cricothyroid muscle, and an internal branch, which enters the larynx through the foramen in the thyrohyoid membrane. This branch supplies sensory innervation to the mucous membrane above the vocal cords. Lesions of the superior laryngeal nerve cause loss of sensation above the vocal cords and a hoarse voice resulting from paralysis of the cricothyroid muscles.

¶ The inferior laryngeal (recurrent laryngeal) nerve innervates all the muscles of the larynx except the cricothyroid. It splits into: (a) an anterior branch that innervates the adductors of the vocal cords (the arytenoids and lateral cricoarytenoid muscles), and (b) a posterior branch that innervates the abductor (the posterior cricoarytenoid).

¶ In removing the thyroid gland great care must be taken to avoid damaging the inferior laryngeal nerves. If the nerves are cut, the vocal cords will assume a paramedian position. If, however, only the posterior branch of the nerve is cut, the abductor of the vocal folds is paralyzed, and the adductors acting as antagonists will close the rima glottidis. Asphyxia will result.

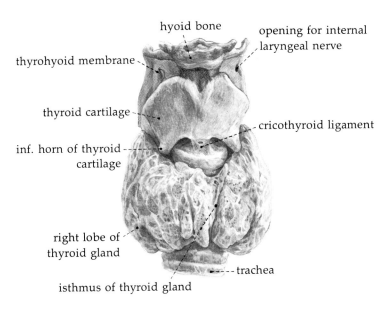

hyoid bone

opening for internal laryngeal nerve

thyrohyoid membrane

thyroid cartilage

inf. horn of thyroid cartilage

cricothyroid ligament

right lobe of thyroid gland

isthmus of thyroid gland

trachea

A. Anterior view of the thyroid gland.
The isthmus is broader than normal.

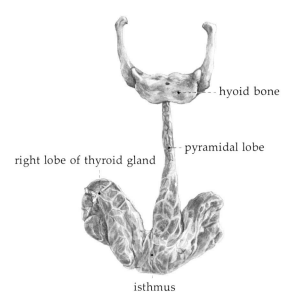

hyoid bone

pyramidal lobe

right lobe of thyroid gland

isthmus

B. Thyroid gland with an abnormally long pyramidal lobe.

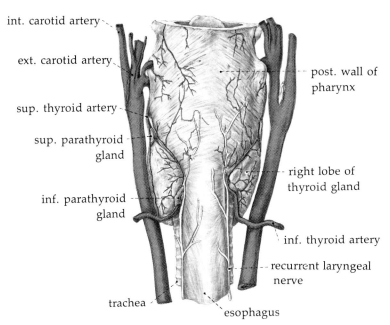

int. carotid artery

ext. carotid artery

sup. thyroid artery

sup. parathyroid gland

inf. parathyroid gland

post. wall of pharynx

right lobe of thyroid gland

inf. thyroid artery

recurrent laryngeal nerve

trachea

esophagus

C. Posterior view of the thyroid gland in relation to the pharynx.

A number of important points should be noted:

¶ The isthmus of the gland extends across the midline in front of the second, third and fourth tracheal rings. Under normal conditions the isthmus can be felt by placing the index finger below the cricoid cartilage and asking the patient to swallow. Since the thyroid gland is connected to the larynx through the pretracheal fascia, the isthmus will be pulled upward and an impression can be gained about its size.

¶ The blood supply of the thyroid comes from two sources: (a) the superior thyroid artery, a branch of the external carotid, is accompanied by the superior laryngeal nerve; (b) the inferior thyroid artery, a branch of the thyrocervical trunk, ascends behind the gland in the tracheoesophageal groove and is accompanied by the recurrent laryngeal nerve. These relationships are important in surgical procedures when the arteries of the gland have to be ligated. Cutting the laryngeal nerves or their branches will result in total or partial paralysis of the laryngeal musculature.

¶ The thyroid gland is surrounded by the pretracheal fascia (see HN81) and its own fibrous capsule. Between the two fasciae are the parathyroid glands and a rich venous plexus.

¶ The pretracheal layer of the fascia around the gland is particularly dense on the anterior aspect but less so on the posterior and medial aspects. Hence, the thyroid often enlarges in a posterior direction and may easily compress the trachea and esophagus. The patient will have difficulty with swallowing and breathing.

¶ Cancers of the thyroid similarly may invade the trachea, esophagus and carotid artery. Sometimes the recurrent laryngeal nerve or even the sympathetic chain may be involved, causing changes in the voice (see HN121) or Horner's syndrome (see HN38).

473

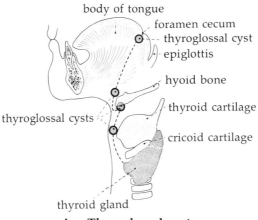

body of tongue
foramen cecum
thyroglossal cyst
epiglottis
hyoid bone
thyroid cartilage
cricoid cartilage
thyroglossal cysts
thyroid gland

A. Thyroglossal cysts.

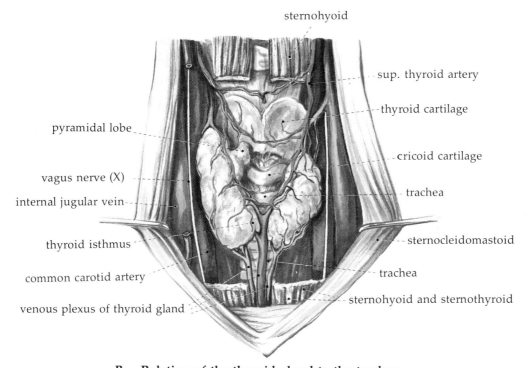

sternohyoid
sup. thyroid artery
thyroid cartilage
cricoid cartilage
pyramidal lobe
trachea
vagus nerve (X)
internal jugular vein
sternocleidomastoid
thyroid isthmus
trachea
common carotid artery
venous plexus of thyroid gland
sternohyoid and sternothyroid

B. Relation of the thyroid gland to the trachea.

¶ The thyroid gland develops as an outgrowth of the epithelium of the floor of the tongue (foramen cecum). The diverticulum descends anteriorly or posteriorly to the hyoid bone and migrates subsequently over the cartilages of the larynx to its final position. The solid cord connecting the tongue with the thyroid gland gradually disappears. Frequently, however, remnants of the cord remain, forming an abnormally long pyramidal lobe or developing as so-called thyroglossal cysts. These cysts are always in the midline, most frequently close to or even behind the hyoid bone. Occasionally, thyroid tissue may be found in the tongue in the region of the foramen cecum.

¶ In patients with acute laryngeal obstructions, tracheotomy is commonly performed, either between the cricoid cartilage and the isthmus of the gland (high tracheotomy) or between the isthmus and the suprasternal notch (low tracheotomy).

High tracheotomy. A vertical incision is made through: (a) the skin; (b) the superficial fascia with the platysmal fibers (watch the anterior jugular veins); (c) the investing layer of the deep cervical fascia; (d) the pretracheal fascia with the sternohyoid muscles, which must be separated; and (e) the trachea, after the isthmus is pulled laterally. Watch for the esophagus.

Low tracheotomy. A vertical incision is made through: (a) the skin; (b) the superficial fascia with the platysmal fibers; (c) the investing layer of deep fascia with the veins; (d) connective tissue containing a rich venous plexus and on occasion a median thyroid artery; (e) the pretracheal fascia; and (f) the trachea. Watch for the brachiocephalic vessels and the upper part of the thymus.

BACK

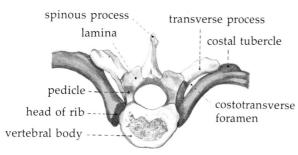

spinous process
lamina
transverse process
costal tubercle
pedicle
head of rib
vertebral body
costotransverse foramen

A. Thoracic vertebra with rib.

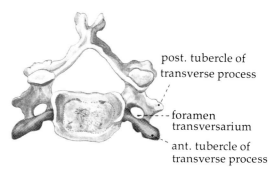

post. tubercle of transverse process
foramen transversarium
ant. tubercle of transverse process

B. Cervical vertebra.

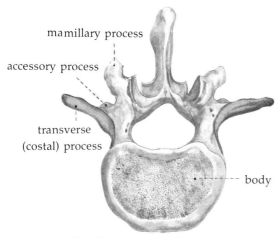

mamillary process
accessory process
transverse (costal) process
body

C. Lumbar vertebra.

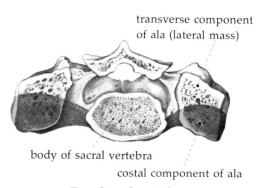

transverse component of ala (lateral mass)
body of sacral vertebra
costal component of ala

D. Sacral vertebra.

When the vertebrae in the various regions of the spine are compared, it is evident that they have a number of homologous components.

¶ The most representative unit of the vertebral column is the thoracic component. These vertebrae are characterized by a body, an arch, a spinous process and two transverse processes. They articulate with the ribs. The head of each rib forms a joint with two adjacent vertebrae at the level of the neurocentral junction, where the arch fuses with the body. In the thoracic region the rib is a free element, and the space between the rib and the vertebra is known as the costotransverse foramen (see T8).

¶ The rib element of the cervical vertebra is represented by the anterior part of the transverse process. Since the costotransverse foramen is now entirely enclosed in the transverse process, it is known as the foramen transversarium. It allows passage of the vertebral artery and a plexus of veins which unite to form the vertebral vein.

¶ In the lumbar region the costal element forms the major (anterior) part of the transverse process. The original transverse process is represented by the accessory process. The mamillary process is related to the articular facet and serves as origin for some of the muscles of the back (for instance, the multifidus—see B15 B).

¶ In the sacral region the costal elements form the anterior part of the lateral mass (ala) of the sacrum. They are completely fused with the original transverse processes of the sacral vertebrae.

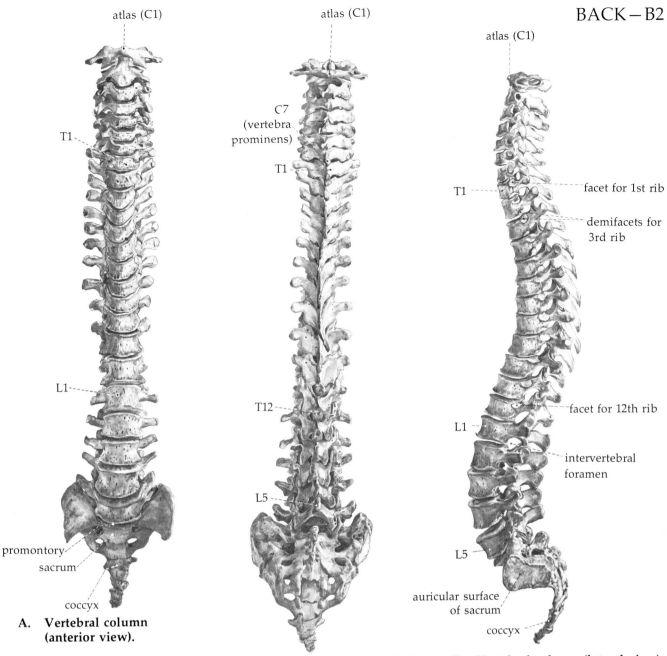

atlas (C1)

T1

L1

promontory

sacrum

coccyx

A. Vertebral column (anterior view).

atlas (C1)

C7 (vertebra prominens)

T1

T12

L5

B. Vertebral column (posterior view).

atlas (C1)

T1

facet for 1st rib

demifacets for 3rd rib

facet for 12th rib

L1

intervertebral foramen

L5

auricular surface of sacrum

coccyx

C. Vertebral column (lateral view).

The vertebral column performs three main functions: (a) it supports the head and trunk and transmits their weight to the lower extremities through the pelvic arch (see P7); (b) it protects the spinal cord (see B23); and (c) it allows considerable movements by the intervertebral joints and discs. Flexion and extension can be achieved in all three regions (cervical, thoracic and lumbar) of the column but are somewhat restricted in the thoracic region. Lateral flexion is extensive in the cervical and lumbar regions, but again is limited in the thoracic region. Rotation is most extensive in the thoracic region.

Considering the functions of the vertebral column, keep in mind:

¶ Diseases of the hip or unequal length of the lower extremities may seriously disturb the normal transmission of weight. Such disturbances are often compensated for by abnormal positions of the vertebral column. For example, lateral deviation (scoliosis) in the thoracic region often results from unequal lengths of the lower limbs.

¶ The normal posterior concavity of the cervical and lumbar regions and the posterior convexity in the thoracic and sacral regions may be accentuated by: (a) muscular diseases and paralysis; (b) structural changes in the bodies and discs; and (c) general bone diseases, such as tuberculosis and rickets. Kyphosis, an exaggeration of the posterior convexity of the vertebral column, is particularly characteristic of the thoracic region (humpback); lordosis, an exaggeration of the posterior concavity, is characteristic of the lumbar region.

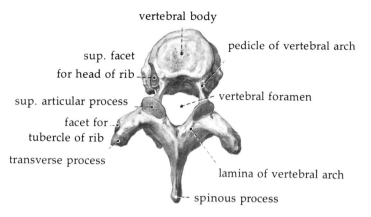

A. Thoracic vertebra seen from above.

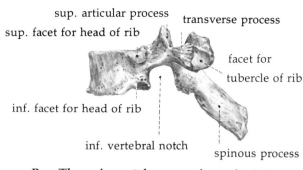

B. Thoracic vertebra seen from the left.

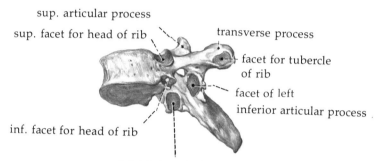

C. Thoracic vertebra seen from the left and below.

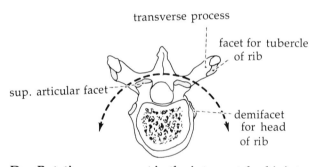

D. Rotation movement in the intervertebral joints.

¶ The thoracic vertebra is the most typical building block of the vertebral column. It consists of a body for weight-bearing and an arch, which together with the body protects the spinal cord in the vertebral canal. The arch is characterized by the pedicles laterally and the laminae posteriorly.

¶ The pedicles are notched at their superior and inferior aspects. The superior notch together with the inferior notch of the adjacent vertebra forms the intervertebral foramen. Through this foramen pass the spinal nerve and blood vessels. Since the canal is relatively narrow, the nerve may easily be compressed, particularly in the cervical region (see B23 and B25).

¶ Each arch carries two superior and two inferior articular processes. The two superior processes articulate with the inferior ones of the adjacent vertebra, thus forming the intervertebral joints. The position of the articular processes determines the type of movement that is possible, and it is evident that the main movement occurring in the thoracic region is rotation (see D).

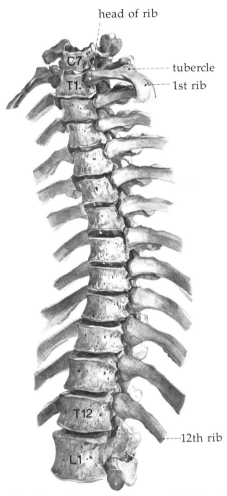

A. **The thoracic part of the vertebral column (see also T8).**

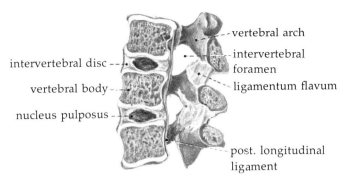

B. **Median section through three successive vertebrae.**

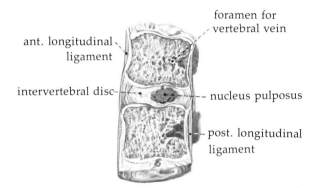

C. **Median section through the intervertebral disc.**

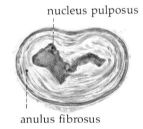

D. **The intervertebral disc seen from above.**

Movements in the vertebral column occur at the intervertebral joints, but the intervertebral discs also play an important role. These discs consist of an anulus fibrosus composed of fibrocartilage and a nucleus pulposus consisting of a gelatinous material that contains much water. The discs serve as shock absorbers and allow the vertebral bodies to move in relation to each other, as in flexion and extension of the spine.

The intervertebral discs are of great clinical importance:

ſ If the discs are exposed to sudden shocks or extreme compression, as in lifting heavy loads, the posterior part of the anulus fibrosus may be ruptured. This occurs most frequently in the lumbar and cervical regions but rarely in the thoracic aea. The nucleus pulposus is then forced through the ruptured area and protrudes either into the vertebral canal or, more laterally, into the intervertebral foramen. The protrusion of the nucleus pulposus is referred to as *herniation of the nucleus pulposus*. Depending on the site of herniation, a spinal nerve or part of the spinal cord may be compressed.

ſ With advancing age, the water content of the nucleus pulposus decreases, and the discs become less elastic. In old age it is sometimes impossible to distinguish between the anulus fibrosus and the nucleus pulposus. As a consequence, the vertebral column loses much of its resilience and elasticity and becomes more rigid.

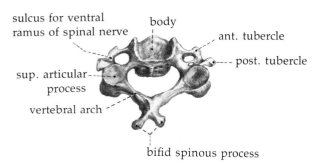

sulcus for ventral ramus of spinal nerve
body
ant. tubercle
post. tubercle
sup. articular process
vertebral arch
bifid spinous process

A. Typical cervical vertebra.
Note the bifid spinous process and the foramen transversarium, which transmits the vertebral vessels.

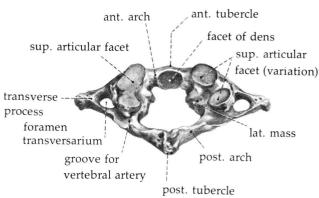

ant. arch
ant. tubercle
facet of dens
sup. articular facet
sup. articular facet (variation)
transverse process
foramen transversarium
lat. mass
groove for vertebral artery
post. arch
post. tubercle

B. Superior aspect of atlas.
Note the lack of the body and spinous process and the articular surfaces for the occipital bone and the axis.

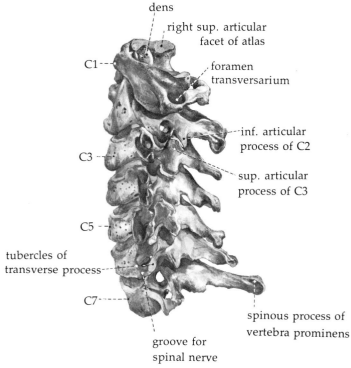

dens
right sup. articular facet of atlas
C1
foramen transversarium
inf. articular process of C2
C3
sup. articular process of C3
C5
tubercles of transverse process
C7
spinous process of vertebra prominens
groove for spinal nerve

C. Cervical part of the vertebral column.

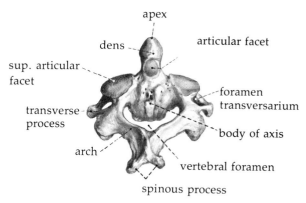

apex
dens
articular facet
sup. articular facet
foramen transversarium
transverse process
body of axis
arch
vertebral foramen
spinous process

D. Posterosuperior aspect of axis.
Note the dens, which represents the body of the atlas.

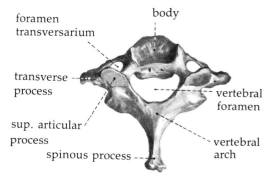

foramen transversarium
body
transverse process
vertebral foramen
sup. articular process
vertebral arch
spinous process

E. Seventh cervical vertebra (vertebra prominens).
Note the long spinous process; the foramen transversarium does not transmit the vertebral vessels and is often absent.

A fall on the head or neck with acute flexion of the neck may cause a fracture or dislocation of the cervical vertebrae. The almost horizontal position of the articular facets allows relatively easy dislocation of the vertebrae without resulting in fractures (see C). Dislocations may even occur after a sudden forward movement, as in car or airplane accidents. In the thoracic and lumbar regions the articular processes have a more vertical position, and in forward dislocations the intervertebral processes are usually fractured. In the cervical region dislocations and fractures of the vertebrae are extremely dangerous because the spinal cord is easily compressed or severed.

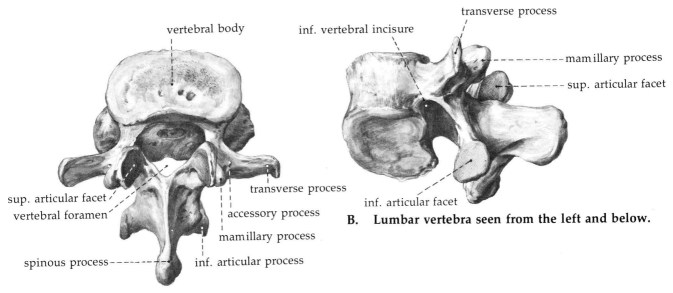

vertebral body

inf. vertebral incisure

transverse process

mamillary process

sup. articular facet

sup. articular facet

vertebral foramen

transverse process

accessory process

mamillary process

inf. articular process

spinous process

inf. articular facet

B. Lumbar vertebra seen from the left and below.

A. Lumbar vertebra seen from above.

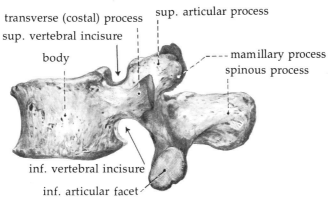

transverse (costal) process

sup. articular process

sup. vertebral incisure

body

mamillary process

spinous process

inf. vertebral incisure

inf. articular facet

C. Lumbar vertebra seen from the side.

Note:

¶ The body of the lumbar vertebra is large in comparison with that of the thoracic and cervical vertebrae. The large size is due to the fact that the lower the position of the vertebra in the column, the greater the weight it has to carry.

¶ The articular facets of the superior articular processes face medially, and those of the inferior ones face laterally. Hence, movement in the lumbar region consists mainly of flexion and extension.

¶ A fall from a great height and landing on the feet or buttocks frequently causes a fracture at the level of T12, L1 and L2 (flexion-compression fracture). Usually the body of a vertebra is compressed and appears wedged on radiographic examination. Sometimes a vertebra is displaced forward on the adjacent lower vertebra, causing fracture or dislocation of the articular facets.

¶ The most frequent site of herniation of the nucleus pulposus is the lower lumbar region. Pressure on the root of the fifth lumbar and first sacral nerves results from this injury, and pain is felt in the back of the thigh, leg and foot along the course of the sciatic nerve. Raising the lower extremity at the hip joint with the knee extended is extremely painful owing to the stretching of the already compressed nerve roots.

¶ Sometimes a herniation of the nucleus pulposus compresses the whole cauda equina, and paraplegia may result (see B25).

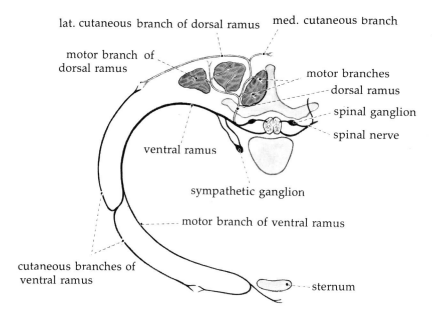

lat. cutaneous branch of dorsal ramus

med. cutaneous branch

motor branch of dorsal ramus

motor branches

dorsal ramus

spinal ganglion

spinal nerve

ventral ramus

sympathetic ganglion

motor branch of ventral ramus

cutaneous branches of ventral ramus

sternum

A.   Diagram of a spinal (thoracic) nerve and its branches.

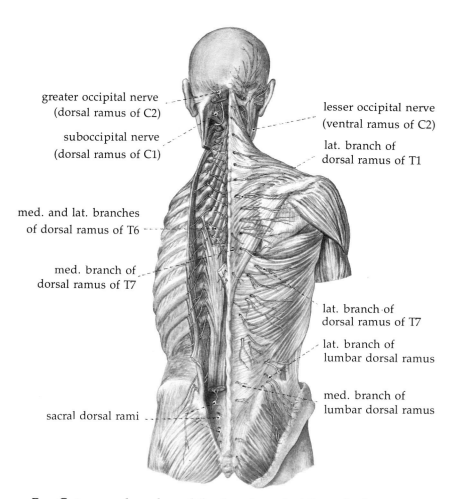

greater occipital nerve (dorsal ramus of C2)

suboccipital nerve (dorsal ramus of C1)

med. and lat. branches of dorsal ramus of T6

med. branch of dorsal ramus of T7

sacral dorsal rami

lesser occipital nerve (ventral ramus of C2)

lat. branch of dorsal ramus of T1

lat. branch of dorsal ramus of T7

lat. branch of lumbar dorsal ramus

med. branch of lumbar dorsal ramus

B.   Cutaneous branches of the dorsal rami of the spinal nerves.

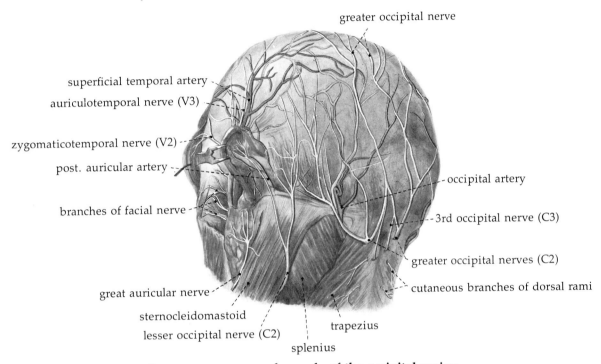

greater occipital nerve

superficial temporal artery

auriculotemporal nerve (V3)

zygomaticotemporal nerve (V2)

post. auricular artery

branches of facial nerve

occipital artery

3rd occipital nerve (C3)

greater occipital nerves (C2)

cutaneous branches of dorsal rami

great auricular nerve

sternocleidomastoid

lesser occipital nerve (C2)

trapezius

splenius

Cutaneous nerves and vessels of the occipital region.

¶ Like the ventral ramus, the dorsal ramus of the spinal nerve contains motor and sensory branches. The motor branches of the dorsal ramus innervate the deep muscles of the neck and back; the sensory branches, consisting of medial and lateral twigs, innervate the skin of the back and neck.

¶ The cutaneous innervation of the occipital and suboccipital regions follows the same pattern as that in the back. The dorsal ramus of the first cervical nerve—the *suboccipital nerve*—is an exception because it fails to divide into medial and lateral branches and usually contains only motor fibers. If the nerve has a sensory component, it accompanies the occipital artery to the scalp and then connects with the greater occipital nerve. The dorsal rami of C2—*the greater occipital nerve,* and C3—the *third occipital nerve,* follow the regular pattern. Both nerves have many sensory branches to the occipital and suboccipital regions and some motor branches to the deep neck musculature. Keep in mind that the *lesser occipital nerve* and the *great auricular nerve* are branches of the ventral rami of C2 and C3.

483

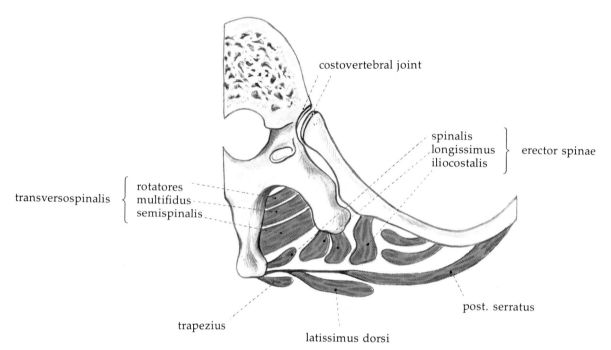

Schematic transverse section through the muscles of the back.

The muscles of the back are divided into: (a) a superficial group; (b) an intermediate group; and (c) a deep group. Note:

¶ The superficial group consists of the trapezius and latissimus dorsi. Both muscles act on the shoulder girdle. The trapezius receives its motor supply from the spinal accessory nerve, and the latissimus dorsi is supplied by the ventral rami of C6 to C8.

¶ The intermediate group consists of the rhomboids (see B11) and the posterior serratus muscles (see B12). They receive their motor innervation through the ventral rami of the cervical and thoracic spinal nerves. Since the muscles of the superficial and intermediate groups are innervated by the ventral rami of the spinal nerves, their precursor cells must have migrated from a ventral position toward the back region at some time during early development.

¶ The deep group is conveniently divided into long superficial bundles, the erector spinae (see B13) and shorter, more deeply placed muscles, the transversospinalis (see B15). Both groups fill the space between the spinous processes of the vertebrae and the angles of the ribs.

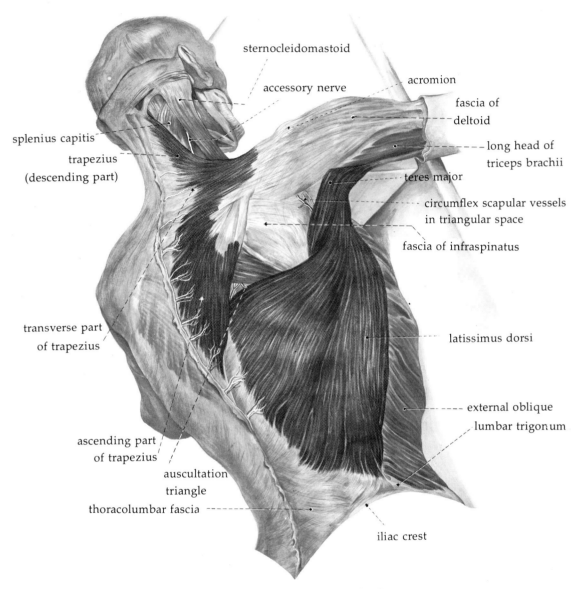

Superficial muscles of the back.
Note the accessory nerve to the sternocleidomastoid and the trapezius.

¶ The triangle bounded by the latissimus dorsi, the trapezius and the rhomboid muscles
is often referred to as the *triangle of auscultation*. Its floor is formed by the muscles of the
sixth intercostal space; hence, it is the most suitable place for auscultation of the lungs
at the back.

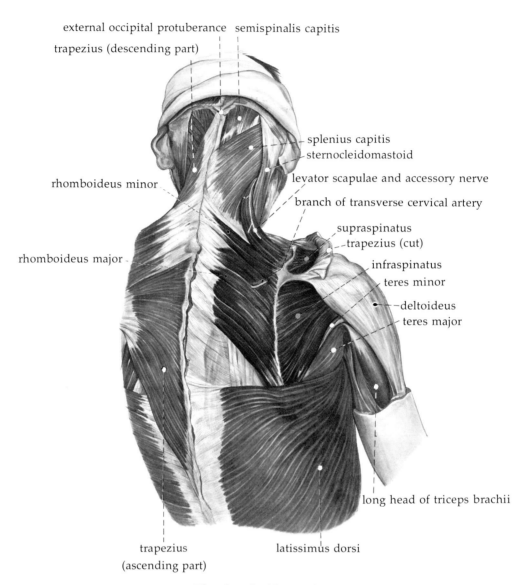

external occipital protuberance   semispinalis capitis

trapezius (descending part)

splenius capitis

sternocleidomastoid

rhomboideus minor

levator scapulae and accessory nerve

branch of transverse cervical artery

supraspinatus

trapezius (cut)

rhomboideus major

infraspinatus

teres minor

deltoideus

teres major

long head of triceps brachii

trapezius
(ascending part)

latissimus dorsi

The rhomboid muscles.

Note:

¶ The rhomboids extend from the spinous processes of C6 to T5 to the vertebral border of the scapula and are essential for movement of the scapula and thus for movements of the shoulder girdle and upper extremity (for details, see UL18 *B*).

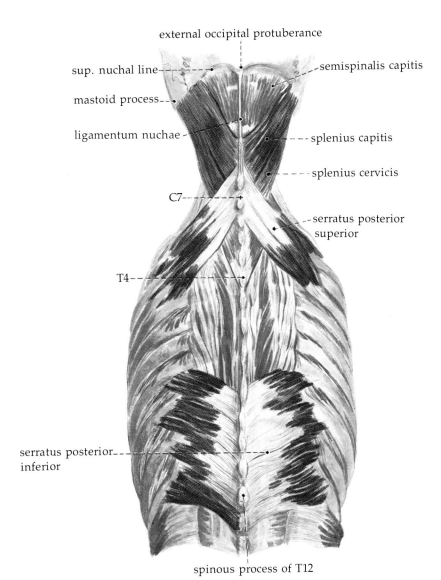

external occipital protuberance

sup. nuchal line

semispinalis capitis

mastoid process

ligamentum nuchae

splenius capitis

splenius cervicis

C7

serratus posterior
superior

T4

serratus posterior
inferior

spinous process of T12

The posterior serratus muscles.

¶ The serratus posterior superior and inferior act on the ribs. The superior muscle can
elevate the ribs, and the serratus inferior can draw the lower ribs downward and backward. The posterior serratus muscles in humans probably play a role in respiration.

(The splenius and semispinalis muscles are shown in B16.)

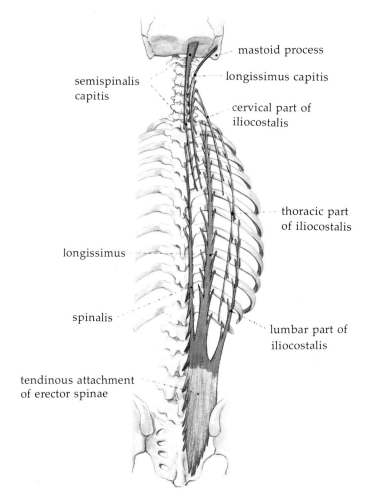

mastoid process

longissimus capitis

semispinalis
capitis

cervical part of
iliocostalis

thoracic part
of iliocostalis

longissimus

spinalis

lumbar part of
iliocostalis

tendinous attachment
of erector spinae

Schematic drawing of the erector spinae musculature.

The erector spinae consists of long muscle bundles that are all innervated by the dorsal rami of the spinal nerves. The muscles are divided into three groups:

¶ The lateral component — *the iliocostalis* — passes from the sacral region somewhat laterally to the angle of the lower ribs (lumbar part); other bundles pass from the lower ribs to the angle of ribs located higher (thoracic part); finally, some bundles pass from the angle of the uppermost ribs to the transverse process of the cervical vertebrae (cervical part).

¶ The intermediate component — *the longissimus* — passes upward and laterally from the sacrum and transverse processes to the angles of the ribs. Its uppermost part, the longissimus capitis, is attached to the posterior aspect of the mastoid process. It is the only portion of the erector spinae that reaches the skull.

¶ The medial component — *the spinalis* — passes from spine to spine from the sacral region to the upper thoracic region.

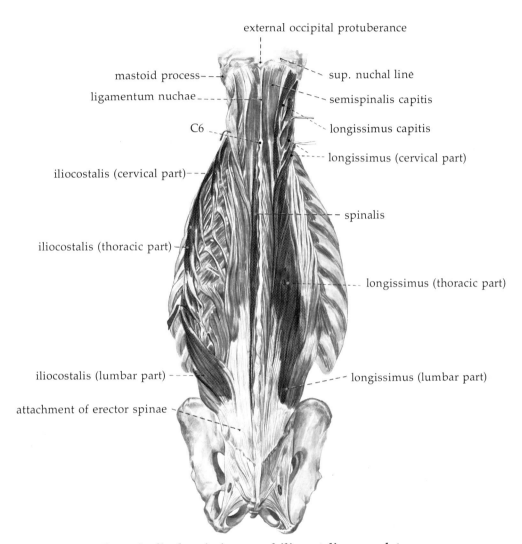

external occipital protuberance

mastoid process

ligamentum nuchae

C6

iliocostalis (cervical part)

iliocostalis (thoracic part)

iliocostalis (lumbar part)

attachment of erector spinae

sup. nuchal line

semispinalis capitis

longissimus capitis

longissimus (cervical part)

spinalis

longissimus (thoracic part)

longissimus (lumbar part)

The spinalis, longissimus and iliocostalis musculature.

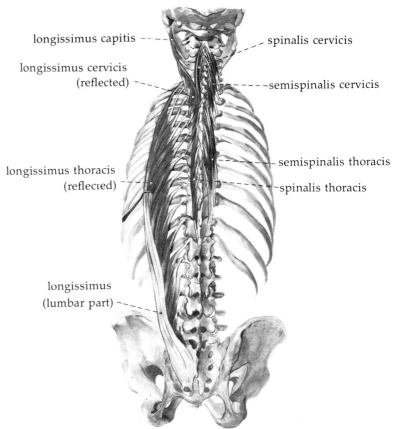

longissimus capitis

spinalis cervicis

longissimus cervicis
(reflected)

semispinalis cervicis

longissimus thoracis
(reflected)

semispinalis thoracis

spinalis thoracis

longissimus
(lumbar part)

A. The semispinalis cervicis and thoracis.
Note also the components of the erector spinae.

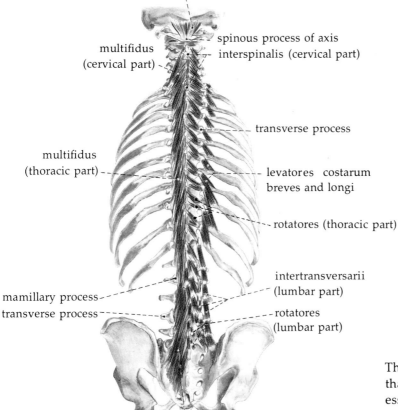

rectus capitis posterior minor

spinous process of axis

multifidus
(cervical part)

interspinalis (cervical part)

transverse process

multifidus
(thoracic part)

levatores costarum
breves and longi

rotatores (thoracic part)

intertransversarii
(lumbar part)

mamillary process

transverse process

rotatores
(lumbar part)

multifidus (sacral part)

B. The multifidus, rotatores, interspinales and intertransversarii.

The second part of the deep back musculature that fills the space between the spinous processes and the angles of the ribs consists of short muscles, together known as the transversospinalis. The main components are: (a) the semispinalis thoracis, cervicis and capitis; (b) the multifidus; (c) the rotatores lumborum, thoracis and cervicis; and (d) a group extending from one spinous process to the next (interspinales) and from one transverse process to the next (intertransversarii). Like the long muscle bundles of the erector spinae, all short muscles are innervated by the dorsal rami of the spinal nerves.

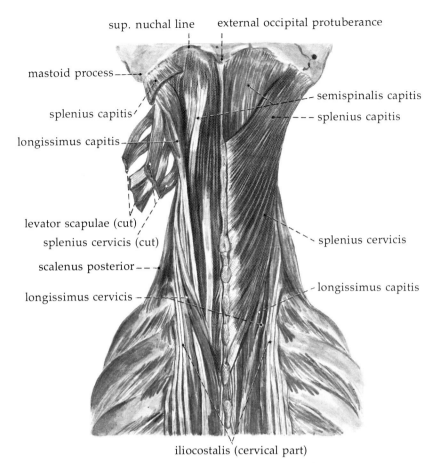

sup. nuchal line   external occipital protuberance

mastoid process

splenius capitis

longissimus capitis

semispinalis capitis

splenius capitis

levator scapulae (cut)

splenius cervicis (cut)

scalenus posterior

longissimus cervicis

splenius cervicis

longissimus capitis

iliocostalis (cervical part)

A. The deep muscles in the neck.

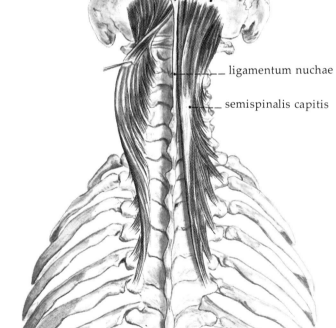

external occipital protuberance   sup. nuchal line

ligamentum nuchae

semispinalis capitis

B. The semispinalis capitis.

The deep musculature of the neck is somewhat more complicated than that of the thorax. This is due to the presence of additional muscles:

¶ The splenius consists of two parts, both of which are innervated by motor branches of the dorsal rami of the spinal nerves and thus belong to the deep musculature. The splenius capitis arises from the lower part of the ligamentum nuchae and the upper four thoracic spines. The muscle is attached to the superior nuchal line of the occipital bone and the mastoid process. The splenius cervicis has a similar origin but inserts into the transverse processes of the upper cervical vertebrae. (Keep in mind that the splenius muscles are superficial to the muscles of the erector spinae (see also B12).

¶ The semispinalis capitis arises from the tips of the transverse processes of C7 to T7 and from the articular processes of C4 to C6. Its tendons pass upward and insert between the superior and inferior nuchal lines of the occipital bone.

491

A. The suboccipital muscles.

external occipital protuberance

rectus capitis posterior minor

rectus capitis posterior major

obliquus capitis superior

transverse process of C1

post. tubercle of C1

spinous process of C2

mastoid process

vertebral artery

obliquus capitis inferior

interspinalis cervicis

rectus capitis posterior
minor and major

occipital artery

post. atlanto-occipital
membrane

greater occipital
nerve (C2)

sup. oblique

B. Schematic drawing of the suboccipital region.

suboccipital nerve
(dorsal ramus of C1)

spinal nerve of C2

dorsal ramus of C1

inf. oblique

vertebral artery

semispinalis cervicis
and capitis

splenius

trapezius

post. atlanto-occipital
membrane

rectus capitis posterior
minor and major

sup. oblique

C. Vertebral artery and first cervical nerve.
The posterior atlanto-occipital membrane has been opened on the right side.

dorsal ramus
of first cervical
nerve

inf. oblique (cut)

vertebral artery

greater occipital nerve

spinous process of C2

The superior and inferior obliques together with the rectus capitis posterior major delineate the suboccipital triangle. In this triangle are found:

¶ The *vertebral artery*. This artery is one of the main arteries supplying the brain. It originates from the first part of the subclavian artery and ascends through the foramina transversaria of the upper six cervical vertebrae. As soon as it has passed through the foramen in the atlas, it winds behind the lateral mass of the atlas in the vertebral groove (see B5 *B*). The artery then passes inferior to the edge of the posterior atlanto-occipital membrane and pierces the dura mater and arachnoid. It subsequently enters the skull through the foramen magnum.

¶ The *first cervical nerve* (suboccipital nerve). This nerve emerges inferior to the edge of the posterior atlanto-occipital membrane and lies between the artery and the atlas. The dorsal ramus emerges below the artery to innervate the two oblique and two rectus muscles. The ventral ramus passes medial and forward to the artery. (Note also the dorsal ramus of the second cervical nerve — the greater occipital nerve.) (see also B8).

¶ The *four pairs of suboccipital muscles.* These muscles extend the head in the atlanto-occipital joints and rotate it in the atlantoaxial joints. (For the movements of these joints, see B19 and B20).

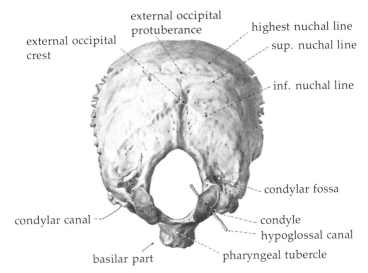

external occipital
protuberance

external occipital
crest

highest nuchal line

sup. nuchal line

inf. nuchal line

condylar fossa

condylar canal

condyle

hypoglossal canal

basilar part

pharyngeal tubercle

A.   External view of the occipital bone.

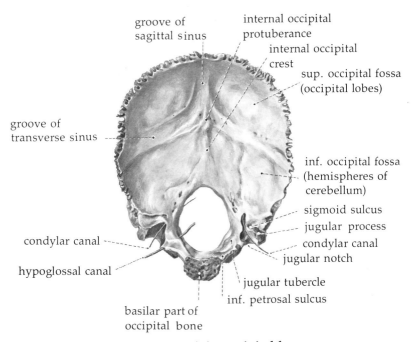

groove of
sagittal sinus

internal occipital
protuberance

internal occipital
crest

sup. occipital fossa
(occipital lobes)

groove of
transverse sinus

inf. occipital fossa
(hemispheres of
cerebellum)

sigmoid sulcus

jugular process

condylar canal

condylar canal

jugular notch

hypoglossal canal

jugular tubercle

inf. petrosal sulcus

basilar part of
occipital bone

B.   Internal view of the occipital bone.
Note the grooves for the venous sinuses.

In examining the occipital bone, note the following points:

¶ On each side of the external occipital crest are three curved lines extending in a lateral direction. The uppermost of the three, the highest nuchal line, is only faintly marked and serves as the attachment of the epicranial aponeurosis. Clinically, this structure is important, since hemorrhages under the galea in the loose areolar tissue cannot descend beyond the line of attachment into the neck (see HN20 B). In the frontal region this attachment of the galea to the bone is absent, and bleeding extends into the orbital region. The superior and inferior nuchal lines serve as attachment for the muscles of the neck.

¶ The hypoglossal canal is sometimes divided by a small bony spicule in two or three foramina. Embryologically, three occipital somites are recognized, and the bony spicules are believed to be remnants of the original segmentation in the occipital region.

¶ The condylar canal is not to be confused with the hypoglossal canal. It serves as a passageway for an emissary vein from the sigmoid sinus to the occipital vein (see HN24).

¶ The foramen magnum provides passage to the medulla oblongata. In addition, the lower parts of the cerebellum (tonsils) may project into the foramen on each side. Under certain conditions the cerebellum may be compressed in the foramen magnum.

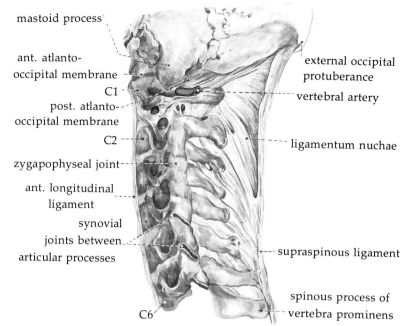

mastoid process

ant. atlanto-occipital membrane

C1

post. atlanto-occipital membrane

C2

zygapophyseal joint

ant. longitudinal ligament

synovial joints between articular processes

external occipital protuberance

vertebral artery

ligamentum nuchae

supraspinous ligament

spinous process of vertebra prominens

C6

A. Cervical vertebral column and atlanto-occipital joint (lateral view).

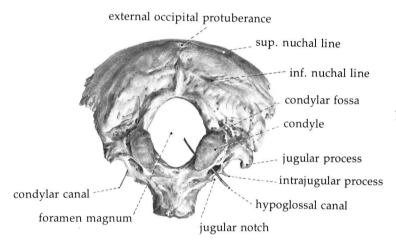

external occipital protuberance

sup. nuchal line

inf. nuchal line

condylar fossa

condyle

jugular process

intrajugular process

condylar canal

foramen magnum

hypoglossal canal

jugular notch

B. Occipital bone with its condylar surfaces seen from below.

sup. articular facet

capsule of atlanto-occipital joint

ant. arch of atlas

transverse ligament of atlas

foramen transversarium

groove for vertebral artery

post. arch of atlas

C. Atlas and its joint surfaces seen from above.

Note:

¶ The posterior atlanto-occipital membrane arches over the vertebral artery. Sometimes the free border of the membrane is ossified, thus providing a bony passageway for the artery. The first spinal nerve also passes through this opening (see B17).

¶ The capsule of the atlanto-occipital joint is strong on the lateral and posterior aspects but weak on the medial side. On this side the joint cavity frequently communicates with the synovial bursa between the dens and the transverse ligament of the atlas.

¶ The two atlanto-occipital joints function as one, and the movements, occurring mainly around a transverse axis, result in flexion and extension of the head. Movement that occurs around an anteroposterior axis results in lateral tilting of the head. (Keep in mind that rotation movements of the head do not occur in the atlanto-occipital joints but in the atlantoaxial joints.)

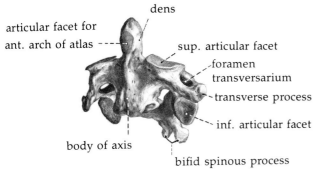

dens

articular facet for
ant. arch of atlas

sup. articular facet

foramen
transversarium

transverse process

inf. articular facet

body of axis

bifid spinous process

A.   The axis with the dens (anterolateral view).

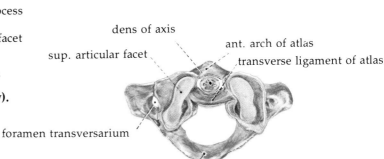

dens of axis

sup. articular facet

ant. arch of atlas

transverse ligament of atlas

foramen transversarium

post. arch of atlas

B.   The atlas and the median atlantoaxial joint (seen from above).

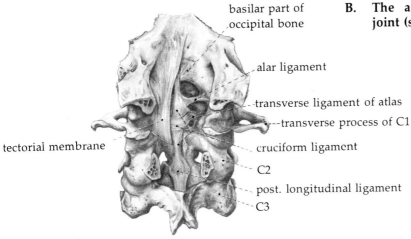

basilar part of
occipital bone

alar ligament

transverse ligament of atlas

transverse process of C1

tectorial membrane

cruciform ligament

C2

post. longitudinal ligament

C3

C.   Ligaments of the median atlantoaxial joint.
The posterior arches of the atlas, axis and
the posterior part of the occipital bone have
been removed.

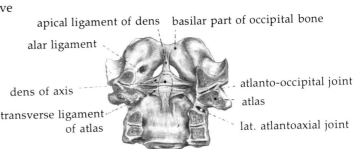

apical ligament of dens   basilar part of occipital bone

alar ligament

dens of axis

atlanto-occipital joint

atlas

transverse ligament
of atlas

lat. atlantoaxial joint

D.   Section through the lateral atlantoaxial joints.

Note:

¶ The atlantoaxial joint consists of three separate synovial joints: (a) two lateral atlantoaxial joints and (b) the median joint between the dens of the axis and the anterior arch and transverse ligament of the atlas. The anterior arch and the transverse ligament together form a ring around the dens. All three joints act as one, and the movement consists of rotation of the atlas on the axis. Since the skull cannot rotate on the atlas, the movement in the atlantoaxial joint results in rotation of the head.

¶ The rotation of the head is restricted by the alar ligaments, which on each side extend from the tip of the dens to the medial sides of the condyles of the occipital bone. They are relaxed on extension of the head but taut on flexion. Hence, rotation of the head is restricted when the head is in a bent position but is much greater when the head is extended.

¶ The apical ligament of the dens and the fibers of the posterior longitudinal ligament together with the transverse ligament of the atlas form the cruciform ligament. The tectorial membrane is an upward extension of the posterior longitudinal ligament (see B21) and covers the cruciform ligament.

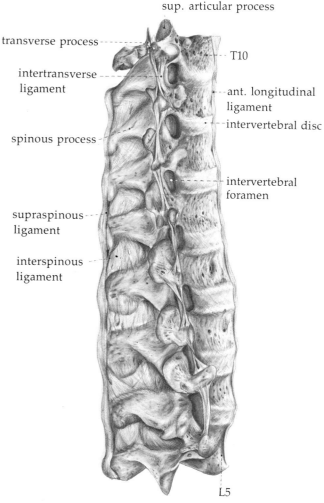

sup. articular process

transverse process

intertransverse
ligament

spinous process

supraspinous
ligament

interspinous
ligament

T10

ant. longitudinal
ligament

intervertebral disc

intervertebral
foramen

L5

A. Ligaments of the vertebral column seen from the right.

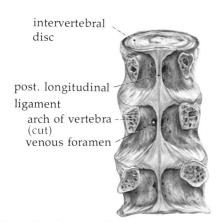

intervertebral
disc

post. longitudinal
ligament

arch of vertebra
(cut)

venous foramen

B. Posterior longitudinal ligament.
The vertebral column is seen from behind; the arches have been removed.

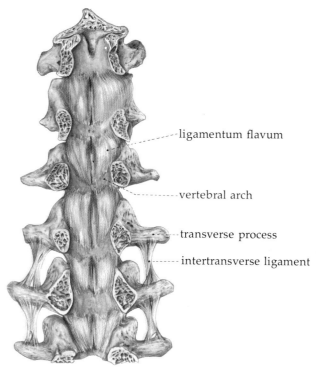

ligamentum flavum

vertebral arch

transverse process

intertransverse ligament

C. Ligamentum flavum and intertransverse ligaments.
The vertebral column is seen from the front; the vertebral bodies have been removed.

The movements of the vertebral column are limited by the shape of the articular facets and also by a number of strong ligaments:

1. The supraspinous and interspinous ligaments extending between the spinous processes restrict flexion of the vertebral column. Both ligaments consist of tough collagenous fibers.

2. The ligamentum flavum connects the vertebral arches, in particular the laminae. It consists mainly of elastic fibers and limits flexion of the column.

3. The anterior and posterior longitudinal ligaments run along the entire length of the ventral and dorsal aspects of the vertebral column. They stabilize the column in its weight-carrying function.

4. Short intertransverse ligaments are found between the transverse processes. They limit the side to side movement of the vertebral column.

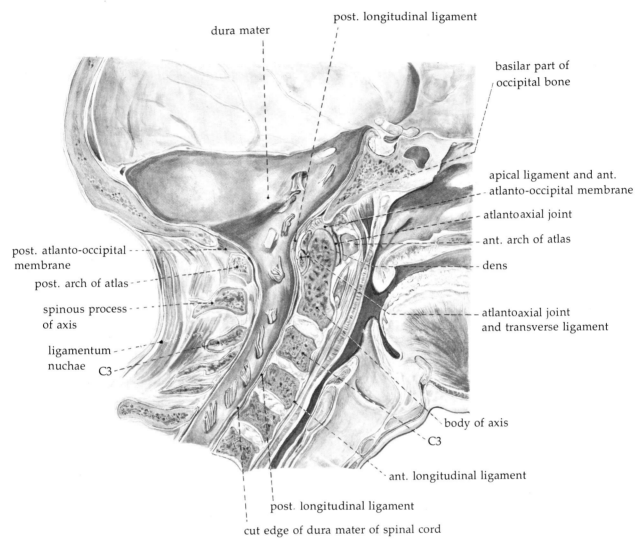

dura mater

post. longitudinal ligament

basilar part of occipital bone

apical ligament and ant. atlanto-occipital membrane

atlantoaxial joint

ant. arch of atlas

dens

atlantoaxial joint and transverse ligament

post. atlanto-occipital membrane

post. arch of atlas

spinous process of axis

ligamentum nuchae

C3

body of axis

C3

ant. longitudinal ligament

post. longitudinal ligament

cut edge of dura mater of spinal cord

Median section through the atlanto-occipital region.
Note the median atlantoaxial joint.

The atlantoaxial region and its relation to the pharynx is clinically important:

⹋ In cases of death by hanging the weight of the body causes the atlas to dislocate from the axis, and the transverse ligament either ruptures or is torn from its attachment. The dens of the axis is then pushed posteriorly with great force and will crush the spinal cord and medulla oblongata. Death results almost immediately.

⹋ Infections of the pharynx and retropharyngeal abscesses sometimes extend posteriorly to the median atlantoaxial joint. The ligaments become edematous and softened. Under such conditions a dislocation of the atlas on the axis may occur.

⹋ If the bony and ligamentous structures of the column are severely damaged by fractures or dislocations, fragments of the vertebrae may penetrate the vertebral canal and compress or cut the spinal cord. It is advisable to be extremely careful with patients who may have broken a cervical vertebra. If a bony fragment cuts the spinal cord in the cervical region, total paralysis results.

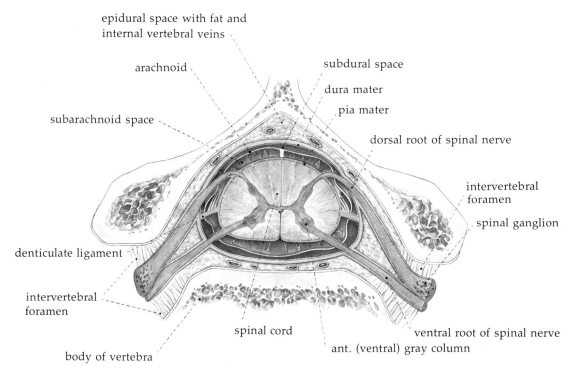

epidural space with fat and
internal vertebral veins

arachnoid

subdural space

dura mater

pia mater

subarachnoid space

dorsal root of spinal nerve

intervertebral
foramen

spinal ganglion

denticulate ligament

intervertebral
foramen

spinal cord

ventral root of spinal nerve

ant. (ventral) gray column

body of vertebra

Transverse section through the spinal cord and membranes.

Note the following important points:

¶ The spinal cord is enclosed in the vertebral canal, and the spinal nerves leave through
the intervertebral foramina. The cord is entirely surrounded by bone: anteriorly by
the vertebral bodies, and laterally and posteriorly by the pedicles and laminae of the
vertebral arches.

¶ After the lamina and the adherent periosteum have been removed, the epidural space
is opened. It contains fatty tissue and the *internal vertebral venous plexus.* This plexus
receives blood from the vertebrae, the meninges and the spinal cord and is drained by
the intervertebral veins. The veins pass through the intervertebral foramina and join
the veins of the external vertebral plexus located on the outside of the vertebral column. This plexus in turn communicates with the intercostal, lumbar and sacral veins.

¶ The veins of the internal and external vertebral plexuses usually have no valves or incompetent valves. The blood flow is, therefore, unrestricted and connects the veins of
the skull and neck with those of the thorax, abdomen and pelvis. The direction of the
flow depends on differences in pressure and may be either upward or downward
When the intra-abdominal pressure is increased, making the return flow through the
inferior vena cava difficult, the blood enters the internal vertebral venous plexus,
which is not subjected to external pressures. Since the internal plexus is connected with
the veins in the skull, this phenomenon may explain why cancer cells from the pelvic
organs metastasize to the vertebral column and even to the cranial cavity.

¶ After removal of the fat and veins the dura mater is visible. This membrane surrounds the spinal cord and also sheathes the dorsal root, the ventral root and the spinal
ganglion of the spinal nerves It extends into the intervertebral foramen and then
blends into the epineurium that covers the peripheral nerves.

¶ After removal of the dura mater, the subdural space is opened, revealing the arachnoid,
a delicate, filmlike membrane. It is separate from the pia mater, which is closely applied
to the spinal cord. The space between the two membranes is the subarachnoid space. In
patients with subarachnoid bleeding in the brain, the blood may descend in this space
to the lumbar region.

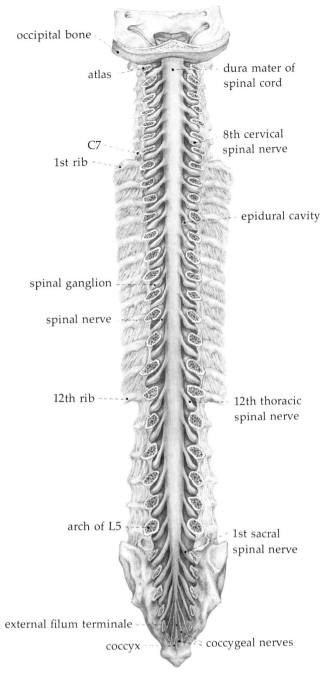

occipital bone

atlas

dura mater of
spinal cord

8th cervical
spinal nerve

C7

1st rib

epidural cavity

spinal ganglion

spinal nerve

12th rib

12th thoracic
spinal nerve

arch of L5

1st sacral
spinal nerve

external filum terminale

coccyx

coccygeal nerves

Spinal cord surrounded by dura mater.
The vertebral arches have been removed.

Note:

¶   The dura mater surrounds the spinal cord and also provides a sheath around the spinal
ganglia. As soon as the spinal nerves leave the intervertebral foramina, the dura mater
blends into the epineurium.

¶   The intervertebral foramen is entirely bounded by bone and cartilage: above and below by the pedicles of two adjacent vertebrae; in front by the vertebral body and intervertebral disc; and posteriorly by the articular processes. This is of great clinical importance, since the spinal nerve, artery and vein, which pass through the foramen, may
easily be compressed by the surrounding structures. This occurs in patients with herniation of the intervertebral discs, fractures of the vertebral bodies and pedicles and
arthritis of the joints of the articular processes.

¶   The dural sac descends into the sacral region and terminates in the external filum terminale in the coccygeal region.

¶   Once the dura is opened and the arachnoid has been removed, the spinal cord is exposed. It terminates with the conus medullaris at the level of L2.

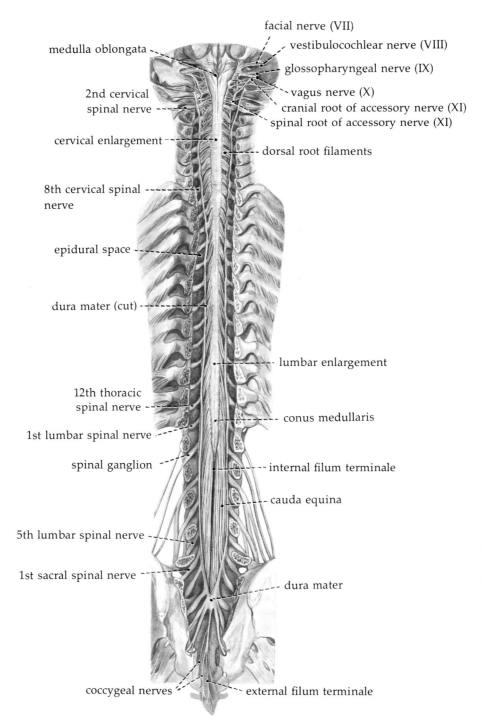

facial nerve (VII)

vestibulocochlear nerve (VIII)

medulla oblongata

glossopharyngeal nerve (IX)

2nd cervical
spinal nerve

vagus nerve (X)

cranial root of accessory nerve (XI)

spinal root of accessory nerve (XI)

cervical enlargement

dorsal root filaments

8th cervical spinal
nerve

epidural space

dura mater (cut)

lumbar enlargement

12th thoracic
spinal nerve

conus medullaris

1st lumbar spinal nerve

spinal ganglion

internal filum terminale

cauda equina

5th lumbar spinal nerve

1st sacral spinal nerve

dura mater

coccygeal nerves

external filum terminale

Spinal cord of a child in the vertebral canal.
The dura mater has been partially removed.

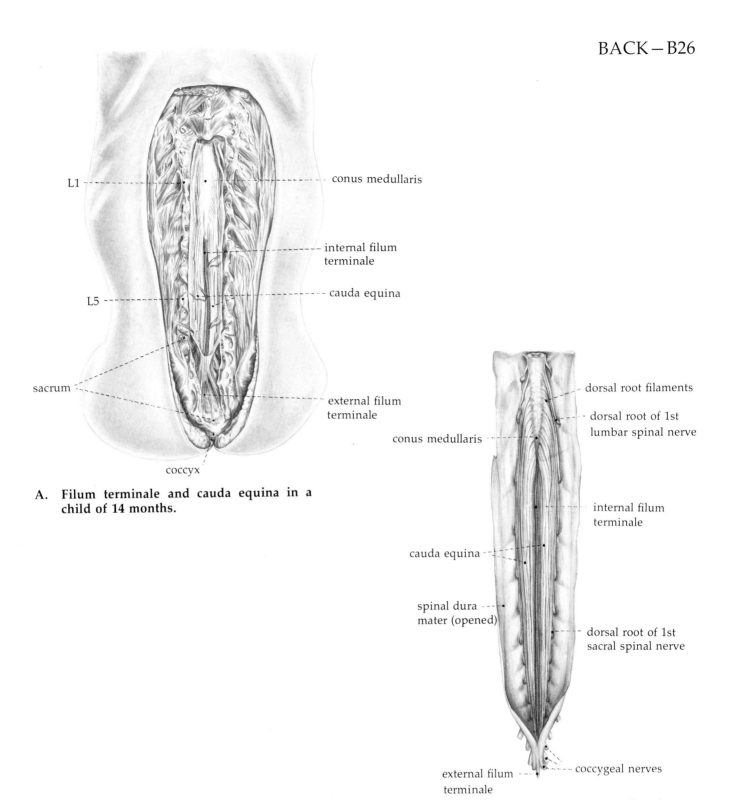

L1 - - - - - - - - - - - - - - - - - - conus medullaris

- - - - internal filum
terminale

L5 - - - - - - - - - - - - - - - - - cauda equina

sacrum - - - - - - - - - - - - - - - - external filum
terminale

coccyx

**A. Filum terminale and cauda equina in a
child of 14 months.**

dorsal root filaments

dorsal root of 1st
lumbar spinal nerve

conus medullaris - - - - - - - -

internal filum
terminale

cauda equina - - -

spinal dura - - -
mater (opened)

dorsal root of 1st
sacral spinal nerve

external filum - - - - - - - coccygeal nerves
terminale

B. Cauda equina of an adult; posterior view.

¶ In the third month of development the spinal cord extends the entire length of the vertebral canal, and the spinal nerves pass through the intervertebral foramina at their level of origin. With increasing age the vertebral column lengthens more rapidly than the neural tube, and the terminal end of the spinal cord shifts from the coccygeosacral region to a higher level. Shortly after birth the terminal end has risen to the level of the third lumbar vertebra. Because of the disproportionate growth, the spinal nerves run obliquely from their segment of origin in the spinal cord to the corresponding level of the vertebral column.

¶ In the adult the spinal cord terminates at the level of L2. Below this point the central nervous system is represented by the internal filum terminale, which marks the tract of regression of the spinal cord. The nerve fibers below the terminal end of the cord are known collectively as the cauda equina.

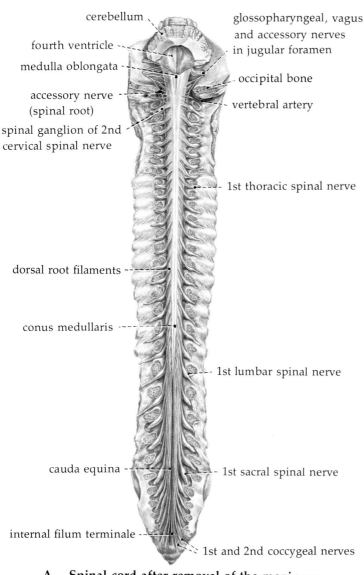

cerebellum

glossopharyngeal, vagus
and accessory nerves
in jugular foramen

fourth ventricle

medulla oblongata

accessory nerve
(spinal root)

spinal ganglion of 2nd
cervical spinal nerve

occipital bone

vertebral artery

1st thoracic spinal nerve

dorsal root filaments

conus medullaris

1st lumbar spinal nerve

cauda equina

1st sacral spinal nerve

internal filum terminale

1st and 2nd coccygeal nerves

A. Spinal cord after removal of the meninges.

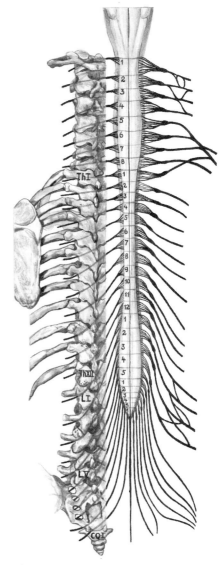

B. Diagrammatic presentation of the spinal cord and nerves.

Note:

¶ The spinal portion of the accessory (XI) nerve arises from the upper four segments of the cervical part of the spinal cord. It ascends in the vertebral canal, passes through the foramen magnum and then joins the cranial portion of the accessory nerve. The two components join and leave the skull through the jugular foramen.

¶ It is clinically important to know that the spinal cord terminates just below the lower level of the first lumbar vertebra and that the subarachnoid space (see B23) extends to about the lower level of the second sacral vertebra. Hence, between L2 and S2 the subarachnoid space contains the cauda equina and the internal filum terminale. In a lumbar puncture the needle is introduced into the subarachnoid space between L3 and L4. The nerves of the cauda equina are usually pushed aside. If a nerve root is touched, either pain will be felt in one of the dermatomes or a muscle will twitch.

¶ Lumbar puncture is carried out to obtain a sample of cerebrospinal fluid, to inject drugs or to induce anesthesia. The patient is placed on his side in a flexed position so that the space between the arches is at its maximum width. The needle is passed above or below the spine of L4. (Remember that the line connecting the highest points of the iliac crests passes over the spine of L4.) After the needle has passed through the skin and fascia, it is pushed through the supraspinous and interspinous ligaments and the ligamentum flavum (see HN21 C). It then enters the epidural space with the internal vertebral venous plexus. At this point blood may escape through the needle, indicating that a vein has been punctured and that the subarachnoid space has not yet been reached. To reach this space, the needle will have to be pushed slightly deeper to pierce the dura mater and the arachnoid (see HN23).

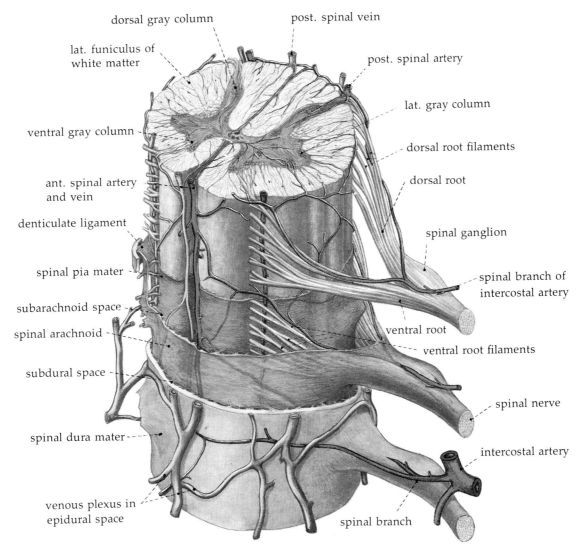

dorsal gray column

post. spinal vein

lat. funiculus of
white matter

post. spinal artery

ventral gray column

lat. gray column

dorsal root filaments

ant. spinal artery
and vein

dorsal root

denticulate ligament

spinal ganglion

spinal pia mater

spinal branch of
intercostal artery

subarachnoid space

spinal arachnoid

ventral root

ventral root filaments

subdural space

spinal nerve

spinal dura mater

intercostal artery

venous plexus in
epidural space

spinal branch

The spinal cord and its meninges.

Note:

⁋ The dura mater encloses the spinal cord and extends along the nerve roots, continuing into the epineurium. Superiorly, it continues into the dura covering the brain (see B22).

⁋ The arachnoid is an impermeable, thin membrane between the dura and the pia mater, from which it is separated by the subdural and subarachnoid space, respectively. It extends along the spinal nerve roots, thus forming small extensions of the subarachnoid space. The subarachnoid space contains: (a) the cerebrospinal fluid; (b) the dorsal and ventral rootlets; (c) the spinal ganglia; and (d) the vessels that supply the spinal cord.

⁋ The pia mater invests the spinal cord. Between the nerve roots it forms the ligamentum denticulatum on either side. These segmental ligaments pass laterally to adhere to the dura mater. In this manner the spinal cord is suspended and fixed in the dural sheath.

⁋ The dorsal and ventral roots consist of a number of fine filaments, which emerge from the cord in a straight line. The two roots join to form the spinal nerve. Since the ventral root conducts motor impulses from the cord to the musculature, and the dorsal root brings sensory impulses from the periphery to the cord, the spinal nerve conducts both motor and sensory impulses. Thirty-one pairs of spinal nerves are attached to the cord.

INDEX

Note: Numbers in boldface indicate legends; numbers in italics indicate labels. Text material is shown in roman type.

INDEX

INDEX

INDEX

INDEX

INDEX

INDEX

INDEX

INDEX

Tubercle (*Continued*)
  mental, *HN87 A*
  of cervical vertebra, *B5 A*
  of humerus, greater, *T16 A*, *UL6 A,B*,
      UL11 B, *UL30 C*, *UL31 A*, *UL34 A,B*
    lesser, *UL6 A*, *UL21 B*, *UL30 C*,
      UL34 A,B
  of iliac crest, *A1*
  of rib, *T7 B,C,D*, *T8 C,D,E*, *T9 A*
  pubic, *A4*, *A11 A*, *A13 A*, *P2 A,B*,
      P5 A,B, *P55 A*, *LL32 A,B*, *LL33 B*,
      LL35 B
  spinous, of sacrum, *P3 B*
  supraglenoid, *UL24 B*, *UL30 A*
  thyroid, *HN117 C*
Tuberosity
  calcaneal, *LL46*, *LL47 A,B*, *LL49 A,B*,
      LL52, *LL61 B*, *LL62 B*, *LL63 A,C,D*,
      LL65 A, *LL68 B*, *LL74*
  clavicular, for costoclavicular ligament,
      UL5 D
  deltoid, *UL6 A*, *UL24 A,B*, *UL28 A*,
      UL29 A
  gluteal, *LL23*, *LL30 B*
  iliac, *P2 B*, *LL32 B*
  ischial, *P2 A*, *P7 A*, *P8 B*, *P20 A*, *P21 A*,
      P23 A, *P36 A*, *P38*, *LL23*, *LL24*, *LL32*
      A,C, *LL34 A,B*, *LL37 A*
  maxillary, *HN85 A*, *HN98 A*
  of cuboid bone, *LL69 B*, *LL70 B*
  of metatarsal, *LL40 A,B*
  of navicular bone, *LL65 A*, *LL69 A*
  of radius, *UL22 E*, *UL24 B*, *UL38*,
      UL61 B, *UL62 B*
  of tibia, *LL7*, *LL17 A*, *LL39 B*, *LL53 A,C*,
      LL54 A, *LL55 A*, *LL60 A,C*
  of ulna, *UL24 B*, *UL62 B*
  pterygoid, *HN84 B*
Tumor(s). See also *Cancer*.
  of parotid gland, *HN13*
  of submandibular gland, *HN82*
  retrobulbar, *HN45*
Tunica albuginea, *P12 B,C*, *P14*,
    P15 A,C,D, *P17 A*
Tunica dartos, *A16*, *P11 A*, *P12 C*
Tunica vaginalis, *A16*, *A18 B,F*, *A21 B*,
    P11, *P12*
Tunnel, carpal, *UL42*, **UL44 A**, *UL48 A*

Ulcer(s)
  from varicose veins, *LL45*
  gastric, *A33*
  of cornea, *HN7*
  peptic, in Meckel's diverticulum, *A35*
Ulna, *UL4 A*, **UL22 C,D**, *UL60 B,C*,
    UL61, *UL63*, **UL64 A,B**, *UL67 A*
Umbilicus, *T12 A,B*, *A7 B*, *A22*, *UL8 B*
Umbo, *HN56 B*, *HN57 B,C*, *HN58 A*,
    HN59
Urachus, *P28 B*, *P42*, *P43*
  obliterated, *A22*
Ureter, *A47*, *A65 A,B*, *A66*, *A67 B,C,D*,
    A68, *A69 A*, *P17 B*, *P25*, *P26*, *P28 B*,
    P29 A, *P30 A,B*, *P32*, *P41*, *P43*, *P44*
  blood supply, **A69 B**
  constrictions, *A68*
  in fetus and newborn *A64 B*, *P13*
  orifice, *P30 A,B*
Urethra, *A21 A*, *P20 B*, *P23 A,B,C*,
    P29 B,C
  female, *P30 B*, *P36 B,C*, *P40 B,C*, *P41*,
    P46 A,B
  internal sphincter, *P30 A*. See also
    Muscle, sphincter vesicae.
  male, *A21 B*, *P17 B*, *P28 B*
    membranous portion, *P15 D*, *P16*
      A,B, *P23*, *P30 A*, *P31 A,B*
    spongy portion, *P15 C,D*
    lymph vessels, *P27*
    prostatic, **P30 A**, *P31 A,C*, *P54 A*

Urethra (*Continued*)
  ruptures of, *P20*, *P23*, *P29*
Urine, in superficial perineal pouch,
    P20 B, *P23*
Urogram, of pelvic calyces and ureter,
    A68 A,B
Uterus, *A21 A*, *P39 A*, *P41*, *P42*, *P43*,
    P46 C, **P47 A**, *P49 A,B*, **P50 A,B**,
    P51 A,B
  anteflexion and anteversion, **P46 C**
  blood supply, **P44 B**
  external os, in multipara, **P50 D**
    in nullipara, **P50 C**
  "genital" ligaments, **P51 B**
  in neonate, *P46 B*
  infections and cancers, *P47*
  innervation, **P58 B**
  lymph drainage, *P53*
  position, *P43*, **P46 A,B**
  pregnant, **P47 C**
  prolapse, *P52*
  retroflexion and retroversion, *P46*
  venous plexus, *P45*
Utricle, prostatic, *P29 B*, *P30 A*, *P31 A*
Uvula, *HN48 A,B*, *HN94 A*, *HN95*, *HN111*
  of bladder, *P30 A*

Vagina, *A21 A*, *P36 C*, *P39 A*, *P40 A,B,C*,
    P41, *P46 A,C*, *P47 C*, **P50 A,B**, *P51 A*,
    P54 B
  cancer of, *P41*
  in neonate, *P36 B*, *P46 B*
  lymph drainage, *P53*
Vallecula, *HN94 B*, *HN95*, *HN96 A*,
    HN97 C, *HN118 B*
Valve(s)
  aortic, *T53 B*, *T54 A*, *T55 B*
  atrioventricular, left *T53 B*. See also
    Valve, mitral.
    right, *T55 A*
  heart, auscultation areas of, *T30*
  ileocecal, *A41 B,C*
  mitral, *T30 A*, *T49 B*, **T53 A**, *T54 A*
  of coronary sinus, *T51 B*, *T55 A*
  of inferior vena cava, *T51 B*, *T55 A*
  of urethra (male), *P15 D*
  of vermiform appendix, **A41 C**
  pyloric, *A33 B*
  semilunar, of aorta, *T49 B*
    of pulmonary trunk, *T49 B*, *T51 B*
  tricuspid, *T30 A*, *T49 B*, *T51 B*
Varicocele, *P14*
Vein(s)
  angular, *HN6 A,B*, *HN16 C*, *HN24*
  at elbow, **UL27 A,B**
  auricular, posterior, *HN6 A*, *HN24*
  axillary, *T4*, *T15 A*, *UL8 A*, *UL11 A*,
    UL14 B, *UL16*, *UL25 B*
  azygos, *T32*, *T36*, *T37*, *T61 A*, *T63*,
    T64 B
  basilic, *UL14 A,B*, *UL23 A*, *UL26 A*
  basivertebral, *A12 B*
  brachial, *UL14 B*, *UL25 B*, *UL26 A*
  brachiocephalic, *T31*, *T32*, *T36*, *T38*,
    T59, *T64 B*, *HN6 A*, *HN75*, *HN80*
  cardiac, *T47 A*, *T48 A*
  caval, and azygos system, **T64 B**
    and portal system, *A5*
  cephalic, *T12 B*, *T13*, *T15 A*, *UL9*,
    UL14 A,B, *UL16*, *UL23 A*, *UL35 A*,
    HN71
  cerebral, *HN23 A*
  cervical, *HN6 A*
  ciliary, posterior, *HN43 B*
  circumflex, femoral, lateral, *LL6 B*, *LL16*
    medial, *LL18 B*
  humeral, *UL14 B*
  iliac, superficial, *T4*, *A13 B*, *LL6 A*,
    LL10
  cochlear, *HN65 D*

Vein(s) (*Continued*)
  colic, *A29*
  collateral, radial and ulnar, *UL14 B*
  cubital, median, *UL14 A*, *UL23 A*
  digital, *UL14 A,B*
  diploic, *HN19 A*, *HN24*
  emissary, *HN19 A*, *HN24*
  epigastric, *P45*
    inferior, *A12 B*, *A17*
    superficial, *T4*, *A5B*, *A13 B*, *P37 A,B*,
      LL6 A, *LL10*
  episcleral, *HN43 B*
  esophageal, *A29*
  extracranial, **HN24**
  facial, *HN6 A,B*, *HN13 A*, *HN24*, *HN70*,
      HN82 B, *HN85 B*
    transverse, *HN6 A,B*, *HN13 A*
  femoral, *T4*, *A13 B*, *P9 B*, *P37 A*, *LL6 A,B*,
      LL14, *LL15*, *LL17 A*, *LL18 A,B*
    deep, *LL6 B*, *LL16*, *LL18 B*
  gastric, *A29*
  gastroepiploic, *A29*
  genicular, *LL6 B*
  gluteal, *P26*, *P45*, *LL26*
  hemiazygos, *T63*, *T64 B*
  hepatic, *A47*, *A57*
  ileal, *A29*
  ileocolic, *A29*
  iliac, external, *A17*, *LL6 B*, *LL11*, *P26*,
      P45
    internal, *P26*
  in urogenital and anal triangles, **P21 B**
  infraorbital, *HN6 B*
  intercostal, *T36*, *T63*, *T64 B*
  interosseous, *UL14 B*
  intervertebral, *A12 B*
  intracranial, **HN24**
  jugular, anterior, *HN6 A*
    external, *HN6 A*, *HN11*, *HN70*
    internal, *T43*, *T59*, *T61 A*, *T64 A*,
      UL14 B, *HN6 A*, *HN13 A*, *HN23 A*,
      HN24, **HN72 B**, *HN73*, *HN76 A*,
      HN80, *HN82 B*, *HN92 A*, *HN107*
  labial, *HN6 B*
  labyrinthine, *HN67 B*
  lingual, *HN6 A,B*, *HN96 C*
  lumbar, *T64 B*, *A12 B*
  maxillary, *HN6 A*, *HN12 B*, *HN13 A*
  meningeal, *HN31 A*
  mesenteric, inferior, *A29*, *A47*
    superior, *A24*, *A29*, *A47*, *A61*
  oblique, of left atrium, *T48 A*
  obturator, *P26*
  occipital, *HN6 A*, *HN24*, *HN105 B*
  of abdominal wall, **A12 B**
  of arm, **UL25 B**, **UL26 A**
  of clitoris, *P45*
  of face, **HN6 B**
  of female pelvis, *P45*
  of head and neck, **HN6 A**
  of kidneys and suprarenal glands, *A63*
  of left ventricle, *T48 A*
  of male pelvis, **P26**
  of penis, deep, *P26*
    dorsal, *P10*, *P14*, *P15 C*, *P19*, *P23 A*,
      P24, *P26*, *P54 A*
    during erection, *P16*
  of prostate, *P26*, *P31*
  of upper limb, **UL14 B**
  of vestibular bulb, *P38*, *P45*
  ophthalmic, *HN23 A*, *HN24*, *HN40 C*
  orbital, *HN6 B*
  ovarian, *A63*, *A65 A,B*, *P45*, *P47 A*,
      P48 A
  pancreaticoduodenal, *A29*
  paraumbilical, *T4*, *A29*
  pericardiacophrenic, *T31*, *T38*
  peroneal, *LL50 A*
  popliteal, *LL6 B*, *LL26*, *LL45*, *LL48 B*
  portal, *A5*, *A27*, *A28*, **A29**, *A47*, *A48 A*,
      A54, *A57*, *A59 A*
    in fetus and infant, *A53 A,B*